Selected Pediatric Cardiovascular Surgery Anesthesia Cases

Jijian Zheng • Mazhong Zhang
Jie Bai
Editors

Selected Pediatric Cardiovascular Surgery Anesthesia Cases

Springer

世界图书出版公司

Editors
Jijian Zheng
The National Children's Medical Center (Shanghai), Department of Anesthesiology of Shanghai Children's Medical Center
Shanghai Jiao Tong University School of Medicine
Shanghai, China

Mazhong Zhang
The National Children's Medical Center (Shanghai), Department of Anesthesiology of Shanghai Children's Medical Center
Shanghai Jiao Tong University School of Medicine
Shanghai, China

Jie Bai
The National Children's Medical Center (Shanghai), Department of Anesthesiology of Shanghai Children's Medical Center
Shanghai Jiao Tong University School of Medicine
Shanghai, China

ISBN 978-981-96-5613-4 ISBN 978-981-96-5614-1 (eBook)
https://doi.org/10.1007/978-981-96-5614-1

Jointly published with World Publishing Shanghai Co., Ltd

The print edition is not for sale in China (Mainland). Customers from China (Mainland) please order the print book from: World Publishing Shanghai Co., Ltd.

The original submitted manuscript has been translated into English. The translation was done using artificial intelligence. A subsequent revision was performed by the author(s) to further refine the work and to ensure that the translation is appropriate concerning content and scientific correctness. It may, however, read stylistically different from a conventional translation.

Translation from the Chinese language edition: "Xiao'er Xinxueguan Shoushu Mazui Bingli Jingxuan" by Jijian Zheng et al., © World Publishing Shanghai Co., Ltd 2023. Published by World Publishing Shanghai Co., Ltd. All Rights Reserved.

This Springer imprint is published by the registered company Springer Nature Singapore Pte Ltd.
The registered company address is: 152 Beach Road, #21-01/04 Gateway East, Singapore 189721, Singapore

Foreword

Pediatric cardiovascular disease, also known as congenital heart disease, or "CHD" for short, not only has a high incidence rate but is also the main cause of death in children under 5 years old due to disease. With the development of surgical, extracorporeal circulation, anesthesia, and intensive care technologies, large pediatric heart centers can now surgically correct congenital heart disease. In this process, anesthetic management plays a very important role in safeguarding the correction of CHD, reducing adverse events, and improving prognosis. Despite this, due to the large age span of children with congenital heart disease, the variety of diseases, the severity of the disease, and the many complications of anesthesia surgery, the management of anesthesia for congenital heart disease surgery is very challenging and individualized management and regulation are crucial.

The department of anesthesiology at Shanghai Children's Medical Center completes nearly 4000 cases of congenital heart disease surgery anesthesia annually. It is currently the Children's Heart Center, which has the most annual cases of congenital heart disease surgery anesthesia in China. It has accumulated much experience in managing critically ill children and has established relatively complete anesthetic management plans and emergency event handling procedures. In 2018, Professors Jijian Zheng, Mazhong Zhang, and Jie Bai led their colleagues in the department to translate and publish "The Pediatric Cardiac Anesthesia Handbook" written by the Department of Anesthesiology at Boston Children's Hospital in the United States, which has played a positive role in promoting the management of CHD anesthesia in China. Although "The Pediatric Cardiac Anesthesia Handbook" succinctly introduces the latest management concepts and principles of CHD anesthesia, it still feels insufficient to guide clinical practice. For this reason, the three professors led their colleagues in the department to carefully select 80 cases, systematically introducing the successful experience of the Department of Anesthesiology at Shanghai Children's Medical Center in the management of CHD anesthesia while also analyzing the existing deficiencies and conducting in-depth discussions in conjunction with the latest management concepts.

The case discussions in this book not only include the anesthetic management of congenital heart disease correction surgery but also include noncardiac surgery and anesthesia and sedation outside the operating room for children with congenital heart disease, covering almost all anesthetic management of congenital heart disease cases. The book's content reproduces daily clinical work and combines the latest congenital heart anesthetic management concepts for in-depth and easy-to-understand discussions. The content is wonderful, the regulations are clear, and it has practical guidance and reference value for the clinical practice of anesthesia for congenital heart disease surgery.

I am honored to be invited to write a preface for this book and happy to recommend it to anesthesiologists nationwide. I hope this book can help physicians engaged in congenital heart anesthesia work and contribute to the perioperative safety of children with congenital heart disease.

Shanghai Jiao Tong University School of Medicine Fan Jiang
Shanghai, China
2022/08

Preface

Previously, we first translated and published the "The Pediatric Cardiac Anesthesia Handbook" from Boston Children's Hospital in the United States, which not only comprehensively expounds on the embryonic development, pathophysiology, extracorporeal circulation and mechanical assisted circulation, and cardiac catheterization of congenital heart disease in children but also outlines the anatomical characteristics, surgical treatment principles, and key points of anesthetic management of more than 20 common congenital heart diseases. The book is published in a handbook format, concise and easy to understand, richly illustrated, and easy to learn. After publication, it is widely welcomed by professionals in pediatric cardiovascular anesthesia and plays an important role in helping cardiologists, cardiac surgeons, and nurses in cardiac care units.

Despite this, when facing complex and critically ill children undergoing cardiovascular surgery, relying solely on the anesthetic management principles in the handbook for specific anesthetic management is still insufficient. Clinical work urgently needs a book based on real cases for reference. The National Children's Medical Center (Shanghai), the department of anesthesiology of Shanghai Children's Medical Center affiliated with Shanghai Jiao Tong University School of Medicine, performs nearly 4000 cases of pediatric cardiovascular surgery anesthesia each year, of which difficult and critically ill cases account for more than half. After thorough exploration and analysis, we have compiled 80 representative anesthesia cases covering pediatric cardiovascular open-heart surgery, catheter interventional treatment surgery, diagnostic and therapeutic operation sedation, and non-cardiovascular surgery into this book, *Selected Pediatric Cardiovascular Surgery Anesthesia Cases*. This book not only realistically reproduces the entire process of anesthetic management of the case but also refers to the latest Chinese and international studies, expert consensus, and guidelines; reviews related knowledge points; and deeply analyzes the experience and lessons or deficiencies in the anesthetic management process, which has a solid clinical reference value.

This book is the result of the joint efforts of all colleagues in the Department of Anesthesiology of Shanghai Children's Medical Center and has received strong support from the Department of Cardiac Surgery and Extracorporeal Circulation. We express our sincere thanks for the hard work of our colleagues! We sincerely thank the cardiovascular patients who have provided us with valuable learning opportunities, and we deeply apologize for any shortcomings! Professors Hao Zhang and Yu Chen gave strong support and guidance and thoroughly reviewed the manuscript, for which we express our deep gratitude!

We know that despite the careful compilation and collective review by all authors, trying to minimize errors, shortcomings are still inevitable, and case discussions are subjective. This book only represents the views of the Shanghai Children's Medical Center's department of anesthesiology and is provided for reference in practice. We kindly ask readers to correct and understand any shortcomings, and we will continue to improve in our future work.

Shanghai, China
2022/08

Mazhong Zhang

Contents

About the Editors and Contributors

About the Editors

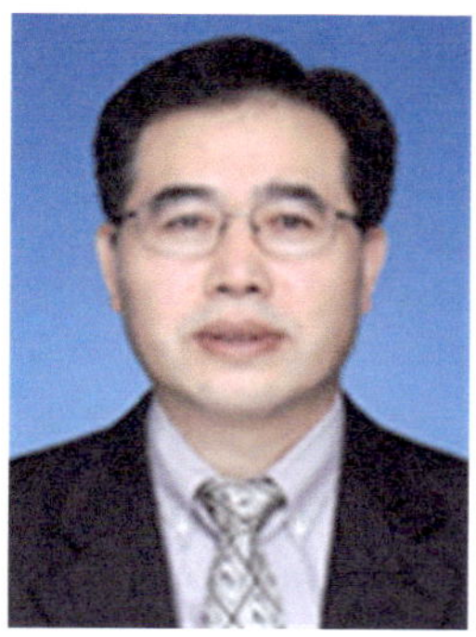

Jijian Zheng, MD PhD, PhD Supervisor, is a Professor and Chair of the Department of Anesthesiology at Shanghai Children's Medical Center affiliated with Shanghai Jiao Tong University School of Medicine. He also acts as the director of the Teaching and Research Section of Anesthesiology and Critical Care Medicine. He graduated with an MD from Weifang Medical College in Shandong, China, in 1990, and earned his PhD from Fudan University in Shanghai, China, in 2001. He currently holds the position of Vice Chair of the Subcommittee on Pediatric Anesthesia at the 14th Chinese Society of Anesthesiology. He is also the Vice Chair of the Pediatric Anesthesia Section at the 12th Shanghai Society of Anesthesiology. Additionally, he is a standing committee member and secretary-general of the Pediatric Anesthesia Subcommittee of the Chinese Society of Cardiovascular and Thoracic Anesthesiology. He serves on the editorial boards of the *Chinese Journal of Anesthesiology* and the *Chinese Journal of Graduate Medical Education*. As the first and corresponding author, he has published over 50 SCI papers in notable journals such as *Nature Neuroscience*, *Neuron*, and *Anesthesia & Analgesia*. Some of the work has been highly evaluated by journals such as Science STKE, *Nature Neuroscience*, *Trends in Neuroscience*, and Faculty1000.

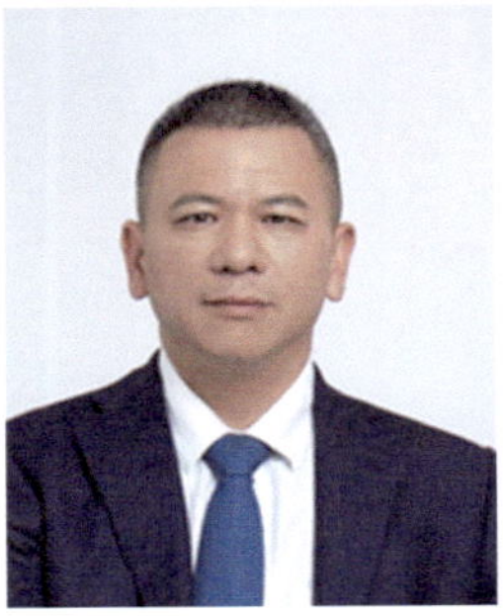

Mazhong Zhang, MD PhD, PhD Supervisor, is a Professor of the Department of Anesthesiology at Shanghai Children's Medical Center affiliated with Shanghai Jiao Tong University School of Medicine. He serves as the Vice President of Shanghai Children's Medical Center/National Children's Medical Center and is the President of Guizhou Hospital of Shanghai Children's Medical Center. He graduated with an MD from Xuzhou Medical College in Jiangsu, China, in 1992, and earned his PhD from Shanghai Jiao Tong University in 2003. He holds several key positions, including Chair of the Subcommittee on Pediatric Anesthesia and Director at the Chinese Society of Cardiovascular Anesthesiology. Additionally, he is the Director of the High-Quality Development Subcommittee of Public Hospitals of the Chinese Health Economics Association. He is a Standing Committee member of the Anesthesia Pharmacology Professional Committee of the Chinese Pharmacological Society. He is the Director of the Anesthesiology Education Research Association of the Medical Education Professional Committee of the Chinese Association of Higher Education. He is also a Standing Committee member of the Anesthesia Professional Committee of the National Cardiovascular Disease Expert Committee. He also acts as the Vice Chairman of the Pediatric Anesthesia Specialized Training Committee of the Chinese Medical Doctor Association, the Standing Director of the Shanghai Hospital Association, and the Vice Chairman of the Quality Control Committee of the Guizhou Hospital Association. He is a Standing editorial board member of the *International Journal of Anesthesiology and Resuscitation*, an Assistant editorial board member of the *Paediatric Anaesthesia*, and an Editorial board member of several journals, including the *Chinese Journal of Anesthesiology*, *Journal of Clinical Anesthesiology*, *Shanghai Medical Journal*, and *Journal of Anesthesia Safety and Quality Control*.

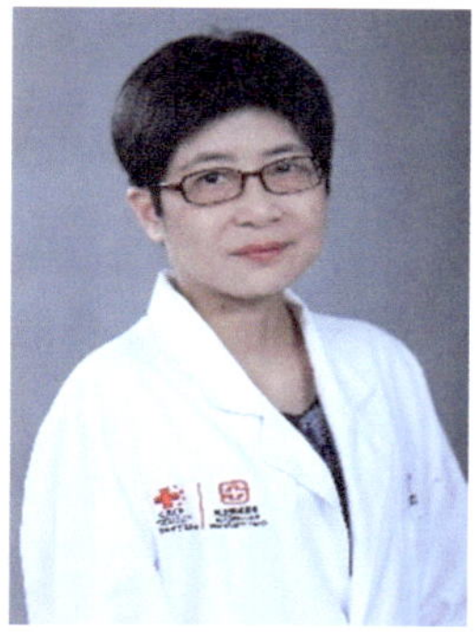

Jie Bai, MD, former Chair of the Department of Anesthesiology at Shanghai Children's Medical Center affiliated with Shanghai Jiao Tong University School of Medicine. She graduated with an MD from the Department of Paediatrics of Shanghai Second Medical University in 1988 and has been engaged in pediatric anesthesia since graduation with rich clinical experience. Her clinical work focuses on the anesthetic management of complex congenital heart disease in infants and children and the management of perioperative pulmonary hypertension in congenital heart disease. In recent years, she has published more than 10 SCI papers as co-author and corresponding author and participated in the translation and writing of several books on pediatric anesthesia.

Editors

Jijian Zheng The National Children's Medical Center (Shanghai), Department of Anesthesiology of Shanghai Children's Medical Center, Shanghai Jiao Tong University School of Medicine, Shanghai, China

Mazhong Zhang The National Children's Medical Center (Shanghai), Department of Anesthesiology of Shanghai Children's Medical Center, Shanghai Jiao Tong University School of Medicine, Shanghai, China

Jie Bai The National Children's Medical Center (Shanghai), Department of Anesthesiology of Shanghai Children's Medical Center, Shanghai Jiao Tong University School of Medicine, Shanghai, China

Associate Editors

Ruidong Zhang The National Children's Medical Center (Shanghai), Department of Anesthesiology of Shanghai Children's Medical Center, Shanghai Jiao Tong University School of Medicine, Shanghai, China

Jie Hu The National Children's Medical Center (Shanghai), Department of Anesthesiology of Shanghai Children's Medical Center, Shanghai Jiao Tong University School of Medicine, Shanghai, China

Yue Huang The National Children's Medical Center (Shanghai), Department of Anesthesiology of Shanghai Children's Medical Center, Shanghai Jiao Tong University School of Medicine, Shanghai, China

Reviewers

Hao Zhang The National Children's Medical Center (Shanghai), Heart Center and Shanghai Institute of Pediatric Congenital Heart Disease, Shanghai Clinical Research Center for Rare Pediatric Diseases, Shanghai Children's Medical Center, Shanghai Jiao Tong University School of Medicine, Shanghai, China

Yu Chen The National Children's Medical Center (Shanghai), Department of Anesthesiology of Shanghai Children's Medical Center, Shanghai Jiao Tong University School of Medicine, Shanghai, China

Contributors

Jie Bai The National Children's Medical Center (Shanghai), Department of Anesthesiology of Shanghai Children's Medical Center, Shanghai Jiao Tong University School of Medicine, Shanghai, China

Yong Bian The National Children's Medical Center (Shanghai), Department of Anesthesiology of Shanghai Children's Medical Center, Shanghai Jiao Tong University School of Medicine, Shanghai, China

Hualin Chen The National Children's Medical Center (Shanghai), Department of Anesthesiology of Shanghai Children's Medical Center, Shanghai Jiao Tong University School of Medicine, Shanghai, China

Yingzhi Dan The National Children's Medical Center (Shanghai), Department of Anesthesiology of Shanghai Children's Medical Center, Shanghai Jiao Tong University School of Medicine, Shanghai, China

Hongbin Gu The National Children's Medical Center (Shanghai), Department of Anesthesiology of Shanghai Children's Medical Center, Shanghai Jiao Tong University School of Medicine, Shanghai, China

Pan He The National Children's Medical Center (Shanghai), Department of Anesthesiology of Shanghai Children's Medical Center, Shanghai Jiao Tong University School of Medicine, Shanghai, China

Huiyan Hou The National Children's Medical Center (Shanghai), Department of Anesthesiology of Shanghai Children's Medical Center, Shanghai Jiao Tong University School of Medicine, Shanghai, China

Jiajia Huang The National Children's Medical Center (Shanghai), Department of Anesthesiology of Shanghai Children's Medical Center, Shanghai Jiao Tong University School of Medicine, Shanghai, China

Yanhui Huang The National Children's Medical Center (Shanghai), Department of Anesthesiology of Shanghai Children's Medical Center, Shanghai Jiao Tong University School of Medicine, Shanghai, China

Yue Huang The National Children's Medical Center (Shanghai), Department of Anesthesiology of Shanghai Children's Medical Center, Shanghai Jiao Tong University School of Medicine, Shanghai, China

Jie Hu The National Children's Medical Center (Shanghai), Department of Anesthesiology of Shanghai Children's Medical Center, Shanghai Jiao Tong University School of Medicine, Shanghai, China

Jing Jiang The National Children's Medical Center (Shanghai), Department of Anesthesiology of Shanghai Children's Medical Center, Shanghai Jiao Tong University School of Medicine, Shanghai, China

Lihong Jin The National Children's Medical Center (Shanghai), Department of Anesthesiology of Shanghai Children's Medical Center, Shanghai Jiao Tong University School of Medicine, Shanghai, China

Wei Ji The National Children's Medical Center (Shanghai), Department of Anesthesiology of Shanghai Children's Medical Center, Shanghai Jiao Tong University School of Medicine, Shanghai, China

Yingying Ji The National Children's Medical Center (Shanghai), Department of Anesthesiology of Shanghai Children's Medical Center, Shanghai Jiao Tong University School of Medicine, Shanghai, China

Bo Li The National Children's Medical Center (Shanghai), Department of Anesthesiology of Shanghai Children's Medical Center, Shanghai Jiao Tong University School of Medicine, Shanghai, China

Jingjing Lv The National Children's Medical Center (Shanghai), Department of Anesthesiology of Shanghai Children's Medical Center, Shanghai Jiao Tong University School of Medicine, Shanghai, China

Ning Ma The National Children's Medical Center (Shanghai), Department of Anesthesiology of Shanghai Children's Medical Center, Shanghai Jiao Tong University School of Medicine, Shanghai, China

Zhezhe Peng The National Children's Medical Center (Shanghai), Department of Anesthesiology of Shanghai Children's Medical Center, Shanghai Jiao Tong University School of Medicine, Shanghai, China

Yang Shen The National Children's Medical Center (Shanghai), Department of Anesthesiology of Shanghai Children's Medical Center, Shanghai Jiao Tong University School of Medicine, Shanghai, China

Yunan Song The National Children's Medical Center (Shanghai), Department of Anesthesiology of Shanghai Children's Medical Center, Shanghai Jiao Tong University School of Medicine, Shanghai, China

Liping Sun The National Children's Medical Center (Shanghai), Department of Anesthesiology of Shanghai Children's Medical Center, Shanghai Jiao Tong University School of Medicine, Shanghai, China

Yanjun Sun The National Children's Medical Center (Shanghai), Department of Cardiothoracic Surgery of Shanghai Children's Medical Center, Shanghai Jiao Tong University School of Medicine, Shanghai, China

Ying Sun The National Children's Medical Center (Shanghai), Department of Anesthesiology of Shanghai Children's Medical Center, Shanghai Jiao Tong University School of Medicine, Shanghai, China

Yingying Tao The National Children's Medical Center (Shanghai), Department of Anesthesiology of Shanghai Children's Medical Center, Shanghai Jiao Tong University School of Medicine, Shanghai, China

Lu Wang The National Children's Medical Center (Shanghai), Department of Anesthesiology of Shanghai Children's Medical Center, Shanghai Jiao Tong University School of Medicine, Shanghai, China

Wei Wang The National Children's Medical Center (Shanghai), Department of Cardiothoracic Surgery of Shanghai Children's Medical Center, Shanghai Jiao Tong University School of Medicine, Shanghai, China

Yanting Wang The National Children's Medical Center (Shanghai), Department of Anesthesiology of Shanghai Children's Medical Center, Shanghai Jiao Tong University School of Medicine, Shanghai, China

Chi Wu The National Children's Medical Center (Shanghai), Department of Anesthesiology of Shanghai Children's Medical Center, Shanghai Jiao Tong University School of Medicine, Shanghai, China

Bin Xue The National Children's Medical Center (Shanghai), Department of Anesthesiology of Shanghai Children's Medical Center, Shanghai Jiao Tong University School of Medicine, Shanghai, China

Wenyan Xu The National Children's Medical Center (Shanghai), Department of Anesthesiology of Shanghai Children's Medical Center, Shanghai Jiao Tong University School of Medicine, Shanghai, China

Wenyin Xu The National Children's Medical Center (Shanghai), Department of Anesthesiology of Shanghai Children's Medical Center, Shanghai Jiao Tong University School of Medicine, Shanghai, China

Yinyu Yang The National Children's Medical Center (Shanghai), Department of Cardiothoracic Surgery of Shanghai Children's Medical Center, Shanghai Jiao Tong University School of Medicine, Shanghai, China

Jianwei Zhang The National Children's Medical Center (Shanghai), Department of Anesthesiology of Shanghai Children's Medical Center, Shanghai Jiao Tong University School of Medicine, Shanghai, China

Jiaping Zhang The National Children's Medical Center (Shanghai), Department of Anesthesiology of Shanghai Children's Medical Center, Shanghai Jiao Tong University School of Medicine, Shanghai, China

Kan Zhang The National Children's Medical Center (Shanghai), Department of Anesthesiology of Shanghai Children's Medical Center, Shanghai Jiao Tong University School of Medicine, Shanghai, China

Mazhong Zhang The National Children's Medical Center (Shanghai), Department of Anesthesiology of Shanghai Children's Medical Center, Shanghai Jiao Tong University School of Medicine, Shanghai, China

Ruidong Zhang The National Children's Medical Center (Shanghai), Department of Anesthesiology of Shanghai Children's Medical Center, Shanghai Jiao Tong University School of Medicine, Shanghai, China

Jijian Zheng The National Children's Medical Center (Shanghai), Department of Anesthesiology of Shanghai Children's Medical Center, Shanghai Jiao Tong University School of Medicine, Shanghai, China

Siyi Zhou The National Children's Medical Center (Shanghai), Department of Anesthesiology of Shanghai Children's Medical Center, Shanghai Jiao Tong University School of Medicine, Shanghai, China

Ming Zhu The National Children's Medical Center (Shanghai), Department of Anesthesiology of Shanghai Children's Medical Center, Shanghai Jiao Tong University School of Medicine, Shanghai, China

Part I

Basic Theory

1 Development of the Heart and Major Blood Vessels

Yanjun Sun

Abstract

Understanding the embryonic development of the cardiovascular system is critical for elucidating congenital cardiovascular malformations. This chapter concisely outlines the key developmental processes of the cardiovascular system based on comparative animal models, with a focus on potential mechanisms driving structural morphogenesis and the pathogenesis of cardiovascular anomalies. During early gastrulation, undifferentiated precursor cells migrate and reorganize to differentiate into cardiac progenitors in the cardiogenic region. These cardiac progenitors subsequently form the primitive cardiac tube through coordinated migration, which further establish the four-chambered heart, conduction system, aortopulmonary septation, and vascular system through looping, septation, and fusion, etc. key processes and form a mature cardiovascular system ultimately. Disruptions in any of these tightly regulated processes may result in congenital cardiovascular malformations.

Y. Sun (✉)
The National Children's Medical Center (Shanghai), Department of Cardiothoracic Surgery of Shanghai Children's Medical Center, Shanghai Jiao Tong University School of Medicine, Shanghai, China
e-mail: sunyanjun@scmc.com.cn

Understanding the developmental process of the heart and major blood vessels during the embryonic period can help understand the pathogenesis of various congenital cardiovascular malformations. In recent years, comparing the heart development models in birds and mice has provided important support for further understanding human heart development and the etiology of congenital heart diseases.

1.1 Cardiac Progenitor Cells

All of the cardiac cells originate from undifferentiated progenitor cells. Progenitor cells enter their final developmental pathway under the influence of external signals. The fertilized egg cell divides repeatedly to form a cell mass and then evolves into two distinct cell layers. The upper embryonic layer separates from the second cell layer, the lower embryonic layer in chickens, or the primitive endoderm in mice and humans. During the gastrula formation, many cells migrate into the blastocyst cavity and rearrange into three embryonic layers: ectoderm, mesoderm, and endoderm, which determine the future body's rudiment by embryonic development.

In the early process of gastrulation, cardiac precursor cells appear. Human gastrulation occurs in the early third week of embryonic development, after which vascular cells immediately appear in the cardiogenic region. During

J. Zheng et al. (eds.), *Selected Pediatric Cardiovascular Surgery Anesthesia Cases*,
https://doi.org/10.1007/978-981-96-5614-1_1

gastrulation, the cardiac precursor cells that migrate through the primitive streak constitute the foremost part of the primitive heart tube. After gastrulation, undifferentiated cardiac precursor cells enter the primitive streak. They then move laterally, meeting with the lateral plate mesoderm at the level of Hensen's node. The lateral plate mesoderm then splits into two layers, the splanchnic layer directly above the endoderm and the somatic layer directly below the ectoderm. The anterior endoderm signals the splanchnic mesodermal cells to promote their differentiation into the cardiac precursor cell lineage.

Cardiac progenitor cells are located at the cephalic end of the epithelial-like splanchnic mesoderm. Cardiac mesodermal cells migrate as a unit instead of a group of individual cells. The cardiac mesoderm on both sides of the embryo moves from the cephalic end to the anterior intestinal portal and reaches the anterior intestinal portal along the midline. When the most cephalic parts of the cardiac mesodermal masses on both sides meet at the midline, the entire group of cardiac precursor cells forms a horseshoe-shaped crescent structure, known as the first (primary) cardiogenic region.

The migration pathway of endocardial precursor cells is similar to that of cardiac precursor cells, but important differences exist. Endocardial precursor cells and endothelial precursor cells are both referred to as angioblasts. Endocardial angioblasts can first be detected in the splanchnic mesoderm. Endocardial angioblasts and cardiac precursor cells move forward to the midline together but migrate as independent cells.

1.2 Heart Tube

1.2.1 Heart Tube Formation

As the precardiac cells from the first cardiogenic region move toward the midline, the endocardial cells form a microchannel network, which then merges into a complex endocardial network covered by myocardial cells. In the normal developmental process, the microchannel network of the endocardium quickly merges to form an endothelial channel located within the muscular duct.

During its formation, the heart tube is connected to the foregut through the dorsal mesocardium. During the looping process, the dorsal mesocardium degenerates, and only the connections at the atrial and arterial poles of the heart tube are retained. The disintegration of the central part of the dorsal mesocardium is the key step in the normal looping process. At this point, the attachments at the arterial and venous ends provide anchoring points for the looping heart tube. The interstitial part of the dorsal mesocardium is called the dorsal mesenchymal protrusion, which protrudes into the atrium from the rear and is a derivative of the second cardiogenic region, which is an important component of the atrioventricular septum and exists as a structure guiding the development of the pulmonary veins. The dorsal mesocardium is also an important pathway for migrating cells that may develop from the abdominal neural tube, including developing neural structures from the neural crest.

After the heart tube is formed, the heartbeat subsequently starts, and blood circulation can be observed (at 20 days of human embryonic age). With the initiation of circulation, the heart becomes the first organ in the embryo to perform its basic mature function.

1.2.2 Segmentation Differentiation of the Heart Tube

Traditionally, the heart tube is considered to include the precursors of all of the cardiac segments. In fact, when the heartbeat starts, the heart tube mainly contains the tissue of the future left ventricle. The looping process adds the outflow tract, right ventricle, atrioventricular connection segment, atrium, and sinus venosus to the heart. In fact, the above structures are involved in most of the complex congenital heart diseases in humans. The primordia of the outflow tract (truncus arteriosus and conus), as well as the right ventricle and most of the ventricular septum and part of the cardiac venous pole, develop from the anterior or second cardiogenic region.

Segmental differentiation produces the physiological function of the embryonic heart. The alternate fast and slow contraction characteristics of different regions of the heart tube ensure unidirectional forward blood flow. The atrium has the fastest spontaneous contraction frequency and is the site of pacemaker activity. The atrium conducts fast, the atrioventricular conducts slowly, the ventricle conducts fast, and the outflow tract conducts slowly. Fast conduction areas show rapid contraction-relaxation mechanical characteristics, while slow conduction areas show slow and sustained contraction. This results in the atrium contracting forcefully first, followed by a sphincter-like contraction of the atrioventricular connection (before the atrioventricular valve matures), which prevents the generation of reverse blood flow during the forceful ejection period of the ventricle. The cardiac cycle of the heart tube ends with a sphincter-like contraction of the outflow tract (before the semilunar valve matures), which also prevents reverse blood flow from the aortic arch.

1.2.3 Heart Tube Looping

As the heart tube extends due to the continuous addition of new cardiac tissue at the arterial and venous poles, the heart tube bends to the right. With the continuation of morphological changes, the heart tube becomes more complex. The left ventricle moves to the front and bottom of the atrium; the right ventricle moves slightly forward to the right of the left ventricle.

The molecular characteristics of the left atrium and right atrium are determined by the left-right signaling mechanism. The molecular differences between the left atrium and right atrium are established early after the appearance of the atrial segments, and their genetic regulation depends on the left-right signaling mechanism. Interestingly, in mouse models with abnormal left-right axis determination, the incidence of transposition of the great arteries usually increases, suggesting that the left-right signaling mechanism is a possible factor affecting normal outflow tract development.

Looping not only determines the left-right positioning of the heart, but it also determines the correct relationship between the various segments of the heart. The looping process includes the initial stages of heart tube growth, bending, and rotation. Looping begins only with the atrioventricular connection connected to the left ventricle and ends only with the outflow tract connected to the right ventricle. The second looping stage is the process of the right atrial inflow tract moving to the top of the right ventricle and the aortic outflow tract moving to the top of the left ventricle. During this process, the outflow tract septum appears as a ridge merging with the primitive muscular septum and atrioventricular cushion. Ventricular septation is a continuous process of closing the primitive interventricular foramen and forming a continuous septum with the conus septum.

1.2.4 Fusion

On the inner surface of the heart cavity, the inwardly curved folds form a small muscular ridge inside the heart, which is located between the atrioventricular connection and the outflow tract, known as the ventricular infundibular rim or ventricular infundibular ridge. Other key landmarks are the two main endocardial cushions of the atrioventricular connection and the two endocardial ridges of the outflow tract. The lower endocardial cushion is attached to the dorsal atrioventricular myocardium, and the upper endocardial cushion is attached to the ventral atrioventricular myocardium. As the fusion process continues, the small right and left lateral atrioventricular endocardial cushions become apparent. The two outflow tract endocardial cushions form an extended spiral ridge extending from the distal end of the arterial trunk to the caudal part of the right ventricular body. The endocardial cushion ridge terminating in the right ventricle in the front is called the septal endocardial ridge. The endocardial cushion ridge terminating in the right ventricle in the back is called the wall endocardial ridge. The wall endocardial ridge contacts the right lateral endocardial cushion, and the right lateral endocardial cushion will form a continuity with the upper endocardial cushion. The septal endocardial ridge will form a continuity with the lower endocardial cushion. As the endocardial cushions fuse during the normal septation process, they, together with the primary atrial septum and dorsal interstitial protrusion, jointly construct the central atrioventricular interstitial complex, which extends from the atrioventricular connection to the distal part of the myocardial outflow tract. Diseases such as complex transposition, persistent arterial trunk, and various types of tetralogy are all derived from deviations in these normal developmental steps. The left ventricular cavity and the right ventricular cavity communicate with each other through the primitive interventricular foramen. Blood enters the outflow tract of the heart from the right ventricle. A cuff-like myocardial structure extends along the outflow tract to the aortic sac located at the height of the pericardial reflection.

1.3 Septation

1.3.1 Development and Myocardialization of the Endocardial Cushions

When the heart is initially formed, the myocardium and endocardial cell layers are separated by an acellular layer, traditionally called cardiac jelly. Cardiac jelly is a type of basement membrane located between two parallel epithelia (myocardium and endocardium) and contains traditional basement membrane proteins. In the early looping heart's outflow tract and atrioventricular area, cardiac jelly undergoes coagulation to form relative protrusions. The resulting endocardial cushions, together with the atrioventricular and outflow tract myocardium with special contraction functions, serve to prevent the generation of reverse blood flow. Atrioventricular endocardial cushions also form cardiac fibrous interstitial tissue, including atrioventricular valves and central fibrous bodies. The embryonic outflow tract endocardial cushions form the aortic-pulmonary septum, semilunar valves, and conus septum. During the endocardial cushions' morphogenesis, interstitial cells that settle into the original acellular cardiac jelly originate from the heart's endocardial cells and a cluster of cells from the epicardium, which migrate into the atrioventricular cushions. Still, they do not enter the outflow tract cushions. Endothelial invasion of cardiac jelly is a true cell differentiation process, which transforms from typical epithelial cells into independently migrating fibroblast-like interstitial cells. Only the endocardium from the outflow tract and atrioventricular cushions has the ability to undergo this transformation and only the myocardium at the junction of the outflow tract and atrioventricular can induce this transformation. Myocardialization is the process of the endocardial cushion interstitium being replaced by myocardium. All septal structures within the heart—the ventricular septum, atrial septum, and conus septum—are to some extent constructed through the fusion of non-myocardial interstitial cushions. Myocardialization undertakes the formation of the muscular conus septum and the inflow and anterior outflow tracts of the muscular ventricular septum. In humans, the atrioventricular membranous septum is the only non-myocardial septal structure originating from endocardial cushion tissue.

1.3.2 Atrial Septation

Atrial septation and the connection of the pulmonary veins to the left atrium are closely related events in normal heart development. At the continuous position of the dorsal mesocardium and the atrium (approximately at the level of the lung bud), there is a protrusion of interstitial cells entering the atrium, namely the "dorsal mesenchymal protrusion." The dorsal mesenchymal protrusion is a derivative originating from the second cardiogenic region, which extends into the atrial cavity and connects with the interstitial cap on the front edge of the primary septum. The two main atrioventricular cushions, the dorsal mesenchymal protrusion, and the interstitial cap are eventually fused together to form the atrioventricular interstitial complex.

The myocardial part of the primary septum originates from the left atrial myocardium. The primary septum grows through the elongation of its myocardial part. The interstitial cap on the front edge of the primary septum belongs to the interstitial tissue, of which the cells originate from the endothelial to interstitial transformation, similar to the cells in the endocardial cushions. As the primary septum continues to grow, the primary septum interstitial cap and the dorsal mesenchymal protrusion come into contact with the two main atrioventricular endocardial cushions. These interstitial tissues fuse to form the atrioventricular interstitial complex, and the primary atrial foramen is closed. Before the primary atrial septum is closed, the secondary foramen appears in the primary septum. Initially, it manifests as small holes appearing on the primary septum, then the number increases, the size enlarges, and finally merges into the final secondary foramen. The secondary septum begins as an atrial fold located between the venous valve on the left side of the sinus venosus and the primary septum. The secondary septum also marks the boundary position between the left and right atrial tissues. The left atrial myocardial surface of the secondary septum shows left atrial markers, while the right atrial myocardial surface of the secondary septum shows right atrial markers.

1.3.3 Ventricular Septation

Because the primary interventricular foramen initially provides all of the inflow blood flow for the right ventricle and all of the outflow blood flow for the left ventricle, its correct closure is crucial for the normal development of the heart. The closure of the primary interventricular foramen is accomplished by coordinating with the growth of the muscular interventricular septum and the fusion of the atrioventricular connection and the outflow tract endocardial cushions.

The original muscular interventricular septum is initially a crescent-shaped structure with its posterior boundary extended to the lower endocardial cushion and its anterior boundary extended to the upper endocardial cushion. Part of the primary interventricular foramen closure process includes the mutual extension of the upper and lower endocardial cushions, which contact and fuse around the sixth week of human gestation. Further growth of the muscular septum leads to fusion between the muscular interventricular septum ridge and the already fused endocardial cushion tissue. The normal development of the inflow tract septum mainly depends on the interaction between the tissue originating from the lower endocardial cushion and the muscular interventricular septum. In contrast, the smooth anterior interventricular septum originates from the interaction between the upper endocardial cushion and the muscular interventricular septum. The membranous septum is the approximate location of the final combination between the muscular septum and the upper and lower endocardial cushions.

1.3.4 Development of the Atrioventricular Connection and Atrioventricular Valves

The electrophysiological and physiological characteristics of the myocardium at the connection between the primitive atrium and ventricle are crucial for the heart before septation. However, the myocardial continuity among the atrioventricular junction, the atrial myocardium, and the ventricular myocardium must be interrupted to allow for the development of crossed cardiac fibers and the correct conduction system function. Apart from the bundle of His, the atrioventricular myocardium and ventricular myocardium are separated by a layer of fibrous insulation called the fibrous ring. The residual part of the atrioventricular junction myocardium in the mature heart is integrated into the final atrial myocardium.

The interstitial cell group of the atrioventricular endocardial cushion in the looped heart and the interstitial cells in the atrioventricular groove on the outer surface of the heart are fused together to cause the fibrous interruption of the atrioventricular myocardial continuity. The interstitial cells of the atrioventricular groove originate from the epicardial cells. The interruption of myocardial continuity in the human heart begins around 52–60 days of gestation and is normally finished by the end of the fourth month of gestation. If the insulating tissue at the atrioventricular junction does not form, it may become the pathological basis of the clinical pre-excitation syndrome.

The development of the atrioventricular valves may be related to the inward growth process of the atrioventricular groove tissue because the final valve attachment point is located between the endocardial cushion tissue and the inward atrioventricular groove tissue under normal circumstances. The atrioventricular valve leaflets are formed by a delamination process that is unclear, separating the endocardial cushion tissue and myocardium from the ventricular wall.

During the delamination process, the atrial surface of the valve leaflet is composed of endocardial cushion tissue, while its ventricular surface is mainly composed of myocardium. The myocardial layer provides continuity with the associated subvalvular tension apparatus. With the evolution of valve leaflet morphology, the myocardial part disappears. Initially, the ends of the atrioventricular valve leaflets are directly connected to the compact ventricular myocardium or connected through the outgrowth of myocardial trabeculae. Papillary muscles originate from two mechanisms: from the initial independent and already existing trabeculae aggregating to form papillary muscles or from myocardial structures separated from the myocardium joining the trabeculae or directly forming papillary muscles themselves. The mitral valve papillary muscles originate from a single large trabecula, which then separates into two independent supporting papillary muscles. Parachute-like mitral valve disease may be caused by the defects in this process. The tricuspid valve papillary muscles are developed independently through different mechanisms. Chordae tendineae are formed by the gradual formation of openings and fiber differentiation in the trabeculae and/or initially solid independent valve leaflets.

1.3.5 Development of the Conduction System

The atrioventricular node can be histologically identified in human embryos around the 33rd day of gestation. It is located at the myocardium below the ventricular edge of the lower endocardial cushion of the atrioventricular canal and is included in the primitive ring. The primitive atrioventricular node is directly continuous with the atrioventricular and ventricular myocardium. From the earliest stages, a bundle of cells that eventually becomes the bundle of His can be seen extending from the main body of the atrioventricular node tissue to the subendocardium of the ventricle. Below the main body of the developing atrioventricular node, the atrioventricular sulcus interstitium will invaginate and contact the endocardial cushion interstitium, and the future bundle of His will be accommodated in the fibrous insulating tissue located at the cross-section of the heart.

The differentiation of conduction tissue in the ventricle seems to be achieved through a process that recruits the "working" myocardium into the conduction system cell lineage. At the same time, it is related to its exit from the cell cycle. Many observations support the argument that the trabeculae of the primitive heart are the initial conduction pathways connecting the proximal bundle of His and the ventricular free wall. In the mature heart, a small portion of the trabeculae may still remain as part of the conduction system. Compared with the central atrioventricular node-His bundle-bundle branch conduction system, the intramural Purkinje fibers are a late-appearing structure. The morphological differentiation of the conduction tissue starts from the atrioventricular node and proceeds outward.

1.4 Morphogenesis of the Outflow Tract

1.4.1 Aorta and Pulmonary Artery Separation

The main pulmonary artery septum's initial formation occurs with the interstitium's coalescence at the top of the aortic sac located between the fourth and sixth aortic arches. This interstitium is a cluster of neural crest cells and the two protrusions formed by the coalescence of the interstitium, which penetrates the endocardial cushion at the end of the arterial trunk of the outflow tract. The separation is directed toward the heart and the separation is completed as the interstitial protrusions originating from the neural crest merge. The septum formation separates the arterial trunk by smooth muscle cells originating from the neural crest. As the separation of the main pulmonary artery progresses toward the heart, the aortic trunk and pulmonary artery trunk become apparent. In the absence of an aortic-pulmonary septum, the cardiac outlet is connected to the common arterial trunk, i.e., the persistent arterial trunk. If the aortic-pulmonary septum is not fully formed, it is the main pulmonary artery window.

1.4.2 Development of the Semilunar Valves

The semilunar valves develop at the junction of the main pulmonary artery septum and the conal septum. They originate from the small crests formed between the wall conal crest and the septal conal crest, the conal endocardial crest, and the interstitial protrusions of neural crest origin, penetrating the conal endocardial crest. The fusion of the endocardial crests is accomplished by the contact between the crests and the subsequent disappearance of endothelial cells at the contact site. These crests are then connected with each other through the spiral or knot-like structure of the main pulmonary artery septum. The development of the semilunar valve leaflets begins immediately after the septum formation. Initially, the solid tip protrusions grow out from the arterial surface of the distal endocardial crest, and the septal cushion will become the leaflet tissue. The valve sinus is formed by active endothelial invagination on the outlet surface of the leaflet. The initial valve leaflets are thickened structures filled with a large amount of extracellular matrix, in which interstitial cells of endocardial origin densely reside. Their arterial surface is composed of cuboidal endothelium, and the ventricular surface is a layer of flat, streamlined endothelium. After the sinus invagination is completed, the leaflets undergo remodeling to form a soft fibrous tissue with mature semilunar valve characteristics.

1.4.3 Conal Septum Septation

The conal septum formation is a multi-step process. Initially, the conal endocardial crest is a "simple" structure composed of cardiac jelly surrounded by endocardium and myocardium. Some endocardial cells differentiate into interstitial cells and invade the cardiac jelly. Subsequently, the conal endocardial crest enlarges and brings together the corresponding endocardial crests, with the conal myocardium contracting like a sphincter each time. The endocardial crests gradually merge from the distal cone toward the base of the heart, forming an initial interstitial conal septum. When the proximal conal cushions merge, they separate the aortic and pulmonary outflow tracts. Then, the endocardial cushion tissue is replaced by myocardial tissue, a process that first occurs in the proximal conal septum and finally in the distal conal septum. The myocardialization of the conal cushions leads to the formation of the atrioventricular crest and the muscular outflow tract septum.

1.5 Morphogenesis of the Great Vessels and Coronary Circulation

1.5.1 Migration of Epicardial Cells and Development of Coronary Arteries

In the process of heart development, the epicardium development is relatively late. Still, its correct formation is essential for the normal development of coronary arteries, valves, and fibroblast clusters in the myocardial interstice. The epicardium development in mammals begins with villous protrusions at the original diaphragm site and migrates outward, which gradually crawls over the surface of the heart. The migrating cells eventually become flat on the myocardial surface and develop morphological characteristics equivalent to the original epithelial cells. The flattening process also allows the cells to occupy a larger surface area and contact adjacent cell clusters until a continuous cell layer is formed. We know very little about this process in human development. These important processes occur in the first two months of embryonic development.

The coronary vessels' precursor vascular plexus originates from the space under the epicardium. During the embryonic heart development, the transport of nutrients to the myocardium includes three sequential and partially overlapping stages. In the first stage, a broad trabecular sinusoidal gap network lined with endocardial cells is generated first, and nutrients may flow to the myocardium through this. The second stage is the formation of the endothelial cell channel network penetrating the myocardium under the epicardium. A small part of these channels will communicate with the trabecular sinusoidal gap. The third stage is the degeneration of the subepicardial vascular network and the formation of muscular arterial channels. After these vascular structures are formed, they will penetrate into the ventricular and atrial wall and establish a network structure in the myocardium. The vessels spread to the ventral side of the heart, then follow the grooves of the heart (especially the atrioventricular groove) to reach the outflow tract and form a vascular plexus in the myocardial sheath surrounding the arterial trunk. These vessels merge with the outwardly growing capillaries originating from the plexus around the arterial trunk, eventually forming the proximal coronary arteries penetrating the aortic wall.

1.5.2 Development of the Aortic Arch

The great vessels are the conduits of blood flow from the heart to all body parts. Therefore, they must be formed and functional when embryonic circulation begins (in humans, this is around 20–22 days of gestation). The embryonic vessels are formed through the process of vasculogenesis, that is, the aggregation of endothelial precursor cells (angiogenic cells) to form a network of small endothelial channels. The dorsal aorta and aortic arch are constructed by the fusion of independently formed local angiogenic networks. When communication is established between these networks, small endothelial channels are merged to form larger channels and form the final lumen. These channels are functional vessels containing only endothelial cells. Interstitial cells in the descending aorta and neural crest cells in the aortic arch region subsequently form smooth muscle cells in the arterial media.

The initial embryonic arterial circulation is morphologically bilateral and symmetrical and includes multiple pairs of aortic arch vessels connecting the cardiac outflow to the paired dorsal aortas. The dorsal aortas are initially paired throughout the length of the embryo. The paired aortas begin to fuse into a single structure from the distal end and proceed in reverse toward the seventh somite. With the degeneration of the first and second aortic arch vessels, they remain open only as capillary structures. The dorsal aorta (carotid duct) located between the third and fourth aortic arch vessels completely degenerates without remnants, making the paired third aortic arch vessels the only blood flow source from the aortic sac/trunk complex to the embryonic head. The third aortic arch vessel becomes the precursor of the final common carotid artery. The right dorsal aorta at the bifurcation of the dorsal aorta completely degenerates, making the right fourth aortic arch vessel a short stalk and connecting the right seventh intersegmental artery (future subclavian artery) to the aortic sac/trunk complex. The right sixth aortic arch vessel becomes the right pulmonary artery. The left sixth aortic arch vessel becomes the left pulmonary artery and the ductus arteriosus; the ductus arteriosus connects the distal pulmonary trunk originating from the pulmonary plexus and the left pulmonary artery at the level of the connection between the left dorsal aorta and the left fourth arch vessel to the left dorsal aorta. The left dorsal aorta is still very patent throughout its length. Still, it undergoes remodeling, so the final left fourth aortic arch vessel, ductus arteriosus, and left seventh intersegmental artery (future left subclavian artery) all connect to the left dorsal aorta within a very small span. The vertebral artery originates from the anastomosis formed between the seven cervical intersegmental arteries. After the continuity between the intersegmental arteries is established, their connections with the dorsal aorta degenerate (except for the connection of the seventh intersegmental vessel of the subclavian artery), making the vertebral artery ultimately originate from the subclavian artery.

1.5.3 Development of Pulmonary Veins

The precursor tissue of the pulmonary trunk vein comes from a bundle of endothelial cells appearing in the embryonic heart dorsal mesentery. The endothelial bundle forms a lumen, initially a midline structure. With the development of the dorsal interstitial protrusion and the intrusion into the atrial cavity on the right side of the original pulmonary vein, the pulmonary vein moves to the left of the midline. During the normal developmental process, the continuous development of the dorsal interstitial protrusion, the myocardialization of this interstitial, and the accompanying development of the primary septum eventually connect the pulmonary veins to the left atrium. Therefore, the development of the pulmonary veins is not a product of the outward growth of the atrial wall. The initial pulmonary trunk vein opening is restructured into four separate pulmonary vein openings in the mature heart. The wall of the pulmonary vein is initially not muscular, but the myocardial sleeves are formed around these veins with the evolution of development.

1.5.4 Development of Systemic Veins

The embryonic systemic veins are also formed through vasculogenesis. Initially, there are three bilateral structures of systemic veins for drainage: the yolk sac vein, the umbilical vein, and the main vein system. The yolk sac vein drains the embryo's gastrointestinal tract and intestinal derivatives. The umbilical vein delivers oxygenated blood from the placenta to the heart. The main vein system receives the return of blood from the head, neck, and embryonic body wall. All these three blood flows drain into the venous sinus of the primitive heart tube. The matured systemic vein system is finally built on the basis of the embryonic vein system through degeneration, reconstruction, replacement, etc., a series of complex changes.

The venous sinus is initially symmetrical on both sides and connects with the left and right superior vena cava, umbilical vein, and yolk sac vein through its left and right "corners." Under normal circumstances, the connections among the left superior vena cava, yolk sac vein, umbilical vein system, and the left corner of the venous sinus degenerate, while the coronary sinus in the heart becomes a major derivative of the left corner of the venous sinus that is preserved. Persistent left superior vena cava can be seen when the degeneration of the connection between the embryonic vein and the left venous corner fails. The right corner of the venous sinus normally accommodates the entire systemic venous drainage, except for part of the cardiac blood flow returning through the coronary sinus. In addition, the tissue located between the openings of the atrium in the mature heart originates from the right corner of the venous sinus.

The left and right yolk sac veins are interconnected through a venous plexus, which will evolve into the hepatic sinus. The left yolk sac vein degenerates after losing its connection with the left corner of the venous sinus. Therefore, the entire venous system of the embryonic gut normally returns to the heart through the right yolk sac vein. The connection from the right yolk sac vein to the right venous sinus, as the terminal part of the inferior vena cava, continues from the fetal stage to the adult stage.

The left umbilical vein also loses its continuity with the left corner of the venous sinus, while the right umbilical vein degenerates as an independent structure. The left umbilical vein forms an anastomosis with the venous duct (originating from the hepatic plexus of the yolk sac vein). The venous duct is closed with life mature. Therefore, no derivative structures of the embryonic umbilical vein system are connected to or persist with the heart.

The main venous system initially includes bilateral anterior and posterior superior vena cava. The anterior and posterior superior vena cava merge at the level of the venous sinus to form the total superior vena cava. The left anterior superior vena cava loses its continuity with the left corner of the venous sinus. Still, it has some remnants on the surface of the heart to serve as a channel for the coronary venous blood flow to enter the coronary sinus, known as the left atrial oblique vein under normal circumstances. Another part of the left anterior superior vena cava is preserved to form the left internal jugular vein. As the left anterior superior vena cava loses its continuity with the heart, it continues with the right anterior superior vena cava through the main venous anastomosis, which forms between the thyroid and thymic veins. This intervascular connection will persist as the left brachiocephalic vein. The right anterior superior vena cava becomes the normal right superior vena cava between the right atrium and the site where the proximal left anterior superior vena cava drains (via the main venous anastomosis).

The posterior superior vena cava is the only structure in the embryonic venous drainage system that can ultimately maintain bilateral symmetry. Most of the two posterior superior vena cava degenerate and lose direct continuity with the venous sinus. The posterior superior vena cava initially drains the body wall, gonads, and kidney structures. The superior vena cava plexus replaces its venous drainage function to the body wall, while the inferior vena cava plexus takes over the venous drainage of the gonads and kidneys.

The posterior vena cava, superior vena cava, and inferior vena cava together form part of the inferior vena cava, which is connected to the inferior vena cava originating from the yolk sac vein, the latter directly connects to the right atrium. In fetal and mature body circulation, the remnants of the posterior vena cava are limited to the farthest part of the inferior vena cava (formed by the anastomosis of the left and right posterior vena cava) and the common iliac vein. The part of the inferior vena cava originating from the posterior vena cava is connected to the superior vena cava segment of the inferior vena cava. The superior vena cava system originates from the azygos vein, and the hemiazygos vein is usually connected to the inferior vena cava between the renal and common iliac veins. The superior vena cava segment of the inferior vena cava is connected to the inferior vena cava segment of the inferior vena cava, and the inferior vena cava segment of the inferior vena cava collects the gonadal vein and renal vein reflux before connecting to the yolk sac vein pathway entering the heart. The initial vascular structure is bilaterally symmetrical in the superior vena cava and inferior vena cava systems. The left pathway degenerates, but the right pathway remains, which forms the typical position of the inferior vena cava on the right side. The mechanism of venous morphogenesis may depend on the correct left-right signal transduction. This is a series of particularly important developmental relationships, which can persist in those children with interrupted inferior vena cava merging with continuous azygos vein, where the hepatic veins directly drain into the right atrium (Yanjun Sun).

Physiological Overview of the Cardiovascular System

2

Jie Bai and Wenyin Xu

Abstract

The cardiovascular system orchestrates blood circulation to deliver oxygen and nutrients while maintaining metabolic homeostasis. This chapter concisely outlines its physiological structure and functional mechanisms, focusing on hemodynamic principles and cardiac pump regulation based on Ohm's and Poiseuille's laws. These laws establish that blood flow depends on pressure gradients, vascular resistance, and blood viscosity. Vascular shear stress and compliance also critically influence blood flow and tissue perfusion. Cardiac output is determined by preload, afterload, contractility, and heart rate. Cardiac contractility hinges on Ca^{2+}-mediated excitation-contraction coupling and sarcomere mechanics, which can be analyzed via pressure-volume loops. Cardiovascular performance is further regulated by neural (sympathetic/parasympathetic) and humoral (e.g., catecholamines, renin-angiotensin system) mechanisms. Understanding these principles is essential for perioperative hemodynamic management and optimizing outcomes in children undergoing congenital cardiac surgery.

J. Bai (✉) · W. Xu
The National Children's Medical Center (Shanghai), Department of Anesthesiology of Shanghai Children's Medical Center, Shanghai Jiao Tong University School of Medicine, Shanghai, China
e-mail: baijie@scmc.com.cn

The cardiovascular system comprises the heart, arteries, veins, and capillaries. The heart pumps blood into the vessels through rhythmic contraction and relaxation to supply sufficient blood to various body parts. The vascular system serves as the conduit of blood circulation and plays a crucial role in regulating the blood flow throughout the body. The heart and vascular system work together to provide enough oxygen and nutrients to the tissues and organs to meet their metabolic requirements and maintain normal life activities. Cardiovascular physiology is an important theoretical basis of perioperative management, which will greatly improve the perioperative management level of anesthesiologists and the postoperative outcomes of patients. This section will introduce the basic principles of hemodynamics, the process of cardiac mechanical movement, and the important factors of regulating cardiovascular function.

2.1 Basic Principles of Hemodynamics

Hemodynamics refers to the kinetics of blood flow in the cardiovascular system, which involves physics and physiology. Based on the basic principles of hemodynamics, it is important for the management of perioperative cardiovascular function to analyze the various factors affecting cardiovascular function.

J. Zheng et al. (eds.), *Selected Pediatric Cardiovascular Surgery Anesthesia Cases*,
https://doi.org/10.1007/978-981-96-5614-1_2

The cardiovascular system, also known as the circulatory system, follows the general physical laws of fluid motion. The formula for flow calculation in physics is V = Q/A (V is velocity, Q is flow, A is pipe cross-sectional area), which reflects the relationship between velocity, flow, and vessel cross-sectional area, i.e., velocity is directly proportional to the flow and inversely proportional to the cross-sectional area of the vessel. When the flow is constant, the velocity in the capillaries is the slowest, while it is the fastest in the aorta because the total cross-sectional area of the capillary bed is the largest, while the cross-sectional area of the aorta is the smallest. Doppler ultrasound technology can estimate the cardiac output (CO) by measuring the velocity time integral of aortic flow and the diameter of aortic annulus, which can be used to guide clinical hemodynamic management.

2.2 Physical Factors Affecting Blood Flow

Ohm's and Poiseuille's physics law can also be applied to the cardiovascular system. The classic Ohm's law: current = voltage/resistance. According to this formula, it can be understood that the blood flow (Q) is directly proportional to the pressure difference at both ends of the vessel (Pi − Po, Pi is the inflow pressure, Po is the outflow pressure), and inversely proportional to the flow resistance (R), i.e., Q = (Pi − Po)/R. Poiseuille's law describes the relationship between various physical factors affecting fluid flow, $Q = (Pi - Po)\pi r^4/8\eta L$ (Q is flow, Pi − Po is the pressure difference at both ends of the pipe, r is the pipe radius, η is the fluid viscosity, L is the pipe length). Combining Ohm's law and Poiseuille's law, the resistance formula can be derived: $R = 8\ \eta L/\pi r^4$, indicating that minor changes in the diameter of vessels can significantly increase the resistance. The pressures in the circulatory system gradually decrease from the arterial to the venous system. In the system, the arteriole system exists in series. When the blood flows to the arterioles, the vascular diameter significantly decreases, the vascular resistance significantly increases, and the vascular pressure decreases due to the arteriole existing in series. During clinical practice, vascular resistance can be regulated by vasoactive drugs that can change the vascular radius by constricting or dilating the peripheral blood vessels. Sodium nitroprusside mainly dilates small arteries, which can significantly reduce peripheral vascular resistance and cardiac afterload while the CO is significantly increased. Although the radius of the single capillary is smaller than that of the single artery, the capillary network exists in parallel, and the total resistance of capillaries is lower than that of a single capillary. Neither the vascular resistance significantly increases nor does the vascular pressure significantly drop from arterioles to capillaries. However, in the terminal stage of pulmonary arterial hypertension, some parallel pulmonary capillaries lose their function and cause further increases in pulmonary capillary resistance and pulmonary arterial hypertension worsening. The increase of blood viscosity is also one of the important factors leading to the increase of peripheral vascular resistance and reducing the blood flow. Children with Tetralogy of Fallot (TOF) are usually accompanied by compensatory erythrocytosis, manifesting as increased hematocrit (HCT). High HCT will significantly increase the blood viscosity, which can further increase the peripheral vascular resistance, decrease the blood flow velocity, and ultimately lead to insufficient perfusion of tissues and organs. The increase of red blood cells is closely related to the increase of viscosity and low perfusion of organs, so attention should be paid to the perioperative management of HCT in children.

2.3 Shear Stress of the Vessel Wall

Many studies have shown that shear stress plays a very important role in maintaining the integrity of vascular endothelial structure and function. It is also an important induction factor of cardiovascular and cerebrovascular diseases. Shear stress refers to the force acting on the vessel wall produced by the friction between flowing blood and the endothelium. It is equivalent to the product of the shear viscosity and the shear rate, i.e., $\tau = \gamma.\eta$, where τ is the shear stress, γ is the shear rate, and η is the shear viscosity. Assuming that the blood vessel is an inelastic cylindrical tube, then the shear rate is the rate of change of the velocity to the radius of the vessel, i.e., $\gamma = du/dr$, where u is the flow velocity, and r is the radius of the vessel, which indicates that the faster the velocity, the greater the shear rate of the vessel wall, and the greater the shear stress of the vessel wall. The Hagen–Poiseuille equation links the shear stress of the vessel wall with the flow: $\tau = 4\ \mu Q/\pi R$ [1]. This formula indicates that the shear stress on the vessel wall is directly proportional to the flow and inversely proportional to the cube of the vessel radius. Shear stress can now be measured relatively easily with the continuous development of technologies such as magnetic resonance imaging, three-dimensional ultrasound vectors, and blood flow imaging over the past 20 years. Shear stress within the normal range can help maintain the integrity of the vascular endothelium, but either too high or too low harms the human body. Congenital heart disease in children can alter the shear stress on the vessel wall after surgery and ultimately affect the endothelial structure and physiological function. Aortic arch surgery or arterial anastomosis can not only increase the shear stress and promote the generation of turbulence, but ultra-high shear stress may also cause vascular intima tearing and form an aneurysm.

2.4 Compliance of the Cardiovascular System

The compliance of the cardiovascular system reflects the ability of transmural pressure to induce changes in organs or vessel volume. The compliances of ventricles and vessels vary dramatically, usually peripheral veins compliance > ventricles > central veins > arteries >arterioles and capillaries. Compared with the left ventricle, the compliance of the right ventricle is higher, so the right ventricle can withstand a large amount of blood return without significantly increasing ventricular pressure. Compared with arteries, the compliance of veins is higher due to their thinner vascular wall, which is about 20–30 times that of arteries. Therefore, most circulating volume is stored in the venous system higher than the arteries. Therefore, the therapeutic volume expansion has a greater impact on the venous capacity.

2.5 Cardiac Pump Function

2.5.1 Special Structure and Function of Cardiomyocytes

The heart is the source power of blood flow, which drives the blood to flow in the circulatory system through cardiac contraction and relaxation. Unlike other tissue cells, cardiomyocytes contain myosin, actin, tropomyosin, troponin complex, and other proteins to form myofilaments, including thin and thick filaments arranged in parallel to form sarcomeres with contractile function. The sarcomere is the basic unit of myocardial contraction. When the sarcomere length is between 2.2 and 3.5 μm, the overlap of myofilaments is optimal. When the sarcomere is too short, the thin filaments bend. When the sarcomere is too long, the overlap of myofilaments decreases, which is not conducive to generating myocardial active tension.

The main component of thick filaments is macromolecular myosin, which is composed of about 300 myosin molecules. The head end of myosin is large and spherical, containing actin-myosin ATPase, which is responsible for ATP hydrolysis and energy release and relaxes the cross-bridge between actin and myosin. The amount of ATP hydrolysis determines the rate of connection and disconnection between actin and myosin, which determines myocardial fibers' contraction speed.

The thin filament is composed of actin, tropomyosin, and troponin. Actin is a spherical molecule composed of a polypeptide chain known as globular actin. Actin is arranged into repeating units to form two strands of α-helices. The forked proteins between the helices are called tropomyosin. The troponin complex comprises Troponin T, Troponin C, and Troponin I subunits, and Troponin T is attached to tropomyosin at certain intervals. Troponin C is a high-affinity calcium-binding site. Troponin I inhibits the interaction between actin and myosin. These proteins play a very crucial role in myofilament sliding. Clinically, the increase of serum troponin reflects the myocardial cell damage and has higher specificity and sensitivity than commonly used myocardial enzyme spectrum detection.

Mitochondria are the power source of cardiomyocytes, which can produce most of the ATP required for contraction. Adult cardiomyocytes contain many mitochondria, which account for more than 30% of the cell volume and provide more than 90% of energy needs through oxidative phosphorylation. Under normal physiological conditions, the oxidation of fatty acids is superior to other nutrients. However, under stress, cardiomyocytes can also obtain energy by oxidizing glucose, lactate, amino acids, and ketone bodies. The glycolysis and lactate production rate in fetal cardiomyocytes is high, but the ATP produced by the fatty acid oxidation pathway is less than 15%. The morphological features and functions of mitochondria in different parts are different. The mitochondria in the myofibrillar interstitium are mainly used for the energy supply to myosin and sarcoplasmic reticulum ATPase, the submembrane mitochondria mainly participate in ion homeostasis, and the perinuclear mitochondria may be related to gene transcription and translation.

The sarcolemma (i.e., cardiomyocyte membrane) is a lipid bilayer structure composed of collagen, glycocalyx, and plasmalemma and includes two major components: intercalated discs and transverse tubules (T-tubules). The intercalated disc is a unique structure at the connection of cardiac fibers, an important feature of the myocardium, formed by the short protrusions of two adjacent cardiac fibers. The intercalated disc has three types of junctional complexes: desmosomes, adherent junctions, and gap junctions. Gap junctions are the basis of chemical and electrical coupling between adjacent cells, composed of connexin family proteins to ensure the electrical and metabolic transmission between cells. In contrast, desmosomes and adherent junctions constitute the mechanical connection between cardiomyocytes. The intercalated disc is the basis for the heart to work synchronously as a whole, and mutations in the component proteins that make up the intercalated disc can cause a variety of cardiomyopathies, including arrhythmia syndromes, myocardial diseases, etc.

The sarcolemma invaginates to form T-tubules to connect with the sarcoplasmic reticulum of cardiomyocytes, quickly transmit the action signals to the inside of cardiomyocytes, and regulate the flow of calcium ions through phospholamban. Phospholamban prevents calcium ions from entering the cytoplasm by inhibiting the interaction of calcium ions with the SERCA (sarcoplasmic reticulum ATPase). In contrast, the phosphorylation of phospholamban can reverse this inhibition, promote the inflow of calcium ions, and cause cardiac contraction. Many studies have shown that the activity of phospholamban in children with heart failure, sepsis, and dilated cardiomyopathy is reduced. Other organelles in cardiomyocytes, such as α-tubulin, β-tubulin, endoplasmic reticulum, nucleus, Golgi apparatus, etc., also play an important role in the contractile process of cardiomyocytes.

Cardiac contraction begins with action potentials and produces mechanical contractions through excitation–contraction coupling. The cardiomyocytes become depolarized when the electrical pulse is transmitted to the myocardium. Then the electrical pulse is conducted along the muscle fiber membrane and the T-tubule system and propagated to adjacent cardiomyocytes through the gap junctions of the intercalated discs. High concentrations of extracellular calcium ions enter the cell through the voltage-gated calcium channels on the muscle membrane and T-tubules and increase the intracellular calcium ion concentration, which further causes the calcium ions to release from the sarcoplasmic reticulum through the ryanodine receptor and the increase of the intracellular calcium ion content. This process is also known as calcium-induced calcium release. During excitation–contraction coupling, the intracellular calcium ion concentration can be increased nearly a hundred times. With the rise of intracellular calcium content, calcium binds to troponin C and causes the conformational change in tropomyosin and troponin to antagonize the action of troponin I, expose the myosin binding site on actin, promote the binding of actin to the head of the myosin to form cross-bridges, which drive the thin filaments to slide into the gap between the thick filaments, the muscle fibers contract, and then the SERCA pumps the intracellular calcium ions back to the sarcoplasmic reticulum against the concentration gradient. At the same time, the cell membrane expels calcium ions through sodium–calcium exchange and calcium pumps, thereby reducing the intracellular calcium ion concentration and promoting the dissociation of actin and myosin. The force and speed of cardiac contraction are directly proportional to the cell's free calcium ions. Neonatal cardiomyocytes are not only small in volume but also lack T-tubules; the development of the sarcoplasmic reticulum is incomplete, and calcium-induced calcium release is limited. The transmembrane movement of extracellular calcium ions plays a more significant role in excitation–contraction coupling. Therefore, neonatal myocardial contraction is more dependent on the concentration of extracellular free calcium ions.

2.5.2 Mechanics of Myocardial Contraction

There are two types of mechanics for myocardial contraction: isometric and isotonic. During isometric contraction, the length of the myocardium remains unchanged while the myocardial tension is increased. The tension produced by stretching the myocardium to different lengths at rest is called resting tension, the exponential relation between myocardial resting tension and length. When the myocardium with a fixed length is activated, it will produce additional tension, called active tension. The total tension is the sum of the resting and active tension. In isometric contraction, the tension created by the myocardium depends on the length during muscle contraction, but neither too short nor too long can produce maximum tension. The tension remains constant in isotonic contraction, but the myocardium becomes short. When the myocardium contracts, the preload (the load when the myocardium is at rest) and the afterload (the load when the myocardium contracts) determine the total load. During myocardial contraction, isometric contraction is initially performed at a fixed length until an isotonic contraction is performed when tension equal to the total load is generated.

2.5.3 Cardiac Cycle

The cardiac cycle refers to a complete process of cardiac contraction and relaxation. The heart chambers' pressure and volume change with the cardiac cycle phase. Understanding the cardiac cycle is of great importance for assessing heart function. The pressure–volume loop (P-V loop) reflects the relationship between ventricular pressure and ventricular volume over the course of the cardiac cycle (Fig. 2.1). The P-V loop can be divided into four phases: isovolumetric contraction, ventricular ejection, isovolumetric relaxation, and ventricular filling. Based on the mechanics of ventricular muscle contraction, each phase corresponds to a specific length-tension relationship. The cardiac cycles of the left and right ventricles are roughly the same, but the performance of the P-V loop differs. For exam-

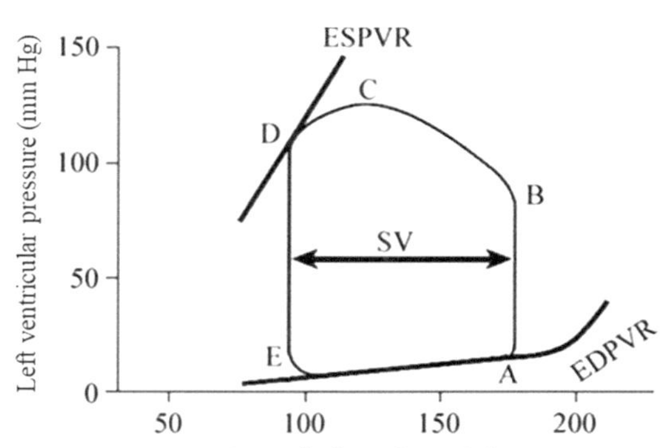

Fig. 2.1 Left ventricular pressure–volume loop. *EDPVR* end-systolic pressure–volume relationship, *ESPVR* end-diastolic pressure–volume relationship

ple, LV pressure and volume change with time-phase changes from A to E during the cardiac cycle.

At the end of diastole, the LV begins to contract, the left ventricular pressure (LVP) rises, the atrioventricular valve closes, and the LVP is still lower than the aortic pressure, the aortic valve has not yet opened, and the blood is in a confined chamber. The left ventricular volume remains unchanged, but the LVP increases rapidly. This brief period is the isovolumetric contraction phase. The P-V loop represents it by the vertical line from point A to B.

When the LVP exceeds the aortic pressure, the aortic valve starts to open, and the LV begins to eject with the pressure and energy gradient development between the LV and the aorta. The ejection process is divided into a brief, rapid ejection period and a longer, slow ejection period. During the rapid ejection period, the pressures in the LV and the aorta rise sharply and terminate after reaching the peak. Thereafter, the ventricular wall tension, ventricular pressure, and ventricular ejection rate all decrease. During the rapid ejection period, the LVP exceeds the aortic pressure, and the ejection volume accounts for more than 80% of the stroke volume (SV). During the slow ejection period, the aortic pressure exceeds the LVP, but the blood can still be ejected from the LV into the aorta with slow velocity even though the pressure gradient has been reversed, which may be due to the potential energy generated by the stretching of the arterial wall. In the P-V loop, it is represented by points B to D. Point C is the highest point of ventricular pressure. The change in left ventricular volume during ejection, i.e., SV, depends on the degree of myocardial contraction. After the aortic valve is closed, the left ventricular contraction ends, and the pressure and volume presented at this point are the left ventricular end-systolic pressure (LVESP) and left ventricular end-systolic volume (LVESV), respectively. The ventricular end-ejection slope, i.e., the end-systolic pressure–volume relationship (ESPVR), reflects myocardial contractility. During ventricular contraction, the contraction of the single myocardial cell is a combination of eccentric, isotonic, and isometric contractions. The ventricular contraction mode is complex and exquisite, with the maximal efficiency of ventricular contraction. The myocardial fibers synergize with each other to generate twisting force during the entire cardiac contraction. The ventricular morphology and structure changes resemble towel-twisting action with minimal energy expenditure. It has been shown that there is no morphological "twisting" in ventricular contraction in patients with single ventricle physiology, which results in more energy expenditure with less efficiency.

The closure of the aortic valve marks the beginning of the left ventricular diastole. At this time, the LVP is higher than that in the atrium, the atrioventricular valve is still closed, the ventricle is in a confined chamber, and the LVP drops rapidly while the volume of the ventricle remains constant. The period from the aortic valve closure to the atrioventricular valve opening is called the isovolumetric relaxation period, which is represented as points D–E in the P-V loop. When the LVP drops below the left atrial pressure, the atrioventricular valve begins to open. The rapid ventricular filling period is initiated, and most of the ventricular filling occurs during this period. The late diastolic period is a slow filling period, the ventricle has fully relaxed at that time. As the ventricular pressure gradually increases, the ventricular compliance begins to reduce, and the filling rate is also gradually decreased. The previous filling was all passive filling, and the ventricular filling caused by atrial contraction is active filling. The atrial contraction causes an increase in atrial pressure, forcing blood to flow into the ventricle. Although the filling caused by left atrial contraction only accounts for 1/10 of the left ventricular filling, when the atrial contraction force becomes weak, such as after congenital heart surgery, junctional ectopic tachycardia (JET), the weakening of atrial ejection can lead to a significant decrease in ventricular filling and CO.

The entire ventricular filling period is represented as points E–A in the P-V loop. At point A, the ventricular volume reaches its maximum, known as the left ventricular end-diastolic volume (LVEDV), i.e., the left ventricular preload, and the pressure at this time is the left ventricular end-diastolic pressure (LVEDP). The slope of the ventricular filling curve during diastole, i.e., the end-diastolic pressure–volume relationship (EDPVR), reflects the LV compliance. When the heart has abnormalities such as hypertrophy, ischemia, infarction, or structural abnormalities, although the LVEDV is the same, the LVEDP can significantly be increased due to decreased ventricular compliance.

The P-V loop width, referred to as the difference between LVEDV and LVESV, is defined as the SV. The ejection fraction (EF) is the ratio of SV to LVEDV. The area surrounded by the P-V loop is the work done by the ventricle. When the myocardial contractility remains constant, the increase in preload can cause the P-V loop to shift to the right and increase SV. The increase of afterload can lift the P-V loop and reduce SV. When children suffer from heart disease or changes in heart function, the P-V loop will also change accordingly. For example, in children with mitral valve insufficiency, blood flows back to the left atrium during left ventricular contraction, impairing isovolumetric contraction function, and points A–B are no longer a vertical line. In addition, volume overload can lead to the ventricular filling volume increase and increase LVEDV. In children with aortic valve stenosis, the resistance to left ventricular ejection is increased, and blood ejection is obstructed, leading to the increase of the pressure gradient across the aortic valve during ejection, a significant increase of the left ventricular contractile peak pressure and a significant increase in point C. At the same time, the wall stress is increased, SV is decreased, and LVESV is increased.

2.6 Factors Affecting Cardiac Output

CO is the basic parameter of cardiac contractile function, which is determined by heart rate (HR) and SV ($CO = HR \times SV$), where the SV depends on the preload, afterload, and contractility. The contraction function reflects the combined effects of various parameters such as ventricular preload, afterload, myocardial contractility, and HR.

2.6.1 Heart Rate

HR is an important factor in regulating CO, which is mainly controlled by the autonomic nervous system. The autonomic nervous system governs the automaticity of the sinus node pacemaker cells through the sympathetic and parasympathetic nerves, thereby changing the HR.

The impact of HR on CO is complex and nonlinear due to the indirect affection on SV. The increase in HR can shorten the ventricular diastolic period, reduce ventricular filling time, and reduce preload. On the other hand, increased HR can also increase the inflow of calcium ions into myocardial cells and enhance myocardial contractility. Studies have shown that too fast or too slow HR and atrioventricular desynchrony will reduce CO. The relationship between CO and HR is an inverted U-shape. After congenital heart correction surgery, a complete atrioventricular block will cause a significant decrease in CO in children. This is because the compensatory increase in SV is insufficient to offset the CO reduction caused by very slow HR and atrioventricular desynchrony.

2.6.2 Stroke Volume and Preload

SV refers to the amount of blood ejected from the ventricle with each heartbeat. It is represented by the difference between the end-diastolic volume and the end-systolic volume, $SV = EDV - ESV$. Changes in EDV and/or ESV will increase or decrease SV. Ventricular preload is an important factor affecting SV, represented by pressure or volume load. Frank and Starling described preload as the initial length of myocardial contraction. The regulation of SV by changing the initial size is called heteromeric regulation. Frank and Starling were the first to describe this phenomenon of cardiac length-dependent autoregulation. The energy produced by myocardial contraction is a function of the initial length of the myocardial fibers, which is the famous Frank–Starling law, a milestone law in cardiovascular physiology. It describes the positive correlation between myocardial contractility and the initial length of myocardial fiber contraction. It clarifies that the increase in ventricular ejection volume is the response to the ventricular diastolic filling increase (preload). The cardiac function curve based on this mechanism is also called the Frank–Starling curve (Fig. 2.2).

When the ventricular contractility, afterload, and ventricular compliance remain constant, the increase in ventricular filling can cause an increase in SV.

As the ventricular preload increases, SV tends to increase. At the beginning of preload increase, SV increases significantly, which forms the steep part of the curve. However, the increase of SV becomes slow and reaches the plateau phase of the curve after some degree of preload increase. The curve does not show a significant decrease when cardiac function is normal, but the curve shows a decline in patients with chronic heart failure or ventricular overexpansion. Regarding the Starling curve and the P-V loop, fluids infusion can increase the preload with subsequent SV increase along the Starling curve, manifesting as an increase of end-diastolic volume on the P-V loop and SV increase without myocardial contractility changes.

Under normal situations, venous return equals CO. Venous return is an important factor affecting preload. Therefore, it is also a determinant of CO. CO can be tripled by venous blood return due to the huge preload reserve in the venous system. Therefore, the regulation of venous blood return is very critical.

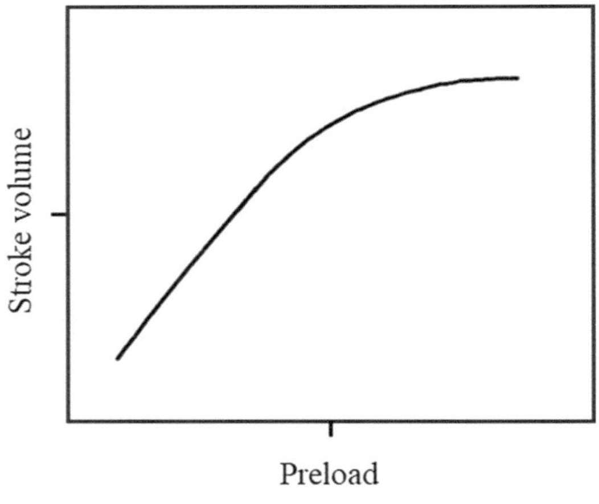

Fig. 2.2 Frank–Starling curve

Various factors, such as mean systemic filling pressure, right atrial pressure, and venous resistance, determine venous blood return. Venous return = (mean systemic filling pressure − right atrial pressure)/venous resistance. The pressure gradient between the mean systemic filling pressure and the right atrial pressure is the driving force for venous return. Any factor that increases this pressure gradient, such as an increase in mean systemic filling pressure (increased volume) or right atrial pressure decrease, can increase venous return and preload. Of these factors, mean systemic filling pressure is, in turn, influenced by blood volume and volume vessels.

The circulatory blood volume is composed of two parts. One part of the circulatory blood volume does not increase the vascular wall tension and only maintains the basic shape of the vessel, which is called non-tension blood volume. The other part produces tension on the vascular wall and increases the tension of the vascular wall, which is called tension blood volume. Tension blood volume accounts for 25%–30% of the total circulating volume, and this ratio will be affected by the changes in vascular wall tension. Tension blood volume is the factor affecting mean systemic filling pressure. Most of the circulating volume belongs to non-tension capacity and has no significant effect on mean systemic filling pressure or venous return.

The venous vascular wall is richly innervated with autonomic nerves, which regulate the interconversion of tension blood volume and non-tension blood volume. Drugs such as dobutamine, sodium nitroprusside, and nitroglycerin can increase vascular compliance, converting some tension blood volume into non-tension blood volume. If the patient is accompanied by insufficient blood volume, it may lead to a decrease in venous return and CO. Pure arterial vasoconstrictors (such as vasopressin) will increase the systemic arterial pressure, but there is no further increase in venous return and CO after the systemic pressure is increased. Vasoconstrictors acting on both arteries and veins (such as norepinephrine) may increase the gradient of venous return and CO.

Intrathoracic pressure changes can affect the preload by the right atrial pressure changes.

During the inspiratory phase of spontaneous breathing, the intercostal space expands, the diaphragm descends, the thoracic cavity expands to produce negative intrathoracic pressure, and the negative intrathoracic pressure is transmitted to the right atrium and vena cava, increases the transmural pressure of the right atrium, expands the right atrium, and decreases the right atrial pressure and vena cava pressure. At the same time, the intra-abdominal pressure is also affected by the diaphragm's descent, leading to the increase of the abdominal vein transmural pressure and the increase of the mean systemic filling pressure. In conclusion, the venous return and preload increase with the increase in the pressure gradient of venous return. The vena cava at the entrance of the thorax can collapse with forceful inhalation due to the negative thoracic pressure and venous return obstruction. At this moment, further lowering the right atrial pressure will no longer affect the venous return.

Unlike spontaneous breathing, the intrathoracic pressure is higher than atmospheric pressure during the inspiratory phase of intermittent positive pressure ventilation. This leads to the pressure increase around the right atrium, compliance decrease, right atrial transmural pressure decrease, and right atrial pressure increase. When continuous positive pressure ventilation is applied, the intrathoracic pressure is higher than atmospheric pressure throughout the respiratory cycle. Under this mode, the right atrial pressure will be increased, and the pressure gradient of venous return will be decreased, leading to systemic venous return decrease, right heart output decrease, and ultimately, left ventricular preload and output decrease.

In children with Fontan physiology, venous return is determined by the pressure gradient between the mean systemic filling pressure and the downstream pressure of caval-pulmonary artery anastomosis. Atrial pressure changes do not affect systemic venous return, but they affect pulmonary venous return. Positive pressure ventilation in Fontan patients increases the intrapleural pressure, reduces the pressure gradient between the mean systemic filling pressure and the pulmonary circulation, as well as the pressure gradient between the pulmonary circulation and the common atrium, and reduces the venous blood return. Early extubation to restore spontaneous breathing and switch from positive to negative pressure ventilation can increase pulmonary blood flow and CO in Fontan patients.

2.6.3 Afterload

Ventricular afterload is also one of the important factors affecting SV. Afterload refers to the resistance the ventricle has to overcome during the ejection process, including any factors preventing the heart ejection. In the absence of stenosis in the ventricular outflow tract and cardiac valves, ventricular afterload mainly depends on the ventricular wall tension and the resistance of the resistance vessels to ejection. When the cardiac contractility and preload are constant, a higher pressure is required for cardiac ejection. If the afterload increases, the Starling relationship becomes weak, with the curve shifting downward. On the P-V loop, the afterload increases lead to a higher pressure during ejection; both ESV and ESP increase under constant preload, ultimately leading to an SV decrease. Afterload is negatively correlated with CO. The cardiac response to afterload change varies with different cardiac functional states. In normal cardiac function, the end-diastolic volume and pressure will be increased if the afterload is suddenly increased. According to the Starling law, the compensatory myocardial work will be increased due to the increase of afterload, the heart can gradually adapt to the increase of afterload, and the myocardial contractility will subsequently increase, and the end-diastolic volume and pressure gradually return to normal levels, CO also returns to its original range. When myocardial function is impaired, the ventricle cannot fully compensate for the increase of afterload through increased myocardial contractility, which can lead to ventricular enlargement and filling pressure increase. Suppose the ventricle works harder according to the Starling mechanism, although CO can still be maintained within the normal range. In that case, increased ventricular filling pressure and afterload will exacerbate myocardial function inhibition. In severe heart failure, the ventricle cannot increase myocardial work through the Starling mechanism, and CO cannot be maintained. In this situation, reducing the ventricular afterload can not only increase CO, but it can also reduce the ventricular filling pressure, which is an important theoretical basis for the clinical treatment of children with heart failure.

The intrapleural pressure affects the left ventricular afterload by affecting the transmural pressure of the intrathoracic arteries. The transmural pressure in the aorta is the difference between the systolic pressure in the aorta and the intrapleural pressure. During spontaneous breathing, the decrease of intrapleural pressure will increase the transmural pressure of the aorta, resulting in higher afterload and smaller left ventricular SV. During positive pressure ventilation, the intrapleural pressure is increased, the aortic transmural pressure is reduced, and the left ventricular afterload is also decreased. Therefore, utilizing positive pressure ventilation to reduce the afterload of children with left ventricular dysfunction can reduce the oxygen consumption of the myocardium and respiratory muscles.

The effect of intrapleural pressure on the right ventricular afterload depends on the relationship between pulmonary vascular resistance and lung volume. The pulmonary vascular resistance is minimized with normal respiration to functional residual capacity and increases with either alveolar expansion or collapse. Increased pulmonary vascular resistance increases the right ventricular afterload. In the continuous positive airway pressure, the alveolar pressure and intrapleural pressure during the inspiratory and expiratory phases are both positive, and the alveolar and extra-alveolar vascular resistance is increased throughout the respiratory cycle.

2.6.4 Myocardial Contractility

Myocardial contractility refers to the ability of the myocardium to contract, which is a parameter independent of HR, preload, and afterload, and reflects the functional status of the myocardium itself. By changing the intrinsic contractility of the myocardium, the CO and stroke work can be changed. This method of cardiac function regulation is unrelated to the initial length, which is also called homometric autoregulation. Myocardial contractility is positively correlated with SV and ventricular work. In the Starling curve, if the contractility changes, the heart will present a new Starling curve. In the corresponding P-V loop, the change of contractility is reflected in the change in ESPVR. When the ESPVR line is shifted upward and to the left, the slope will be increased, and the EF and SV will increase while EDPVR remains unchanged. If the ESPVR line is shifted to the right and downward, then it indicates a decrease in myocardial contractility, EF, and SV, while EDPVR remains unchanged.

Myocardial contractility is affected by many factors. Any step in the excitation–contraction coupling can affect myocardial contractibility. However, from the perspective of the myocardium contraction mechanism, the strength of myocardial contractility is mainly determined by the intracellular Ca^{2+} concentration, and the key factor determining the shortening speed is the cross-bridge ATPase activity, which controls the conversion rate of chemical energy into mechanical energy at cross-bridge, thereby affects the myocardial contractile velocity and amplitude. Under appropriate initial length, the overlap of thick and thin myofilaments is the pre-requirement of activated cross-bridge formation, but the formation of activated cross-bridges depends on the degree of intracellular Ca^{2+} concentration increase and the affinity of troponin for Ca^{2+}. Any factor that can increase the intracellular Ca^{2+} concentration or the affinity of troponin with Ca^{2+} can increase the formation of activated cross-bridges and enhance myocardial contractility. For example, catecholamines can activate β receptors, increase intracellular cAMP concentration, and then increase Ca^{2+} channels opening on the cell membrane and Ca^{2+} release from the sarcoplasmic reticulum, thereby increasing the intracellular Ca^{2+} concentration. Calcium sensitizers can increase the affinity of troponin with Ca^{2+} to form a stable conformational relationship and promote cross-bridge binding to thin filaments, enhancing myocardial contractility. Autonomic nerve activity and various humoral factors can also affect myocardial contractility.

The heteromeric regulation and home metric regulation of myocardial contraction often coexist. When the myocardial contractility is evaluated, it is impossible to rule out the influence of preload, afterload, etc. In clinical practice, parameters such as SV, cardiac index, ejection fraction, and maximum slope at the end of ventricular contraction are commonly used to reflect myocardial contractility.

2.6.5 Ventricular Compliance and Diastolic Function

Cardiac diastolic function refers to the ability to increase ventricular volume at the end of cardiac diastole. Clinically, it is usually represented by the trend of changes in ventricular volume and pressure. Ventricular compliance refers to the change of volume caused by a unit pressure change ($\Delta V/\Delta P$). Within the normal ventricular functional range, the pressure–volume relationship is linear, but ventricular compliance is affected by volume load. As the ventricular volume gradually increases, the ventricular compliance correspondingly decreases. At this time, further increasing the volume will cause a significant increase in pressure, and the pressure–volume relationship becomes a curve. Therefore, when the volume load is adjusted, not only the inherent cardiac compliance should be considered, but the change of ventricular compliance caused by the volume load change should also be considered. Neonates have poor cardiac compliance and cannot tolerate excessive preload. Excessive increases in preload tend to result in increased EDP and venous pressure, so neonates are more susceptible to volume-related heart failure, limiting the effectiveness of neonatal volume infusion. Therefore, when the preload tolerance has reached the maximum contractility, neonates can only increase CO by increasing HR, which is one of the reasons why neonatal and infant CO depend on HR.

The myocardial structure of the left and right ventricles differs, and their compliance is not exactly the same. The right ventricular myocardium is thin and highly compliant. Therefore, it can withstand relatively large volume loads. When adjusting preload, the different compliance of ventricles should be considered. In the case of left ventricular dysfunction, infusing a small amount of fluid may lead to excessive preload and the occurrence of pulmonary edema. When adjusting the preload of children with left ventricular dysfunction, the main goals should be to reduce the venous return and vascular tension; for children with right ventricular dysfunction, dehydration or vasodilator drugs should be used cautiously in order to maintain a certain level of right CO and to ensure adequate left heart preload.

2.7 Regulation of Cardiovascular Function

Cardiovascular function is regulated by neural and humoral factors to maintain relatively stable HR, CO, arterial pressure, and tissue perfusion, which can meet the metabolic requirements of various organs and tissues under different conditions.

2.7.1 Neural Regulation

The sinus node, atrioventricular junction, and bundle of His of the heart are dually innervated by the sympathetic and parasympathetic (vagus) nerves, while the ventricular muscle is mainly innervated by the sympathetic nerve. When the sympathetic nerve is excited, the postganglionic fibers of the sympathetic nerve release norepinephrine, which binds to myocardial β_1-adrenergic receptors to increase HR, myocardial contractility, and CO. Excitation of the cardiac vagus nerve releases acetylcholine from the postganglionic fiber terminals, which binds to the cardiac M-type cholinergic receptors to slow HR and atrioventricular conduction.

The nerves innervating the vascular smooth muscle can be divided into two major categories: vasoconstrictor nerves and vasodilator nerves. Most vascular smooth muscles are only innervated by sympathetic vasoconstrictor nerve fibers, while a small portion of vessels (such as skeletal muscles) receive dual innervation from sympathetic vasoconstrictor nerve fibers and vasodilator nerve fibers. Capillary smooth muscles are mainly influenced by local tissue metabolites. The main effect of sympathetic vasoconstrictor nerve fibers excitation is to constrict blood vessels, sympathetic vasodilator nerves cause skeletal muscle vessels to dilate during intense exercise.

2.7.2 Humoral Regulation

Humoral regulation refers to the regulatory effects of certain chemicals in the blood and interstitial fluid on the myocardium and vascular smooth muscle functions.

2.7.2.1 Epinephrine and Norepinephrine

The adrenal medulla secretes epinephrine and norepinephrine. Epinephrine accelerates the HR and strengthens myocardial contraction. Different vascular smooth muscles are dominated by different adrenergic receptors. In the vascular smooth muscles of organs such as the skin, kidneys, and gastrointestinal tract, α receptors dominate, and the binding of epinephrine presents a vasoconstrictive effect. In the vessels of skeletal muscles and the liver, β_2 receptors dominate, small doses of epinephrine cause vasodilation, and large doses also excite α receptors and cause vasoconstriction. Norepinephrine causes widespread vasoconstriction in all body organs.

2.7.2.2 Renin–Angiotensin–Aldosterone System

The renin–angiotensin–aldosterone system is one of the important humoral regulation systems composed of a series of peptide hormones and corresponding enzymes, which includes renin, angiotensin I, angiotensin II, angiotensin III, aldosterone, etc., which are widely present in the myocardium, vascular smooth muscle, skeletal muscle, brain, kidney, and other organ tissues. Among them, angiotensin II has a strong vasoconstrictive and hypertensive effect, while the vasoconstrictive effect of angiotensin III is weaker. Angiotensin I stimulates the adrenal medulla to secrete epinephrine and norepinephrine. Aldosterone can induce Na^+ and water retention effects. Clinically, angiotensin-converting enzyme inhibitors and angiotensin receptor antagonists are commonly used drugs for hypertension, improvement of cardiac function, and prevention and treatment of coronary heart diseases.

Other vascular active substances include vasopressin, vasodilatory, and vasoconstrictive substances produced and released by vascular endothelial cells, the kinin system, cardiovascular active peptides, gas signal molecules, prostaglandins, cytokines, and some systemic hormones, etc., and all of them play important roles in the regulation of cardiovascular function.

The factors affecting cardiovascular physiological function are complex and interrelated, which should be comprehensively considered in clinical practice. The basic principles of hemodynamics are the foundation of perioperative hemodynamics management. Furthermore, the normal cardiovascular physiological functions and their regulatory mechanisms are the theoretical basis for identifying and intervening in pathological states. Understanding these basic theories will help manage perioperative hemodynamics, prevent and intervene in perioperative cardiovascular adverse events, and improve the safety of perioperative anesthesia in pediatric patients (Jie Bai, Wenyin Xu).

Reference

1. Lai YC, Potoka KC, Champion HC, et al. Pulmonary arterial hypertension: the clinical syndrome. Circ Res. 2014;115(1):115–30.

Pathophysiology of Congenital Heart Disease

3

Yue Huang and Wenyan Xu

Abstract

Understanding the pathophysiological changes in congenital heart disease (CHD) is crucial for perioperative anesthesia management in pediatric CHD patients. This chapter concisely outlines the key pathophysiological mechanisms, including shunting, obstructive, mixed, and regurgitant lesions, alongside myocardial ischemia and pulmonary hypertension (PH). Left-to-right shunts increase pulmonary blood flow and volume load, while right-to-right shunts cause hypoxemia. Obstructive lesions may lead to pressure overload and myocardial ischemia. Mixing lesions rely on intercirculatory blood mixing regulated by systemic-to-pulmonary vascular resistance ratios. Regurgitant lesions can lead to cardiac volume overload and progressive functional decline. Coronary anomalies or supply-demand imbalance may result in myocardial ischemia, while increased pulmonary vascular resistance or elevated pulmonary blood flow can cause PH. Therefore, perioperative anesthetic management requires balancing systemic and pulmonary vascular resistances, maintaining cardiac output, optimizing oxygenation, and tailoring individualized strategies to optimize outcomes.

Children with congenital heart disease (CHD) not only exhibit specific anatomical changes in the heart, but they are also associated with a series of pathophysiological alterations and functional reserve changes in multiple organs. Therefore, it is crucial to fully understand these abnormal changes, which is essential for perioperative anesthetic management. The basic pathophysiologic changes that cause hemodynamic abnormalities in children with CHD include shunting, mixing, obstruction, and regurgitation. In addition, myocardial ischemia may also be present in children with CHD. In some more complex cases, these basic pathologic changes may coexist.

3.1 Shunting Lesions

Shunting refers to the process by which the venous return from a circulatory system is recirculated by the same circulatory arterial system, which includes physiological and anatomical shunts. Recirculation of systemic venous blood occurs when blood flows from the systemic venous atrium (right atrium) to the aorta, which results in a physiologic right-to-left shunt. Similarly, recirculation of pulmonary venous blood occurs when the blood flows from the pul-

Y. Huang (✉) · W. Xu
The National Children's Medical Center (Shanghai), Department of Anesthesiology of Shanghai Children's Medical Center, Shanghai Jiao Tong University School of Medicine, Shanghai, China
e-mail: huangyue@scmc.com.cn

J. Zheng et al. (eds.), *Selected Pediatric Cardiovascular Surgery Anesthesia Cases*,
https://doi.org/10.1007/978-981-96-5614-1_3

monary venous atrium (left atrium) to the pulmonary artery (PA), which results in a physiologic left-to-right shunt. Anatomic shunting refers to the blood flowing from one circulatory system into another via openings at the level of the heart chambers or great vessels. Shunting can be simple or complex. The direction and magnitude of anatomic shunting depend on the size of the opening, the resistance ratio of both sides of the shunt, i.e., systemic vascular resistance (SVR) and pulmonary vascular resistance (PVR), ventricular compliance, and the presence of anatomic obstructions. Physiological shunting can occur without anatomic shunting (no abnormal shunt openings), such as in children with transposition of the great arteries (TGA), who have physiologic shunts without anatomic shunts.

Left-to-right shunting is the most common CHD, which is characterized by the oxygenated blood from the systemic flowing into the pulmonary circulation due to shunt lesions. The common left-to-right shunt lesions include atrial septal defect (ASD), ventricular septal defect (VSD), atrioventricular septal defect (AVSD), patent ductus arteriosus (PDA), and partial anomalous pulmonary venous return (PAPVR). All of these left-to-right shunts increase the cardiac preload, which is influenced by the location and size of the orifice. When the pulmonary blood flow (PBF) exceeds systemic blood flow (Qp:Qs > 1), the additional increase in blood flow cannot further increase arterial oxygen content but increases the volume load on the heart instead, leading to the dysfunction of cardiac systole and diastole and the decrease of cardiac output (CO). The increased PBF may also further decrease pulmonary compliance, increase airway resistance, and increase the work of breathing. A progressive increase in PVR may lead to pulmonary vascular obstructive disease (PVOD). Shunting at the level of the great arteries increases PBF, which further increases the blood return from the pulmonary veins to the left atrium and increases left ventricular end-diastolic volume (LVEDV). According to the Frank–Starling principle, increased work per beat in the left ventricle can result in the dilation of left ventricular chambers and myocardial hypertrophy. In addition, the oxygenated blood can be shunted into the low-pressure pulmonary circulation when the aortic valves are closed during diastole and result in the decrease of systemic diastolic pressure and inadequate coronary artery perfusion. With the increase of ventricular hypertrophy and oxygen consumption, myocardial ischemia can occur due to the insufficiency of oxygen delivery, which can ultimately result in pulmonary venous congestion and pulmonary edema due to left heart failure. As PVR increases, the right ventricular pressure (RVP) overload can occur and lead to right heart failure. The left-to-right shunt in ASD mainly occurs during the atrial systole, and the magnitude of the shunt mainly depends on the relative compliance of the left and right ventricles during diastole. The magnitude of left-to-right shunt in VSD mainly depends on the size of the defect and the PVR/SVR ratio. If the VSD is small, the left-to-right shunt belongs to the restricted shunting because the amount of shunting mainly depends on the size of the VSD instead of the PVR/SVR ratio. However, the left-to-right shunt in large VSDs usually belongs to unrestricted shunting since the amount of left-to-right shunting mainly depends on the PVR/SVR ratio. The lower the PVR/SVR ratio, the greater the amount of left-to-right shunting. In addition to the hemodynamic effects described above, significant atrial or ventricular shunting is also characterized by increased right ventricular preload. The long-term increase of blood flow and pressure in the pulmonary circulation can result in a significant increase of PVR. When PVR exceeds SVR, shunting reverses, and a right-to-left shunt develops, which can result in cyanosis and erythrocytosis. When the changes in PVR are irreversible, it is known as Eisenmenger's syndrome.

Although the anesthetic management of children with left-to-right shunts should be individualized, fully understanding the effects of anesthetics on PVR and SVR shares some common grounds. All of the anesthetics can dose-dependently inhibit the function of the myocardial contract, with infants less than 6 months of age being most sensitive. Therefore, it is more helpful to maintain CO and hemodynamic stability by the combination of small doses of different anesthetics instead of large doses of a single anesthetic. In addition, regulation of inspired oxygen concentration and ventilation parameters can maintain adequate oxygenation, but they cannot increase left-to-right shunting via PVR reduction.

Obstructive lesions in the right ventricle (RV) or pulmonary circulation resistance greater than systemic circulation resistance can cause the recirculation of systemic venous blood and physiologic right-to-left shunting, which reduces PBF, causes the deoxygenated mixing of blood into the systemic circulation, and finally results in hypoxemia and cyanosis. In addition, the right ventricular ejection obstruction can significantly increase the right ventricular pressure overload, ultimately leading to right heart failure. When the defect size or shunt approaches or exceeds the diameter of the aortic root (non-restrictive defect), right ventricular pressures are equal to the systolic pressures of the great artery vessels. RVP may reach the level of systemic circulation. Physiologic shunting is usually the result of anatomic shunting, but it can also occur in the absence of anatomic shunting, such as in TGA.

3.2 Obstructive Lesions

The pathophysiology of obstructive lesions depends on the anatomic locations and the obstructive severities. Obstructions can occur at the valves, supra- and/or subvalvular levels, such as pulmonary stenosis (PS), aortic stenosis (supra- and/or subvalvular), coarctation of the aorta (CoA), and mitral stenosis. Atresia is an extreme form of obstruction. The bicuspid aortic valve may be the left heart obstructive lesion with the least hemodynamic impact, whereas aortic atresia and hypoplastic left heart syndrome (HLHS) may be the worst left heart obstructive lesions with the most significant hemodynamic effects. A variety of congenital heart defects can cause right heart obstruction with a variety of clinical signs and symptoms, but all of these defects can be accompanied by right-to-left shunting. The severities of right heart obstruction depend on the degree of structural malformation of the heart and/or great vessels. In mild cases, only exercise intolerance or mild fatigue may be observed. However, severe right heart obstruction in the newborn may present with significant cyanosis or congestive heart failure (CHF). Dynamic obstruction can also occur during ventricular contraction, such as Tetralogy of Fallot (TOF).

Left ventricular obstruction can cause systemic circulatory hemodynamic disturbances, which may be caused by single-level obstruction, such as hypertrophic cardiomyopathy, CoA, interruption aortic arch (IAA), aortic stenosis (supra- and/or sub-valvular), or multi-level obstructions, such as Shone's syndrome. Left ventricular obstruction can lead to varying degrees of pulmonary hypertension (PH) and/or inadequate coronary perfusion. In neonates with severe left ventricular outflow tract obstruction (LVOTO), the left ventricular afterload is significantly increased, and the left ventricular ejection fraction is dramatically decreased, which results in ① Systemic hypotension and hypoperfusion. If the ductus arteriosus stays patency, the systemic perfusion mainly depends on the blood flow of the right ventricular and pulmonary artery. If the ductus arteriosus is closed, the patient often shows signs of severe shock, such as systemic hypotension, acidosis, and severe respiratory distress. ② Increased ventricular-wall tension and decreased myocardial perfusion pressure can lead to myocardial ischemia. ③ Hypoxemia, the deoxygenated blood flows from the RV into the systemic circulation through the patent ductus arteriosus (PDA) and even retrograde perfusion of the coronary arteries. ④ Elevated left ventricular end-diastolic pressure (LVEDP) and left atrial pressure (LAP) cause left-to-right shunting through the patent foramen ovale (PFO), which increases pulmonary blood flow (Qp). Therefore, the key to anesthetic management is maintaining adequate CO and diastolic pressure to ensure coronary perfusion. It is difficult for children with increased LVEDP to tolerate fluid overload and elevated SVR.

Congenital cardiac malformations in one or more anatomic regions, such as the right atrioventricular (AV) valves, right ventricular outflow tract (RVOT), pulmonary valve, main pulmonary artery (MPA), and/or branches of the PA can obstruct the blood flow from the right heart. Congenital cardiac malformations are usually caused by abnormal tissue displacement during development, which can directly lead to cardiac malformations. Furthermore, the anatomical irregularities can also cause hemodynamic impairment, which indirectly leads to cardiac malformations. Thus, both of them contribute to the occurrence of cardiac malformations. Therefore, it is very likely that obstructive lesions occur in several anatomic regions. Most right cardiac obstructive lesions are accompanied by right-to-left shunting, which further results in cyanosis. For example, the right-to-left shunts through ASD or PFO in children with severe Ebstein's anomaly or the right-to-left shunts through VSD in children with TOF. Complete pediatric obstruction of right heart outflow, such as severe pulmonary stenosis (PS) or pulmonary atresia (PA), is characterized by reduced PBF, hypoxemia, and right heart failure. The pulmonary perfusion in these children depends on the patency of ductus arteriosus, which provides blood flow to the PA from the aorta. Atrioventricular valve stenosis blocks the return flow of the vena cava or pulmonary veins, resulting in signs of systemic or pulmonary circulation congestion. Therefore, critically ill newborns with right ventricular obstruction require an infusion of prostaglandin E_1 (PGE_1) to keep ductus arteriosus patency. Otherwise, as the PDA closes, cyanosis worsens and may even lead to death.

3.3 Mixed Lesions

Cyanotic CHD is often accompanied by mixed lesions. When the intracardiac communication is very large, the two ventricles actually become a common chamber, and the arterial and venous blood are completely mixed at the level of the atria or ventricles before being pumped into the systemic and pulmonary circulations. At this point, the mixed lesions with bidirectional shunting can cause or exacerbate cyanosis. The ratio of CO distributed to the systemic and pulmonary blood flow depends on the SVR, PVR, and the presence or absence of obstruction. If there exists LVOTO, then the left-to-right shunting (Qp:Qs > 1) dominates, which increases PBF and decreases systemic perfusion. If there exists right ventricular outflow tract obstruction (RVOTO), then the right-to-left shunt dominates (Qp:Qs < 1), which significantly reduces PBF and causes hypoxemia. In the absence of outflow tract obstruction, the blood flow to the systemic or pulmonary circulation depends on the PVR/SVR ratio. Generally, PVR is lower than SVR with predominant left-to-right shunting and increased PBF (Qp:Qs > 1). When PVR is greater than SVR, the right-to-left shunting predominates, and PBF decreases (Qp:Qs < 1). It is more beneficial to maintain the balance of oxygen delivery between the systemic and pulmonary circulations by decreasing SVR rather than increasing PVR. It is particularly dangerous to increase SVR in those neonates with HLHS after stage I palliative operation, which can potentially lead to the increase of systemic steal and PBF. Previous research has shown that permissive hypercapnia is more beneficial for those patients with single ventricle physiology than reducing the fraction of inspired oxygen (FiO_2) in balancing the blood flow of systemic and pulmonary circulation because it can minimize the impact on systemic oxygenation while PBF is reduced. In those children, after the bidirectional Glenn procedure, hypoventilation-induced $ETCO_2$ increase can increase the blood return to the heart and improve blood oxygenation due to cerebral vasodilation. However, high $ETCO_2$ can also carry the risk of PVR elevation. So, the associated risks must be carefully balanced. Negative pressure ventilation can significantly increase CO in children after the Fontan procedure and improve systemic oxygen delivery. In those children with Fontan fenestration, measures must be taken to reduce PVR and the right-to-left shunting, and then the systemic oxygenation is ultimately improved. Given the low baseline arterial oxygen saturation in children with cyanotic CHD, systemic oxygen delivery heavily relies on the increase of hemoglobin concentration to improve the oxygen-carrying capacity of the blood.

Inter-circulatory mixing is a unique situation in patients with TGA. The atrioventricular connections in children with TGA are concordant, but the ventricular–arterial connections are discordant, which results in a parallel circulation. In other words. The deoxygenated blood returning to RA from the systemic circulation enters RV, which then is ejected directly into the systemic circulation via the aorta and subsequently returns to RA. The vital organs and tissues, such as the brain and heart, are thus perfused with deoxygenated blood. Conversely, oxygenated blood returning to LA from the pulmonary circulation enters LV, then passes through PA and returns to LA. This results in completely independent systemic and pulmonary circulations and coexists in parallel with pulmonary venous blood recirculating within the pulmonary circulation and systemic venous blood recirculating within the systemic circulation. Oxygen saturation in the PA is significantly higher than that in the aorta, which is the basis of transposition physiology. At this point, the child must depend on the blood mixing between the parallel circulations to survive. Inter-circulatory mixing can occur at multiple levels, including intracardiac communications at the level of the atrium (ASD and PFO) or the ventricle (VSD) and extracardiac communications at the level of the great arteries (PDA). Effective inter-circulatory mixing is critical for those children with TGA to survive. The effectiveness of mixing is not only determined by the hemoglobin oxygenation and the severities of clinical manifestations, but it is also influenced by numerous anatomic and physiologic factors, which include the number, location, and restriction of inter-circulatory communications. Mixing at the atrial level is most effective because the LAP is always higher than right atrial pressure (RAP). Throughout the cardiac cycle, the direction of blood flow is consistently from left to right (oxygenated pulmonary venous blood to deoxygenated systemic venous blood), resulting in increased oxygen content in the RV and increased oxygen saturation in the aorta. Bidirectional shunting is likely to occur (blood from aortic shunts to PA via PDA, blood from RV shunts to LV via VSD), so mixing at the ventricular septum or PDA level is often ineffective. The most common inter-circulatory mixing in d-TGA is usually from PFO only, which often requires atrial septostomy to increase inter-circulatory mixing and alleviate cyanosis. The efficiency of mixing is also affected by Qp. Various factors decreasing PBF can also reduce mixing and worsen cyanosis, such as PS or total CO reduction due to hypovolemia or anesthetics that inhibit myocardial contractility.

The oxygenated blood from the inter-circulatory mixing is delivered to the entire body through effective systemic circulation, while the deoxygenated blood from inter-circulatory mixing is delivered to the lungs through effective pulmonary circulation. Effective blood flow refers to the volume of venous blood that comes from one circulatory system and enters into the other circulatory system, i.e., effective pulmonary blood flow refers to the volume of systemic venous blood that enters into the pulmonary circulation and effective systemic blood flow refers to the volume of the pulmonary venous blood that enters into the systemic circulation. Effective blood flow is usually the result of blood flowing through the heart along normal pathways, but it may also be the result of anatomic right-to-left or left-to-right shunts. Both effective pulmonary and systemic blood flow are essential to maintain survival. Total pulmonary circulation blood flow is the sum of effective pulmonary blood flow and recirculated pulmonary blood flow. Total systemic blood flow is the sum of effective systemic blood flow and recirculated systemic blood flow. Regardless of the complexities of lesions, effective pulmonary and systemic blood flows are always equal, but the total pulmonary and systemic blood flows are not necessarily equal. Therefore, recirculating blood flow (physiologic shunt) is an additional ineffective blood flow. Due to the parallel existence of the systemic and pulmonary circulations in TGA, the effective blood flow is only a small fraction of the total pulmonary or systemic blood flow, while the recirculating blood flow accounts for the largest fraction. The greater the proportion of effective blood flow to total pulmonary or systemic blood flow, the higher the arterial oxygen saturation.

Cyanosis is the most common clinical manifestation of TGA. Neonates with TGA and intact ventricular septum (TGA/IVS) combined with small PDAs or PFOs usually develop severe cyanosis, acidosis, and heart failure on the first day of life. Children with TGA/IVS combined with a large PDA or PFO/ASD, or TGA combined with VSD, have more effective inter-circulatory mixing and higher PaO_2, but the risk of CHF is also higher.

3.4 Regurgitant Lesions

Apart from Ebstein's anomaly, isolated primary valvular regurgitation is relatively rare in children with CHD. Children with Ebstein's anomaly not only have tricuspid valve (TV) issues, but they also have right ventricular (RV) myocardium issues. The pathophysiological changes and clinical manifestations of children with Ebstein's anomaly vary with the severity of the anatomical anomaly. In children with types C and D Ebstein's anomaly, the TV is significantly shifted toward the apex, which significantly reduces RV volume, even in a nonfunctional RV chamber. In addition, RVOTO and severe valvular regurgitation can also occur. So, most of the regurgitant systemic venous blood is shunted through an ASD and causes cardiac hypertrophy and pulmonary hypoplasia, which further leads to PVR increase and cyanosis. Persistent elevation of PVR can impede the blood ejection from the hypoplastic RV into the pulmonary circulation and cause the pulmonary circulation perfusion to depend on PDA. RV can establish effective forward blood flow as PVR decreases in relatively mild cases, such as type A and B.

Although congenital pulmonary valve regurgitation is rare, severe pulmonary regurgitation may occur postoperatively in children with TOF and others who require placement of a conduit between the RV and PA. Aortic regurgitation (AR) and mitral regurgitation (MR) are the more significant valvular regurgitant lesions. Regurgitation can cause ventricular volume overload, leading to progressive dilatation and CHF. In cases with severe regurgitation, both the proximal and distal chambers of the regurgitant valve dilate, which further causes volume overload. In children with MR, both LV and LA are dilated. In children with AR, LV is enlarged, and the aorta is dilated or pulsatile.

Isolated MR is quite rare in children with CHD. Although atrioventricular regurgitation of the systemic ventricle is relatively common in children with AVSD, single ventricle (SV), and congenitally corrected transposition of the great arteries (ccTGA), these situations are not usually considered as MR. MR is associated with abnormalities of the mitral valve annulus, leaflets, chordate tendineae, or papillary muscles. Left ventricular volume overload caused by aortic incompetence or dilated cardiomyopathy can lead to annular dilation. Cleft mitral valve or leaflet expansion may also cause regurgitation. Leaflet expansion may be caused by congenital structural abnormalities, connective tissue disorders like Marfan's syndrome, or inflammatory diseases like rheumatic fever. Papillary muscle dysfunction may also lead to MR, such as dilated cardiomyopathy. Factors that increase left ventricular afterload and volume overload will also worsen mitral incompetence. Other rare causes include valve apparatus deformation caused by tumors.

The mitral valve incompetence gradually worsens as time goes by. It usually requires a larger LVEDV to maintain sufficient CO and compensate for the blood regurgitating from the mitral valve during systole. The increase of LVEDV, in turn, further exacerbates annular dilation, leading to progressive worsening of ventricular dysfunction and, ultimately, leading to cardiovascular decompensation. MR can cause LA dilation and associated atrial arrhythmias (such as atrial fibrillation), which can also cause cardiovascular decompensation. In those patients with persistent severe MR, especially when they are associated with ventricular dysfunction and elevated LVEDV, severe PH can occur, which may potentially compromise the right ventricular function. The rightward septal shift may also compromise right ventricular function due to left ventricular dilatation.MR can be reduced by decreasing SVR and correcting the aortic valve abnormalities (stenosis or regurgitation). Increased coronary blood flow can reverse papillary muscle dysfunction due to myocardial ischemia.

3.5 Myocardial Ischemia

The causes of subendocardial ischemia in children with CHD include myocardial ischemia induced by congenital or acquired coronary artery abnormalities and localized myocardial ischemia caused by an imbalance of oxygen supply/consumption with normal coronary arteries. The main types of coronary artery malformations include: ① anomalous origin of the coronary arteries from the PA; ② anomalous origin of the coronary artery from the aorta; ③ congenital atresia of the left main coronary artery; ④ coronary arteriovenous fistula; ⑤ myocardial bridging of the coronary arteries; ⑥ coronary artery aneurysms; and ⑦ coronary artery stenosis.

Subendocardial perfusion not only depends on the coronary perfusion pressure (CPP), referring to the difference of the aortic diastolic pressure minus the LVEDP, but it also depends on the effective perfusion time, namely diastolic dominance. Therefore, the relationship between heart rate, diastolic pressure, and ventricular end-diastolic pressure determines the occurrence of subendocardial ischemia. Aortic diastolic pressure is typically low in normal neonates and infants. In patients with single ventricle physiology, the systemic blood flow depends on the supply of ductus arteriosus. In patients with persistent truncus arteriosus, the aortic diastolic pressure is relatively lower because more blood flow enters into the pulmonary circulation with low resistance during the diastolic period. Impaired ventricular systolic and diastolic function and/or increased ventricular end-diastolic volume can increase end-diastolic pressure, which is particularly harmful to subendocardial perfusion. During tachycardia, higher diastolic pressure is required to maintain sufficient subendocardial perfusion. Otherwise, myocardial ischemia may occur due to the reduced effective coronary perfusion time caused by the shortened diastolic period. Coronary artery anomalies caused by conditions such as Kawasaki disease, anomalous left coronary artery arising from the pulmonary artery (ALCAPA), and Williams syndrome can complicate the management of CHD.

ALCAPA is one of the most refractory coronary artery anomalies. The pathophysiology of ALCAPA is complex and changes with the growth and development of the neonate and the reduction of pulmonary vascular resistance and pressure since the anatomical structures and physiological environments constantly change In neonates with ALCAPA, the left ventricle can still be well perfused from the left coronary artery originating from the PA and maintain sufficient left ventricular function due to the high PVR and pulmonary artery pressure, even though the oxygen saturation of mixed venous blood is relatively low. As PVR and pulmonary artery pressure decrease after birth, the blood flow in the left coronary artery may reversely flow into the PA and cause "coronary steal," which further affects the left ventricular perfusion and results in myocardial ischemia and ventricular dysfunction. The left coronary artery perfusion primarily depends on the diastolic period because it can be obstructed during the systolic period. The increase in LVEDP can further reduce coronary perfusion pressure. If significant collateral circulation is formed, the "coronary steal" may also affect right ventricular perfusion during systole and diastole, but as in normal coronary physiology, systolic perfusion of some right ventricular myocardium is protective. The potential unique advantage of ALCAPA reversing coronary blood flow into the pulmonary circulation is that it may help maintain PVR and pulmonary artery pressure, which delays the onset of symptoms. Left heart failure is related to left ventricular dilatation. Mitral valve insufficiency can result from both mitral annular dilatation and ischemia or dysfunction of the papillary muscles, which can lead to LV volume overload and LV function deterioration, usually manifesting as pulmonary congestion, CO decrease, and severe dilated cardiomyopathy due to ischemia.

3.6 Pulmonary Hypertension

Pulmonary hypertension (PH) is elevated pulmonary artery pressure from any cause. A resting mean pulmonary artery pressure (mPAP) of ≥25 mm Hg is considered PH. Pediatric PH can arise from a variety of causes and pose a threat to children of all ages. Physiologic PH is defined as the thickening of the small pulmonary arteries' smooth muscle, narrowing of the small pulmonary arteries' lumen, and increasing pulmonary resistance in neonates. With the growth and development, the muscular layer of small pulmonary arteries degenerates and becomes thin, the lumen becomes larger, and pulmonary resistance decreases. Hypoxia, acidosis, and infection can cause the small pulmonary artery spasm in neonates, which continuously increases PVR, and the transition from fetal to adult circulation is impaired, which results in right-to-left shunting at the level of the atrium and/or ductus arteriosus and clinically manifests as severe hypoxemia, namely, persistent pulmonary hypertension of the Newborn (PPHN).

PH in children with CHD is usually secondary to the left-to-right shunting or left heart obstructive disease. According to the formula $P = R \times Q$, pulmonary artery pressure is the product of pulmonary resistance (Rp) and pulmonary blood flow (Qp). Thus, abnormalities of resistance and flow in the pulmonary circulation (intrauterine or postnatal) may lead to the development of PH in children with CHD. Increased pulmonary resistance may be pre-capillary, post-capillary (pulmonary veins, left atrium, or mitral valve), or both. In children with biventricular circulation, if the resting mPAP ≥25 mm Hg, pulmonary artery wedge pressure (PAWP) ≤15 mm Hg, and pulmonary vascular resistance index (PVRI) >3 WU/m^2, it is defined as pre-capillary PH; if the resting mPAP ≥25 mm Hg and PAWP ≥15 mm Hg, it is defined as post-capillary PH.

Pre-capillary PH is usually caused by the narrowing of small pulmonary arteries. The children with CHD and the left-to-right shunts can lead to PH due to increased PBF. The progression of pre-capillary PH depends on the size and location of shunts. Post-tricuspid shunts, such as VSD, PDA, aortopulmonary window, various types of arterial truncus, and surgery intended to increase PBF, are commonly associated with the development of PH. PH caused by post-tricuspid shunts usually occurs in childhood, whereas complex lesions such as AVSD or truncus arteriosus can lead to PH in early life. Pre-tricuspid shunts, such as ASD, are less commonly associated with PH and usually occur very late if PH does occur since ASD mainly increases PBF instead of a significant increase of pressure overload. The pathophysiology of CHD-related PH may be associated with pulmonary vasoconstriction, intimal wall hypertrophy, and remodeling of the pulmonary vascular bed. The mechanism of injury may relate to the high flow and pressure-induced pulmonary vascular endothelium damage, activation of elastase and matrix metalloproteinases, which degrades the extracellular matrix and releases FGF, TGF-β_1, etc. factors, and further leads to the proliferation and hypertrophy of pulmonary vascular smooth muscle cells, neointimal formation. In the end, histologic changes occur, such as smooth muscle cell extension into the pulmonary arterioles, medial hypertrophy, endothelial hyperplasia and fibrosis, plexiform lesions, and thinning of the pulmonary arterial tree. Endothelial dysfunction and pulmonary vascular remodeling ultimately lead to progressive and irreversible PVR and pulmonary artery pressure increases and reduced PBF.

Post-capillary PH can be caused by pulmonary vein stenosis, anomalous pulmonary venous return, obstruction of pulmonary venous blood return to the left atrium in cor triatriatum, or elevated LAP due to congenital mitral stenosis, congenital aortic stenosis, severe coarctation of the aorta, severe left ventricular systolic or diastolic dysfunction. Such patients with PH typically present with signs of pulmonary venous hypertension, such as pulmonary edema and Kerley B-lines. Echocardiography and cardiac catheterization can usually identify the site and degree of obstruction. Over time, patients with post-capillary PH may also develop "pre-capillary" PH due to reactive pulmonary artery constriction, which further increases the pulmonary artery pressure. Since the dilation of pulmonary vasculature can increase the PBF and worsen the pulmonary edema in the presence of downstream obstruction, any treatment approach related to the dilation of pulmonary vasculature is contraindicated in this situation. The best treatment for these patients is to relieve the obstruction (Yue Huang, Wenyan Xu).

4 Anesthetic Management of Children with Congenital Heart Disease

Ning Ma

Abstract

Perioperative anesthesia management for children with congenital heart disease (CHD) requires multidisciplinary collaboration and precise understanding of anatomical anomalies and pathophysiological changes. This chapter outlines key perioperative strategies, including preoperative assessment (medical history, genetic background, comorbidities, physical examination, cardiopulmonary reserve, lab tests, imaging evaluation, and cardiac catheterization) and preparation for fasting, premedication optimization, and determinization of individualized anesthesia protocols tailored to shunt direction, obstruction severity, and mixing physiology. Intraoperative management integrates invasive blood pressure monitoring, transoesophageal echocardiography, cerebral oxygenation assessment, and temperature, while modulating pulmonary-to-systemic vascular resistance ratios and maintaining oxygen delivery-consumption balance. During cardiopulmonary bypass, prioritize perfusion pressure optimization and metabolic homeostasis. Postoperative care focuses on cardiopulmonary recovery, coagulation management, and multimodal analgesia, with early detection of complications. Complex CHD cases necessitate coordinated teamwork to optimize surgical-anesthesia-ICU transitions, improving outcomes.

N. Ma (✉)
The National Children's Medical Center (Shanghai), Department of Anesthesiology of Shanghai Children's Medical Center, Shanghai Jiao Tong University School of Medicine, Shanghai, China
e-mail: maning@scmc.com.cn

Surgery is indeed an effective method for congenital heart disease (CHD). With the rapid development of medical technologies, the surgical treatment of CHD has been greatly improved. Most children with CHD can recover to normal children's levels, and their growth and development will not be affected if they receive timely surgical treatment. The surgical treatment of complex CHD requires the joint efforts of a medical team, including cardiac surgeons, cardiologists, anesthesiologists, perfusionists, intensivists, and nurses. In addition to the quality of surgical procedures, the effect of cardiopulmonary bypass (CPB), and postoperative management, perioperative anesthetic management is also very important to the prognosis of CHD patients. Therefore, this brings great challenges and demands to pediatric cardiac anesthesiologists.

For the anesthetic management of children with CHD, it is not only the patients' abnormal circulatory physiology and comorbidities, but also the surgical procedures, CPB, and many other factors need to be considered. It requires a deep understanding of the pathophysiology of CHD, disease diagnosis and treatment, pediatrics, cardiac anesthesia, and intensive care.

J. Zheng et al. (eds.), *Selected Pediatric Cardiovascular Surgery Anesthesia Cases*, https://doi.org/10.1007/978-981-96-5614-1_4

4.1 Preoperative Visit and Assessment

4.1.1 Medical History

1. History of Present Illness.
   Be familiar with the main symptoms of heart disease.

   There are many types of CHD. Their clinical manifestations mainly depend on the severity and complexity of cardiovascular malformations. Complex and severe malformations will show severe symptoms shortly after birth, even threatening life, while some simple malformations such as ventricular septal defect (VSD), atrial septal defect (ASD), and patent ductus arteriosus (PDA) may not have any obvious symptoms during the early stage, but the diseases still have the potential of developing and worsening, so they need to be diagnosed and treated in time to avoid missing the opportunity of surgical treatment. The main symptoms of CHD include ① Recurrent upper respiratory tract infections, which are prone to turning into pneumonia. ② Poor growth and development, thinness, excessive sweating. ③ Weak sucking when feeding, dystopia, or the baby refuses to eat, coughs, and breathes rapidly. ④ Children often complain of fatigue and poor physical strength. ⑤ Cyanosis of the lips and nails, cyanosis after crying or activity, or clubbing of fingers/toes. ⑥ History of squatting, fainting, and hemoptysis.

   Recurrent pulmonary infections may be caused by increased pulmonary blood flow, commonly seen in asymptomatic children with CHD. The differentiation between heart failure and upper respiratory tract infection can be very difficult, both of which can present as mild shortness of breath, wheezing, and upper respiratory tract congestion. Activity levels that match the children's ages can help assess cardiac function and reserve capacity. Infants with heart failure may have symptoms of low cardiac function reserve during breastfeeding, and they may also manifest as sweating, fatigue, dyspnea, and cyanosis around the mouth. The inability of children with CHD to keep up with the paces of other siblings is often a very reliable clinical sign of deteriorating cardiac function.
2. Family History.
   If parents have CHD, the probability of their children having CHD is 3–5%, while this probability is only 0.8% in the general population. Genetic diseases are divided into five categories: monogenic diseases, polygenic diseases, chromosomal diseases, mitochondrial diseases, and somatic cell genetic diseases. Except for somatic cell genetic diseases, which are mainly related to tumors, the other four genetic diseases may be related to cardiovascular diseases.
   (a) Monogenic diseases include autosomal dominant inheritance, autosomal recessive inheritance, X-linked inheritance, etc. Currently, about 120 kinds of monogenic diseases are accompanied by cardiovascular system defect syndromes, some of which have already been determined by the gene location and gene mutation of the genetic defect, such as Marfan syndrome, Noonan syndrome, long QT syndrome (LQTS) without deafness, and supravalvular aortic stenosis (present as autosomal dominant inheritance), as well as Ellis–Van syndrome and LQTS with deafness, etc. (present as autosomal recessive inheritance).
   (b) Polygenic inherited diseases refer to genetic diseases related to more than two pairs of genes. The onset of diseases is related to genetic factors, but they are also affected by environmental factors, so they are also called multifactorial inheritance disorders, such as Tetralogy of Fallot (TOF), etc.
   (c) Chromosomal diseases are the diseases caused by chromosomal abnormalities. About 50 kinds of human chromosomal diseases are accompanied by cardiovascular abnormalities. The frequency of cardiovascular system involvement in children with Down syndrome is 40–50%, mainly shown as endocardial cushion defects, VSD, and ASD, while TOF and

transposition of the great arteries (TGA) have also been reported. The frequency of cardiovascular involvement in children with Edwards syndrome is close to 100%. VSD and PDA are most frequently seen, ASD is also commonly seen, and other cardiac abnormalities include aortic valve and/or pulmonary valve malformation, pulmonary stenosis (PS), aortic stenosis (AS), TGA, TOF, dextrocardia, and vascular abnormalities. The frequency of cardiovascular involvement in children with Patau syndrome is about 80%, commonly shown as PDA, VSD, ASD, PS, AS, TGA, etc. Most of these three syndromes are thought to be caused by chromosomal non-separation. In addition, the childbirth age of the mother may also be involved as well.

(d) Mitochondrial diseases are caused by mitochondrial DNA mutations, mainly involving the nervous and neuromuscular systems. Some cardiomyopathies belong to mitochondrial diseases.

3. Mother's Pregnancy History.
   Ask if the mother had any viral infections during the first three months of pregnancy and whether she took any drugs and chemical toxins that might affect fetal development or was exposed to radiation, etc.
4. Previous History of Surgical and Interventional Treatments.
   Children with CHD, especially of complex types, may need to undergo multiple palliative surgeries, interventional treatments, or radical surgeries. It is necessary to understand their previous cardiac surgery procedures, surgical effects, sequelae, and whether there is a history of rescue and resuscitation.
5. Be Familiar with Whether the Pediatric Patients Have Other Malformations or Whether the Heart Diseases Are Due To Some Congenital Syndromes.
   About 8% of children with CHD will have other malformations. In addition to congenital heart malformations, some syndromes may also have other problems: ① Malformations of the airway and its surrounding tissue structures. For example, CHARGE syndrome, Edwards syndrome, and Turner syndrome often combine with micrognathia. Noonan syndrome often combines with a short-webbed neck and macrognathia. Hurler syndrome may combine with macroglossia and short neck. These combined malformations may cause difficulty in tracheal intubation or even in mask ventilation. In addition, children with DiGeorge syndrome may have shorter tracheas, and the endotracheal tube can easily go to one bronchus during tracheal intubation. ② Metabolic abnormalities. For example, DiGeorge syndrome often combines with hypocalcemia, etc. ③ Cardiac arrhythmias. Children with LQTS are prone to torsades de pointes and sudden cardiac death (SCD). Children with Brugada syndrome are prone to ventricular tachycardia (VT), ventricular fibrillation (VF), and SCD. Common syndromes in children and their combined CHD are shown in Table 4.1.
6. Be Familiar with the Children's Internal Medicine Treatment.
   Including medicine treatment, such as diuretics, angiotensin-converting enzyme inhibitors (ACEI), digoxin, etc. Some medications need to be terminated before cardiac surgery. Common perioperative medications and precautions are shown in Table 4.2.

4.1.2 Physical Examination

1. General Information.
   Includes height, weight, nutritional status, blood pressure, pulse, etc.

   As the children grow up, their heart rates (HR) gradually decrease, but blood pressures gradually increase, so the interpretation of their vital signs should be age-dependent. In congestive heart failure, children with CHD often cannot achieve weight, height, and head circumference growth that matches their ages. On the contrary, cyanotic children often do not show growth retardation.

   The availability of vascular access and monitoring sites must also be assessed. If a

Table 4.1 Common syndromes in children and their combined CHD

Syndrome	Combined CHD
CHARGE syndrome (ocular defects, congenital heart defects, choanal atresia, renal malformation, genital hypoplasia, and ear malformations)	65% of patients have conotruncal malformation or aortic arch malformation
DiGeorge syndrome (22nd chromosome deletion, CATCH 22 syndrome)	Interruption of the aortic arch, persistent truncus arteriosus (PTA), VSD, PDA, TOF
Duchenne muscular dystrophy	Cardiomyopathy
Ehlers–Danlos syndrome	Aortic aneurysm, carotid aneurysm
Ellis–van Creveld syndrome (chondroectodermal dysplasia)	50% of patients have common atrium
Fetal alcohol syndrome	25–30% of patients have VSD, PDA, ASD, TOF
Friedreich's ataxia	Cardiomyopathy
Type II glycogen storage disease (Pompe disease)	Cardiomyopathy
Holt–Oram syndrome	ASD, VSD
Leopard syndrome (cardio-cutaneous syndrome)	Pulmonary atresia (PA), PR interval prolongation, cardiomyopathy
LQTS	Long QT interval
Jervell and Lange Nielsen syndrome Romano–Ward syndrome	Ventricular arrhythmias
Marfan syndrome	Aortic aneurysm, aortic valve regurgitation, and/or mitral valve regurgitation
Mucopolysaccharidosis	Aortic valve regurgitation and/or mitral valve regurgitation, coronary artery disease, cardiomyopathy
Noonan syndrome	PA (valve dysplasia), left ventricular hypertrophy, interventricular septal hypertrophy
Tuberous sclerosis	Cardiac rhabdomyoma
Shprintzen syndrome (velocardiofacial syndrome, 22q deletion)	conotruncal malformation, TOF
VACTERL syndrome	VSD, conotruncal malformation (TOF, PTA)
Williams syndrome	Supravalvular aortic stenosis, PA
Zellweger syndrome (cerebrohepatorenal syndrome)	PDA, VSD, ASD

Table 4.2 Common perioperative medications and precautions

Classification of cardiac drugs	Interactions	Precautions
Angiotensin-converting enzyme inhibitors	Hypotension induced by general anesthesia	Cancel the morning dose or reduce the dose in children with hypotension; avoid using drugs with significant vagomimetic effects; avoid fixed-dose induction schemes
β-blockers	Acute withdrawal accelerates tachycardia and arrhythmias; enhances the hypotensive effect of volatile anesthetics; reduces the reactivity of positive inotropic drugs	Can continue medication perioperatively
Calcium channel blockers	May enhance the negative inotropic and chronotropic effects of volatile anesthetics	Can continue medication perioperatively
Diuretics	Hypovolemia and hypokalemia; may enhance the effect of neuromuscular blocking agents	Discontinue medication before surgery

(continued)

Table 4.2 (continued)

Classification of cardiac drugs	Interactions	Precautions
Antiarrhythmic drugs	Can cause arrhythmia if cardiotonic drugs are administrated and electrolyte imbalance is present; high catecholamine state; interaction with other antiarrhythmic drugs can lead to bradycardia	Avoid electrolyte imbalance; avoid arrhythmogenic drugs; close monitoring
α_2 receptor agonists	Reduce perioperative shivering, ischemia, and the need for anesthetics and analgesics	Continue use perioperatively under close monitoring

child with CHD has previously undergone palliative subclavian artery shunt surgery, it may be difficult to measure the pulse and blood pressure in that arm. Some children may have very poor peripheral vascular development, and only very small capillaries can be seen in superficial parts. Children who have undergone multiple surgeries often have difficulty establishing peripheral venous access. These will all affect the choice of induction method of anesthesia.

2. Cardiac Status.
   Includes heart size, heart sounds, and heart murmurs, etc.
   (a) Inspection: Presence or absence of a precordial bulge, chest deformity, diffuse precordial pulsation, etc.
   (b) Palpation: Whether fine tremors can be felt (pay attention to the location and whether they occur during systole or diastole), sometimes a lifting impulse of the apex can also be felt.
   (c) Percussion: Can roughly estimate the size and position of the heart.
   (d) Auscultation: Pay attention to the strength of the first and second heart sounds and the characteristics, timing, loudness, location, and transmission direction of murmurs, etc.
3. Peripheral Vascular Signs.
   In cases of severe aortic valve insufficiency, diastolic pressure decreases, pulse pressure increases, and peripheral vascular signs such as De Musset's sign, pistol shot sound of femoral artery (Traube's sign), and capillary pulsation sign can often be observed.
4. Check for Symptoms and Signs of Cardiac Insufficiency.
   The symptoms and signs of cardiac insufficiency include changes in breathing patterns, limited activity, jugular vein distension, pleural and abdominal effusion, and liver enlargement.
5. Airway Conditions.
   Including teeth, tongue, mouth opening degree, and whether there is tracheal stenosis or other difficult airway-related anatomy alterations. If the child has been intubated, the reasons and timing of intubation and the type, size, and depth of the endotracheal tube should be clarified, and the oxygen concentration, airway pressure, and other mechanical ventilation parameters should be known.

4.1.3 Laboratory Tests and Other Auxiliary Examinations

1. Laboratory Tests.
   Routine tests include complete blood count, electrolytes, liver and kidney function, coagulation function, etc.
   (a) Complete blood count: For patients with CHD and normal blood volume, the hematocrit increase can indicate the severity and progression of hypoxemia. When the hematocrit exceeds 60%, capillary stasis and secondary end-organ damage (including stroke) can occur. Despite these risks, if the guidelines for preoperative fasting are relaxed, allowing the children to drink clear liquids up to 2 h before the induction of anesthesia, these patients

generally do not need preoperative intravenous fluids.

(b) Fluid, electrolytes, and acid-base balance: Plasma electrolyte concentration screening should be performed, especially for patients with CHD who have been on long-term treatment with digitalis and diuretics. Potent diuretics can cause hypokalemia and hyponatremia, while hypocalcemia can also be observed in patients with congestive heart failure and 22q11.2 microdeletion syndrome. Severe congestive heart failure can be accompanied by restlessness and irritability. It is important to rule out the possibility of hypoglycemia, which can also cause such manifestations.

(c) Liver and kidney function: It is very important to select sedative-hypnotics, analgesics, and muscle relaxants by determining the preoperative status of liver and kidney function.

(d) Coagulation function: Cyanosis can affect the coagulation function of patients with CHD and lead to prolonged prothrombin time (PT), partial thromboplastin time (PTT), and bleeding time (BT). In addition, the platelet count and function may also decrease.

(e) Specific tests may sometimes be required depending on the types of CHDs.

2. Electrocardiogram (ECG).
   ECG can accurately reflect the position of the heart and indicate whether there is hypertrophy in the atrium and ventricle. In addition, it can also accurately determine whether there is arrhythmia and the function of the cardiac conduction system.
3. Transthoracic Echocardiography (TTE).
   Preoperative TTE examination is very important for children with CHD, which can be used to clarify cardiac anatomy and function and provide great help for improving preoperative preparation, evaluating the impact of surgery on pathophysiology, formulating surgical plans, and predicting the occurrence of intraoperative accidents or special events.
4. Chest X-Ray and Computed Tomography (CT).
   Chest X-rays can be used to confirm clinical manifestations and diagnoses, such as whether there is cardiac enlargement, the amount of pulmonary blood flow, previous surgical treatment, and whether there is currently pulmonary edema, infiltration, or acute pulmonary infection, etc. For aortic and other major vascular surgeries and multiple thoracotomies, further CT or other examinations are needed to clarify the location of vascular lesions and whether there is tracheal compression and significant adhesions, etc.
5. Magnetic Resonance Imaging (MRI) of the Heart and Great Vessels.
   MRI is a very useful non-invasive imaging tool for children with CHD, often used for the segmental description of cardiac abnormalities, evaluation of thoracic aortic abnormalities, assessment of truncus arteriosus deformities, determination of systemic-pulmonary venous abnormalities, and non-invasive detection and quantification of shunts, stenosis, and regurgitation. MRI is also useful in quantifying ventricular function, local ventricular wall motion, valve function, flow velocity, and flow volume and is particularly useful for imaging the aortic arch, pulmonary artery, and mediastinal vessels in complex CHD. MRI can provide accurate and useful information for certain lesions, including aortic stenosis, pulmonary artery abnormalities, abnormal pulmonary venous connections, residual left superior vena cava, and intracardiac septal defects, conduits, and shunts. For some children with CHD, it can replace cardiac catheterization and non-invasively evaluate coronary artery abnormalities, myocardial perfusion defects, and conditions related to myocardial scarring (such as arrhythmogenic right ventricular dysplasia). Nowadays, newer MRI images can be used for 3D printing, reconstruction of complex lesions, and establishment of cardiac models to help plan the surgical process. Cardiac adenosine stress MRI can be used to delineate the induced ischemic areas.

MRI scan usually takes a relatively longer time, and it often requires pediatric patients to be absolutely immobilized or to control breathing to obtain the best image. So, sedation or anesthesia may be needed. During anesthesia, the children need MRI-compatible anesthesia machines and monitors.

6. Cardiac Catheterization Lab.
Cardiac catheterization lab remains the gold standard for anatomical and physiological assessment of CHD. Although many anatomical issues can now be non-invasively addressed, the cardiac catheterization lab remains an important tool for understanding physiological data or the complexity of anatomy. It is divided into right and left heart catheterization examination, which is performed under X-ray fluoroscopy with the placement of a radiopaque plastic catheter through the brachial or femoral vein into the right atrium via the superior or inferior vena cava, and then sequentially to the right ventricle and pulmonary artery.
It is crucial to carefully review the cardiac catheterization lab data and to be familiar with its potential impact on surgical and anesthetic plans. The cardiac catheterization lab data that are important to anesthesiologists are listed as follows:
(a) The children's response to sedative drugs.
(b) The pressure and oxygen saturation of all heart chambers and major blood vessels.
(c) The location and size of intra- and extracardiac shunts.
(d) Pulmonary vascular resistance (PVR) and systemic vascular resistance (SVR).
(e) The size and function of heart chambers.
(f) Valve anatomy and function.
(g) Systemic and pulmonary artery malformations related to previous surgeries.
(h) The anatomy of coronary arteries.
(i) The anatomy, location, and function of previously established palliative cardiac shunts.
(j) Acquired or congenital anatomical variations that may affect vascular access or surgery.

4.2 Preoperative Preparation

4.2.1 Drugs Preparation

1. Intravenous Sedatives.
(a) Propofol: Propofol can be used in children with CHD and sufficient cardiovascular reserve. The intravenous bolus injection of propofol for the induction of anesthesia can cause a slight decrease in myocardial contractility. The intravenous infusion can cause a slight decrease in preload, but mean arterial pressure (MAP) and HR are significantly reduced. Propofol can cause the reduction of preload, afterload, and myocardial contractility, so it should be used with caution in patients with significantly impaired ventricular function and left ventricular outflow tract obstruction. Propofol infusion has little effect on pulmonary vascular pressure and resistance, but it can reduce SVR and increase right-to-left shunting.

Propofol has no significant effect on sinus node or atrioventricular node conduction, which makes it an ideal sedative during electrophysiological studies and radiofrequency ablation. However, propofol can suppress ectopic atrial tachycardia, which may be disadvantageous for mapping during ectopic atrial tachycardia radiofrequency ablation. Although propofol is very useful for short-term sedation after cardiac catheterization and surgery, it should not be used for long-term sedation in the ICU because of the potential for propofol infusion syndrome.

(b) Ketamine: Ketamine can cause a significant increase in HR, MAP, and cardiac output (CO) by stimulating the sympathetic nervous system and inhibiting the reuptake of catecholamines through the mediation of the central nervous system. Ketamine has good hemodynamic stability with few complications, which is suitable for various patients with CHD, including TOF. The recognized adverse reactions associated with the use of ketamine do not differ in patients with CHD, including delirium, drooling, an increase in brain metabolism, intracranial pressure, cerebral blood flow, and cerebral oxygen consumption. This drug has become one of the main drugs for general anesthesia induction in patients with CHD. Ketamine can be either intravenously or intramuscularly administrated. The induction dose is 1–2 mg/kg intravenous or 5–10 mg/kg intramuscular injection, and the maintenance dose is 1–5 mg/(kg·h). Ketamine, supplemented with small doses of midazolam and (or) morphine, can be used for interventional cardiac catheterization and postoperative analgesia in pediatric cardiac surgery. If oxygenation and ventilation are well maintained, ketamine can be safely used in children with pulmonary hypertension. Ketamine can also be used as a preoperative medication, with the most common oral dose being 5–6 mg/kg.

Ketamine can increase HR, blood pressure, and myocardial contractility when the hemodynamic reserve is well maintained. However, when the children's cardiac reserves are severely limited or myocardial contractility is low, their own endogenous sympathetic nervous systems have been maximally stimulated, and they may have been treated with β-adrenergic drugs for a long time, which results in down-regulation of β-receptors and weakened response to endogenous catecholamines. Then, the inhibitory effect of ketamine on the myocardium will dominate, and care must be taken to use it.

(c) Etomidate: It is an imidazole derivative introduced into clinical practice in 1972. It does not significantly affect hemodynamics and mainly produces hypnotic and sedative effects through interaction with γ-aminobutyric acid receptors. It has almost no effect on spontaneous respiration. It does not release histamine and change airway smooth muscle tension. It can also reduce cerebral blood flow, cerebral oxygen consumption, metabolism rate (30–50%), and intracranial pressure.

Clinical doses of etomidate have no direct inhibitory effect on the myocardium and the systemic or pulmonary hemodynamics in patients with intracardiac shunting (including those with pulmonary hypertension), so etomidate is the first choice of induction drug for patients with poor ventricular function. Even a single induction dose of etomidate may have adrenal function inhibitory effect, so for patients receiving corticosteroid treatment or at risk of long-term adrenal suppression, additional supplementation with corticosteroids should be considered.

(d) Dexmedetomidine: Dexmedetomidine was first introduced in the United States in 1999 as a highly selective α_2 receptor agonist. The sedative effect of dexmedetomidine is produced by the α_2 receptors binding in the locus coeruleus of the brain. In contrast, the analgesic effect of dexmedetomidine is produced by the α_2 receptor binding in the spine. By reducing the sympathetic nerve activity of the central nervous system, dexmedetomidine can lead to a dose-dependent reduction in HR and MAP. Moreover, it can also enhance the effect of opioids. Therefore, it is more suitable for pediatric cardiac surgery as an effective auxiliary drug for intraoperative general anesthesia and a component of postoperative sedation protocol. In preterm infants and full-term newborns less than 30 days old undergoing CHD surgery, the clearance rate of dexmedetomidine is significantly reduced, and the elimination half-life of preterm infants is significantly increased up to 7.6 h. Therefore, the dose needs to be reduced for this age group, and monitoring for adverse reactions should be strengthened.

Dexmedetomidine not only has a relatively small impact on spontaneous respiration, but it can also reduce the reactivity of the trachea and reduce the dose of opioids, which is beneficial for tracheal intubation and early smooth removal of the tracheal tube. Although dexmedetomidine can inhibit supraventricular and ventricular arrhythmias, sinus bradycardia, junctional bradycardia, and sinus arrest are uncommon. Rapid infusion of dexmedetomidine can cause transient hypertension, and continuous infusion can cause hypotension and bradycardia.

(e) Midazolam: Midazolam has good sedative and anterograde amnesic effects, and it is often used to prevent intraoperative awareness. Although its impact on hemodynamics is mild, the use of large doses of midazolam (or other benzodiazepines) in infants may increase the demand for positive inotropic drugs.

2. Inhalational Anesthetics.

All of the inhalational anesthetics can reduce the resting tension of arterial smooth muscle by decreasing the calcium ion content, thereby reducing blood pressure and SVR. Still, the degree of reduction varies with the different anesthetics. When the end-tidal concentration reaches 1.5 MAC, halothane causes the greatest inhibition on myocardial contractility, and CO, sevoflurane, isoflurane, and desflurane cause the least inhibition. The younger the age, the greater the inhibitory effect. The greatest risk is in infants who are less than 6 months old.

Isoflurane can improve cardiac reserve by reducing SVR. Still, it has a strong irritating smell and can cause coughing, laryngospasm, and decreased pulse oxygen saturation (SpO_2) if isoflurane is used to induce anesthesia alone. So, it is rarely used for anesthesia induction in children with CHD.

The effects of desflurane on heart and lung function are similar to isoflurane. Furthermore, it has the lowest blood-gas partition coefficient and tissue solubility, which allows for rapid equilibrium between the inhaled gas and the alveolar concentration and the rapid decrease of alveolar concentration after discontinuation. Therefore, the depth of anesthesia can be easily adjusted when it is used for pediatric cardiac anesthesia. Desflurane is highly irritating, and laryngospasm is higher during inhalational induction. So, desflurane cannot be used alone for inhalational anesthesia induction. In addition, desflurane can cause catecholamine release if its concentration is rapidly increased. So, it is not suitable to use desflurane as the only anesthetic for children with ischemic heart diseases.

Sevoflurane has an aromatic smell with little respiratory irritation. It is more tolerable for children, which makes it the preferred drug for pediatric inhalational induction of anesthesia. The blood-gas partition coefficient and tissue solubility of sevoflurane are slightly higher than those of desflurane, so anesthesia induction and recovery are also fast. Inhalation of high concentrations (6–12%) of sevoflurane can lead to arrhythmias in some children, mainly atrial or junctional arrhythmias. Sevoflurane can also cause tachycardia, especially in older children, but the systemic arterial pressure can be well maintained. Sevoflurane induction can develop bradycardia (less than 80 beats per minute) in 20% of infants. During sevoflurane anesthesia in infants, the decrease in HR and MAP is less than that of halothane, and echocardiography suggests that contractility and cardiac index are normal.

3. Narcotic Analgesics.

Fentanyl and sufentanil are commonly used narcotic analgesics during pediatric CHD surgery, which have mild effects on heart rate and blood pressure and good hemodynamic stability. Fentanyl 25 μg/kg can eliminate the increase in pulmonary artery pressure and resistance during suctioning in the postoperative recovery period in infants with CHD. High doses of fentanyl can effectively improve the increase in HR, MAP, and stress hormones caused by harmful stimuli. The efficacy of sufentanil is 5–10 times more potent than fentanyl, with a large safety margin and high liposolubility. It can quickly distribute into all body tissues. The effects of sufentanil on hemodynamics, recovery time, and extubation time are similar to those of fentanyl.

Remifentanil is a synthetic ultra-short-acting anesthetic. It is metabolized by plasma esterase with a half-life of 3–5 min, which is unrelated to the infusion duration. It's very conducive to rapid postoperative recovery and especially suitable for short, highly stimulating, non-cardiac surgeries. Larger doses of remifentanil can prolong sinus atrial conduction and recovery time but do not prolong atrial His interval. If used for electrophysiological research, the impacts of these drugs on electrophysiological effects should be considered. Because the half-life of remifentanil is short and there is no accumulation, it plays a very important role in fast-track pediatric cardiac anesthesia.

4. Muscle Relaxants.
   (a) Succinylcholine: Succinylcholine is currently rarely used for anesthesia in children with CHD because it is associated with malignant hyperthermia, hyperkalemic cardiac arrest, and bradycardia. Succinylcholine acts faster than non-depolarizing muscle relaxants. It is currently only used for emergency full-stomach patients, laryngospasm treatment, and as part of muscle injection induction.
   (b) Rocuronium: Rocuronium is currently the fastest-acting medium-duration non-depolarizing muscle relaxant. The common dose for endotracheal intubation is 0.6–1.2 mg/kg via intravenous bolus injection. Suppose the dose is increased to more than three times the ED_{95}. In that case, the onset time of rocuronium will be further shortened, approaching that of succinylcholine, and it can replace succinylcholine for modified rapid sequence induction. Although rocuronium has little cardiovascular effect, it still has a weak vagolytic effect, and an increase in HR can usually be observed after use. When rocuronium is injected into the deltoid muscle at 1.8–2 mg/kg, appropriate intubation conditions can be achieved within 3–4 min.
   (c) Atracurium and Cisatracurium: Both are non-depolarizing muscle relaxants that are eliminated independently of organ function and are more suitable for children with liver and kidney dysfunction. High doses of atracurium often cause histamine release and cause hypotension. Therefore, there are more concerns when they are used in children with CHD. Cisatracurium is a stereoisomer of atracurium, which the Hoffman elimination reaction can also degrade, but it rarely causes histamine release and has less impact on the cardiovascular system.
5. Commonly Used Vasoactive Drugs and Antiarrhythmic Drugs Are Shown in Table 4.3.
6. Others.

Vasodilators (nitroglycerin, prostaglandin E_1, prostacyclin, etc.), diuretics (furosemide, mannitol, etc.), hemostatics (aminocaproic acid, batroxobin, etc.), anticoagulants (heparin), etc.

4.2.2 Preoperative Mental Preparation and Preoperative Medications

Preoperative visits help to understand the patient's mental state preliminarily. Children's psychological reactions and behaviors at different developmental stages vary: ① Infants under 6 months old easily accept anyone's kindness and rarely experience separation anxiety. ② Toddlers from 6 months to 3 years old develop quickly and have a certain understanding of the environment, language, disease, and surgery, but their abilities are limited. They have not yet learned to get along with peers or adults, and their separation anxiety from parents is very obvious, which can easily lead to regressive behavior after surgery. ③ Children aged 3–7 years old know they are sick, but they can easily remember and exaggerate adverse events. Separation from parents is a mental trauma, especially for those who have undergone multiple surgeries. ④ Children aged 7–12 years old enjoy playing various roles. They are of school age and used to being separated from their parents. They can not only understand what will happen but also can describe the surgery and the expected effects. They will actively participate in the entire preoperative process. ⑤ Patients over 12 years old can participate in discussions and make some decisions, which include choices of anesthetic induction, infusion methods, and postoperative pain relief methods.

Table 4.3 Commonly used vasoactive drugs and antiarrhythmic drugs

Drug	Single dose	Infusion speed	Remarks
Atropine 0.5 mg diluted to 5 mL (0.1 mg/mL)	20 μg/kg IV		Maximum dose: Children 1.0 mg, Adolescents 3.0 mg
Amiodarone 150 mg diluted with 5% glucose to 50 mL (3.0 mg/mL)	5.0 mg/kg Slow IV bolus over 15–30 min	5.0–15 μg/(kg·min)	
Calcium gluconate 100 mg/mL	30–60 mg/kg IV		
Dopamine 40 mg diluted to 40 mL (1 mg/mL)		3.0–10 μg/(kg·min)	Titrate to effect
Epinephrine 1 mg diluted to 10 mL (0.1 mg/mL); when infused intravenously, 0.03 × kg(mg) diluted to 50 mL	In case of hypotension, 1.0 μg/kg IV; in case of cardiac arrest, 10 μg/kg IV; if necessary, repeat every 3–5 min	0.02–0.1 μg/(kg·min)	Titrate to effect
Isoprenaline When infused intravenously, 0.03 × kg(mg) diluted to 50 mL		0.01–0.1 μg/(kg·min)	Tachycardia, palpitations, angina, pulmonary edema, hypertension, hypotension, ventricular arrhythmias, and rapid arrhythmias
Lidocaine Diluted to 1.0 mg/mL	1.0 mg/kg IV	20–50 μg/(kg·min)	
Norepinephrine When infused intravenously, 0.3 × kg(mg) Diluted to 50 mL		0.05 μg/(kg·min)	Titrate to effect
Phenylephrine When infused intravenously, 0.3 × kg(mg) Diluted to 50 mL	0.5 μg/kg	0.1 μg/(kg·min)	Titrate to effect
Terlipressin When infused intravenously, 0.03 × kg (mg) diluted to 50 mL		0.005–0.03 μg/(kg·min)	Titrate to effect

Affected by trauma, pain, and various physiological and psychological diseases, mental and behavioral problems in children during the perioperative period are very common and require appropriate prevention and intervention. The best results can be achieved by adopting individualized intervention methods according to the children's surgery/anesthesia histories, adverse medical experiences, and combinations of psychological reactions and behaviors at different developmental stages. Prevention and intervention methods include both drug and non-drug measures.

There are various non-drug measures. For infants and young children, parents can hold them all the way to the operating room. Our hospital allows older children to accompany their family members in the waiting area and provides books, toys, etc. We also try to use brightly colored toy cars to transport preschool children aged 2 to 5 years old, and they can "drive" into the operating room. Compared with traditional trolleys, the mYPAS anxiety score of children transported by toy cars is significantly reduced, and the effect of relieving pre-anesthesia induction anxiety is comparable to the effect of preoperative medication. The anxiety level of their parents is also reduced with increased satisfaction evaluation. All these methods are not only simple and easy to implement with a small investment, but they also have good practical effects.

For those children who may have difficulty separating from their parents, administration of preoperative sedatives in advance can be considered. Midazolam and α_2 adrenergic receptor agonists are commonly used preoperative separation drugs in recent years. Taking midazolam 0.5–0.75 mg/kg orally or dexmedetomidine 2.0–3.0 μg/kg intranasally 15–30 min before surgery can effectively alleviate preoperative anxiety in children, facilitate mother-child separation, and do not prolong recovery time. Since the process of taking medication can also cause tension and stress in children, it should be combined with non-drug intervention measures. If the children are unwilling to take oral or nasal medications, they can be changed to intramuscular injections of ketamine 2–3 mg/kg and midazolam 0.1 mg/kg. The dosage of preoperative medication should be individualized to avoid respiratory depression. For smaller children and those with congestive heart failure, the dose should be reduced, and the anesthesiologist should be present. To older children, medication can be administered after venous catheterization.

4.2.3 Preoperative Fasting

The fasting time for infants and children before surgery is generally defined as follows: ① No clear liquids 2 hours before surgery. ② No breast milk 4 hours before surgery. ③ No formula milk 6 hours before surgery. ④ No solid food intake 8 hours before surgery.

The American Society of Anesthesiologists revised the preoperative fasting guidelines in 2010, and these guidelines are also applicable to children with CHD. The principle of preoperative fasting should maintain a certain degree of flexibility, and the fasting time for children with CHD should be shortened as much as possible, especially for small infants and some high-risk patients. On the morning of the surgery, allowing the children to drink clear liquids until 2 h before surgery can result in lower clinical dehydration levels (manifested as dry mucous membranes and delayed capillary refills). Still, the gastric volumes or gastric acids are not increased. This is especially important for children with CHD who have cyanosis, polycythemia, outflow tract obstruction (such as hypertrophic cardiomyopathy and aortic stenosis), cavopulmonary anastomosis, and shunt-dependent physiology. In addition, relaxing the restriction of preoperative fasting time can reduce the risk of hypoglycemia in high-risk patients, especially infants under 6 months whose glycogenolysis and gluconeogenesis are impaired and whose glycogen storage function is immature. If the surgery is postponed, children should be allowed to drink water according to the postponed time.

4.2.4 Others

The perioperative management of complex CHD cases requires the joint efforts of a team of doctors (surgeon, anesthesiologist, cardiologist, and ICU doctors), nurses, and perfusionists. Cardiac surgeons, cardiologists, and anesthesiologists must discuss the children's current situations and surgical plans before surgery, determine the necessity for further evaluations or treatments of the children, and discuss special situations that may be encountered during surgery. Reasonable communication and cooperation will optimize patient care and promote perioperative clinical management.

4.3 Intraoperative Anesthetic Management

4.3.1 Anesthetic Monitoring

It is best to place various non-invasive monitoring devices before the induction of anesthesia in CHD surgery. Still, when the anesthesiologist faces the crying children, it may be postponed until after the induction of anesthesia. If the patients' conditions are relatively stable, the induction of anesthesia can be initiated under SpO_2 and ECG monitoring only to reduce stress and stimulation. Then other monitoring devices can be quickly added once the patients are sedated or after the induction.

1. Respiratory Function Monitoring.

Respiratory function monitoring includes tidal volume, ventilation frequency, airway pressure, and end-tidal carbon dioxide ($ETCO_2$). Good ventilation management is the basis of anesthetic management for children with CHD. After the induction of anesthesia, the airway should be quickly controlled, and ventilation management should be carried out to optimize the ratio of pulmonary ventilation to pulmonary blood flow in the children. Blood gas analysis should be performed as soon as possible to evaluate the ventilation effect, which includes arterial partial pressure of oxygen (PaO_2), arterial partial pressure of carbon dioxide ($PaCO_2$), pH, etc.

SpO_2 monitoring is conducted by placing the oxygen saturation probe on the upper or lower limbs. If it is required by surgery, two probes can also be placed in the related areas proximal and distal to the PDA. SpO_2 and $ETCO_2$ monitoring can quickly reflect ventilation and oxygenation conditions, help guide ventilation and hemodynamic regulation, and help optimize the ratio of pulmonary/systemic blood flow (Qp/Qs) before and after shunt and pulmonary artery banding surgery. The variation of physiological dead space in children with CHD is relatively large. When there is a right-to-left intracardiac shunt or hypoxic spell of TOF, the pulmonary blood flow decreases, leading to an increase in physiological dead space, and $ETCO_2$ may be significantly lower than the actual value of $PaCO_2$, leading to a rise in the pressure difference between $PaCO_2$ and $ETCO_2$. In addition, the reliability of the SpO_2 probe can be reduced when peripheral blood vessels constrict at deep hypothermia or when peripheral vascular pulsatility disappears during circulatory arrest. For newborns, a tongue sensor can be used to monitor central oxygen saturation to reduce temperature-related variability.

2. Cardiovascular Function Monitoring.
   (a) ECG: ECG electrodes should be placed on the children's chests and limbs far away from the surgical preparation area to monitor HR, rhythm, and ST segment changes. Five-lead ECG needs to be observed during the induction of anesthesia and surgery. Most ECG monitors can now perform automatic ST segment analysis. Leads II and V_5 are most suitable for detecting arrhythmias and myocardial ischemia.
   (b) Blood Pressure Monitoring: The arterial catheterization not only allows for continuous monitoring of arterial blood pressure invasively, but also allows to draw blood samples at any time for blood gas analysis, which is beneficial for regulating the internal environment. It is an important monitoring method during the anesthetic process of CHD surgery. The radial artery and femoral artery are the most commonly used sites. For young children, a 22 G or 24 G catheter is frequently used in the radial artery, while a 20 G catheter can be used for older children and adolescents. Try to avoid brachial artery puncture and catheterization, as it carries a higher risk of ischemia in the distal limb. Consideration should be given when surgeries that have been performed or are about to be performed may affect arterial blood pressure monitoring on the same side, such as modified B-T shunt surgery. During surgeries of coarctation of the aorta, aortic arch/isthmus obstruction, or PDA ligation, it is best to simultaneously monitor the arterial blood pressure of the upper and lower limbs. The femoral artery is often used for lower limb arteries, which is convenient and easy, but when the puncture site is high, bleeding is not easy to compress. There is a risk of hematoma and bleeding rupture into the abdominal cavity. The posterior tibial artery and dorsal foot artery can also be used. For those surgeries requiring CPB, try to avoid arterial blood pressure only monitored in the distal lower limb since they often cannot reflect the aortic pressure in newborns and infants

during hypothermic CPB and immediately after weaning.

In some cases where it is difficult to conduct direct intra-arterial pressure measurement on upper and lower limbs, non-invasive cuff blood pressure monitoring or SpO_2 monitoring can be used as a partial substitute.

(c) Central Venous Pressure (CVP): Percutaneous central venous catheterization can provide many benefits. Central venous access can be reliably established even in newborns with lower body weight. Using real-time ultrasound assistance can increase the success rate of central venous catheterization in newborns to 90–95%. In some children who need strict postoperative assessment of pulmonary artery pressure (PAP), surgeons can also place a transthoracic pulmonary artery catheter. For a concise guide to the types of central venous and arterial catheters, see Table 4.4.

(d) Transesophageal Echocardiography (TEE): Two-dimensional echocardiography combined with pulsed Doppler ultrasound and color blood flow imaging can provide detailed morphological and physiological information for most children with CHD and has now become the standard management of pediatric CHD surgery. TEE overcomes many limitations of TTE imaging, including poor window quality due to obesity, mechanical ventilation, and recent cardiac surgery. Still, TEE should be a good supplement to TTE during operation rather than completely replacing it.

Table 4.4 Concise guide to central venous and arterial catheter types

Age/Weight	Central vein	Artery
Infants <5 kg	4 Fr—5 cm	Radial artery 24 G Radial artery 2.5 Fr 2.5 cm Femoral artery 2.5 Fr 5 cm
Infants <10 kg	4 Fr—5 cm	Radial artery 22–24 G
Toddlers	5 Fr—5 cm	Radial artery 2.5 Fr 2.5 cm
<20–25 kg Preschool children	5 Fr—8 cm	Femoral artery 2.5 Fr 5 cm Radial artery 20–22 G
Older children	7 Fr triple lumen	Femoral artery 3 Fr 5 cm Radial artery 20–22 G

The main indications for TEE include diagnosis, perioperative evaluation, and percutaneous intervention. In most cases, TEE can provide detailed features of cardiovascular malformations in children with CHD and is particularly useful for the repair of the aortic valve or atrioventricular valve, complex ventricular outflow tract reconstruction, and complex anatomical structures that preoperative TTE cannot fully determine. In the late stage of CPB, TEE helps to identify surgical risk factors and improve prognosis. TEE can assess right or left ventricular contraction abnormalities (based on wall motion or changes in systolic thickness); thereby, TEE can be used to guide the administration of vasoactive drugs and help children to wean off CPB as soon as possible. TEE can also be used to assess the quality of surgical repair and cardiac function. It can promptly prompt residual structural defects that must be repaired immediately and avoid re-operation later. During routine intraoperative TEE examination, about 15% of treatment decisions after CPB are affected by the results of TEE examination (such as re-CPB and repair of residual defects), but TEE is not helpful for evaluating residual obstruction of the aortic arch because the imaging of this part is not good. Although TEE can help detect whether there is residual gas in the heart chamber, its role in optimizing the exhaust process still needs to be further explored, especially for newborns and infants.

The potential risk of TEE is that when the probe size is relatively large or the probe is bent, it may compress the descending aorta, reducing the perfusion of its distal part, or compress the left atrium, affecting ventricular filling. Moreover, it may cause twisting of the endotracheal tube or entry into one side of the main bronchus and compress the trachea and bronchus during the insertion of the TEE probe. If the probe is pulled out too hard, it may cause accidental slippage of the endotracheal tube. When the body temperature and the flow rate are low, the TEE probe can cause esophageal injury due to heat production, so most hospitals choose to suspend probe imaging, disconnect the probe from the machine, or remove it during CPB.

3. Central Nervous System Function Monitoring.

The goal of brain function monitoring is to enhance the understanding of brain function during cardiac surgery and help develop effective brain protection strategies. Various techniques have been used for intraoperative brain monitoring in children with CHD to prevent secondary brain injury caused by hypoxia, ischemia, emboli, and electrophysiological disorders. They mainly include the following three methods used separately or in combination.

(a) Near-Infrared Reflectance Spectroscopy (NIRS): It's mainly used to monitor regional tissue oxygen saturation (rSO_2) and is a noninvasive monitoring technology that can reflect the overall hemodynamics and the perfusion status of tissue and organs. When NIRS is used for brain function monitoring, it mainly reflects the balance of oxygen supply and consumption in brain tissue. Similar to the principle of pulse oximetry, NIRS works by measuring the difference in absorption of near-infrared light by oxygenated and deoxygenated hemoglobin when used for brain oxygen saturation monitoring. Since near-infrared light can penetrate the skull, this technique can examine superficial areas of brain tissue. Although this technique was initially developed to monitor brain tissue oxygenation, it can also monitor the oxygenation of body tissues by placing the probe on the abdominal wall, quadriceps femoris, or the kidney area. This rSO_2 value is usually expressed as a percentage, not an absolute value of tissue oxygenation. Therefore, it is better to determine the baseline values before the induction of anesthesia or before CPB for trend determination. Brain NIRS mainly reflects venous blood oxygen saturation, and the value is related to jugular venous bulb saturation. Studies have shown that the decrease of NIRS values (especially below 50–60%) is associated with poor neurodevelopmental prognosis in infants with hypoplastic left heart syndrome undergoing stage I Norwood surgery. Although the correlation is not linear, it suggests that NIRS can be used to evaluate the harmful consequences of hypoxia clinically. Immediately after the operation, the oxygen saturation of the body and brain can predict overall complications and mortality. The time (in minutes) when brain oxygen saturation is below 50% can be used to predict morbidity and can serve as an early warning of hypoxia, bleeding, and/or low cardiac output states. Kidney NIRS monitoring found that the children need longer mechanical ventilation and ICU recovery time if kidney oxygen saturation decreases by more than 20% and lasts for 20 min.

Regarding the application of NIRS during CHD surgery, there have been quite a few prospective studies. However, current evidence still cannot provide clear thresholds for brain or body NIRS (i.e., complications increase below this threshold), nor has it been proven that differences in NIRS values lead to different long-term cardiac, renal, or neurodevelopmental prognoses. Generally speaking, checking for correctable related causes is necessary if the NIRS value drops by more than 20%.

(b) Transcranial Doppler Sonography (TCD): TCD can measure cerebral blood flow velocity and detect cerebral microemboli. It is also an effective method for continuously monitoring cerebral blood flow insufficiency or cerebral venous obstruction during CPB. Furthermore, it is suitable for newborns and infants.

TCD technology applies the Doppler principle to detect the frequency shift of blood signals in the middle cerebral artery (MCA)to calculate blood flow velocity. The low-frequency ultrasound waves can be transmitted into the brain tissue with relatively small signal attenuation in newborns/infants due to their thin skulls. Since the diameter of the MCA is relatively constant, blood flow velocity can be used to roughly estimate cerebral blood flow. TCD has many advantages: ① Non-invasive. ② No radiation. ③ Continuous monitoring. ④ It can capture rapid changes in blood flow velocity caused by changes in temperature or perfusion. The disadvantages include ① Poor reproducibility, especially at low flow rates; minor movements of the children's heads can significantly change the signals. ② There is a lack of effective research during hypothermic CPB. At this time, reduced body temperature, slower flow rate, and non-pulsatile laminar perfusion may limit the accurate cerebral blood flow velocity measurement.

(c) Electroencephalography (EEG): Used to monitor the changes in cortical electrical activity.

Although classical EEG monitoring can detect cerebral ischemia or can be used to evaluate the physiological functions of the central nervous system, it is rarely used for intraoperative monitoring due to factors such as multiple electrode placements, significant electrical interference, and high requirements of signal analysis processing. The most commonly used intraoperative EEG monitoring devices, such as Bispectral Index (BIS), brain state, and entropy index, etc. are all processed EEGs and converted into dimensionless values, which are convenient for quickly reflecting the functional status of the brain and mainly used for monitoring the depth of anesthesia. Factors such as hypothermia, cerebral ischemia, and epilepsy can also have a significant impact on depth monitoring. Postoperative EEG analysis found that many high-risk patients have shown sub-epileptic seizure activity, and these abnormalities may be related to poorer neuropsychological prognosis. The value and clinical significance of intraoperative EEG monitoring after CPB still need further clarification.

4. Temperature Monitoring.

Hypothermia is the main measure for heart and brain function protection during CHD surgery. Reasonable cooling and rewarming management are crucial for the intraoperative management of patients with CHD. Accurate and continuous monitoring of body temperature changes in different body areas can help make reasonable judgments and take effective measures. All CPB patients need both peripheral and core temperature monitoring. Rectal temperature represents the peripheral temperature, and esophageal and nasopharyngeal temperatures represent core temperatures, which usually reflect the brain temperature changes. The balance between rectal and esophageal temperatures is the best indicator of uniform body cooling and rewarming. The change in rectal temperature is slower than the change in esophageal and nasopharyngeal temperatures, whether during cooling or rewarming. The brain temperature is estimated through the esophagus and nasopharynx temperature during the cooling and rewarming process. The overestimation or underestimation error can reach 5 °C. Before initiating low-flow CPB or deep hypothermic circulatory arrest (DHCA), it is very important to provide enough cooling time to reduce the core temperature.

A bladder temperature probe can be installed on the Foley catheter, but newborns and low-weight patients have physical size limitations. Although tympanic temperature monitoring can better reflect brain temperature, there is a possibility of tympanic membrane rupture when the probe is inserted and is rarely used.

5. Others.

When surgery requires CPB or may cause renal ischemia, or when anesthetic management may lead to urinary retention, a Foley catheter should be placed to monitor urine output. Recording the total urine output and urine production rate before, during, and after CPB can help evaluate renal function, balance input and output, maintain the effective blood volume, etc.

4.3.2 Anesthesia Selection, Induction, and Maintenance

When children with CHD undergo heart surgery, a variety of anesthesia plans can be used. All these plans aim to provide sufficient sedation or general anesthesia while maintaining cardiac output (CO) and oxygen delivery. Many children with CHD have limited cardiac reserves, and the probability of successful resuscitation is lower than in normal children if cardiac arrest or other adverse cardiac events occur. Therefore, it is crucial to choose the anesthesia plan and anesthetic dosage wisely and comprehensively understand the unique pathophysiology of different types of CHD and the anesthesia requirements for specific surgery.

1. Choice of Anesthesia Plan.
   To choose the optimal anesthesia plan, the anesthesiologists should fully consider not only the pathophysiological changes of children with CHD, CPB, body temperature, etc. but also the differences in pharmacokinetics and pharmacodynamics under special situations in children with CHD.
   (a) Intracardiac shunt: The presence of a right-to-left intracardiac shunt can slow down the rising rate of inhalational anesthetics in arterial blood since part of the CO bypasses the lungs and dilutes the concentration of inhalational anesthetics in the systemic arterial blood. Inhalational anesthetics with lower solubility (such as sevoflurane and desflurane) are more easily affected, while those with higher solubility (such as halothane) are less affected.

When there is a significant right-to-left shunt, drugs administrated intravenously can directly enter the left side of the heart and are less diluted by systemic venous blood; thus, some medications (such as lidocaine, intravenous induction drugs, and muscle relaxants) may reach higher concentrations in the arteries, brain, and heart in a short time.

Left-to-right intracardiac shunt has almost no effect on the induction speed of inhalational anesthetics. Increased pulmonary blood flow can increase the absorption of inhalational anesthetics and cause the concentration of anesthetics in the pulmonary capillary blood to rise. Still, the concentration gradient between the alveoli and pulmonary capillaries is thereby decreased, then the absorption of anesthetics is reduced and these two effects cancel each other out ultimately. Only in the case of severe congestive heart failure accompanied by significant interstitial and alveolar edema, a left-to-right shunt may cause an increase in ineffective alveolar ventilation due to the combined effects of diffusion limitation and ventilation/perfusion ratio imbalance. At this time, the new anesthetic drugs are no longer absorbed; thereby, the induction of inhaled anesthesia may slow down.

(b) Changes in body temperature: Both animal experiments and clinical trials have found that hypothermia can reduce the MAC value of inhalational anesthetics and can also slow down the metabolism of all drugs by decreasing the reaction rate of drug metabolizing enzymes, whether these enzymes are in the liver (cytochrome P450 system), kidneys or plasma. Rewarming can significantly increase the metabolic rate of intravenous drugs.
(c) CPB: The effect of CPB on the pharmacokinetics and pharmacodynamics of anesthetics varies greatly depending on the type of oxygenator, flow rate, temperature, and ultrafiltration. After the initiation of CPB, many different mechanisms can affect the plasma levels of intravenous drugs. The priming solution of the CPB circuit can dilute the patient's blood volume by 50–300% and cause an immediate decrease in drug plasma levels. Many drugs can also bind to the membrane oxygenator and other CPB pipeline components, further reducing plasma levels. The degree of this effect depends on the patient's age and body size, the type of drug and its lipophilicity, the type of pipelines used, the patient's plasma albumin concentration, etc. Compared with other commonly used intravenous anesthetics, muscle relax-

ants have greater fluctuations in efficacy during hypothermic CPB, so if early reversal of muscle relaxation is needed, it is recommended to use a muscle relaxation monitor to assess the degree of neuromuscular blockade.

The ideal anesthesia plan can make the patient quickly reach a state of amnesia, analgesia, and muscle relaxation and has no significant effects on the hemodynamics. There is currently no ideal anesthesia plan, and anesthetic management strategies must be implemented individually according to patient condition changes. Therefore, it is not only necessary to comprehensively review the patient's medical history, physical examination, laboratory results, and imaging data (especially echocardiography) but also to fully consider the surgical procedures, duration, extracorporeal perfusion, and possible emergencies. Individualized anesthetic management plans should be proposed. For example, it is very important to maintain sufficient preload and afterload for patients with severe left ventricular outflow tract obstruction. Hemodynamic goals include avoiding tachycardia and increased myocardial contractility. At this time, the plan to use a large dose of propofol is risky. For patients with dilated cardiomyopathy and decreased ventricular function, drugs that may further reduce myocardial contractility or significantly change preload and afterload should not be used. In addition, for patients with severe pulmonary hypertension, an anesthesia plan that reduces harmful stimuli leading to a large amount of catecholamine secretion should be adopted to avoid the occurrence of a pulmonary hypertension crisis.

Because there are many types of CHD, the pathophysiology is complex and changeable, and the surgical procedures are different and changeable, so anesthesiologists must understand the advantages and disadvantages of varying anesthesia plans in various CHD surgeries and carefully design safe and effective individualized anesthesia plans. In addition, anesthesiologists sometimes need to prepare some alternative anesthesia plans and the strategy should be changed according to the situation when the hemodynamic goal is not achieved. Sometimes, certain vasoactive drugs and positive inotropic drugs need to be prepared to offset the adverse effects of the selected anesthesia plan.

2. Induction of Anesthesia.

   There is no ideal induction technique of anesthesia suitable for all patients with CHD. The patient's age, cardiopulmonary function, degree of cyanosis, emotional state, etc., will all affect the choice of anesthesia technique. The degree of cardiac dysfunction in the patient, defects, sedation level of preoperative drugs, and whether a venous catheter has been placed, etc. need to be balanced during the induction of anesthesia. The other factors which need to be considered include pulmonary hypertension, arrhythmia, complications, etc.

   (a) Intravenous induction: It provides more flexible drug choices and titration-based administration methods and can help to control the respiratory tract more quickly. For children with severe ventricular contraction impairment and pulmonary artery pressure approaching or exceeding aortic pressure, intravenous induction should be prioritized. Before anesthetic induction, the patients should be oxygenated first via a face mask to denitrogenate and increase oxygen reserves. The commonly used induction protocol of general anesthesia in our hospital: intravenous bolus injection of midazolam 0.05–0.2 mg/kg, etomidate 0.3 mg/kg, sufentanil 1.0–2.5 μg/kg, and rocuronium 0.6–1.2 mg/kg.

   (b) Inhalational induction: For CHD children without significant heart and lung function impairment, inhalational induction of anesthesia can be safely applied by mask. Sevoflurane is the preferred choice for inhalational induction of anesthesia, especially when peripheral venous access is difficult to establish quickly. However, for cyanotic patients with reduced pulmonary blood flow, the time for inhalational induction of anesthesia is prolonged.

3. Maintenance of Anesthesia.
   The maintenance of anesthesia depends on the children's ages, conditions, surgical characteristics, CPB time, and whether mechanical ventilation is required postoperatively. Our hospital usually adopts a combined intravenous and inhalational protocol: intravenous continuous infusion of propofol 4–6 mg/(kg·h), sufentanil 1–2.5 μg/(kg·h), and rocuronium 0.6–1.2 mg/(kg·h) and intermittent inhalation of sevoflurane. BIS is often used to monitor the depth of anesthesia during the maintenance of anesthesia.

For some children with simple CHD and good general conditions, sometimes a fast-track anesthesia protocol is adopted to speed up turnover and reduce hospital stays and overall costs. In this situation, it is necessary to agree with the surgeon, the anesthesiologist in the PACU, and the ICU doctor in advance and formulate a complete handover process. The maintenance protocol of anesthesia also needs to be adjusted accordingly. For example, suppose the plan is to extubate the endotracheal tube in the operating room after surgery. In that case, remifentanil can be used to replace sufentanil to avoid excessive residual opioids, which can affect the children's breathing recoveries after surgery. In addition, the management of sedatives and muscle relaxants also needs to be more precise, considering the timing of medication, surgery time, CPB, and other factors.

4.3.3 Management Before CPB

After the induction of anesthesia and endotracheal intubation, the position of the endotracheal tube must be carefully verified and properly secured; then, the ventilator parameters are properly set up according to the patient's required minute ventilation. When there is a large amount of physiological dead space, attention should be paid to the difference between $ETCO_2$ and $PaCO_2$. The arterial and venous pressure waveforms should be carefully confirmed, and the venous infusion line should be kept unobstructed. In addition, arterial blood gas analysis should be performed routinely. The baseline values of activated clotting time (ACT) value, NIRS value, etc. should be measured for comparison.

Additional sedatives, analgesics, and muscle relaxants can be administered as needed, supplemented with inhalational anesthetics such as sevoflurane. In addition, Vasodilators can also be intravenously given if it is necessary. Hypotension often occurs after induction and before skin incision. So, circulatory support should be in a timely manner (including volume support and appropriate administration of inotropic and vasoactive drugs). During sternum splitting, ventilation should be suspended, and the lungs should be kept at the end of exhalation with the APL valve opened to prevent pleural rupture. After the pericardium is opened, heparin 3 mg/kg is given through the internal jugular vein (it is required to confirm with the surgeon before administration). ACT should be rechecked 3–5 min after heparin administration to ensure ACT is more than 480 s. Tranexamic acid should be continuously infused intravenously.

The process of mediastinum dissection and cannulation by the cardiac surgeon is dynamic. To identify anatomical structures and get full exposure, the heart is often pressed slightly and dissected vascular structures. This may cause arrhythmia and a temporary decrease of preload and CO, which further leads to hypotension, transient hypoxemia, or even VF. During the process of aortic cannulation, the posterior wall of the aorta may be compressed, which may possibly cause a temporary disappearance of the arterial waveform, especially for low-weight newborns. Therefore, anesthesiologists should be vigilant about this. They must be able to identify these temporary, unavoidable, and essentially benign arrhythmias caused by cardiovascular surgical procedures and be able to distinguish them from more serious arrhythmias that persistently interfere with physiological status. It is crucial to communicate with the surgeon now, and the surgeon should be reminded to pause the procedures if necessary.

For children with a history of median sternotomy, there is a possibility of heart and major blood vessel rupture and massive bleeding during re-thoracotomy due to the lack of pericardial protection and the varying degrees of adhesion between the heart and major blood vessels. The risk of malignant arrhythmia is also significantly increased. Therefore, it should be very careful during splitting the sternum again. The chest CT imaging should be reviewed carefully before surgery to understand the adhesion situation as much as possible. If severe adhesion is suspected, cannulations of the femoral artery and vein can be performed in advance, or just vessel separation is preset for standby. In our hospital, for children undergoing secondary median sternotomy, the right femoral artery and vein are routinely examined by ultrasound to confirm their diameters and structure and whether there exists stenosis, thrombosis, etc. The cannula sizes also need to be discussed with the perfusionist. From skin incision to the establishment of CPB, attention should always be paid to the progress of the surgery with preparation for a large amount of blood transfusion and fluid replacement. In addition, external defibrillation electrode pads can be placed in advance to deal with external cardiac defibrillation in emergencies.

4.3.4 Management During CPB

Once CPB begins, the anesthesiologist must quickly determine whether venous drainage and arterial perfusion are sufficient. Insufficient venous drainage can cause venous distension, cyanosis, bulging of the infant's fontanelle, sudden increase of internal jugular vein pressure, or dramatic drop of cerebral rSO_2. Increased superior vena cava pressure caused by kinking or clamping of the cannula tip is one of the factors that need to be ruled out. The decrease of cerebral rSO_2 measured by NIRS or the decrease of cerebral blood flow velocity detected by TCD suggests possible obstruction of cerebral venous return. The increase of pressure in the arterial pipeline accompanied by a decrease in MAP often suggests arterial cannula obstruction, displacement, or aortic dissection.

It is usually beneficial for surgical operations to adjust respiratory parameters. If there is no PDA or other pulmonary shunt after the occlusion of the vena cava, mechanical ventilation can be stopped. Mechanical ventilation with a smaller VT can also be retained during parallel circulation. After the initiation of CPB, venous fluid replacement and the use of vasoactive drugs should be suspended, and the adjustment of hemodynamics and internal environment will be temporarily handed over to the perfusionist. Anesthesiologists should keep communicating with the perfusionist during CPB, strengthen monitoring, maintain appropriate perfusion pressure and flow, and keep rectal/nasopharyngeal temperature, hematocrit, urine volume, electrolytes, acid-base balance, etc., within the normal range. The internal environment disorders should be corrected in time. If DHCA is adopted, pay attention to its duration. When the CPB continues, ACT should be reviewed once every hour, and additional heparin should be added as appropriate. During CPB, analgesics, sedatives, and muscle relaxants can be continuously pumped to maintain anesthesia at a moderate level. Anesthesiologists should ensure sufficient neuromuscular blockade to avoid chills at low temperatures, which will significantly increase the body's oxygen consumption.

After hypothermic CPB and circulatory cessation, it is very important to avoid hyperthermia in order to reduce oxygen consumption and prevent possible ischemia/reperfusion injury. After the surgeon has completed the main operation procedure inside the heart, the body temperature can be gradually increased based on real situations, so that the body temperature rises evenly and avoids excessive high brain temperature. The goal of rewarming is to reach a core temperature of 35–37 °C. In order to prevent heat redistribution and heat loss after CPB withdrawal, the surface temperature should be kept roughly the same as the core temperature before CPB terminates. Once the pediatric patients are fully rewarmed, using a warming water blanket and warm air blanket under the body can help prevent hypothermia and maintain normal body temperature. During the rewarming stage, the concentration of anesthetic drugs will be changed, and it is unpredictable. The children may experience intraoperative awareness, especially when anesthesia is getting light. Therefore, many anesthesiologists used to give benzodiazepines such as midazolam at the beginning of rewarming to avoid intraoperative awareness in children.

Before aortic declamping, the patient should be kept in the Trendelenburg position, and the lungs should be inflated for air exhaust from the left heart until the aorta is declamped. Most children with CHD can automatically resume heartbeat a few minutes after the aorta is declamped. Our hospital routinely starts pumping dopamine or dobutamine 5.0 μg/(kg·min) after the aorta is declamped. After the vena cava is declamped (or communicated with the surgeon), mechanical ventilation can be restarted, with the respiratory parameters being adjusted as needed. If VF occurs, defibrillation should be conducted immediately with the power of direct cardiac defibrillation 0.5–2 J/kg. Epinephrine and lidocaine can be administrated if necessary. For those with difficult resuscitation, the cause should be carefully identified, especially hypothermia, coronary artery air embolism, hyperkalemia, acidosis, etc. Pay attention to whether the rhythm is sinus and whether there is a conduction block or ST segment change. If necessary, a small amount of isoproterenol can be given, or a pacemaker can be installed. In addition, if the heart contraction is weak, epinephrine 0.02–0.3 μg/(kg·min) can be added on the basis of pumping dopamine/dobutamine. If the peripheral resistance and perfusion pressure are considered insufficient, norepinephrine 0.02–0.3 μg/(kg·min) or vasopressin can be used as appropriate.

At this stage, the anesthesiologist must systematically evaluate body temperature, internal environment, and various respiratory and circulatory parameters to ensure successful weaning off CPB. Common causes of dynamic changes in cardiopulmonary function after CPB include heart and lung ischemia/reperfusion injury, inflammation caused by CPB, and myocardial injury caused by surgical procedures and sutures. Therefore, anesthesiologists must be vigilant, must be able to predict organ-specific dysfunction and failure, and must provide rapid treatment measures. When the CPB duration is very long, the supporting time of parallel circulation should be extended as appropriate until cardiac function recovers.

Before CPB separation, the anesthesiologists must confirm the following one more time: ① Hemodynamics is stable, heart rhythm is regular or stable, reliable pacing rhythm is present, and arterial blood pressure and CVP are within the appropriate range. ② Endotracheal tube is suctioned, mechanical ventilation parameters are carefully adjusted as well as PEEP is applied if necessary. ③ Central venous access is available, and the syringe pump runs normally. ④ Nasopharyngeal temperature > 36 °C. ⑤ Arterial blood gas results are stable. ⑥ Appropriate blood volume is assessed by directly viewing the heart and monitoring the filling pressure of the right or left atrial.

After complex CHD surgery, it may be difficult to separate the children from CPB. In this case, the anesthesiologist should analyze the causes with the surgeon and perfusionist together. Common causes in this situation include ① Poor surgical results or residual defects that must be repaired. ② Pulmonary hypertension. ③ Right or left ventricular dysfunction. There are two common methods for assessing the structure and function of the heart after surgery, which can be used alone or in combination: ① Directly measure the pressure of each major blood vessel and heart chamber through a pressure catheter. ② Intraoperative use of TEE can provide structural or functional images to help assess cardiac condition after repair. If structural abnormalities are found, CPB should be restarted, and the residual defects should be repaired before the pediatric patients leave the operating room.

4.3.5 Management After CPB Separation

1. Management of Circulatory Function.

After weaning off CPB, the patients may experience left or right heart failure and pulmonary hypertension, especially when the cardiac defect is complex and the operation time is too long.

After CHD surgery in children, the left ventricular contractile state may decrease due to local ischemia caused by surgery, preoperative myocardial condition, the impact of DHCA on myocardial compliance, and the changes of left ventricular load caused by repair. Treatment strategies for left ventricular dysfunction include optimizing preload, increasing HR, increasing coronary perfusion pressure, correcting ion calcium levels, and administration of positive inotropic drugs. Positive inotropic drug support usually starts from dopamine 3–10 μg/(kg·min) or epinephrine 0.03–0.05 μg/(kg·min). ① Effects of dopamine in children are age-related. After CHD surgery, the increase of CO caused by dopamine is more related to the increase of HR rather than stroke volume in children, while dopamine can significantly increase stroke volume in young adults. In addition, infants and newborns respond well to epinephrine and dopamine infusion with the increase of both systemic arterial blood pressure and CO. ② In cases of pediatric left ventricular dysfunction, early supplementation of calcium after CPB may be helpful, but attention should be paid when using calcium in slow sinus or junctional rhythms to prevent significant slowing of atrioventricular conduction. ③ For children with severe left ventricular dysfunction, such as low blood pressure, high left atrial filling pressure, or decreased contractility or local ischemia indicated by echocardiographic Doppler imaging, epinephrine treatment at 0.02–0.2 μg/(kg·min) may be helpful. ④ Milrinone, a potent phosphodiesterase III inhibitor, is an effective inotropic and vasodilator drug for infants and children. After neonatal open-heart surgery, milrinone can increase stroke volume, reduce SVR and PVR, and finally increase cardiac index. ⑤ Dobutamine is a relatively weak positive inotropic drug in children, which can sometimes cause rapid arrhythmias, possibly related to its structural similarity to isoproterenol. Dobutamine is used in children after CHD surgery mainly for its effects on increasing HR and CO.

After TOF repair, pre-existing right ventricular hypertrophy, right ventricular incision, and right ventricular outflow tract patching across the valve ring can lead to acute pulmonary valve regurgitation and right ventricular volume overload, which manifests as postoperative right heart dysfunction. The therapeutic goal is to reduce PVR and maintain coronary perfusion but not dilate the right ventricle. It is necessary to maximize preload up to the highest part of the Starling curve due to the decrease in right ventricular contractility, but excessive volume load can cause serious diastolic dysfunction, tricuspid regurgitation, etc. If right ventricular dysfunction is severe, sternal closure should be delayed to maintain the sternum in an open state, which can eliminate the impedance of the chest wall and mechanical ventilation, thus allowing the right ventricular end-diastolic volume to reach its maximum. Another strategy for neonates, infants, and children with right ventricular dysfunction after CPB is to allow right-to-left shunting at the atrial level. If right heart dysfunction persists, even leading to impaired systemic CO, extracorporeal membrane oxygenation (ECMO) can be considered. In some children with severe ventricular dysfunction, the myocardium may have suffered from temporary damage, i.e., myocardial stunning, which may gradually recover over time and it is the theoretical basis for ECMO used in circulatory support. ECMO helps to reduce ventricular wall tension, increase coronary perfusion, and maintain systemic perfusion of oxygenated blood. It's more effective than left ventricular failure when ECMO is used for right ventricular dysfunction or pulmonary hypertension. When pulmonary artery pressure is suspected to be high, it can be directly measured and compared with systemic blood pressure, so to analyze the cause. If necessary, treprostinil will be administrated at 0.01–0.05 μg/(kg·min) to reduce pulmonary artery pressure.

2. Respiratory Management.

The damage to lung tissue from CPB involves multiple factors, including pulmonary edema, decreased pulmonary compliance, reduced functional residual capacity (FRC), decreased vital capacity, and lack of alveolar surfactant, which ultimately result in increases in alveolar-arterial oxygen pressure difference and pulmonary shunting and dysfunction of ventilation and gas exchange. During CPB, mechanical ventilation is stopped, and lung tissue cannot exchange gases effectively as well a large amount of secretion accumulates in the airway, which can cause a collapse of lung segments or lobes. The first step of restoring ventilation after CPB separation is to ensure the correct position of the endotracheal tube, manually ventilate to observe whether both lungs are inflated, and appropriately adjust the mechanical ventilation parameters. Ventilation parameters should be adjusted based on arterial blood gas analysis rather than $ETCO_2$ because there is often a significant difference between $PaCO_2$ and $ETCO_2$ in children with CHD. $PaCO_2$ can reflect the true level of carbon dioxide inside the body, while $ETCO_2$ is also affected by pulmonary blood flow and mechanical ventilation. The trend of $ETCO_2$ changes is more helpful in detecting acute changes in pulmonary blood flow. Some children with CHD may have a tendency for pulmonary hypertension before and after surgery. If hypoxia, carbon dioxide accumulation, and acidosis are present at the same time, they may exacerbate pulmonary vasoconstriction and even affect systemic hemodynamics, so special attention should be paid to the adjustment of ventilation parameters.

The ventilation mode must be selected to match the children's hemodynamic status to achieve sufficient CO and gas exchange. PEEP can increase FRC, promote lung re-expansion, and redistribute lung water from the alveolar septal area to the more compliant hilar area, improving gas exchange and reducing pulmonary vascular resistance, which is beneficial for children with left ventricular dysfunction. However, too high PEEP levels can increase right ventricular afterload and will be harmful. Usually, PEEP of 3–5 cm H_2O can help maintain FRC and redistribute lung water, but it does not cause hemodynamic damage. Although the effect of lung re-expansion alone is limited, it can significantly reduce atelectasis, improve oxygenation and lung function after CPB, and increase SaO_2 when it is used in conjunction with PEEP.

3. Coagulation Management.

After CPB, it is necessary to use protamine to neutralize the anticoagulant effect of heparin. The ratio of protamine to heparin dosage is 1.0–1.5:1 (considering CPB duration and the total amount of heparin used in CPB), and calcium agents can be used at the same time. Before the infusion of protamine, the anesthesiologist must confirm again with the surgeon and perfusionist, and this communication can avoid catastrophic thrombosis in the CPB circuit. Protamine allergy can cause pulmonary artery constriction, leading to non-cardiogenic pulmonary edema, airway spasm, and peripheral vasodilation. Therefore, protamine should be injected slowly. If the allergic reaction occurs, protamine should be terminated immediately, and calcium agents, methylprednisolone, antispasmodic, and diuretics can be given intravenously. The doses of vasoactive drugs should be adjusted to maintain hemodynamic stability. Once protamine is administered, the perfusionist should promptly stop intracardiac suction to ensure that the blood in the circuit is still fully heparinized so that emergency or unexpected CPB support can be immediately re-established when surgery needs to be continued or when hemodynamics is decompensated.

The volume of the CPB circuit often exceeds the estimated blood volume of infants and children, which can lead to a decrease in coagulation factors and platelets in circulation, thereby causing dilutional coagulation dysfunction. Regardless of the degree of dilution, the resulting coagulation disorder needs to be treated after CPB. The activation of the coagulation cascade during CPB and the subsequent hyperfibrinolysis are the main reasons for the occurrence of bleeding and coagulation dysfunction after CPB, so antifibrinolytic treatment is used as a supplementary means to promote hemostasis. In our hospital, tranexamic acid is routinely used, with 10 mg/kg primed in the CPB circuit and then with 10–20 mg/kg titrated intravenously after endotracheal intubation and before CPB. Sometimes, an additional dose can be given later for CHD surgeries with long duration and heavy bleeding. After CPB has been weaned off, hemostatic drugs can be given intravenously as appropriate, and hemocoagulase is commonly used.

It is important for surgeons to conduct surgical hemostasis carefully. If there is obvious bleeding in the surgical field after CPB separation, the cause should be actively sought. ACT should be routinely reviewed and protamine can be added as needed, but excessive protamine can also cause increased exudation of blood, so careful identification is important. If necessary, blood samples can be tested through Sonoclot or Thromboelastogram (TEG) to assess coagulation and fibrinolysis status and guide further treatment accurately.

Once the cause of bleeding is identified, targeted transfusion of fresh plasma, platelets, prothrombin complex, fibrinogen complex, and cryoprecipitate can correct coagulation dysfunction. Anesthesiologists need to understand the differences in components, indications, timing of application, and efficacy of different blood products. Component transfusion after CPB begins with platelet transfusion, with the goal of normalizing postoperative platelet count. Because stored platelets are suspended in plasma, transfusion of platelets can also transfuse coagulation factors. Cryoprecipitate contains high concentrations of fibrinogen, factor VIII, von Willebrand factor, and factor XIII, and its transfusion after CPB can correct secondary hypofibrinogenemia caused by CPB. For newborns and patients with low body weight, it is important to control the total volume of different blood products, and concentrated coagulation factors should be given if necessary, such as recombinant activated factor VII (rFVIIa). It can bind to the tissue factor exposed to the endothelium and activate factors IX and X, leading to the production of thrombin and the formation of blood clots. It can reduce blood loss, transfusion requirements, and cases of rethoracotomies in children undergoing CHD surgery with CPB, but it is expensive and not suitable for routine prophylactic use.

4. Others.

Near the end of the surgery, it is still crucial to closely observe changes in the children's vital signs and make full use of this relatively stable period for further adjustments as follows: ① Review arterial blood gas analysis, routine blood tests, ACT, etc., and correct acid-base balance disorders and electrolyte disturbances. ② Pay attention to the degree of cardiac filling and exudation of blood and urine output, as well as maintain effective blood volume and hemodynamic stability, especially for surgeries like Glenn or Fontan procedures that are more dependent on preload. ③ When the surgeon is performing surgical hemostasis, placing chest drainage tubes, and suturing the sternum, the anesthesiologist should pay attention to changes in HR, CVP, MAP, and ECG. If there are signs of cardiac compression, pericardial tamponade, and pneumothorax, they should remind the surgeon to deal with the problems in time and delay the sternal closure if necessary. ④ Pay attention to the changes of various ventilator parameters, $ETCO_2$, and SpO_2, before and after the sternum is closed. Changes in thoracic and lung compliance may cause insufficient effective ventilation of the lungs, especially when pressure-controlled mechanical ventilation is adopted. ⑤ Continue to keep warm to prevent the children's body temperatures from being too low (keep body temperature ≥ 35 °C).

4.4 Postoperative Anesthetic Management

4.4.1 Transfer to the Cardiac Intensive Care Unit (CICU) After Surgery

After operation, the fast-track anesthesia process can be adopted with the endotracheal tube being removed in the PACU of the operating room for some milder patients whose operation time is shorter, while to most patients, the endotracheal tube will be kept in the CICU, and the respiratory and circulatory support treatment will continue to be used, so it is necessary to transfer the patient safely and quickly from the operating room to the CICU. Although the journey is generally short, the transfer process undoubtedly increases the risk of complications and death for those critically ill patients. Measures must be taken to minimize these risks, including meticulous planning, reasonable allocation of personnel and equipment, continuous monitoring of the patient's vital signs during the transfer process, and uninterrupted support for the function of important organs.

The transfer of the patient from the operating room to the CICU can be briefly divided into the preparation stage, the transfer stage, and the post-transfer stabilization stage.

1. Preparation Stage.

Before preparing to leave the operating room, the anesthesiologist must contact the relevant personnel in the CICU in advance and inform them of the following: ① The surgical method, including whether the final choice is radical surgery or palliative surgery, whether to delay closing the sternum, etc. ② Important events that occurred during surgery/anesthesia, such as whether there was major bleeding, severe allergic reactions or major rescues during operation. ③ The main facilities currently in use, including temporary pacemakers, ECMO, etc. ④ The types, doses, and speeds of vasoactive drugs, etc.

Before the transfer, ensure that the transfer ventilator or simple breathing bag works well to fully meet the patient's ventilation needs during the transfer process. Insufficient ventilation can lead to hypoxemia and hypercapnia, which can increase the PVR of some patients, but over-ventilation can also be harmful in some cases. The cylinder gas source must be sufficient. Generally pure oxygen is adopted, but for newborns or some children patients who need fine adjustment for the balance between the systemic and pulmonary circulation, an air-oxygen mixer is needed to set the appropriate oxygen concentration and flow rate. In addition, appropriate emergency resuscitation drugs should be prepared, and the battery of the syringe pump must be sufficient. For newborns and small infants, special attention should be paid to keeping warm during the transfer process.

2. Transfer Stage.

The process of moving the patient from the operating table to the transport bed carries significant risks, and it is essential to avoid the dislodging of drainage tubes, infusion pathways, and pump lines of vasoactive drugs. After moving the patient to the transport bed, the anesthesiologist should immediately check as follows: ① Make sure the endotracheal tube is not twisted or loose, the chest is rising and falling well, and if manual bag ventilation is used, its amplitude and frequency are kept close to the level before transport. ② Recalibrate the zero point of the pressure transducer and confirm that the heart rate and blood pressure have not fluctuated violently. ③ Properly fix monitoring equipment and syringe pumps on the transport bed to prevent them from falling. ④ Chest drainage tube can be briefly clamped, but if there is suspicion of excessive bleeding or cardiac tamponade, it should be unclamped as soon as possible. The transport phase requires all medical personnel to work together to deliver the patient to the CICU smoothly and as quickly as possible.

3. Post-transport Stabilization Phase.
   (a) After being transported to the CICU, the patients should be immediately ventilated with adjusted respiratory parameters, and their hemodynamic parameters should be quickly checked after the monitors are connected and calibrated. Make sure the syringe pumps are connected to the power source. The dosages and speeds of vasoactive drugs should be re-verified. In addition, the drainage tube should be unclamped and kept patent, and the volume of drainage should be measured.
   (b) The anesthesiologist should finish all of the relevant anesthesia records and medical documents.
   (c) The anesthesiologist should hand in details to the CICU doctor at the bedside, including the patient's vital signs, important events during the operation, volume of blood transfusion and fluid replacement, special cardiovascular medication, etc.

4.4.2 General Principles of Postoperative Management

Postoperative management is one of the important factors determining the outcome of CHD surgery. Although this work is now basically handled by the CICU team, as a member of the team, the anesthesiologist needs to understand and participate in it immediately after the operation. At the same time, understanding the general guiding principles and methods of postoperative management will bring many benefits to improving the perioperative management level.

The characteristic of the postoperative phase is that the patient gradually recovers from the abnormal condition of CPB and cardiac surgery, accompanied by a series of pathophysiological and pharmacological changes. During this period, the effects of cardiac surgery, potential diseases, hypothermic CPB, and the effects of special techniques such as DHCA may all cause special related problems. Immediately after operation, it is necessary to promptly identify abnormal conditions and special problems and apply appropriate treatment. Even if it is a normal recovery, the physiological changes secondary to load changes, surgical trauma, and CPB are still ongoing.

CHD patients have very different postoperative conditions due to factors such as potential diseases, preoperative conditions, postoperative sequelae, CPB duration, and intraoperative complications. Complications include insufficient blood volume, residual structural defects, left and right ventricular failure, hyperdynamic circulation, pulmonary hypertension, cardiac tamponade, arrhythmia, cardiac arrest, pulmonary dysfunction, oliguria, seizures, hypercoagulable state, thrombosis, brain dysfunction, etc. When these abnormalities occur, they usually indicate the need for closer observation, invasive monitoring, drug administration, and increased cardiopulmonary support. These abnormal recoveries should be detected and actively treated in a timely manner.

4.4.3 Postoperative Pain Management

Pain and postoperative agitation are the most common issues during CICU management. Once the anesthetic and analgesic effects wear off, analgesics must be used immediately after surgery. The administration of potent opioids can alleviate postoperative stress responses, thereby reducing complications. In most cases, postoperative pain can be treated with small doses of opioids intravenously, which is very important for taking off the ventilator earlier postoperatively in children. When long-term intubation and ventilation support are needed, continuous infusion of benzodiazepines and opioids can provide adequate sedation and analgesia until the start of ventilator withdrawal. The quantitative pain management of children is highly subjective and not very accurate, which brings certain difficulties to pain monitoring and the implementation of safe and effective pain treatment. By meeting the different needs of the patients and then providing multidisciplinary, personalized care, great progress has been made in the pain management of children. In the hospital where the author works, sufentanil is routinely used by a patient-controlled analgesia pump (PCA) with continuous small-dose intravenous infusion in children with CHD, and the doctors and nurses in the CICU can add the supplementary dose according to the actual situation. If the children are going to undergo unilateral thoracotomy, the medical staff can also use regional anesthesia to control the pain, which mainly includes ultrasound-guided unilateral paravertebral nerve block and intercostal nerve block. Through this method, the pressing numbers of PCA are significantly reduced with less respiratory suppression, better arterial oxygenation, earlier ventilator withdrawal, and fewer postoperative respiratory complications. It's especially suitable for those children who need early extubation after surgery. (Ning Ma).

Cardiopulmonary Bypass and Extracorporeal Membrane Oxygenation

5

Yinyu Yang and Wei Wang

Abstract

Cardiopulmonary bypass (CPB) and extracorporeal membrane oxygenation (ECMO) serve as vital extracorporeal circulatory technologies. This chapter concisely overviews both technologies, with a focus on pediatric CPB management. CPB core components include roller/centrifugal pumps, membrane oxygenators, and temperature-modulated circuits. Key aspects of CPB management emphasize adult-pediatric distinctions in flow parameters and temperature control, perfusion flow adjustment by body metrics, ACT-guided heparin titration, anesthesia management, hemodilution targets, ultrafiltration, α-stat/pH-stat blood gas management, deep hypothermic strategies, and protamine reversal. ECMO uses simplified circuits with centrifugal pumps and oxygenators to offer medium-to-long-term cardiopulmonary support with veno-venous mode for respiratory support and veno-arterial mode for cardiorespiratory support. While CPB facilitates surgical intervention, ECMO sustains critically ill patients during recovery, both demand meticulous anticoagulation and monitoring. Despite risks like bleeding and thrombosis, these technologies remain pivotal in modern cardiac and critical care.

Cardiopulmonary bypass (CPB) is a technique of extracorporeal circulation that temporarily replaces the function of the heart and lungs with an artificial heart–lung machine during surgery to maintain the patient's blood circulation and oxygen supply. CPB is performed by professional perfusionists who manage intraoperative perfusion and vital signs. Generally, CPB is a type of extracorporeal circulation utilized for short-term support during surgical procedures, particularly cardiac surgeries. On the other hand, extracorporeal membrane oxygenation (ECMO) is a type of extracorporeal circulation primarily utilized for medium to long-term support and treatment.

CPB supports hemodynamics and oxygenation by suspending the heart and lungs during surgery. Typically, surgeons need to perform surgery in a bloodless surgical field, and CPB requires the use of an artificial heart–lung machine to replace the function of the heart and lungs. Surgeons place a cannula into the right atrium, vena cava, or femoral vein to drain blood from the venous system. This blood is then filtered, cooled or heated, oxygenated, and returned to the body by a mechanical pump. The perfusion cannula is often inserted through the ascending aorta, but it can also be inserted into the femoral artery, axillary artery, or

Y. Yang (✉) · W. Wang
The National Children's Medical Center (Shanghai), Department of Cardiothoracic Surgery of Shanghai Children's Medical Center, Shanghai Jiao Tong University School of Medicine, Shanghai, China
e-mail: yangyinyu@scmc.com.cn

J. Zheng et al. (eds.), *Selected Pediatric Cardiovascular Surgery Anesthesia Cases*,
https://doi.org/10.1007/978-981-96-5614-1_5

brachiocephalic artery to perfuse the whole body with oxygenated blood.

Heparin is typically used for systemic anticoagulation before CPB, and protamine is usually administered to neutralize the anticoagulative effects of heparin after CPB. During surgery, cooling is generally used to suppress the patient's metabolism, reduce oxygen consumption, and improve the surgical field. However, low temperatures can increase the blood viscosity. So, it is also necessary to dilute blood by crystalloid fluids.

CPB is commonly used in cardiac surgeries. This technique substitutes the heart and lung functions and allows the surgeons to operate on the heart. In many surgeries, such as coronary artery bypass grafting (CABG), it is difficult to operate on a beating heart, so a cardioplegic solution is used to stop the heart. In surgeries requiring to open cardiac chambers, such as mitral valve repair or replacement, it is necessary to use extracorporeal circulation to avoid systemic air intake and provide a bloodless surgical field to assist the surgeon in completing the surgery. The heart–lung machine continuously pumps blood into the systemic circulation, which effectively substitutes the function of the heart. At the same time, the returned venous blood is oxygenated, and the carbon dioxide is removed by the oxygenator, which effectively substitutes the function of the lungs.

During the CPB process, the patient's body temperature can be reduced to deep hypothermia. The patient can survive for up to 45 min without perfusion in hypothermia. Permanent brain damage usually occurs if blood flow stops at normal temperature for 3–4 min, even leading to death. Similarly, CPB can also be used to rewarm hypothermic patients. Literature reports that CPB technology can successfully resuscitate patients with body temperatures above 16 °C.

ECMO is a simplified artificial heart–lung circuit mainly composed of a centrifugal pump and an oxygenator, which can replace the function of the heart and lungs in the medium to long term. When traditional conservative treatment is ineffective, ECMO technology can be used to save the lives of critically ill children with post-cardiac surgery, heart and lung dysfunction, acute respiratory failure, massive pulmonary embolism, lung injury caused by infection, and a series of other conditions that damage heart and lung function. Although ECMO does not provide any therapeutic effect, it can provide precious extra time to recover heart and lung function. For children with terminal diseases, cancer, severe neurological damage, uncontrollable sepsis, and other irreversible diseases, ECMO cannot save their lives.

5.1 Cardiopulmonary Bypass

Normally, one or more venous cannulas are used to drain blood from the patient by gravity during the CPB process. Whether the drainage is sufficient plays an important role in the operation. Factors affecting drainage mainly include the size of the venous cannula, the height difference between the child and the venous reservoir, the length and inner diameter of the venous drainage cannula, the continuity of blood flow, the characteristics of the venous reservoir, and the child's volume status. Venous cannulation is usually conducted at the superior and inferior vena cava (two cannulas) or the right atrium (one cannula). If the drainage is unsatisfactory, a vacuum-assist venous drainage device (VAVD) can be used to increase venous drainage. It is generally believed that ≥ -40 mm Hg negative pressure is relatively safe during congenital heart disease surgery while using excessive negative pressure will increase the risk of red blood cell lysis and air entering the venous line.

During the CPB process, despite adequate venous return, blood may still flow back to the left heart through alternative pathways (such as bronchial arteries, small cardiac veins, etc.), leading to congestion in the surgical field. Children with cyanotic congenital heart disease often exhibit a highly developed bronchial circulation. In children with left-to-right shunts, a large part of the pulmonary blood flow may be provided by communications between the systemic and pulmonary arteries caused by anatomical (patent ductus arteriosus, major-pulmonary artery collateral vessels) or surgical operations (Blalock–Taussig operation, Waterston operation, Potts operation, central shunt operation). If these shunts are not ligated or controlled before CPB, the blood from these shunts blood will enter the pulmonary artery, and then enter the left atrium and left ventricle. In addition, aortic valve insufficiency can also result in blood to flow back to the left ventricle. In these cases, the blood perfused by the aortic cannula may flow retrogradely into the left ventricle, and this retrograde filling will cease once the aorta is cross-clamped. To prevent myocardial damage and subendocardial ischemia caused by left ventricular dilation, it is necessary to incise the left atrium or place a left ventricular drainage cannula. During operation, a drainage cannula is often placed at the junction of the left atrium and the right upper pulmonary vein for drainage.

Cardiac suction devices are used to clear the blood from the surgical field, enhancing visibility and improving surgical exposure. Most cardiac suction devices use roller pumps to drive suction. This part of the blood needs to be filtered by the filter in the venous reservoir before returning to the reservoir to remove particulate impurities from the surgical field, thereby playing a role in blood protection. To avoid clotting and blockage of the CPB circuit, the patient must be fully heparinized before CPB or, more accurately, before cannulation and the use of cardiac suction.

5.1.1 Equipment and Composition

The CPB system consists of two main functional components: the pump and the oxygenator. The relatively low-oxygen venous blood is first drained into the oxygenator. Then the oxygenated blood by the oxygenator is perfused into the arterial system through aortic cannulation by the pump. The heat exchanger controls body temperature by heating or cooling the blood in the circuit (Fig. 5.1).

1. Pump.

During the CPB process, the pump substitutes for the heart, transporting blood from the venous reservoir to the oxygenator and heat exchanger. The pump can be either a roller pump or a centrifugal pump. The current roller pump is characterized by a small amount of priming and convenient adjustment of the arterial pump head position to close to the venous blood reservoir and oxygenator. Therefore, in most pediatric CPB cases, the perfusionist typically chooses the roller pump as the arterial perfusion pump.

Heart–lung machines have multiple roller pumps, and each drive pump's speed can be adjusted through the central console. The working principle of the axial flow pump is to squeeze the pipeline by the rotor rotation to promote blood perfusion. The advantages of a roller pump include accurate flow and low cost, so it is widely used in CPB. However, there is a risk of folding and rupture for the roller pumps since they are blocking.

Centrifugal pumps can also be used for blood perfusion during CPB. The working principle of a centrifugal pump is to generate centrifugal force by changing the speed of the pump head to promote blood perfusion. Since the centrifugal pump is a non-blocking pump, it is safer when folding and rupture of the circuit occur, and it will also reduce the occurrence of hemolysis events. So, some scholars believe that the centrifugal pump is superior to the roller pump. However, the flow control of the centrifugal pump is more difficult in pediatric patients because the flow is low during pediatric CPB. So, the centrifugal pump is only used in some older and heavier patients.

2. Oxygenator.

The oxygenator serves as an artificial lung by performing gas exchange (oxygen and carbon dioxide) through a solid membrane or microporous membrane. Currently, the membrane oxygenators used in pediatric cardiac surgery include the microporous membrane lungs and non-porous membrane lungs. The heat exchanger is integrated with the oxygenator to heat or cool the blood by convective heat exchanger. After the blood is oxygenated and temperature-adjusted by the oxygenator and heat exchanger, the oxygenated blood first passes through the microthrombus filter on the arterial line to reduce the microthrombus. Then it enters the patient's circulatory system via the aortic cannula. Furthermore,

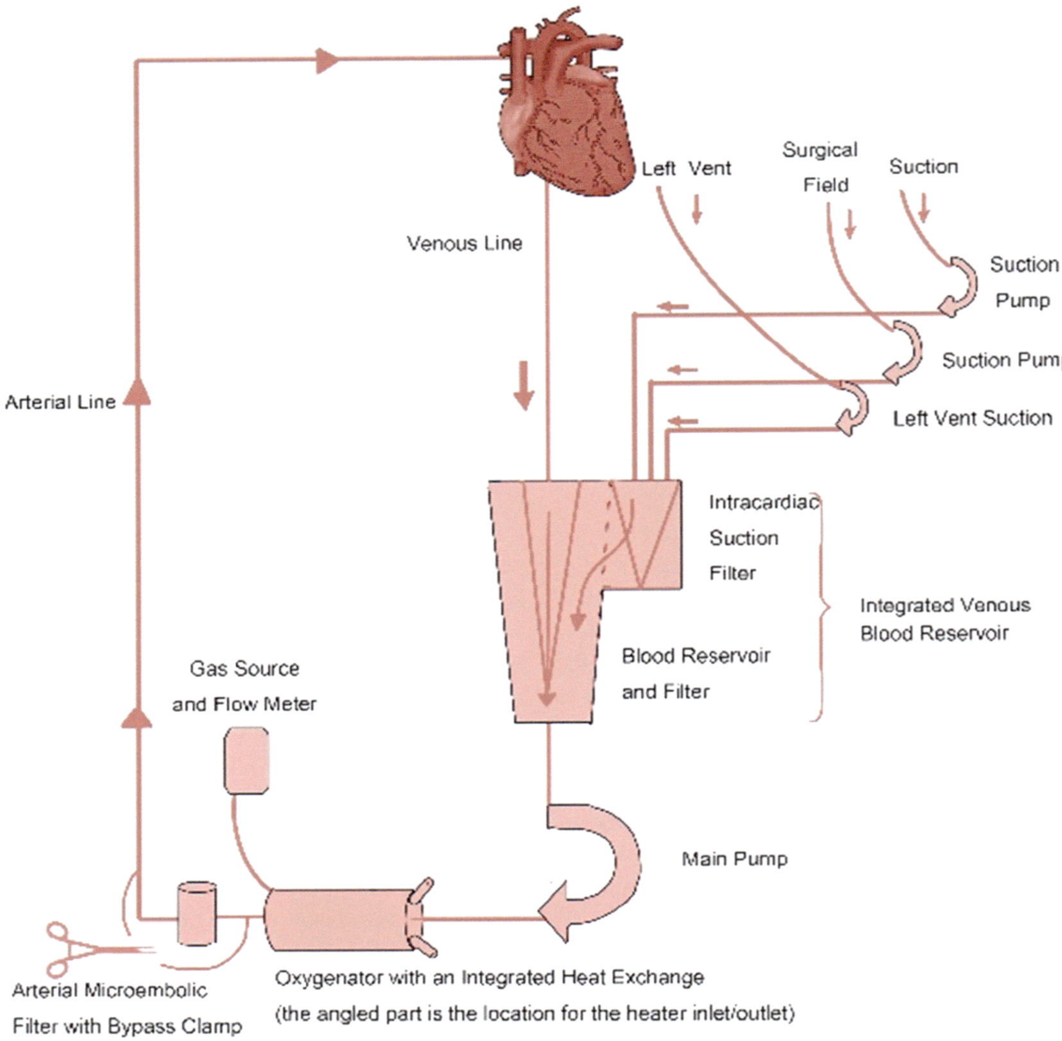

Fig. 5.1 Simplified diagram of the CPB circuit

it is often necessary to reduce the metabolism of the heart and the whole body by cooling during CPB. Intraoperative warming and cooling effects are achieved by changing the water temperature in the heat exchanger (water tank) connected to the oxygenator. It should be noted that the heat exchanger should be cleaned regularly to ensure relatively sterilized.

The location and type of cannulation may vary depending on the type of surgery. Due to the significant differences in weights and growth and development statuses among pediatric patients, it is necessary to adjust the size and position of the cannula according to the real situation to ensure sufficient perfusion and drainage during surgery.

In order to successfully complete pediatric congenital heart surgeries, it is necessary to stop the heartbeat in most situations. The cardioplegic solution is usually used to stop the heartbeat and protect myocardial cells. It is administered into the coronary arteries (usually through the aortic root) and/or cardiac veins (through the coronary sinus) via a catheter, a process known as antegrade and retrograde perfusion. The main types of cardioplegic solutions currently used include crystalloid cardioplegia, blood-containing crystalloid cardioplegia, and HTK solution. Their mechanisms of cardiac arrest and myocardial protection vary to some extent.

5.1.2 Management During CPB

1. Differences Between Adult and Pediatric CPB.

Pediatric CPB has many unique characteristics due to the different physiological characteristics of children at various developmental stages. In addition, children with congenital heart disease often have varying degrees of developmental delay, which requires an individualized CPB plan based on the specific condition. It's worth noting that children are not simply miniaturized adults. The differences between adult and pediatric CPB are summarized in Table 5.1. It can be seen that pediatric CPB has a greater degree of blood dilution compared to adults, so it is often necessary to add concentrated red blood cells to the priming fluid to reduce blood dilution. Using an appropriate circuit and oxygenator can also effectively reduce the priming and achieve the effect of reducing blood dilution. Due to the large differences in pediatric weights, preparing 3–4 different types of oxygenators and 3–5 different sizes of CPB circuits in advance is necessary. The surgical needs of pediatric patients at different ages and stages of growth and development can be met through personalized combinations.

Table 5.1 Differences between adult and pediatric CPB systems

	Adult	Child
Estimated blood volume	65 mL/kg	<10 kg: 85 mL/kg
Effect of blood dilution	25–33%	Up to 100–200%
Adding concentrated red blood cells or whole blood to priming fluid	Rarely	Usually
Oxygen consumption	2–3 mL/(kg·min)	6–8 mL/(kg·min)
Total flow at 37 °C CPB	50–75 mL/(kg·min)	150–200 mL/(kg·min)
Lowest temperature during CPB	Room temperature or mild hypothermia	Mild hypothermia or lower
Total circulation arrestor local brain perfusion	Rarely	Often used in the following diseases: HLHS, aortic arch hypoplasia
Perfusion pressure	50–80 mm Hg	30–50 mm Hg
Acid–base balance management	Mainly α-stability	Mainly pH stability at <30 °C
Difference in $PaCO_2$ measurement results	30–45 mm Hg	20–80 mm Hg

2. CPB Flow.

During the CPB process, the primary task should be to ensure sufficient venous drainage and adequate arterial perfusion and then adjust the parameters to achieve the expected flow, temperature, and acid–base balance.

The choice of flow in CPB mainly depends on the balance of oxygen supply and demand. A decrease in temperature can significantly reduce oxygen consumption. For every 1 °C of decrease in body temperature, the oxygen consumption of the whole body and brain will decrease by 5–6%. Oxygen consumption can be reduced to a certain extent by using the controlled cooling technique. At the same time, the CPB flow can also be reduced, which will be of great help for surgeons to complete surgery in a bloodless surgical field. Whole-body hypothermia is usually used during pediatric CBP, and many operations are conducted at a body temperature of 28–32 °C. The CPB flow of infants, children, and adults is generally maintained at 1.8–2.5 L/(min·m^2) under mild to moderate hypothermia. When the flow is expressed in mL/(kg·min), the flow of newborns will be significantly higher than that of adults because the relationship between weight and body surface area varies with age (Table 5.2). Under low body temperature conditions of 18–22 °C, the perfusion flow of newborns and infants should adopt a low flow rate, generally 50–75 mL/(kg·min) or 0.7–1.2 L/(min·m^2) (Table 5.3).

Table 5.2 Flow during total CPB related to weight

Patient's weight (kg)	Flow during total CPB [mL/(kg·min)]
<3	150–200
3–10	125–175
10–15	120–150
15–30	100–120
30–50	75–100
>50	50–75

Table 5.3 CPB flow at different temperatures

Patient's temperature (°C)	Flow (min·m^2)
≥35	≥2.5
32	2.2
30	2.0
28	1.8
26	1.6
24	1.4
22	1.2
20	1.0
18	0.7

3. Anticoagulation Management.

Unfractionated heparin is commonly used for anticoagulation during CPB, and the activated clotting time (ACT) should be monitored. Most centers determine the amount of heparin before CPB based on age or weight, considering that the priming fluid at the start of CPB will reduce the level of plasma heparin, so heparin should be added to the priming fluid. The routine dose of heparin to be given in the body is usually 300–400 u/kg, and the target ACT before CPB should be greater than 480 s. Some centers use the heparin management system (HMS), i.e., a heparin dose response test (HDR), to determine the patient's ACT reactivity to heparin. The required dose of heparin is determined based on the patient's estimated blood volume to achieve the anticoagulation target (ACT ≥480 s).

Heparin should be administered via a central vein to ensure that the drug can quickly return to the heart. In infants or newborns, it is common for the surgeon to administer heparin directly through the heart (usually the right atrium). It is essential to ensure that heparin reaches central circulation. The ACT result can be determined a few minutes after the heparin injection. The arterial ACT reaches its peak within 30 seconds after injection, and the peak of venous ACT is within 60 s.

4. Anesthetic Management During CPB.

During CPB, anesthesiologists will give perfusionists different doses of sedatives, analgesics, and muscle relaxants. Some centers also blow inhalational anesthetics into the oxygenator.

5. Monitoring During CPB.

Standard monitoring during CPB includes:

(a) Standard ASA monitoring (ECG, temperature, blood pressure, pulse, end-tidal carbon dioxide monitoring).
(b) Twelve-lead ECG monitoring.
(c) Temperature monitoring at two sites: nasopharynx, oropharynx, esophagus, and rectum.
(d) Arterial catheterization for invasive artery pressure monitoring (Mean Arterial Pressure, MAP).
(e) Central venous pressure monitoring (CVP): If CVP is elevated, consider the possibility of improper venous catheterization.
(f) Urine output monitoring.
(g) Recently, some cardiac centers have recommended using near-infrared cerebral oxygen monitors and/or transcranial Doppler ultrasound monitoring.

6. Blood Dilution.

Due to the small blood volume of children, the priming volume of the CPB circuit often exceeds the child's own blood volume, so the degree of blood dilution in children is much higher than in adults. For example, the estimated blood volume of a 70 kg adult is 5250 mL (70 kg × 75 mL/kg). Using 1000 mL of priming fluid to perfuse the CPB circuit, the degree of blood dilution is only about 20%.

On the contrary, the estimated blood volume of a 3 kg newborn is 255 mL (3 kg × 85 mL/kg). Currently, the CPB circuit volume in most China centers is about 350 mL, with a dilution degree of about 150%. Some international centers can control the CPB pipeline volume to about 200 mL, but the blood dilution degree is still over 80%.

7. Priming Fluid.

For adult CPB, crystalloid fluid is usually used for priming due to the relatively low blood volume dilution. To alleviate anemia caused by blood dilution, a suitable amount of concentrated red blood cells or whole blood should be added to the priming fluid for children. There is a huge difference in priming volume, which mainly depends on the CPB equipment used (oxygenator, circuit, etc.).

When only crystalloid/colloid fluid is used for priming, the following formula can be used to determine the hematocrit (HCT) of the child during the CPB process:

$$\text{HCT during CPB} = \begin{bmatrix} \text{Estimated Blood Volume}(\text{EBV}) \\ \times \text{HCT}/(\text{EBV} + \text{priming volume}) \end{bmatrix}.$$

Suppose the calculated HCT is within an acceptable range. In that case, adding red blood cells to the priming fluid is unnecessary, and CBP can be initiated by simply adding the necessary buffer solution. If the calculated HCT is low, a suitable amount of red blood cells should be added to the priming fluid to achieve the desired HCT during CPB. The volume of blood to be added to the priming fluid can be calculated using the following formula:

Volume of blood to be added to the priming fluid (mL).

$$= \begin{bmatrix} (\text{EBV} + \text{circuit volume}) \\ \times (\text{desired HCT during bypass}) \\ -(\text{EBV} \times \text{HCT}) \end{bmatrix} / (\text{HCT of priming blood}).$$

$$\text{EBV} = \text{child's weight}(\text{kg}) \times \text{unit weight blood volume}(\text{mL}/\text{kg}).$$

The circuit priming volume is calculated from the components used.

HCT of blood products: stock whole blood is 35–40%, and concentrated red blood cells are 65–75%.

Medical institutions add different types of blood products to the priming fluid (concentrated red blood cells or whole blood) and have acceptable minimum HCT values. Although concentrated red blood cells are usually used by most centers when priming is needed for the cardiopulmonary circuit, when the priming volume and the child's blood volume dilution are large, the use of whole blood or plasma can prevent the dilution of coagulation factors caused at the start of CPB.

8. Ultrafiltration.

Children undergoing cardiac surgery will experience blood dilution and severe systemic inflammatory response due to the CPB circuit, which leads to tissue edema and organ dysfunction and increases the incidence of complications and mortality. In the 1980s, conventional ultrafiltration (CUF) was applied clinically to filter out excess fluid during the CPB rewarming stage. However, CUF, postoperative diuresis, and even peritoneal dialysis have no significant improvement effect on postoperative fluid overload, complication incidence, and mortality. In 1991, Naik and other scholars proposed the concept of modified ultrafiltration (MUF), which can efficiently remove a large amount of excess fluid, increase postoperative HCT, and effectively improve clinical prognosis.

CUF is commonly used in almost all pediatric CPB surgeries (Fig. 5.2). It can remove as much excess volume from the venous reservoir as possible. This excess volume comes from the crystal components in the cardioplegia solution, valve reflux test fluid, or simply the blood volume overload. CUF uses a roller pump to actively or passively drive blood into the ultrafilter and filter out excess fluid.

MUF is ultrafiltration that continues after weaning from CPB. MUF can concentrate the patient's blood and the blood in the CPB circuit while the CPB circuit retains priming. The direction of blood flow in MUF can be carried out in two ways: from the arterial to the venous or from the venous to the arterial. Arterial end to venous end method (Fig. 5.3a): Blood in the aortic cannula is driven to the inlet of the ultrafilter by the roller pump, and the blood at the outlet of the ultrafilter is delivered to the right atrium through the venous cannula. Venous end to arterial end method (Fig. 5.3b).

The blood in the right atrium is driven into the ultrafilter by the roller pump, and the blood, after

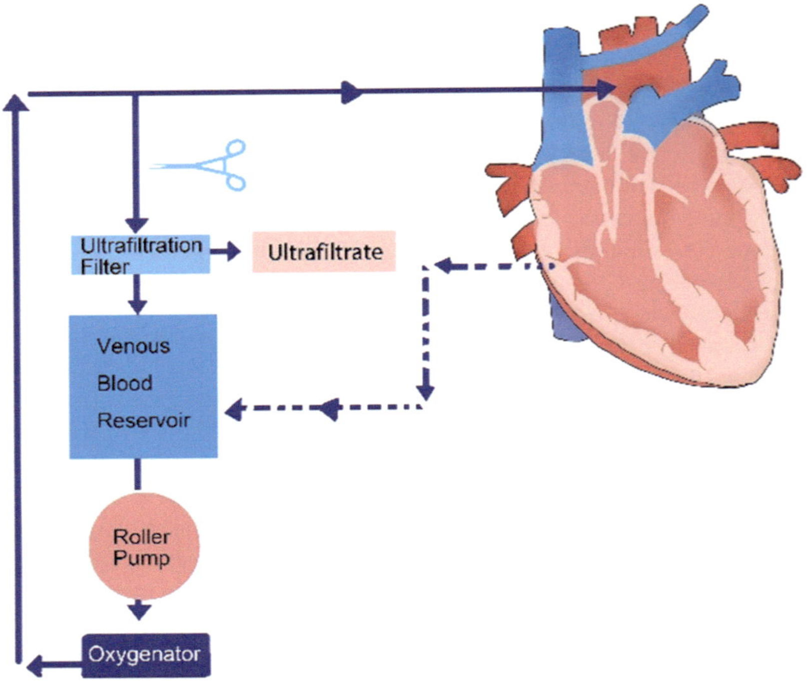

Fig. 5.2 Schematic diagram of conventional ultrafiltration

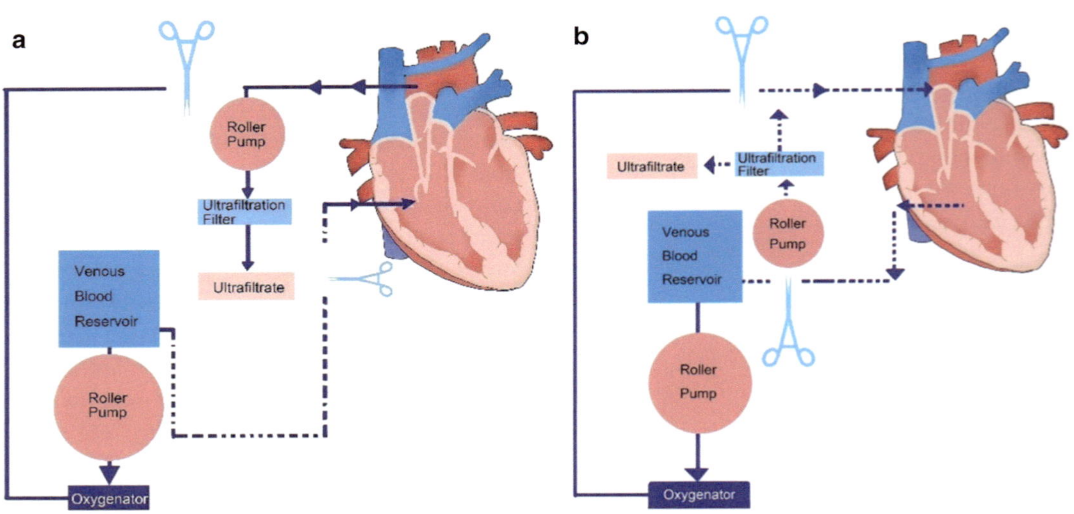

Fig. 5.3 Schematic diagram of modified ultrafiltration. (**a**) arterial to venous; (**b**) venous to arterial

ultrafiltration, enters the aorta through the arterial cannula. As the fluid is filtered out via these two methods, the remaining blood in the CPB circuit can replenish the fluid filtered out in the ultrafiltration circuit to maintain the patient's blood volume stability. There is no uniform regulation on when to stop MUF, and it can generally depend on the ultrafiltration time (10–15 min), target HCT value (40%), or the amount of filtered fluid (750 mL/m^2).

The main advantage of MUF compared with CUF is that it can continue to concentrate blood after CPB weaning off. The degree of blood concentration is much greater than that of CUF, especially in small infants. Since the two ultrafiltration methods do not exclude each other, many centers often use CUF + MUF for fluid management during CPB.

9. Blood Gas Management.

Blood gas management also plays an important role in CPB. The electrochemical neutral state plays an important role in preserving cellular protein and enzymatic structures and maintaining a constant transmembrane hydrogen ion (H^+) gradient, which is necessary for many cellular metabolic processes. In addition, optimizing the function of the body's imidazole buffering system also depends on maintaining intracellular electrochemical neutrality. The imidazole group of histidine is widely present in blood and cellular proteins, which is a very important buffering system. It is in a state of electrochemical neutrality when the concentration of H^+ is equal to that of OH^-. As the temperature decreases, the dissociation constant (PK) of water in cells increases, and the decrease in temperature will lead to a decrease in the concentration of OH^- and H^+ ions. Electrochemical neutrality can be maintained as long as OH^- and H^+ maintain the same concentration. Therefore, to maintain the state of electrochemical neutrality, the pH must be increased when the temperature decreases. In cells at 37 °C in electrochemical neutrality, the measured cell pH is 7.40; in cells at 20 °C in electrochemical neutrality, the measured cell pH is 7.80. $PaCO_2$ regulates the change in cell pH at low temperatures. When the temperature decreases, the solubility of CO_2 in blood increases. If the total CO_2 content in the blood remains stable, the increase in CO_2 solubility will cause a decrease in $PaCO_2$. For example, if the total CO_2 content remains stable, the blood $PaCO_2$ measured at 37 °C is 40 mm Hg, and when measured at 20 °C, the $PaCO_2$ is 16 mm Hg. To maintain electrochemical neutrality, the pH will increase as the temperature decreases.

pH homeostasis and α homeostasis are two different ways of managing acid–base balance, which directly affect the blood supply to the brain and other organs. Although the management of acid–base balance in pH homeostasis and α homeostasis often involves whether temperature correction is needed, it must be emphasized that these are two completely different concepts. The interpretation of blood gas analysis test results (whether temperature corrected or not) does not determine the method of acid–base management (pH homeostasis or α homeostasis). It should be noted that in children at 37 °C, there is no difference in the management of pH homeostasis and α homeostasis. As the child's body temperature gradually decreases, the differences between the two management strategies will become more and more obvious, until the temperature is below 30 °C, the management of the two methods has clinical relevance.

When the blood sample of a child with hypothermia is sent to the laboratory for examination, the blood is heated to 37 °C before measurement. The result measured at 37 °C is the "uncorrected value," which is then converted to the temperature-corrected result through the nomogram. The nomogram explains the changes in blood pH, O_2, and CO_2 solubility caused by temperature in a closed system. When the pH and $PaCO_2$ measured at 37 °C are corrected to a lower temperature, compared with the results at 37 °C, the pH will increase, and the $PaCO_2$ will decrease. Therefore, the state of electrochemical neutrality is maintained by keeping the pH alkaline in the blood gas after low-temperature correction and normal in the uncorrected blood gas. This is also known as α homeostasis management. In practical operations, it is easier to apply uncorrected results and maintain pH, $PaCO_2$ At 37 °C, it is considered within the normal range. When α-steady-state management is applied, cerebral blood flow and cerebral oxygen consumption are appropriately coupled together. The only exception is during deep hypothermia, when the brain's automatic regulation function is lost, and the changes in cerebral blood flow directly follow changes in arterial blood pressure.

pH steady-state regulation refers to maintaining the results of blood gas tests within the normal range after temperature correction. If temperature correction is not performed, the results of blood gas tests will be acidic. During hypothermic CPB, $PaCO_2$ is increased by blowing in CO_2, lowering the pH. Unlike the CO_2 total content remaining stable in α-steady-state regulation, pH steady state will cause an increase in CO_2 content. During hypothermic CPB, cerebral blood vessels remain responsive to changes in different $PaCO_2$. This response is maintained during moderate hypothermia, but it is weakened during deep hypothermia, and the brain's autonomous regulation of cerebral blood flow is completely lost during deep hypothermia. When moderate hypothermia uses pH steady-state management, the cerebral blood flow and metabolism will be uncoupled, and the brain's automatic regulation of cerebral blood flow is lost. Therefore, there is a linear correlation between cerebral blood flow and arterial pressure, and the brain is in a state of high perfusion because the cerebral blood flow is much greater than the cerebral blood flow related to the brain's metabolic rate. This high perfusion state results from the combined effect of reduced cerebral oxygen consumption caused by hypothermia and cerebral vasodilation caused by higher $PaCO_2$ at low temperatures. In addition, pH steady-state management inhibits the brain's metabolic rate and extends the time that oxygen is available to brain tissue during circulatory arrest. pH steady-state also reduces pulmonary blood flow and pulmonary blood flow still exists even during total bypass due to the presence of collateral circulation, which is beneficial to prevent the effects of blood steal on cerebral circulation and improve heat exchange during warming and cooling periods. The cerebral over-perfusion may increase the probability of microemboli entering the cerebral circulation.

The risk of embolism in adults is higher than in children because adult arteries are prone to form calcified plaques, so α-steady-state blood gas management is commonly used in adult cardiac surgery. Children rarely have embolisms due to vascular disease. However, children often use hypothermic bypass and often have uneven brain cooling due to stealing blood from the brain's blood flow due to collateral circulation. Therefore, pH steady-state blood gas management is often used in this type of pediatric CPB.

10. Deep Hypothermic Circulatory Arrest and Regional Perfusion Techniques.

Deep hypothermic circulatory arrest (DHCA) is a technique in which the patient's body temperature is lowered to below 20 °C, the supply of blood flow to the aorta is stopped, and the patient's blood volume is drained into the venous reservoir. This technique provides surgeons with an almost ideal surgical field, which can be used for complex aortic arch repair, total anomalous pulmonary venous connection correction, or when the patient's age and/or anatomy hinder the venous return during the surgical repair process.

The application of regional cerebral perfusion (RCP) technology can limit or even eliminate the need for deep hypothermic circulatory arrest (DHCA). RCP refers to reversing arterial pump blood flow direction, usually through the innominate artery, directly perfusing only the right subclavian and common carotid arteries. Different institutions have different methods for managing the flow, acid–base balance, and temperature of RCP. Some centers use a higher flow rate (60–70 mL/kg·min), but usually, a flow rate of 20–40 mL/kg·min can provide appropriate perfusion for cerebral circulation. Some centers will precisely control the flow by monitoring transcranial Doppler ultrasound and near-infrared cerebral oxygen.

11. Protamine Neutralization.

After CPB, if the hemodynamics are stable and the surgical repair is satisfactory, protamine can be given to neutralize heparin. Protamine can be given once it is confirmed that CPB will not be used again. Once protamine neutralizes heparin, the intracardiac suction should be stopped to prevent blood clot formation and blockage of the CPB circuit (especially the oxygenator). It is necessary to conduct systemic heparinization again before CBP initiation. The venous cannula is usually removed before protamine is intravenously administered. The arterial cannula can be removed only after sufficient hemostasis is achieved, and there is no further need for blood to return through the circuit.

There are various methods for using protamine to neutralize heparin, all of which have achieved good clinical results. Some centers neutralize with 1.0–1.3 mg of protamine per 100 IU of heparin after CPB. This is based on the ratio of protamine to heparin neutralization in vitro experiments being 1.3:1. The ACT value determines the amount of heparin during CPB, and the heparin level related to the ACT value is calculated by reverse calculation of the heparin dose–response curve. Some centers do not consider the dose of heparin and simply give a fixed dose of protamine based on the child's weight (3–4 mg/kg). Other centers give 1–1.3 mg of protamine per 100 IU of heparin used. Some centers perform heparin tests and calculate the amount of protamine based on the child's blood volume, with a neutralization ratio of 1:1–1:3.

Regardless of the method used, the ACT value should be retested after heparin neutralization by protamine. In addition to the prolonged ACT caused by residual heparin, platelet reduction, dilution of coagulation factors, and other factors can also cause ACT prolongation after heparin neutralization, especially in infants and young children,

5.2 Extracorporeal Membrane Oxygenation

ECMO, or extracorporeal life support (ECLS), is a core technology derived from CPB. It is an extracorporeal circulation technology that provides circulatory and respiratory support for children with heart and/or lung failure, which can provide medium- to long-term support for patients.

The working principle of ECMO is similar to CPB, which temporarily drains venous blood from the body, oxygenates the red blood cells, removes the blood carbon dioxide, and then reinfuses it into the patient's arterial/venous system. Currently, ECMO is widely used in the treatment of critically ill children with acute heart failure after cardiac surgery, fulminant myocarditis, acute respiratory distress syndrome (ARDS), septic shock, etc. It is worth noting that ECMO itself has no therapeutic effect; the main purpose is to win valuable time for recovering a patient's cardiopulmonary function, clinical diagnosis, and treatment.

ECMO has achieved good results in rescuing critically ill children in emergencies in the past decade. The literature reports that cardiopulmonary resuscitation (CPR) by ECMO (ECPR) has a better survival rate than traditional CPR. ECPR combined with mild hypothermia treatment can have a better prognosis for the nervous system.

In 2020, with the continuous increase of children infected with the novel coronavirus worldwide, ECMO also played the role of the last line of defense in the treatment of critically ill children. Many pediatric patients who were ineffective in traditional treatment were successfully saved.

5.2.1 Indications and Contraindications

The Extracorporeal Life Support Organization (ELSO) has issued ECMO indications and clinical guidelines. However, the timing of ECMO initiation varies slightly from center to center in actual medical work. Still, the indications for ECMO usually include the following reversible diseases and acute severe circulatory and respiratory failure that are unresponsive to conventional treatment:

1. Acute respiratory failure, despite optimizing ventilator settings including fraction of inspired oxygen (FiO_2), positive end-expiratory pressure (PEEP), and inspiratory to expiratory (I:E) time ratio, but the ratio of arterial oxygen pressure to inspired oxygen concentration (PaO_2 /FiO_2) is less than 100 mm Hg.
2. Hypercapnic respiratory failure, arterial blood gas pH less than 7.20.
3. Cardiogenic shock.
4. Cardiac arrest.
5. Unable to wean off CPB after cardiac surgery.
6. As a bridge to heart transplantation or a ventricular assist device placement.

7. As a bridge before lung transplantation.
8. Septic shock (still controversial).
9. Hypothermia, i.e., core temperature is 24–28 °C, circulation is unstable, or core temperature is below 24 °C.

During the COVID-19 epidemic, Chinese intensivists were also the first to use ECMO for respiratory support in children with low blood oxygen levels after mechanical ventilation and unable to maintain oxygenation. Early reports showed that ECMO significantly improved oxygenation in children and reduced mortality by about 3%. For critically ill children, the mortality rate dropped from 59% to 71% of conventional treatment to 46%.

Currently, there are fewer and fewer absolute contraindications for ECMO, and the benefits and risks of the patient should be weighed before ECMO initiation. Relative contraindications for ECMO include the following:

1. Irreversible disease or inability to recover.
2. Existence of severe conditions affecting survival treatment (neurological damage, terminal illness, etc.).
3. Age and weight.
4. Severe birth defects or chromosomal abnormalities (13, 18-chromosome deformities, etc.).

5.2.2 ECMO Support Modes

The typical ECMO circuit includes a centrifugal pump, membrane oxygenator, perfusion/drainage cannula, and other devices (Fig. 5.4). In addition, the circuit can be connected to a three-way connector for pressure monitoring and continuous venous oxygen saturation monitoring as needed clinically.

The main ECMO support modes include veno-venous (V-V) and veno-arterial (V-A).

Veno-venous (V-V) ECMO: Generally speaking, vascular access can be established through percutaneous puncture of the internal and femoral jugular veins. It is mainly used for children with respiratory failure whose heart function is still acceptable for long-term lung support. Blood flows back from the venous system to the oxygenator for oxygenation and carbon dioxide removal and then returns to the venous system. In addition, there is also a type of double-lumen cannula (Fig. 5.5), which can drain the blood flow of the superior and inferior vena cava and perfuse back to the right atrium after being inserted into the jugular vein.

Veno-arterial (V-A) ECMO: Generally, ECMO can be established through the cervical arterial and venous or femoral arterial and venous pathways. Infants and young children need to expose the blood vessels under direct vision for a surgical incision. The vascular pathway is generally established directly from the right atrium to the aorta for children after cardiac surgery. VA-ECMO can provide substitute support for both the heart and lungs. Blood returns from the venous system to the oxygenator, where it is oxygenated, carbon dioxide is removed, and the temperature is adjusted. The blood is then delivered to the arterial circulation.

The cardiac output of patients with ECMO consists of ejection from their own heart and ECMO flow. It is necessary to maintain appropriate alveolar ventilation since part of the venous blood flow can still enter the pulmonary circulation. When all venous blood is drained, VA-ECMO is equivalent to complete CPB. When only part of the venous blood is returned, VA-ECMO is equivalent to parallel circulation during CPB.

The operational differences between VA-ECMO and VV-ECMO are shown in Table 5.4, and the changes in physiological functions are shown in Table 5.5.

5.2.3 Precautions

1. Special attention must be paid to prevent tube slippage and tube folding when transferring in or out of the operating room.
2. Due to systemic heparinization, platelet reduction, and lack of coagulation factors, the child may have a tendency to bleed more and need to ensure sufficient vascular access and blood products.

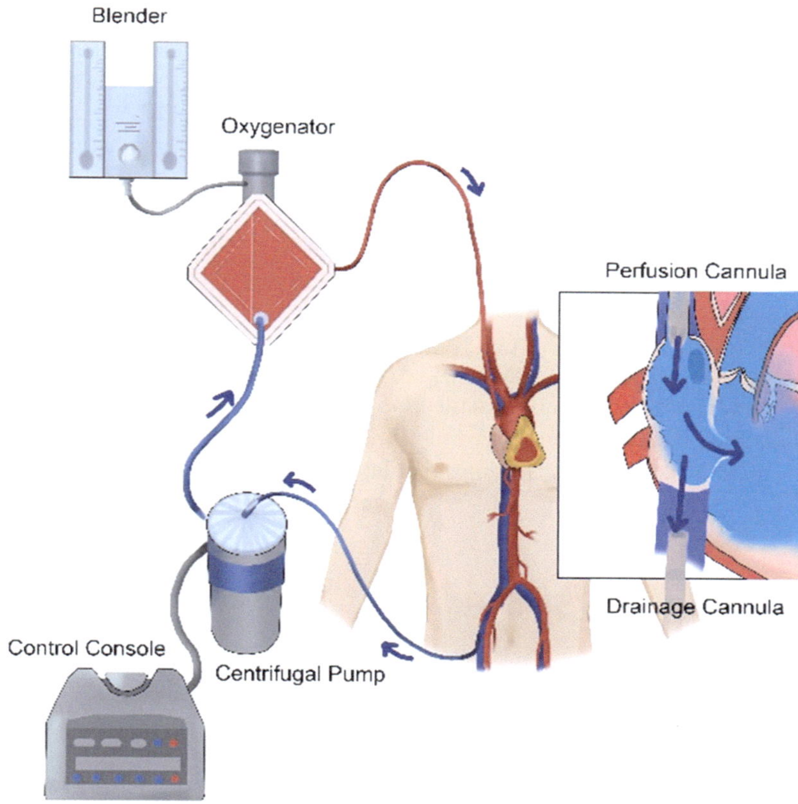

Fig. 5.4 ECMO circuit composition diagram

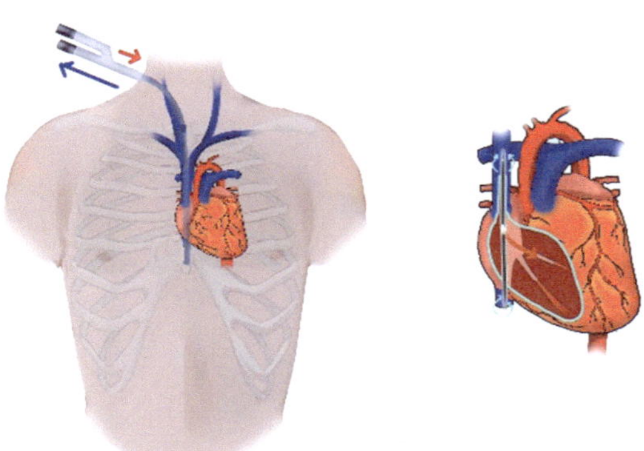

Fig. 5.5 VV-ECMO double-lumen cannula diagram

Table 5.4 Operational differences between VA-ECMO and VV-ECMO

	VA-ECMO	VV-ECMO
Support type	Heart and lung	Lung
Circulatory support	Partial or full	None
Intubation location	Vein and artery	Vein

Table 5.5 Physiological differences between VA-ECMO and VV-ECMO

	VA-ECMO	VV-ECMO
Preload of the heart	Decreased	Unchanged
Afterload of the heart	Increased	Unchanged
Pulmonary blood flow	Decreased	Unchanged
Pulse pressure difference	May decrease	Unchanged
Source of coronary blood flow	Left ventricular ejection or ECMO blood flow	Left ventricular ejection

3. The pharmacodynamics of inhaled drugs used by ECMO patients will change, and the reduction of alveolar ventilation will reduce the effect of inhaled anesthetics.
4. The hemodynamic stability of VV-ECMO patients depends on their own heart function, such as vasoconstrictor drugs sometimes, and

(or) positive inotropic drugs if needed for support.

5. Children on VA-ECMO often use vasoconstrictor inotropic drugs before assistance and need to be continued during ECMO support.
6. Unlike CPB, the arterial pressure in ECMO is pulsatile due to left ventricular ejection. In VA-ECMO, if the pulse wave becomes flat, the most possible reason may be that most of the blood flow enters the ECMO circuit. In addition, if the left ventricle is completely bypassed or the aortic valve cannot open, it is also manifested as non-pulsatile blood flow.
7. During the operation of VA-ECMO and VV-ECMO, the lower level of lung ventilation can help to reduce barotrauma and volumetric trauma to the lowest level. (Respiratory rate < 10 times/min, FiO_2 < 40%, PIP <25 mm Hg, PEEP 5–15 mm Hg).
8. The anticoagulation, in this case, is achieved by intravenous administration of unfractionated heparin. The anticoagulation test varies according to the situation of each center. Some measure heparin content (anti-Xa) and activated clotting time (ACT).
9. When using drugs, consider that the ECMO circuit increases the child's total blood volume and the possibility of drugs being adsorbed by the pipeline and oxygenator (Yinyu Yang, Wei Wang).

Part II

Discussion of Anesthesia Cases for Surgery of Congenital Cardiovascular Diseases

Anesthetic Management of One-Lung Ventilation for Atrial Septal Defect Repair via a Small Axillary Incision

6

Hualin Chen

Abstract

A 4-year-old boy with an atrial septal defect underwent minimally invasive repair via a small axillary incision. A bronchial blocker was used to occlude the right main bronchus, and one-lung ventilation was performed, which provided a better surgical field of view for the surgeons. Compared with adults, children, especially infants, have softer ribs and functional residual volume close to residual volume level, making them prone to hypoxemia during one-lung ventilation. In anesthetic management for such children, we should consider the pathophysiological changes caused by one-lung ventilation and the impact of left-right cardiac shunt.

With the development of minimally invasive concepts and techniques, an increasing number of pediatric patients with congenital heart defects have undergone minimally invasive surgeries, achieving favorable treatment outcomes. Compared with the traditional sternotomy atrial septal defect (ASD) repair, small axillary incision ASD repair has less trauma and rapid recovery and also offers a more aesthetically pleasing, less exposed incision. However, lateral thoracotomy ASD repair presents challenges such as deep operation site, limited operative field, and difficult exposure due to dilated lungs. Traditional bilateral lung ventilation technology is not conducive to optimal surgical field exposure, and repeated lung tissue compression can cause lung injury. While one-lung ventilation (OLV) technology can collapse the lung on the operative side, eliminate the need for lung compression, significantly improve the operative field visibility, and reduce lung tissue damage. OLV can be achieved through double-lumen endotracheal tubes, single-lumen bronchial tubes, Univent tubes, and bronchial blockers (BBs). Compared to other tools, BBs have the advantages of simple operation, less trauma, and lack of age and endotracheal tube size restrictions. They can be placed both within and outside the endotracheal tube. Therefore, more and more infant patients use BBs to complete OLV. This article describes the anesthetic management of ASD repair via a small axillary incision in OLV.

6.1 Case Presentation

A 4-year-old boy with 15 kg in weight, G1P1, was born at full term without an asphyxia history. He was diagnosed with ASD by hearing a heart murmur 2 years ago, and an echocardiographic

H. Chen (✉)
The National Children's Medical Center (Shanghai), Department of Anesthesiology of Shanghai Children's Medical Center, Shanghai Jiao Tong University School of Medicine, Shanghai, China
e-mail: chenhualin@scmc.com.cn

J. Zheng et al. (eds.), *Selected Pediatric Cardiovascular Surgery Anesthesia Cases*,
https://doi.org/10.1007/978-981-96-5614-1_6

examination recommended surgical treatment. The child has good feeding habits, normal activity tolerance, and no significant cyanosis of the lips. Echocardiography showed: ASD (secondary hole type) 2.0 cm, central location, left-to-right shunt; normal atrioventricular valve activity; mild mitral regurgitation, mild tricuspid regurgitation. ASD repair via a small axillary incision was planned under general anesthesia.

Physical examination: The patient was conscious with stable breathing. Auscultation: the breath sounds of both lungs were slightly coarse without dry or wet rales; the heart sounds were strong with regular rhythm, and II/VI systolic murmur could be heard at the left 2–3 intercostal spaces.

Laboratory tests: Routine blood tests, coagulation, and liver and kidney function were normal.

Electrocardiogram: Sinus rhythm, incomplete right bundle branch block with right ventricular hypertrophy, left axis deviation.

6.2 Anesthetic Management

The child received oral midazolam syrup 0.5 mg/kg in the waiting area 20 min before the anesthesia. After entering the operating room, routine monitoring was given: non-invasive blood pressure (NIBP) at 100/60 mm Hg, heart rate (HR) at 110 bpm, and pulse oxygen saturation (SpO_2) at 98%. Anesthesia was induced with intravenous bolus doses of 1.0 mg midazolam, 4.5 mg etomidate, 30 μg sufentanil, and 10 mg rocuronium. An ID 5.0 mm cuffed tracheal tube was intubated under a visual laryngoscope and a fixed depth of 14 cm. A 5F BB was placed in the tracheal tube, guided by a bronchoscope to the appropriate position in the right main bronchus. Left radial artery puncture catheterization was established for invasive arterial pressure measurement; right internal jugular vein puncture catheterization was used for central venous pressure (CVP) measurement, fluid infusion, blood transfusion, drug application, etc. General anesthesia was maintained by intravenous infusion of 5.0 mg/(kg·h) propofol, 2.5 μg/(kg·h) sufentanil, and 0.6 mg/(kg·h) rocuronium combined with sevoflurane inhalation to maintain appropriate anesthesia depth according to bispectral index (BIS). After placing the child in the left lateral decubitus position, the BBs position was adjusted and confirmed again under a bronchoscope. During the operation, pressure control ventilation was used with respiratory parameters set as oxygen flow rate of 2 L/min and FiO_2 of 60%. During bilateral lung ventilation, VT of 120 mL, I:E ratio of 1:2, RR was adjusted to maintain end-tidal carbon dioxide pressure ($ETCO_2$) around 35 mm Hg; during one-lung ventilation, the BBs cuff was inflated, VT of 90 mL, I:E ratio of 1:2, positive end-expiratory pressure (PEEP) of 5 cm H_2O, RR was adjusted to maintain $ETCO_2$ around 40 mm Hg. After occlusion of the superior and inferior vena cava, the mechanical ventilation was stopped, and continuous positive airway pressure (CPAP) of 10 cm H_2O was given to the dependent (lower) lung. The heart automatically resumed beating and sinus rhythm after aortic cross-clamp release. Dopamine was infused at 5.0 μg/(kg·min). After the vena cava cross-clamp release, the BBs cuff was deflated and removed, bilateral lung ventilation was resumed, manual lung re-expansion was performed, and ventilation settings were the same. During the preparation for modified ultrafiltration on cardiopulmonary bypass (CPB), the child suddenly developed ventricular fibrillation. It was difficult to place the internal defibrillation electrode plate due to the child undergoing a lateral thoracotomy. External defibrillation electrodes were immediately adhered to the left apex and right scapular area, and wet gauze was stuffed inside the thoracic cavity. After biphasic shock of 2 J/kg (30 J) was delivered, successfully restoring sinus rhythm. Following the completion of modified ultrafiltration, protamine was slowly infused intravenously to neutralize heparin. Arterial blood gas after heparin neutralization showed pH 7.4, $PaCO_2$ 39.6 mm Hg, PaO_2 244.2 mm Hg, HCT 28.1%, Na^+ 140 mmol/L, K^+ 4.1 mmol/L, Cl^- 106 mmol/L, Ca^{2+} 1.1 mmol/L, Lac 1.4 mmol/L, BE −0.73 mmol/L.

6.3 Postoperative Outcome

The entire procedure lasted 90 min, with mild hypothermic bypass for 28 min, aortic clamping for 20 min, and subsequent parallel circulation for 5 min. The intraoperative urine output was 200 mL, and 60 mL of autologous blood was reinfused. The patient was transferred to the Cardiac Intensive Care Unit (CICU) with an endotracheal tube and removed 3 h after the operation. The patient was discharged from the CICU on the second day and from the hospital on the fourth day.

6.4 Review of Knowledge Points

6.4.1 Atrial Septal Defect (ASD)

ASD is a congenital heart defect characterized by a communication between the left and right atria due to a defect in the atrial septum, accounting for approximately 6% to 10% of all congenital heart diseases. ASD is mainly divided into ostium secundum type (80%), ostium primum type, sinus venosus type, and coronary sinus type. ASD is a simple shunt. Small ASDs are restrictive shunts, allowing only a small amount of blood to enter the right atrium through the defect from the left atrium. Large ASDs (diameter reaching 1.0 cm or more) are usually non-restrictive, and the direction and volume of shunting depend on the compliance of the left and right ventricles, which in turn are influenced by systemic and pulmonary vascular resistances. Although large ASDs can significantly increase pulmonary blood flow, the pressure of the pulmonary artery can be maintained within the normal range for a prolonged period because the pressure from the systemic circulation in ASD patients does not transmit to the pulmonary vasculature, leading to an increase in pulmonary blood volume only. Therefore, children with isolated ASDs usually have no symptoms in the early stage. Only a murmur can be heard. With age, they may experience fatigue, decreased exercise tolerance, atrial arrhythmias, right ventricular dysfunction, and pulmonary hypertension.

Although percutaneous transcatheter closure of ASD is a frontline treatment choice in many medical centers currently, open-heart surgical repair remains the classic treatment method for non-ostium secundum ASDs, large ostium secundum ASDs, cases with inadequate tissue at the defect margins, or patients with a small left atrium. With the development of minimally invasive concepts and techniques, minimally invasive open-heart surgical repair for ASD repair has also been widely used, especially the vertical small incision under the right axilla, which is not only safe and effective, but also minimizes trauma, promotes rapid recovery, offers a more concealed and aesthetically pleasing incision, and avoids the potential defect of asymmetric breast development in females caused by the right anterior lateral incision. The advantages of minimally invasive ASD repair with partial sternotomy through the mid-chest have not yet been confirmed in pediatric patients. Thoracoscopic-assisted and robotic minimally invasive surgery methods are limited due to the size of the child's chest and the diameter of peripheral blood vessels.

6.4.2 Pediatric One-Lung Ventilation

OLV includes absolute and relative indications. Absolute indications refer to the conditions that require lung isolation, such as massive hemorrhage, lung infection, empyema, bronchopleural or bronchocutaneous fistulas, etc.; relative indications are primarily aimed at improving surgical visibility and maintaining lung isolation, such as lung lobectomy, thoracoscopic procedures, and certain pediatric heart surgeries performed in partial lateral decubitus positions. The factors causing children more prone to hypoxemia during OLV include ①Due to the softness of the ribs, the dependent lung is easily affected by gravity, surgeon's pressure, and abdominal pressure, leading to decreased compliance and ventilation of the dependent lung. ② Children have a smaller physique, the hydrostatic gradient from the non-dependent lung to the dependent lung is reduced, and blood shunting is reduced, leading to ventilation/blood flow mismatch.

Pediatric OLV techniques include double-lumen endotracheal tubes, Univent tubes, single-lumen endotracheal tubes, and BBs. Due to technical limitations, double-lumen endotracheal tubes and Univent tubes are only suitable for children aged 8 and above. A single-lumen endotracheal tube can perform OLV by inserting into one bronchus. Tube depth adjustment is required when switching ventilation mode, making management more complex. Although BBs have the risk of displacement, they are suitable for patients of any age, offering simplicity in operation and ease of management.

The placement of BBs includes two methods: inside and outside of the endotracheal tube, neither of which is superior or inferior. Both require bronchoscope guidance and confirmation. The choice of BBs placement method: <2 years old, 5F placement outside the endotracheal tube; 2–6 years old, 5F placement inside or outside the endotracheal tube; 6–8 years old, 7F placement inside or outside the endotracheal tube; 8–10 years old, 9F placement inside or outside the endotracheal tube. During OLV, it is generally recommended to use low tidal volumes and apply PEEP to maintain the $SpO_2 \geq 90\%$. Children often have hypercapnia during OLV, even with sufficient ventilation, but it usually disappears after resuming two-lung ventilation. If hypoxemia occurs, notify the surgical team first, increase the FiO_2 to 1.0, and perform lung recruitment maneuvers on the ventilated lung to reduce intrapulmonary shunting caused by lung atelectasis. Other measures include checking the position of BBs, clearing the airway, increasing the PEEP of the ventilated lung by 1–2 cm H2O, provide CPAP to the non-ventilated lung by 5–10 cm H_2O. If these measures still cannot improve the child's hypoxemia, it should be changed to two-lung ventilation. After one-lung ventilation, the collapsed lung should be fully re-expanded, but airway pressure > 30 cm H_2O should be avoided.

6.5 Discussion

The management of OLV in children with ASD via a small axillary incision mainly includes: ① choosing the appropriate OLV technique; ② the mutual influence between increased pulmonary blood flow due to left-to-right shunting and one-lung ventilation.

6.5.1 Preoperative Evaluation

The majority of children with ASD have good cardiac reserve and can tolerate inhalation anesthesia induction. Children with atrial enlargement are prone to atrial arrhythmias but usually can tolerate it well. It is recommended to pre-place external defibrillation electrodes for children with a lateral thoracic small incision. In this case, the boy developed ventricular fibrillation upon weaning from CPB, which was successfully cardioverted with external defibrillation electrodes, restoring sinus rhythm. The preoperative visit should focus on assessing the child's respiratory system, whether there are recent upper respiratory tract infections, airway malformations, tracheobronchial or other factors that make it difficult to implement OLV and make full preparations.

6.5.2 Intraoperative Anesthetic Management

The goals of intraoperative anesthetic management include ① maintaining age-appropriate heart rate, myocardial contractility, and preload to sustain cardiac output and perfusion of the systemic circulation; ② avoiding an increase in the PVR:SVR ratio, as an increased PVR:SVR ratio can lead to right-to-left shunting, resulting in decreased oxygen saturation; ③ avoiding a decrease in the PVR:SVR ratio, as a decreased PVR:SVR ratio can increase left-to-right shunting, leading to increased pulmonary blood flow and potential inadequate perfusion or oxygen delivery to the systemic circulation.

Atelectasis is closely related to postoperative pulmonary complications. Although there is no consensus on the management of OLV during congenital heart surgery, the current common protective lung ventilation strategies are to use low tidal volumes, appropriate PEEP, and lung recruitment maneuvers and give a certain CPAP to the non-ventilated lung. In this case, we applied 10 cm H_2O CPAP during the CPB period. In adult cardiac surgery, applying 10 cm H_2O CPAP during CPB can improve postoperative alveolar-arterial oxygen gradient, but whether applying 10 cm H_2O CPAP during pediatric lateral position cardiac surgery has a lung protective effect has not been clearly reported. In this case, the child was ventilated with a small tidal volume of 6 mL/kg plus 5 cm H_2O PEEP during OLV, 10 cm H_2O CPAP was used during CPB, lung recruitment maneuver was given after the recovery of bilateral lung ventilation. Throughout the entire surgical procedure, there were no occurrences of hypoxemia, and hemodynamics remained stable. The oxygenation index was 406 after ultrafiltration.

6.5.3 Anesthetic Management after CPB

Except for very few ASD patients with increased PVR who may have increased reactivity of the pulmonary vascular bed after CPB, there are usually no problems in ASD patients during the process of weaning from CPB support after repair surgery. Therefore, for ASD patients with increased PVR, it is necessary to adopt a hyperventilation strategy and/or combine drugs that reduce PVR after CPB to prevent right ventricular dysfunction secondary to increased afterload. There are various reasons for ventricular fibrillation occurring upon cessation of CPB support, including low body temperature, heart failure, electrolyte disorder, or coronary air embolism. The body temperature of the boy, in this case, was 36.0 °C; there was no change in the T-wave on the electrocardiogram, and sinus rhythm was immediately restored after defibrillation, which basically ruled out the possibility of ventricular fibrillation caused by low body temperature, electrolyte disorder, and coronary air embolism. The aortic cross-clamp time for this case was 20 min, with a subsequent parallel circulation time of 5 min, which was only one-fourth of the aortic cross-clamp time. In this case, the insufficient parallel circulation time with incomplete recovery of myocardial function upon weaning from CPB support may be the primary reason for ventricular fibrillation.

Most ASD patients do not require prolonged mechanical ventilation support postoperatively. Through precise perioperative management, early extubation and fast-track anesthetic management are feasible. Fast-track or ultra-fast-track anesthetic management is also a hot spot and development direction in the field of congenital heart disease. In this case, the boy was extubated 3 h after surgery and successfully completed fast-track anesthetic management.

6.6 Conclusion

OLV technique can provide excellent surgical field exposure for congenital heart disease correction surgery through a thoracotomy, expedite the surgical process, and enhance the safety of surgical procedures. However, the optimal ventilation mode still requires further research. It is recommended to routinely place external adhesive defibrillation electrodes preoperatively to ensure perioperative safety for the child in case internal defibrillation is not feasible (Hualin Chen).

7 Anesthetic Management of Ventricular Septal Defect Repair Surgery in an Infant with Conal-Septal Ventricular Septal Defect

Lihong Jin

Abstract

A 6-month-old male infant with a heart murmur for over 4 months was diagnosed with ventricular septal defect (VSD) (conal-septal type) by echocardiography. He was scheduled to undergo VSD repair surgery under cardiopulmonary bypass (CPB). The conal-septal VSD causes a significant increase in pulmonary blood flow due to the left-to-right shunt. Furthermore, the higher pressure of the systemic circulation is directly transmitted to the pulmonary vascular bed, which can easily cause pulmonary arteriole spasm, pulmonary hypertension, and right heart failure in the child. In addition, recurrent respiratory infections are also common in infants with conal-septal VSD due to increased pulmonary blood flow. Notably, the aortic valve leaflet of children with conal-septal VSD is prone to prolapse into the defect area and cause aortic insufficiency. Therefore, once the patients are diagnosed with conal-septal VSD, early surgery is necessary. The anesthetic management of these children needs to pay special attention to the preoperative cardiac function status, pulmonary artery pressure, closure of the aortic valve, and upper respiratory tract infection.

Ventricular septal defect (VSD) is the most common congenital heart disease, accounting for about 20% of all congenital heart diseases. It either exists alone or coexists with other structural abnormalities. Van Praagh classifies VSD as Atrioventricular Canal, Muscular, Membranous, Conoventricular, and Conal types. The surgical procedures and the keys of anesthetic management vary with the location and size of the VSD. The right coronary cusp of the aortic valve often lacks support in patients with conal-septal VSD, which can easily cause the right coronary cusp to prolapse into the aortic valve orifice and inadequate closure of the aortic valve leaflets. These patients usually need early surgery after diagnosis to better protect the aortic valve and cardiac function. The number of conal-septal VSD repairs accounts for about one-third. This article reports the anesthetic management of a child with conal-septal VSD undergoing VSD repair surgery under cardiopulmonary bypass (CPB).

L. Jin (✉)
The National Children's Medical Center (Shanghai), Department of Anesthesiology of Shanghai Children's Medical Center, Shanghai Jiao Tong University School of Medicine, Shanghai, China
e-mail: jinlihong@scmc.com.cn

J. Zheng et al. (eds.), *Selected Pediatric Cardiovascular Surgery Anesthesia Cases*,
https://doi.org/10.1007/978-981-96-5614-1_7

7.1 Case Presentation

A 6-month-old boy was born full-term with a weight of 6 kg. A heart murmur was heard for over 4 months during a physical examination. Echocardiography indicated: VSD (conal-septal type). He was scheduled for elective VSD repair surgery. There were no other disease histories or food or drug allergies. There was also no history of surgery or trauma. He was vaccinated on schedule.

Physical examination: The patient was conscious and had a normal mental response. Clear lung sounds, regular heart rhythm, strong heart sounds, II–IV systolic murmur at the left 3rd–fourth intercostal space, accentuated P2. The liver was not palpable below the ribs, and there was no cyanosis or edema in the limbs.

Laboratory tests: Normal routine blood tests, coagulation, and liver and kidney function.

Chest X-ray: Enlarged heart shadow, increased lung markings.

Echocardiography: Pulmonary artery widening (mild), normal pulmonary valve activity with transvalvular flow speed 2.3 m/s, VSD (conal-septal) 0.75 cm, left-to-right shunt, shunt bundle width 0.37 cm (near the septal crest), shunt speed 4.2 m/s. Normal aorta, with part of the valve leaflet embedded in the ventricular septal defect, mild right aortic valve cusp prolapse and regurgitation, left aortic arch.

Electrocardiogram (ECG): Sinus rhythm, left atrial enlargement (possible).

Chest CT: VSD (conal-septal), 4.1 mm × 8 mm, a small amount of exudate in the lower lobe of the left lung.

Preoperative diagnosis: VSD (conal-septal type), elective VSD repair surgery with CPB support.

7.2 Anesthetic Management

The child took 3.0 mg of midazolam syrup orally in the waiting area 20 min before surgery for preoperative sedation. When the Ramsay sedation score reached 4, the child was brought into the operating room. Then, routine ECG, non-invasive blood pressure (NBP), and pulse oxygen saturation (SpO_2) were monitored. The peripheral vein in the back of the right hand was accessed. Basic vital signs were as follows: the heart rate (HR) 153 beats/min, SpO_2 95%, BP 85/45 mm Hg. Anesthesia was induced with intravenous bolus doses of 1.2 mg etomidate, 12 μg sufentanil, and 3.6 mg rocuronium. An ID 3.5 mm cuffed endotracheal tube was intubated with a depth of 11 cm at the incisors. General anesthesia was maintained by continuous intravenous infusion of 5.0 mg/(kg·h) propofol, 2.5 μg/(kg·h) sufentanil, and 0.6 mg/(kg·h) rocuronium and combined with sevoflurane intermittent inhalation. The ventilator parameters were set as follows: pressure-controlled ventilation (PCV) mode, oxygen flow rate 2 L/min, fraction of inspired oxygen (FiO_2) 50%, peak inspiratory pressure (PIP) 15 cm H_2O, respiratory rate (RR) about 26 times/min, inspiratory time to expiratory time (I:E) 1:2, end-tidal carbon dioxide partial pressure ($ETCO_2$) about 40 mm Hg. The right radial artery was catheterized with a 24 G catheter under ultrasound guidance for continuous invasive arterial pressure (ABP) monitoring. The right internal jugular vein was catheterized with a 4F, 5 cm double-lumen venous catheter under ultrasound guidance for central venous pressure (CVP) monitoring and infusion of fluids, blood products, and drugs. Before skin incision: ABP 95/55 mm Hg, HR 120 beats/min, CVP 10 cm H_2O. Before aortic cannulation, 18 mg of heparin was intravenously injected. When ACT >480 s, CPB began. After the VSD was repaired and the aortic cross-clamp was released, dopamine 5.0 μg/(kg·min) was intravenously infused, and the heart automatically resumed to sinus rhythm. The dosage of dopamine was adjusted according to the blood pressure. When the vena cava cross-clamp was released, PCV ventilation was resumed with the ventilation parameters set as follows: oxygen flow rate 2 L/min, FiO_2 50%, PIP 15 cm H_2O, RR 20 times/min, I:E 1:2. Transesophageal echocardiography showed: no obvious VSD residual shunt, mild aortic valve regurgitation. CPB was gradually weaned off. After modified ultrafiltration, 57 mg of protamine was given to neutralize heparin (total heparin dosage was 38 mg). Artery blood gas analysis: hematocrit 31%, no other obvious abnormalities. At the end of the operation, ABP 100/65 mm Hg, HR 110 beats/min, CVP 12 cm H_2O, and dopamine 5.0 μg/(kg·min) were intravenously infused. The patient was transferred to the cardiac surgery intensive care unit (CICU) with mechanical ventilation assistance.

7.3 Postoperative Outcome

The operation lasted 90 min, with 30 min of CPB time. Fifty milliliter of autologous blood was reinfused, and 100 mL of urine was output. The endotracheal intubation was removed 4 h after surgery. The patient was transferred back to the general ward on postoperative day 4 and discharged from the hospital on postoperative day 7.

7.4 Review of Knowledge Points

7.4.1 Ventricular Septal Defect (Classification and Main Pathophysiology)

VSD refers to the incomplete development of the ventricular septum during the embryonic period, leading to abnormal blood flow between the left and right ventricles at the ventricular level. VSD is the most common congenital heart disease, accounting for 1.5–3.0% of full-term newborns. The incidence rate is even higher in premature infants, up to 7%. Van Praagh classifies the ventricular septal defects as Atrioventricular Canal, Muscular, Membranous, Conoventricular, and Conal types. According to the size of the defect, VSD can be divided into large, medium, and small types. Small VSD: defect <0.5 cm; Medium VSD: defect 0.5–1.0 cm; Large VSD: defect >1.0 cm. The size of the shunt in VSD is related to the size of the defect, the pressure difference between the left and right ventricles, and the relative resistance between the systemic and pulmonary vascular beds (SVR:PVR). Under normal circumstances, SVR is significantly higher than PVR, which causes left-to-right shunting in VSD. In some cases, SVR:PVR decreases, or even PVR is higher than SVR, which causes bidirectional shunting or right-to-left shunting. Unlike atrial septal defect, children with VSD not only have increased pulmonary circulatory blood flow but also suffer from direct transmission of systemic pressure, which can easily cause pulmonary artery spasms and early onset of pulmonary hypertension. Therefore, the preload and afterload of the right ventricle are both significantly increased, which causes right ventricular hypertrophy. With the increase in pulmonary hypertension, the amount of blood flowing back to the left ventricle can be significantly increased, which results in the left ventricle preload increase and the left atrium and left ventricle dilation.

7.4.2 Conal-Septal VSD Repair Procedures

Prolapse of the right coronary cusp of the aorta and aortic valve insufficiency often accompany conal-septal VSD. To better protect the function of aortic valves and cardiac function, early surgical closure of Conal-septal VSD is required. The operation usually involves a transverse incision at the root of the pulmonary artery and VSD closure with a patch rather than directly suturing. Direct suturing can easily cause deformation of the aortic and pulmonary valves, resulting in postoperative aortic and pulmonary regurgitations.

7.5 Discussion

7.5.1 Preoperative Assessment and Preparation

Children with VSD usually have left-to-right shunting, but bidirectional shunting can also occur in children with large and nonrestrictive VSDs. Left-to-right shunting can significantly increase pulmonary blood flow and the risks of preoperative recurrent pulmonary infections, which results in an increase in airway reactivity, a decrease in pulmonary compliance, and postoperative complications. Therefore, it is necessary to prevent and control preoperative pulmonary infections proactively. The pulmonary vascular bed in children with large VSD is affected by both high pulmonary blood flow and high systemic circulatory pressure, which cause early onset of pulmonary arterial hypertension. Severe pulmonary arterial hypertension can reach or approach the level of systemic circulatory pressure, leading to bidirectional shunting. Once bidirectional shunting occurs, VSD closure is unsuitable because it will significantly increase the right ventricular afterload and cause a mismatch between the right ventricular function and afterload. Therefore, for older children with large VSD and increased pulmonary artery pressure, preoperative cardiac catheterization is required to determine whether there is bidirectional shunting and whether the VSD can be closed. In addition, the location and type of VSD are also important aspects of preoperative assessment and surgical timing selection, especially for conal-septal VSD, which can easily lead to aortic valve prolapse and embedding in the defect area, and further result in aortic valve damage and regurgitation.

In this case, the right aortic valve prolapsed into the conal-septal VSD and was partially embedded in the interventricular septum, which caused mild aortic valve regurgitation. The defect size was 0.75 cm, a medium-sized VSD with left-to-right shunting. Therefore, the surgeons decided to repair the VSD early to avoid the aortic valve damage and the pulmonary artery pressure increase. The child had no obvious preoperative symptoms such as dyspnea, sweating, feeding difficulties, and recurrent pulmonary infections. The ASA grade was II–III with good compensatory cardiac and pulmonary functions. Routine preoperative preparation was carried out without special treatment. Therefore, preoperative assessment and preparation should focus on the patient's cardiac function status, pulmonary artery pressure, aortic valve closure condition, upper respiratory tract infection, etc.

7.5.2 Intraoperative Anesthetic Management

Children without congestive heart failure can well tolerate the induction of both intravenous anesthesia and inhalational anesthesia. For newborns and children with congestive heart failure, it is recommended to use the opioid-based induction of intravenous anesthesia to maintain hemodynamic stability. Anesthetic management should focus on maintaining the sinus rhythm, myocardial contractility, and cardiac preload as much as possible to ensure sufficient cardiac output. Maintaining a PVR:SVR ratio is relatively constant to balance the systemic and pulmonary circulation blood flow and avoid exacerbating pulmonary arterial hypertension.

In this case, the patient had mild aortic regurgitation. Therefore, it was necessary to avoid bradycardia and the significant increase in systemic vascular resistance to prevent the aggravation of aortic regurgitation during the anesthesia. In addition, the decrease in diastolic pressure can cause an increase in cardiac preload and the insufficiency of myocardial blood supply. Atropine and vasoactive drugs can be prepared and used during the operation to increase heart rate and peripheral vascular resistance appropriately. The induction of anesthesia should be titrated and the changes of electrocardiogram ST segment should be closely monitored. The invasive arterial monitoring should be established as soon as possible. If hypotension occurs, vasoconstrictor drugs and/or heart rate-increasing drugs should be used promptly. In addition, these children usually undergo surgery at a younger age and have a lower body weight. The process of aortic or venous cannulation often leads to hypotension and arrhythmia. It is necessary to monitor the changes in hemodynamics closely, communicate with the surgeon in a timely manner, temporarily stop the operation, and/or use short-acting vasoactive drugs to maintain blood pressure stability when necessary. In this case, the child patient had no obvious preoperative pulmonary infection, pulmonary hypertension, or heart failure, so there were no special requirements for respiratory management. PCV ventilation, FiO_2

around 50%, tidal volume 8–10 mL/kg or small tidal volume + PEEP, and maintaining $ETCO_2$ at 35–45 mm Hg can meet the requirements of surgical anesthesia. In addition to routine monitoring, for children with recurrent pulmonary infections and heart failure or severe pulmonary hypertension, pulmonary artery pressure also needs to be monitored.

7.5.3 Anesthetic Management After Extracorporeal Circulation

After the VSD is repaired, the pulmonary artery pressure in patients with small or medium to large VSD, who have not yet developed obvious pulmonary hypertension, can drop rapidly. These children rarely need positive inotropic drugs to support them after the operation. Sometimes, vasodilators such as nitroprusside, milrinone, etc., might be needed to dilate peripheral vessels due to the occurrence of hypertension after CPB. Pulmonary hypertension after CPB can be reduced by the increase of FiO_2 and mild hyperventilation to reduce pulmonary vascular resistance or direct dilation of pulmonary blood vessels by milrinone or nitric oxide, all of which can help to reduce or prevent the occurrence of pulmonary hypertension crisis. After the VSD is repaired, routine transesophageal echocardiography should be conducted to assess the residual shunts, pulmonary artery pressure, and the condition of the pulmonary and aortic valves. Special attention should be paid to the condition of the aortic valve in children with conal-septal VSD after surgery. For those patients with severe aortic insufficiency, valvuloplasty should also performed. If recurrent arrhythmia or low cardiac output occurs after sternal closure, delayed sternal closure is recommended to relieve cardiac compression and ensure the child's safety.

7.6 Conclusion

In summary, special attention should be paid to the cardiac function status, pulmonary artery pressure, aortic valve closure status, and upper respiratory tract infection in children with conal-septal VSD for surgical VSD repair. During anesthesia, bradycardia, hypotension, and myocardial ischemia should be avoided. The vascular resistance of the systemic and pulmonary circulation should be carefully evaluated and regulated after the VSD is closed. To prevent recurrent arrhythmias or low cardiac output after sternal closure, delayed sternal closure may be an alternative to ensure the perioperative safety of the child with conal-septal VSD. (Lihong Jin).

Anestheti Management for Surgical Repair of Atrial and Ventricular Septal Defects in an Infant with Severe Pulmonary Hypertension

8

Yang Shen

Abstract

A 2-month-old girl was admitted to the hospital due to "congenital heart disease, heart failure with shortness of breath." Echocardiography suggested "ventricular septal defect (VSD), atrial septal defect (ASD), and severe pulmonary hypertension (PAH)." After admission, the child's respiratory distress deteriorated. She underwent endotracheal intubation, mechanical ventilation, and supportive treatments such as anti-infection and diuresis and was then scheduled to undergo VSD and ASD repair under general anesthesia. This case was very challenging for anesthetic management due to the child's young age, low weight, large defect size, severe PAH, and large intracardiac shunt. According to infants' physiological and pathophysiological characteristics, adjusting the balance of systemic-pulmonary circulation resistance, rational use of positive inotropic drugs, and maintaining appropriate heart rate, myocardial contractility, and preload are the key points of anesthetic management in this case.

Y. Shen (✉)
The National Children's Medical Center (Shanghai), Department of Anesthesiology of Shanghai Children's Medical Center, Shanghai Jiao Tong University School of Medicine, Shanghai, China
e-mail: shenyang@scmc.com.cn

Ventricular septal defect (VSD) is the most common congenital heart disease, with an incidence rate of 1.5–3.0% in full-term newborns. Children with large VSDs, especially those whose VSD diameter is close to the aortic valve annulus diameter, may experience recurrent respiratory infections, heart failure, and pulmonary arterial hypertension during infancy. These children need timely surgical treatment. In addition to the large VSD, this case also has a large atrial septal defect (ASD), further increasing the left-to-right shunt at the atrial and ventricular levels. This chapter describes the experience of anesthetic management for surgical repair of large atrial and ventricular septal defects in an infant with severe pulmonary hypertension (PAH).

8.1 Case Presentation

A 2-month-old girl with 4.1 kg in weight was admitted to our hospital due to "rapid breathing, heart failure, and congenital heart disease." She was delivered by cesarean section at full term without asphyxia. Echocardiography at another hospital demonstrated VSD, ASD, and severe PAH. After admission, the girl's heart rate (HR) was 180 beats/min, respiratory rate (RR) 65 breaths/min, blood pressure (BP) 85/55 mm Hg, pulse oxygen saturation (SpO_2) 92% at room air, and 97% under oxygen mask. The girl was lethar-

J. Zheng et al. (eds.), *Selected Pediatric Cardiovascular Surgery Anesthesia Cases*,
https://doi.org/10.1007/978-981-96-5614-1_8

gic, had difficulty breathing, and had coarse, wet rales in both lungs. She was intubated with mechanical ventilation support as well as symptomatic and supportive treatments such as anti-infection and diuresis. PC-AC (pressure control-assist control) ventilation mode: fraction of inspired oxygen (FiO_2) 25%, end-expiratory pressure (PEEP) 5.0 cm H_2O, RR 30 breaths/min, inspiratory pressure (PIP) 22 cm H_2O.

Physical examination: The girl was malnourished. Blowing murmurs could be heard at the left edge of the sternum between the II and IV intercostal spaces.

Laboratory test: Hemoglobin 80 g/L, hematocrit 25%, normal liver, kidney, and coagulation function.

Echocardiography: VSD (perimembranous) 0.8 cm, left-to-right shunt speed 2.0 m/s, ASD two bundles (bundle width 0.58 cm and 0.23 cm, respectively), mild to moderate regurgitation with an ultrasound beam width of 0.33 cm and speed of 4.33 m/s, pressure difference 75 mm Hg, PAH.

Electrocardiogram (ECG): Right ventricular enlargement, right atrial enlargement, left atrial enlargement (possible).

Chest X-ray: Pneumonia in both lungs, heart shadow enlargement.

8.2 Anesthetic Management

The child was smoothly transported to the operating room with tracheal intubation. Upon entering the operating room, HR was 150 beats/min, BP was 85/49 mm Hg, and SPO_2 was 98%. Pressure control ventilation (PCV) was used with respiratory parameters set as 30% FiO_2, 16 cm H_2O PIP, 35–40 mL tidal volume (VT), 22 breaths/min RR, 1:2 inhalation to exhalation ratio (I:E), 4.0 cm H_2O PEEP, and 35–40 mm Hg end-tidal carbon dioxide ($ETCO_2$). Anesthesia induction was performed with intravenous bolus of etomidate 1.2 mg, sufentanil 8.0 μg, and rocuronium 2.5 mg. Anaesthesia was maintained by propofol 4.0 mg/(kg·h), sufentanil 2.0 μg/(kg·h), rocuronium 0.5 mg/(kg·h), and combined with 1–2% sevoflurane inhalation.

After anesthesia induction, arterial (left femoral artery) and central venous (right internal jugular vein) catheterization were performed under ultrasound guidance to continuously monitor invasive blood pressure (ABP) and central venous pressure (CVP). The right femoral vein was also catheterized for rapid fluid replacement and blood transfusion. VSD and ASD repairs with median sternotomy incision were performed under cardiopulmonary bypass support. The heart automatically resumed beating and sinus rhythm after the aortic cross-clamp was released; dopamine was infused at 5.0 μg/(kg·min) via a central venous pump, maintaining systolic pressure 70–80 mm Hg, HR 130–150 beats/min. After the cross-clamp of the vena cava was released, pressure control ventilation was resumed with respiratory parameters set as FiO_2 60%, $ETCO_2$ around 30 mm Hg. It is beneficial for reducing pulmonary vascular resistance(PVR) by maintaining mild hyperventilation. No residual shunt was found by transesophageal echocardiography. Modified blood ultrafiltration was conducted after cardiopulmonary bypass was gradually weaned off. After modified blood ultrafiltration, protamine 45 mg and thrombin 0.5 U were infused through the femoral vein. Blood gas analysis: pH 7.4, PaO_2 62.4 mm Hg, $PaCO_2$ 38.1 mm Hg, BE -0.5, HCT 30.9%, Hb 10.1 g/dL, K^+ 3.6 mmol/L, Ca^{2+} 1.2 mmol/L, Cl^- 99.1 mmol/L, Lac 1.7 mmol/L. The respiratory parameters were adjusted: FiO_2 increased from 60% to 70%, PEEP increased to 6.0 cm H_2O, and manual lung recruitment was performed.

8.3 Postoperative Outcome

The surgery lasted approximately 90 min in total, with a cardiopulmonary bypass time of 40 min. 40 mL of autologous salvaged blood was transfused during the surgery. After the operation, the child was smoothly transferred to the Cardiac Intensive Care Unit (CICU) under ECG, SpO_2, and ABP monitoring, ABP 100/61 mm Hg, HR 123 bpm, SpO_2 99%, CVP 10 cm H_2O, rectal temperature 36.5 °C, stable hemodynamics, lactate level within normal range. On the postoperative day 2, blood pressure dropped, heart rate increased, lactate 2.8 mmol/L, N-terminal pro-brain natriuretic peptide (NT-proBNP) >45,000 pg/mL, LVEF was 37.7%, and no significant residual shunt was found. Epinephrine and milrinone were intravenously infused. On postoperative day 3, LVEF was 38.4%, lactate was 0.7 mmol/L, and intravenous norepinephrine was added to maintain blood pressure. On postoperative day 5, heart function gradually recovered with LVEF 52.5%, and the endotracheal tube was successfully removed. On the postoperative day, the infant was transferred from the CICU to a normal ward. The infant was discharged from the hospital 2 weeks later.

8.4 Review of Knowledge Points

8.4.1 Pulmonary Arterial Hypertension Related to Congenital Heart Disease

Pulmonary hypertension (PH) is defined as an increase of mean pulmonary arterial pressure $\geq$ 25 mm Hg at rest, which is evaluated by right heart catheterization. Based on the evaluation of pulmonary wedge pressure, pulmonary vascular resistance, and cardiac output, PH can be hemodynamically classified into pre-capillary(pulmonary wedge pressure $\leq$ 15 mm Hg), post-capillary (pulmonary wedge pressure > 15 mm Hg), or combined. Pre-capillary PH is also often known as PAH due to increased pulmonary blood flow and arterial pressure in the pulmonary circulation. Many children with congenital heart disease have PAH. Newborns with large VSD may have normal pulmonary blood flow due to the relatively high PVR. However, PVR will be quickly reduced to normal at 2–3 months after birth and significantly lower than SVR. Since then, early PAH is easily developed in children with large VSD because the high pressure from systemic circulation can be directly transmitted to the pulmonary vascular system through VSD, and the pulmonary blood flow is significantly increased from left to right shunt. Although large ASD can significantly increase the pulmonary blood flow, the high pressure from the systemic circulation cannot be transmitted to the pulmonary vascular system through ASD. The development of pulmonary hypertension in patients with ASD is usually slow. Post-capillary PH is mainly caused by pulmonary venous drainage obstruction and increased pressure in the left atrium, where the blood of the pulmonary veins returns.

8.5 Discussion

8.5.1 Preoperative Assessment and Preparation

During preoperative assessment of children with VSD, special attention should be paid to the children's condition at birth, history of growth and development, nutritional status, location and size of VSD, pulmonary artery pressure, heart failure, lung infection, and accompanied malformations. These factors significantly increase the incidence of adverse events during the perioperative period. The nutritional status in this case was poor before surgery. Therefore, improving the child's nutritional status before surgery is better if conditions permit. The VSD and ASD sizes, in this case, were both about 0.8 cm, which belonged to relatively large VSD and ASD with left-to-right shunting at the atrial and ventricular levels and resulted in increased pulmonary blood flow and pulmonary artery pressure. Increased pulmonary blood flow tends to cause recurrent upper respiratory and lung infections, significantly increasing the incidence of postoperative respiratory-related adverse events and the time of mechanical ventilation and hospital stay at CICU. The tricuspid valve pressure difference + 5 mm Hg can estimate the pulmonary artery pressure. The pulmonary artery pressure in this case was about 80 mm Hg, belonging to severe pulmonary hypertension. The risk of anesthetic management is significantly increased.

For those children with VSD and/or ASD who have recurrent upper respiratory infections, refractory pneumonia, heart failure, or severe pulmonary hypertension, early surgical repair of

VSD and/or ASD should be considered. Efforts should be taken to treat lung infections, optimize cardiac function, and reduce or avoid further increases in pulmonary artery pressure before surgery. After mechanical ventilation, inotropic support, diuresis, vasodilation, anti-infection treatment, and nutritional support, the cardiac function was significantly improved, and the lung infection was well controlled. In addition, the preoperative ventilation mode and ventilator parameters settings should also be noted. Positive inotropic drugs, such as dopamine, epinephrine, and norepinephrine, should be prepared in advance.

8.5.2 Induction and Maintenance of Anesthesia

High-dose sufentanil combined with etomidate, a sedative-hypnotic with minor circulatory effects, and rocuronium, a fast-acting non-depolarizing muscle relaxant, was chosen in this case to reduce or avoid the significant suppression of systemic circulation and the increase of pulmonary vascular resistance caused by harmful stimuli. The hemodynamics were stable during the induction of anesthesia. The anesthesia method, mainly based on high-dose opioids, not only has a minor effect on the circulatory system but also can effectively suppress the increase in pulmonary vascular resistance caused by harmful stimuli, reducing or avoiding the occurrence of a pulmonary hypertension crisis.

Anesthesia was maintained with propofol 4.0 mg/(kg·h), sufentanil 2.0 μg/(kg·h), rocuronium 0.5 mg/(kg·h) intravenous infusion, and combined with intermittent inhalation of 1–2% sevoflurane. The whole anesthetic process was stable. In addition to the satisfactory depth of anesthesia, the inhibitory effect on systemic circulation was minor. The pulmonary vascular resistance also did not increase.

8.5.3 Intraoperative Anesthetic Management

The goal of intraoperative anesthetic management is to maintain heart rate, myocardial contractility, and preload while avoiding the occurrence of a pulmonary hypertension crisis. This child has a large VSD and ASD, a large amount of left-to-right shunting, significantly increased pulmonary blood flow, and severe pulmonary artery hypertension. Therefore, it is useful to appropriately adjust FiO_2, maintain a slightly low to normal $ETCO_2$, and avoid a significant decrease or increase in the PVR:SVR ratio before the closure of VSD and ASD. The substantial reduction in the PVR:SVR ratio will aggravate left-to-right shunting, increase the pulmonary blood flow, and reduce forward blood flow from the left ventricle, which results in insufficient systemic circulation blood volume, low blood pressure, inadequate perfusion of important organs, and even cardiac arrest. On the contrary, the significant increase in the PVR:SVR ratio can exacerbate pulmonary artery hypertension, leading to right-to-left shunting or the occurrence of a pulmonary hypertension crisis. Therefore, during anesthesia, the respiratory parameters should be adjusted based on the results of blood gas analysis to avoid significant changes in the PVR:SVR ratio due to respiratory factors.

The child, in this case, was young, the thermoregulatory center was not yet mature, the ability to regulate body temperature was poor, and the operating room temperature should be maintained at 25–30 °C as much as possible before the start of cardiopulmonary bypass to avoid circulatory disorders caused by too low room temperature. Infants with congenital heart disease may have many characteristics of fetal myocardium, which are immature in structure, function, metabolism, etc. The increase of ventricular load in this child resulted in the decrease of ventricular function before surgery, making it easy to have low cardiac output postoperatively. Therefore, for those children with immature myocardium, special attention should be paid to reduce/avoid the direct damage to the myocardium caused by surgical operation, fluid overload, cardiopulmonary bypass, and postoperative residual shunting.

8.5.4 Anesthetic Management After Cardiopulmonary Bypass

After the cardiopulmonary bypass support was weaned off, it was necessary to fully reassess the child's pulmonary artery pressure and cardiac function. Closure of VSD can eliminate the effects of high blood flow and high pressure from the left ventricle on the pulmonary vessels. Usually, the pulmonary artery pressure will rapidly reduce to some extent after VSD surgery. For those children with small VSD or large VSD and pulmonary hypertension has not yet developed, closure of VSD can restore pulmonary artery pressure to near the normal range. However, for those children with large VSD and severe pulmonary artery hypertension, preoperative severe pulmonary hypertension can cause hypertrophy of the middle layer of the pulmonary vessel wall. Even if the VSD is closed, these children's pulmonary vascular bed maintains high reactivity to vasoconstrictive stimuli. In addition, the infant's pulmonary vascular endothelium is not yet mature; cardiopulmonary bypass can easily damage it and increase postoperative pulmonary vascular resistance. To avoid postoperative mismatch between right ventricular afterload and myocardial contractility, PVR can be reduced by increasing FiO_2 and hyperventilation. In addition, drugs that directly dilate the pulmonary vessels can reduce PVR. In this case, FiO_2 and ventilation frequency increased after surgery to reduce PVR.

Although positive inotropic drug support is rarely necessary for children without pulmonary hypertension after VSD surgery, we still chose to continuously infuse dopamine at 5.0 μg/(kg·min) to increase myocardial contractility and maintain hemodynamic stability since this child had a lung infection and heart failure before surgery. In addition, we need to keep vigilance to the hypotension caused by the anticoagulant effect of protamine-reversing heparin or pulmonary hypertension triggered by an allergy to protamine.

8.6 Shortcomings and Limitations

After the withdrawal of the cardiopulmonary bypass in this case, the pulmonary artery pressure had significantly decreased compared to preoperative, which was based on the surgeon's experience instead of monitoring the changes of pulmonary artery pressure through the pulmonary artery catheterization. There was a lack of references and guidance for the anesthesiologists to optimize the treatment measures. It is recommended to routinely monitor pulmonary artery pressure before the withdrawal of cardiopulmonary bypass. For children with severe pulmonary hypertension, it is recommended to place a pulmonary artery catheterization to guide subsequent pulmonary hypertension treatment better.

8.7 Conclusion

Children with large atrial and ventricular defects often experience severe pulmonary hypertension, recurrent lung infections, and heart failure before surgery. The primary objective of anesthetic management is maintaining heart rate, myocardial contractility, and preload to ensure cardiac output. Before the intracardiac shunt is closed, the PVR:SVR ratio should be kept constant to maintain systemic circulation blood flow or avoid the increase of right-to-left shunting and the occurrence of pulmonary hypertension crisis. After withdrawal of cardiopulmonary bypass, it is reasonable to reduce PVR by adjusting the ventilation strategy and optimizing the pulmonary vasodilator drugs. It is also beneficial to use positive inotropic drugs to improve heart function (Yang Shen).

Anesthetic Management of Pulmonary Artery Banding Surgery in an Infant with Multiple Ventricular Septal Defects

9

Jiajia Huang

Abstract

A 2-month-old infant was diagnosed with multiple ventricular septal defects upon an echocardiographic evaluation after birth. Subsequently, symptoms of difficulty in feeding, shortness of breath, etc. gradually deteriorated. To protect the normal development of pulmonary vascular beds and alleviate the symptoms of congestive heart failure, pulmonary artery banding (PAB) surgery was proposed. The key points of anesthetic management for PAB are to control heart failure before surgery, choose the best time of operation, avoid the increase of left-to-right shunt due to excessive ventilation before banding, and stay alert to acute right heart failure caused by increased right ventricular afterload after banding.

Infants with multiple ventricular septal defects (VSDs) are prone to pulmonary hypertension (PH) and cardiac insufficiency in the early stage of life due to the presence of large amounts of left-to-right shunt. These infants often cannot tolerate radical surgery, which makes PAB the first surgical choice to protect the normal development of pulmonary circulation. This case report introduced the anesthetic management of a 2-month-old infant with multiple VSDs who underwent PAB surgery.

J. Huang (✉)
The National Children's Medical Center (Shanghai), Department of Anesthesiology of Shanghai Children's Medical Center, Shanghai Jiao Tong University School of Medicine, Shanghai, China
e-mail: huangjiajia@scmc.com.cn

9.1 Case Presentation

The patient was a 2-month-old infant with 48 cm in length and 3 kg in weight. After birth, a heart murmur was found during auscultation, and multiple VSDs were found during echocardiographic examination. The infant was recently brought to our hospital for the treatment of gradual deterioration of difficulty in feeding and shortness of breath, etc., symptoms and was admitted to the department of cardiology for further treatment.

Physical examination: The infant was conscious without obvious abnormalities in mental response. The infant had physical development lag, wheezing, shortness of breath, and positive three-concave signs. Auscultation: The heart rate (HR) was 160 beats/min, regular rhythm. A grade III/VI rough systolic murmur was audible at the third to fourth intercostal spaces along the right margin of the sternum.

Laboratory tests: No significant abnormalities were found in routine blood tests. The liver, kidney, and coagulation functions were normal.

Echocardiography: The right atrium and right ventricle were significantly enlarged, the right

J. Zheng et al. (eds.), *Selected Pediatric Cardiovascular Surgery Anesthesia Cases*,
https://doi.org/10.1007/978-981-96-5614-1_9

ventricular wall was slightly thickened, and the left ventricular systolic activity was normal. The aorta had a tricuspid valve. The pulmonary artery was significantly widened with the inner diameter of the main trunk 1.44 cm. The atrial septal defect (ASD) was 1.28 cm, extending posteriorly and downwardly from the central part. VSD (muscle), cheese-like, with multiple shunts visible from above the regulatory fasciculus to the apex of the heart, with a range of approximately 2.08 cm, and three wider bundles: 0.33 cm (located above the regulatory fasciculus), 0.19 cm (lower edge of the regulatory fasciculus), 0.28 cm (near the apex), bidirectional shunting at the ventricular level, with a left-to-right shunting velocity of 1.6 m/s. Left aortic arch.

Cardiac CT: ASD 1.08 mm, right atrium enlargement, multiple VSDs 12.4 mm in the muscular part below the bundle with small muscular trabeculae blocking in the middle, right ventricular enlargement, main pulmonary artery dilation, acceptable development of the left and right pulmonary arteries.

In the cardiology department, the infant received treatment with furosemide and spironolactone as diuretics, digoxin as a cardiotonic, and captopril as a vasodilator. After 1 week of treatment, the infant was transferred to the cardiac surgery department.

Preoperative diagnosis: VSD (multiple), ASD (ostium secundum type), PH, PAB surgery was scheduled to be performed under general anesthesia.

9.2 Anesthetic Management

The infant was transferred to the operating room with noninvasive blood pressure (NBP) 95/51 mm Hg, HR 176 beats/min, and pulse oxygen saturation (SpO_2) 96%. A peripheral vein was accessed, and anesthesia was induced by intravenous injection of midazolam 0.5 mg, etomidate 1.0 mg, sufentanil 6.0 μg, and rocuronium 2.0 mg. After the disappearance of the eyelash reflex, a cuffed endotracheal tube with an inner diameter of 3.5 mm was intubated under a visible laryngoscope. The pressure-controlled ventilation-volume guaranteed (PCV-VG) mode was used, and the respiratory parameters were set as follows: oxygen flow rate 2 L/min, fraction of inspired oxygen (FiO_2) 50%, tidal volume (VT) 30 mL, respiratory rate (RR) 25 times/min, inspiratory time to expiratory time (I:E) ratio 1:2, peak inspiratory pressure(PIP) 15 cm H_2O with positive end-expiratory pressure (PEEP) 4 cm H_2O. During the operation, end-tidal carbon dioxide ($ETCO_2$) was maintained within the range of 40–50 mm Hg.

Following the induction of anesthesia and endotracheal intubation, the left femoral artery and the right internal jugular vein were quickly catheterized for invasive arterial pressure (ABP) and central venous pressure monitoring, respectively. The right femoral vein was accessed for rapid fluid replacement. Intraoperative blood gas analysis was performed (Table 9.1). According to the blood gas analysis results, FiO_2 was reduced to 40%, and the respiratory rate was decreased to 20 times/min. Anesthesia was maintained by continuous infusion of sufentanil 2.0 μg/(kg·h), propofol 4.0 mg/(kg·h), and rocuronium 0.5 mg/(kg·h). After induction of anesthesia, the ABP dropped from 92/50 mm Hg to 63/35 mm Hg, which was enhanced by ventilation control and intravenous infusion of dopamine. After the PAB surgery, the mean pulmonary artery pressure dropped from 39 mm Hg to 15 mm Hg, and ABP rose from 62/30 mm Hg to 81/42 mm Hg. Due to the reduction of pulmonary blood flow after banding, SpO_2 dropped from 100% to 88%, and PaO_2 dropped from 224 mm Hg to 59.4 mm Hg under the unchanged condition of FiO_2 40% (Table 9.2).

Ten minutes after banding, the infant's ABP transiently dropped to 56/27 mm Hg. Dopamine 7.5 μg/(kg·min) and norepinephrine 0.05 μg/(kg·min) were infused intravenously to maintain the blood pressure at around 85/40 mm Hg. Arterial blood gas analysis tests were conducted before and after the PAB to assess the surgical effect (Table 9.2). After the PAB, the patent ductus arteriosus (PDA) ligament was ligated. Intraoperative body temperature was monitored, and active warming measures such as warm air blankets and liquid warming were given, maintaining the body temperature above 36.5 °C.

Table 9.1 Intraoperative blood gas test results

Time point	Hb (g/dL)	pH	PaO_2 (mm Hg)	$PaCO_2$ (mm Hg)	BE (mmol/L)	Na^+ (mmol/L)	K^+ (mmol/L)	Cl^- (mmol/L)	Ca^{2+} (mmol/L)	Lac (mmol/L)
After induction	9.8	7.59	306	24.4	3.1	135	4.0	99	1.16	1.7
Before PAB	9.3	7.44	224	37.3	1.6	135	4.0	101	1.19	1.3
After PAB	9.5	7.41	59.4	40.9	1.8	135	3.7	100	1.20	1.0

Table 9.2 Changes in various indicators before and after pulmonary artery banding

Time point	Pulmonary artery flow speed (m/s)	Pulmonary artery pressure gradient (mm Hg)	HR (times/minute)	SpO_2 (%)	PaO_2 (mm Hg)	Pulmonary artery pressure (mm Hg)	Aortic pressure (mm Hg)
Before PAB	1.6	11	136	100	224	58/27(39)	62/30(42)
After PAB	3.4	46.7	134	88	59.4	19/11(15)	81/42(53)

9.3 Postoperative Outcome

The PAB surgery was conducted without cardiopulmonary bypass (CPB) support. The total duration of PAB surgery was 75 min. The estimated intraoperative blood loss was about 5 mL. The urine output was 10 mL. In addition, 30 mL of lactated Ringer's solution and 20 mL of red blood cells were transfused during the operation. After surgery, the patient was transferred to the Cardiac Intensive Care Unit (CICU) with endotracheal intubation. Bedside echocardiography was used to evaluate pulmonary artery pressure and flow velocity at the banding level during the first 2 days after the operation. The flow velocity and pressure gradient at the banding level were 3.85 m/s, 59.2 mm Hg (day 1), and 3.72 m/s, 55.2 mm Hg (day 2). The patient was extubated on postoperative day 3, transferred to the general ward of cardiology the next day, and discharged from the hospital 1 week later.

9.4 Review of Knowledge Points

9.4.1 Pathophysiology of VSDs

The size and number of VSDs are the key factors in determining the volume of the shunt flow. Multiple VSDs refer to two or more locations of VSD, usually a single perimembranous VSD combined with muscular or other types of VSD. The typical muscular VSD presents as a "Swiss-cheese" type defect containing 4 or more small defects. Depending on different factors such as the location, number, and size of the VSD, the surgical plan for multiple VSD includes direct radical treatment, staged surgery, and hybrid closure. Because the ratio of pulmonary vascular resistance (PVR) to systemic vascular resistance (SVR) is usually 1:10–1:20, children with multiple VSD usually have a large left-to-right shunt, and the pulmonary blood flow is significantly increased. At the same time, the pulmonary vascular bed is affected by high blood flow and systemic pressure, which can easily lead to pulmonary arterial hypertension (PAH). Children with severe PAH and significantly increased PVR (Eisenmenger syndrome) are usually not suitable for VSD closure, as closing the VSD will dramatically increase the post-load of the right ventricle and cause right ventricular dysfunction. Therefore, infants with multiple VSDs always cannot tolerate radical surgery. It was recommended to perform pulmonary artery banding (PAB) to protect the development of a pulmonary vascular bed and alleviate the symptoms of congestive heart failure before performing biventricular radical surgery. In addition, some muscular VSDs need to be closed through a left ventricular incision which will seriously affect the myocardial function of the infant. Therefore, for some infants with multiple muscular VSDs, pulmonary artery banding is a better palliative treatment.

9.4.2 Standards of Pulmonary Artery Banding

1. The diameter of the pulmonary artery trunk is similar to the ascending aorta.
2. The aortic pressure rises by 10–20 mm Hg. The distal total pulmonary artery systolic pressure should be reduced to less than 50% of the aortic systolic pressure measured before banding for children who will eventually undergo biventricular repair. For those undergoing univentricular repair, the distal pulmonary artery pressure should be reduced as much as possible at an acceptable oxygen saturation level. 30% of the systemic arterial pressure or ≤ 20–25 mm Hg was recommended.
3. Regarding oxygen saturation, the recommended values for children undergoing biventricular and univentricular repair are 90% and 80–85%, respectively, at room air.

9.5 Discussion

Those patients with multiple VSDs undergoing pulmonary artery banding surgery are often very young and low in weight. They may already have heart failure and increased pulmonary artery pressure before surgery, which brings certain challenges to anesthetic management. Perioperative management should focus on:

9.5.1 Preoperative Evaluation and Preparation

Children with multiple VSDs often have a large left-to-right shunt, which significantly increases the pulmonary blood flow and blood stasis in the vascular bed. They are often complicated with preoperative heart failure and pulmonary infections. Therefore, preoperative optimal measures should include furosemide and/or spironolactone as a diuretic and digoxin as a cardiotonic to enhance heart failure, anti-infection, and selection of the best surgical timing. In addition, this infant was in malnutrition and physical development lag. Preoperative high-energy milk powder was supplemented after consultation with the nutrition department to create good surgical conditions.

9.5.2 Anesthetic Management

Children with multiple VSDs often have a large left-to-right shunt and increased pulmonary artery pressure before surgery. Before the establishment of CPB, it is necessary to avoid the increase of left-to-right shunt caused by the decrease of pulmonary vascular resistance and hypoxia and acidosis at the same time. The patient should also be fully sedated to reduce hemodynamic changes caused by various stress responses. Meanwhile, anesthesiologists should avoid using anesthetics that severely inhibit myocardial contractile function.

Infants and children without congestive heart failure can well tolerate inhalational anesthesia. However, for newborns and infants with congestive heart failure, large-dose opioid intravenous induction was recommended rather than inhalational anesthesia, which can not only provide good hemodynamic stability but also effectively suppress hemodynamic fluctuations caused by surgical stimulation. This child was induced with 2.0 μg/kg sufentanil and maintained with sufentanil 2.0 μg/(kg·h) combined with propofol and sevoflurane. The entire anesthesia process went smoothly.

It is necessary to continuously monitor ECG, ABP, CVP, and $ETCO_2$ changes during the operation. The pulmonary artery pressure and arterial blood gas analysis should also be regularly checked. The mean arterial pressure (MAP) should be maintained at ≥40 mm Hg to ensure systemic circulatory perfusion during the operation. Appropriate fluid replacement and/or vasoactive drugs can be used. In addition, it is also recommended that red blood cell suspension be transfused to improve the oxygen-carrying capacity of children with preoperative Hb less than 8 g/dL. The surgeon should be reminded to operate gently to avoid damaging the pulmonary artery.

Ventilation adjustment is one of the most reliable ways to regulate PVR. To maintain systemic circulatory blood flow and reduce the left-to-right shunt, decreasing the PVR:SVR ratio should be avoided. Hyperventilation should be avoided as much as possible to prevent the decrease of PVR. An appropriate increase in the blood carbon dioxide level is recommended for the effects of increasing PVR and reducing the left-to-right shunt. The FiO_2 should also be controlled below 50%. Pure oxygen ventilation should be avoided because it can reduce pulmonary circulation resistance.

9.5.3 Postoperative Considerations

After PAB surgery, the right ventricular afterload will be significantly increased, which can lead to bradycardia, tachycardia, hypoxemia, hypotension, etc. right heart failure symptoms, and even cardiac arrest. A moderate amount of vasopressor drugs (milrinone, dopamine, epinephrine, etc.) can be used to improve right heart function.

9.6 Shortcomings and Limitations

In this case, the child's ABP transiently dropped from 92/50 mm Hg to 63/35 mm Hg after the induction of anesthesia, which might be due to pure oxygen ventilation and manual hyperventilation during the induction of anesthesia. Once the pulmonary vascular resistance was reduced to a certain extent, the left-to-right shunting was significantly increased, and the systemic circulatory volume was significantly reduced, which led to the transient blood pressure drop. The blood gas analysis after induction showed a significant increase in blood oxygen partial pressure (PaO_2 306 mm Hg) and hypocapnia ($PaCO_2$ 24.4 mm Hg), which confirmed this phenomenon. The hemodynamics became stable after adjusting the respiratory parameters and using vasopressor drugs.

9.7 Conclusion

In summary, PAB surgery is an effective option for infants with multiple VSDs. The key point of anesthetic management during the surgery necessitates comprehensive monitoring, appropriate ventilation management, and support of myocardial contractility (Jiajia Huang).

10 Anesthetic Management of Complete Atrioventricular Canal Defect Repair in a Child with Down Syndrome

Jiajia Huang

Abstract

A 19-month-old female was admitted to our hospital due to her distinctive facial features. She was diagnosed with Down syndrome based on a chromosomal examination. She was also diagnosed with a complete atrioventricular canal defect accompanied by a large atrial (1.08 cm) and ventricular (1.88 cm) septal defect by echocardiography. The blood flow velocity and pressure gradient at the level of the common valve were 4.2 m/s and 70 mm Hg, respectively. The child has had difficulty feeding recently. An elective surgical repair was planned to improve her heart function. In this case, the key points of anesthetic management include preoperative assessment of the possibility of airway obstruction and difficult intubation, intraoperative vigilance for the occurrence of conduction block, and the prevention and control of perioperative pulmonary hypertension crisis.

Complete atrioventricular canal defects (CAVC) involve a large septal defect (atrial septum and part of the ventricular septum) and common atrioventricular valves connecting the two atria and ventricles. A large amount of left-to-right shunt and severe atrioventricular valve regurgitation can cause irreversible pulmonary vascular resistance and refractory heart failure in infants and young children. There is a close relationship between Down syndrome and CAVC. In those children with Down syndrome and CAVC, severe pulmonary artery hypertension may occur very early. This chapter reports the anesthetic management in a patient with both CAVC and Down syndrome.

10.1 Case Presentation

A 19-month-old girl was 7 kg in weight and 78 cm in height. She was brought to our hospital due to her distinctive facial features and aggravated difficulty feeding in the past few weeks.

Physical examination: Distinctive facial features, wide interocular distance, narrow palpebral fissures, and low nasal bridge. The heart rate (HR) was 140 beats/min, regular rhythm. A grade III/VI systolic murmur was heard in the precordial area. No thrill was palpated.

Laboratory test: No significant abnormalities in routine blood tests. Normal liver, kidney, and coagulation function.

Echocardiography: Right atrium and ventricle enlargement, pulmonary artery widening, and pulmonary artery main trunk inner diameter 2.24 cm. The common atrioventricular valve, the

J. Huang (✉)
The National Children's Medical Center (Shanghai), Department of Anesthesiology of Shanghai Children's Medical Center, Shanghai Jiao Tong University School of Medicine, Shanghai, China
e-mail: huangjiajia@scmc.com.cn

J. Zheng et al. (eds.), *Selected Pediatric Cardiovascular Surgery Anesthesia Cases*,
https://doi.org/10.1007/978-981-96-5614-1_10

anterior bridge leaf, was divided, and the tendons were mainly attached to the crest of the ventricular septum. On the left side of the common valve: The forward blood flow speed was 1.2 m/s, moderate regurgitation with bundle width 0.4 cm. On the right side of the common valve: The forward blood flow speed was 1.0 m/s, mild to moderate regurgitation with multiple regurgitation bundles, the widest bundle was 0.32 cm, with a regurgitation speed of 4.2 m/s, and a pressure gradient of 70 mm Hg. Atrial septal defect (ASD, type I) 1.08 cm, left to right shunt. Ventricular septal defect 1.88 cm (VSD atrioventricular canal type), bidirectional shunt. Left aortic arch. Patent ductus arteriosus (PDA) with the pulmonary artery end 0.4 cm and the left to right shunt speed was 1.0 m/s.

Electrocardiogram (ECG): Incomplete right bundle branch block.

Cardiac catheterization: When fraction of inspired oxygen (FiO_2) was increased from 21% to 60%, the SpO_2 and the superior vena cava (SVC) mean pressure was changed from 69.3% and 11 mm Hg to 84.2% and 13 mm Hg, respectively. Pulmonary artery wedge pressure 13 mm Hg, left ventricular pressure 63/6 mm Hg, left pulmonary artery pressure 59/24/41 mm Hg, and main pulmonary artery pressure 61/6/30 mm Hg.

Preoperative diagnosis: CAVC, PDA, ASD (type I), pulmonary hypertension, and Down syndrome. After discussion with the cardiologist and cardiac surgeon team, it was decided to perform complete atrioventricular canal defect correction surgery (double flap method) under general anesthesia.

10.2 Anesthetic Management

The child drank 0.5 mg/kg midazolam syrup 30 min before anesthesia. She was transferred to the operating room after falling asleep. Basic vital signs were monitored: noninvasive blood pressure (NBP) 63/30 mm Hg, HR 120 beats/min, and SpO_2 99%. After the peripheral vein was accessed, the induction of anesthesia was initiated with intravenous administration of etomidate 2.0 mg, sufentanil 15 μg, and rocuronium 4.5 mg. A cuffed endotracheal tube with an inner diameter of 4.0 mm was intubated under direct laryngoscopy with a depth of 12 cm. Pressure-controlled ventilation-volume guaranteed (PCV-VG) mode was used with ventilator parameters set as oxygen flow rate 2 L/min, FiO_2 30%, tidal volume (VT) 60 mL, respiratory rate (RR) 25 times/min, inspiratory time to expiratory time (I:E) ratio 1:2, positive end-expiratory pressure (PEEP) 4 cm H_2O.

After intubation, the left radial artery and right internal jugular vein were catheterized for invasive arterial blood pressure (ABP) and central venous pressure (CVP) monitoring. The left femoral vein was accessed for rapid fluid replacement. Arterial blood gas analysis was checked after induction of anesthesia. The respiratory parameters were adjusted to maintain the PaO_2 at 80 mm Hg and $PaCO_2$ at 40–50 mm Hg. During the operation, propofol 4.0 mg/(kg·h), sufentanil 2.0 μg/(kg·h), and rocuronium 0.5 mg/(kg·h) were intravenously infused and combined with sevoflurane intermittent inhalation to maintain BIS value between 40 and 60.

Hemodynamics was stable during the operation. Cardiopulmonary bypass (CPB) was established after administration of heparin 3.0 mg/kg. Repair was performed using a double-patch technique after aortic cross-clamp and cardiac arrest. After the aorta cross-clamp was released, the sinus rhythm of the heartbeat was automatically resumed with HR 130 beats/min. Continuous infusion of dopamine 5.0 μg/(kg·min) and epinephrine 0.05 μg/(kg·min) was used to maintain ABP around 85/40 mm Hg. Transesophageal echocardiography (TEE) was used to evaluate surgical outcomes and cardiac function, which showed mild regurgitation around the mitral and tricuspid annulus and no residual shunt around the patch. Protamine was given at a ratio of 1.2:1 to antagonize heparin after ultrafiltration. Intraoperative body temperature was monitored, and active warming measures such as warm air blankets and liquid warming were used with the body temperature above 36.5 °C.

10.3 Postoperative Outcome

The CAVC repair surgery was performed with CPB support under mild hypothermia. The two-patch technique was used for CAVC repair. The operation lasted a total of 185 min, with a CPB time of 110 min and an aortic cross-clamping time of 86 min. After the operation, the patient was transferred to the Cardiac Intensive Care Unit (CICU) with ABP monitoring and intubated. In addition to the continuous use of dopamine and epinephrine, milrinone 0.5 μg/(kg·min) was added to maintain cardiac function and reduce pulmonary vascular resistance in CICU. Chest X-ray showed atelectasis or consolidation in the upper left lung. C-reactive protein and white blood cells were significantly elevated the day after the operation. The child was successfully extubated on postoperative day 7 and discharged from the hospital on postoperative day 10.

10.4 Review of Knowledge Points

10.4.1 Characteristics of Down Syndrome and Anesthesia-Related Issues

Down syndrome was first reported by John Langdon Down of Britain in 1866 and officially named by the World Health Organization (WHO) in 1965. Autopsies have found that 60% of children with Down syndrome have heart disease. Endocardial cushion defects are the most common heart disease, accounting for about 40%.

Difficult airways, atlantoaxial instability, and immune deficiencies associated with Down syndrome can make anesthesia more challenging. Airways: These children have underdeveloped mid-facial areas, enlarged tongues, increased secretions, and excessive enlargement of the tonsils and adenoids, which can easily lead to airway obstruction. Congenital subglottic stenosis is also common. Atlantoaxial ligament laxity: These children have widespread hypotonia joint laxity and atlantoaxial instability. The process of intubation and positioning should be particularly careful and gentle because of this. Immune deficiency: The incidence of perioperative infection is high, especially as respiratory infections.

10.4.2 Pathophysiology of CAVC

The pathophysiological manifestation of CAVC is regurgitating a single set of atrioventricular valves and a large amount of left-to-right shunting. The severe atrioventricular valve regurgitation increases ventricular volume load and pulmonary artery pressure, which can lead to ventricular enlargement and heart failure. Children present with difficulty in feeding, dyspnea, fatigue, recurrent respiratory infections, and developmental delay. The degree of atrioventricular valve regurgitation affects children's onset of heart failure. As regurgitation worsens, shunting can directly enter the right atrium, and the accompanying pulmonary vascular disease will rapidly worsen in the first year of the child.

10.4.3 Surgical Treatment of CAVC

Research from the University of Michigan Medical School shows that the median age of surgery for children with CAVC is 4.8 months. Due to the presence of large shunts, children with CAVC are prone to have pulmonary arterial hypertension (PAH) early on. Therefore, the surgical age for these children should be 3–6 months, as the atrioventricular valve tissue is sufficiently mature at this time, which is more conducive to surgical repair before changes in the pulmonary vascular bed and the formation of PAH. Early surgery is crucial because the possibility of an irreversible increase in pulmonary vascular resistance greatly increases over time. About half of the children die within 6 months, and 80% die within 2 years if untreated.

10.5 Discussion

10.5.1 Preoperative Assessment and Preparation

In addition to assessing cardiac function and the degree of PAH, airway evaluation is also a key point of the preoperative assessment in children with CAVC and Down syndrome.

Oral midazolam can be considered for preoperative sedation to make separation from parents easier since most children with Down syndrome have developmental delays and certain cognitive and cooperation obstacles. Vital signs should be closely monitored during the sedation process.

The presence of immune deficiency greatly increases the incidence of perioperative infections in these patients. Therefore, antibiotics should be used preventively before surgery, and invasive operations such as central venous puncture should actively follow aseptic principles to reduce the chance of infection.

10.5.2 Intraoperative Anesthetic Management

Children with Down syndrome are very sensitive to inhalational anesthetics and are prone to bradycardia, which may be related to the lower sympathetic excitability of these patients. Therefore, intravenous induction is more suitable for these patients.

Cardiac conduction block may occur after surgery since the atrioventricular node is close to the patch position. Therefore, the anesthesiologist should closely monitor the changes in ECG after CPB. If a cardiac conduction block occurs, it is necessary to remind the surgeon to repair the patch again or to place an epicardial A-V sequential pacemaker to assist in weaning from CPB.

The prevention of perioperative pulmonary hypertension crisis is essential. Children with CAVC usually have PAH before surgery and even after surgery. Mechanical hyper-ventilation should be used to maintain $PaCO_2$ 35–40 mm Hg and PaO_2 above 100 mm Hg. Milrinone, treprostinil, iloprost, and inhaled nitric oxide are all beneficial. Pulmonary artery catheter monitoring of pulmonary artery pressure is helpful for postoperative management of patients with PAH. The goals of anesthetic management of CAVC repair surgery are summarized in Table 10.1.

10.5.3 Postoperative Anesthetic Management

After weaning off CPB, transesophageal echocardiography should be conducted to detect the residual VSDs and the condition of the mitral valve. After CAVC repair surgery, sufficient sedation, analgesia, and hyperventilation should be given to patients with CAVC to avoid the risk factors that can trigger pulmonary hypertension crises such as hypoxia, hypercapnia, acidosis, pain, and hypothermia. Any children with residual pulmonary hypertension should be actively treated. Routine infusion of low-dose dopamine, dobutamine 2.5–5.0 μg/(kg·min), and (or) milrinone 0.5–0.7 μg/(kg·min) can help optimize these children's cardiac output. Postoperative blood pressure should be controlled as high blood pressure can lead to tearing of the mitral valve repair sutures and exacerbate regurgitation. In addition, fluid balance should be strictly controlled, as excessive fluid administration can increase left atrial pressure and cause mitral valve annulus dilation and regurgitation to worsen.

Table 10.1 Goals of anesthetic management for CAVC repair surgery

During surgery	After CPB
Maintain heart rate, contractility, and preload in order to maintain cardiac output	Maintain age-appropriate heart rate and sinus rhythm
Avoid a decrease in the PVR:SVR ratio	Lower PVR, especially in children with PAH, consider using drugs such as milrinone, iloprost, and inhaled nitric oxide
Avoid a significant increase in the PVR:SVR ratio; avoid an increase in right-to-left shunt volume	Positive inotropic drug support such as dopamine 5.0–10 μg/(kg·min), milrinone 0.5–1.0 μg/(kg·min)

10.6 Conclusion

The anesthetic management of children with CAVC and Down syndrome should consider a variety of issues related to the respiratory, circulatory, and immune systems. Active treatment of pulmonary hypertension during the perioperative period and maintenance of normal cardiac rhythm and function can effectively reduce the perioperative mortality rate in these children with CAVC and Down syndrome (Jiajia Huang).

11 Anesthetic Management of Surgical Correction of Scimitar Syndrome in a Child with Cardiopulmonary Insufficiency

Yong Bian

Abstract

A 7-month-old female infant with paroxysmal dyspnea and cyanosis of the limbs was diagnosed with anomalous right pulmonary venous drainage (Scimitar syndrome) by echocardiography. Wet rales were heard in both lungs by physical examination. She was admitted into our hospital with a preliminary diagnosis of "Scimitar syndrome and lung infection." During the symptomatic treatment in the medical ward, respiratory distress and progressive worsening of cyanosis occurred and caused secondary congestive heart failure and respiratory failure. Emergency surgery was required to correct the anomalous pulmonary venous drainage. Once multiple pulmonary veins were affected by Scimitar syndrome and accompanied by congenital pulmonary dysplasia, the risk of heart and lung failure was significantly increased. Pulmonary vein obstruction may be life-threatening in a small number of children. Early surgery is the key to reversing this condition. Anesthetic management of these children should focus on respiratory management, regulating pulmonary vascular resistance, aggressive cardiac support, and treating pulmonary hypertension.

Scimitar syndrome (SS) is a rare congenital cardiopulmonary vascular disease with partial anomalous venous connection of the right pulmonary veins to the infra-diaphragmatic inferior vena cava (IVC) via the confluence, right lung hypoplasia, and a variable systemic arterial blood supply to the right lung. The name derives from its "scimitar" shape of the anomalous pulmonary venous connection to the inferior vena cava in the radiologic appearance, which resembles a curved Turkish sword. SS may also be accompanied by underdevelopment of the lung, abnormal development of the right pulmonary artery, isolated right lower lung, diaphragmatic and musculoskeletal deformities, etc. The anomalous drainage of the right pulmonary vein to the systemic vein causes left-to-right shunting. In most cases, the symptoms of SS are mild. However, the symptoms will be very severe if the entire right pulmonary veins are involved and accompanied by poor lung tissue development or other deformities. They can cause a mismatch of pulmonary circulation blood and secondary cardiac insufficiency. Surgical correction is the principal approach to save these children's lives. Precise and timely perioperative anesthetic management plays a vital role in the successful surgical correction and the prognosis of the children. This chapter reports on the

Y. Bian (✉)
The National Children's Medical Center (Shanghai), Department of Anesthesiology of Shanghai Children's Medical Center, Shanghai Jiao Tong University School of Medicine, Shanghai, China
e-mail: bianyong@scmc.com.cn

J. Zheng et al. (eds.), *Selected Pediatric Cardiovascular Surgery Anesthesia Cases*,
https://doi.org/10.1007/978-981-96-5614-1_11

perioperative management of a child with Scimitar syndrome accompanied by cardiopulmonary insufficiency.

11.1 Case Presentation

The patient was a 7-month and 10-day-old girl weighing 6.5 kg. She was born full-term without asphyxia. A heart murmur was detected during auscultation at a local hospital due to paroxysmal dyspnea more than a month ago. Five days later, the dyspnea worsened, so she was brought to our hospital for further diagnosis and treatment.

Physical examination: Auscultation of both lungs revealed moist rales and a III/VI systolic murmur was heard in the precordial area between the third and fourth ribs. The second heart sound of the pulmonary valve was accentuated.

Laboratory tests: Blood routine Hb 94 g/L, TBIL 38.0 μmol/L, AST 68 U/L, no obvious abnormality in coagulation function.

Echocardiography: Right pulmonary vein abnormal drainage, right pulmonary artery underdevelopment, flow velocity of the right pulmonary artery 2.8 m/s, right atrium and right ventricle enlargement, left ventricular ejection fraction (LVEF) 46%.

Chest CT: Scimitar syndrome, anomalous right pulmonary veins connection to inferior vena cava, underdeveloped right pulmonary volume, and artery, the right lower lung blood supply from the abdominal aorta via side branches.

Chest X-ray: Cardiac silhouette enlargement, the right lower pleural effusion.

Electrocardiogram: Sinus rhythm, T wave top-notch, right atrial and right ventricular hypertrophy.

After admission, the girl received symptomatic treatment of anti-infection, diuresis cardiotonic, and enhancement of cardiac function. Three days later, acute respiratory distress occurred with a respiratory rate (RR) of 52 times/min and pulse oxygen saturation (SpO_2) of 69%. Physical examination revealed the presence of emotional blunting, limb cyanosis, and hepatosplenomegaly by abdominal percussion. The blood pressure progressively reduced, with the lowest value being 45/32 mm Hg. The chest X-ray showed uneven transparency of both lungs, suggesting a possible infection in the right lower lung. Norepinephrine at 0.05 μg/(kg·min) and epinephrine at 0.1 μg/(kg·min) were intravenously infused to maintain blood pressure. Continuous positive airway pressure (CPAP) support was also used. SpO_2 was maintained around 85%. After discussion, it was determined that emergency surgery was required to save the girl's life due to the imbalance of pulmonary ventilation to blood flow ratio caused by the primary disease and secondary congestive heart failure.

Preoperative diagnosis: Scimitar syndrome, heart failure. Emergency right pulmonary vein anomalous drainage correction surgery was required.

11.2 Anesthetic Management

The girl was transported to the operating room with an intravenous infusion of norepinephrine 0.05 μg/(kg·min) and epinephrine 0.05 μg/(kg·min). The ABP was 82/41 mm Hg, HR was 161 beats/min, and SpO_2 was 86% before induction of anesthesia. 0.5 mg midazolam, 1.5 mg etomidate, 6.5 μg sufentanil, and 4.0 mg rocuronium were intravenously administrated for anesthesia induction. Endotracheal intubation was conducted with an ID 3.5 mm cuffed tube. Pressure-controlled ventilation-volume guaranteed (PCV-VG) mode was chosen with the following settings: oxygen flow rate 2 L/min, fraction of inspired oxygen (FiO_2) 70%, tidal volume (VT) 50 mL, RR 28 times/min, inspiratory-to-expiratory ratio (I:E) 1:2, positive end-expiratory pressure (PEEP) 6 cm H_2O. During the operation, the respiratory rate was adjusted to maintain the partial pressure of end-tidal carbon dioxide ($ETCO_2$) at 40–45 mm Hg.

After induction of anesthesia, a central venous catheter was placed into the right internal jugular vein to monitor central venous pressure (CVP). In addition, cerebral oxygen

Table 11.1 Intraoperative blood gas test results

Time point	pH	Hb (g/dL)	HCT (%)	PaO_2 (mm Hg)	$PaCO_2$ (mm Hg)	BE (mmol/L)	Na^+ (mmol/L)	K^+ (mmol/L)	Cl^- (mmol/L)	Ca^{2+} (mmol/L)	Lac (mmol/L)
Admission	7.23	9.5	27.8	55	51.3	−3.8	136	3.71	111	1.21	3.2
Discharge	7.38	11.2	33.2	101.5	40	−1.76	135	3.48	108	1.3	4.3

saturation was continuously monitored. During the operation, propofol 4.0 mg/(kg·h), rocuronium 0.5 mg/(kg·h), and sufentanil 2.0 μg/(kg·h) were intravenously infused and combined with intermittent 1–2% sevoflurane inhalation to maintain anesthesia. Before the establishment of cardiopulmonary bypass (CPB), ABP was maintained at (60–70)/(35–45) mm Hg, SpO_2 at 85%–90%, CVP around 10 cm H_2O, and cerebral oxygen saturation at about 70%. After systemic heparinization and establishment of CPB, reimplantation of the anomalous right pulmonary vein was performed under deep hypothermic circulatory arrest (DHCA). The total time of DHCA was 41 min. The lowest cerebral oxygen saturation during DHCA was 52%. After restoring circulation, the proximal right pulmonary artery was enlarged with patch repair. Once the aortic cross-clamp was removed, automatic rewarming was initiated. After rewarming to 32 °C, dopamine 5.0 μg/(kg·min) and epinephrine 0.08 μg/(kg·min) were initially infused, and mechanical ventilation was resumed after the vena cava clamp was released. Postoperative transesophageal echocardiography showed unobstructed pulmonary vein anastomosis with the blood pulmonary vein flow rate at 0.8 m/s, the pulmonary artery flow rate at 2.0 m/s, proximal right pulmonary artery flow rate at 2.5 m/s, and no residual shunt at the atrial and ventricular levels. After reducing the perfusion flow rate, CPB was successfully weaned off with ABP at 82/43 mm Hg, HR at 161 beats/min, CVP at 9 cm H_2O, SpO_2 at 95%, and brain oxygen saturation at 63%. The systemic heparinization was antagonized by protamine sulfate at a ratio of 1.2 mg of protamine per 100 IU of heparin. Then, 50 mL of autologous blood was transfused back to the patient. Postoperative blood gas analysis showed lactate at 4.3 mmol/L (Table 11.1), which is considered to be related to the prolonged DHCA. No specific treatment was given. The girl was transferred to the CICU with endotracheal intubation after surgery.

11.3 Postoperative Outcome

The operation lasted 3 h and 5 min, CPB time was 2 h and 15 min, and DHCA time was 41 min. During the operation, 75 mL of Ringer's acetate solution and 50 mL of autologous blood were infused. The urine output was 12 mL. Fentanyl was continuously infused for 2 days after surgery. The girl's blood pressure and pulse oxygen saturation decreased on postoperative day 2, which was considered to be related to pulmonary hypertension. Then, intravenous administration of milrinone was supplemented. On postoperative day 4, the girl's hemodynamics became stable, and the positive inotropic drugs and milrinone were reduced. The endotracheal tube was removed on postoperative day 6, and she was discharged from our hospital on postoperative day 25.

11.4 Review of Knowledge Points

11.4.1 Pathophysiology of Scimitar Syndrome

The incidence of SS is 1/100,000 to 3/100,000 in live births. It is a syndrome characterized by congenital pulmonary vascular malformations, including all or part of the right pulmonary veins abnormally draining into the systemic venous circulation, underdevelopment of the right lung, underdeveloped ipsilateral pulmonary artery, rightward shift of the mediastinum, and anomalous systemic arterial supply to the right lower lung (Fig. 11.1).

The pathophysiological changes of SS are similar to those of partial pulmonary venous drainage. Left-to-right shunting causes oxygenated venous blood to re-enter the pulmonary artery and produce blood recirculation. Left-to-right shunting reduces the adequate forward blood flow of the left ventricle and leads to overload volume of the right atrium and right ventricle. The size of the left-to-right shunt depends on the number of abnormal pulmonary veins draining to the right lung and whether there are other cardiac malformations. A large amount of left-to-right shunting can lead to pulmonary hypertension and right heart failure.

In addition, children with SS are more prone to lung infections, cyanosis exacerbation, and pulmonary vascular disease due to the left to right shunting-associated pulmonary blood flow increase. It can lead to severe pulmonary hypertension in children of SS with abnormal systemic arterial collateral formation, underdeveloped lungs with reduced pulmonary vascular bed, pulmonary vein stenosis, and obstruction.

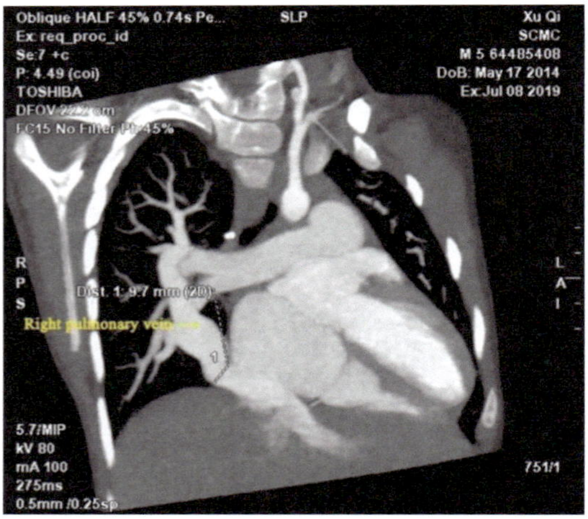

Fig. 11.1 CT showing the right pulmonary veins draining into the inferior vena cava, consistent with the presentation of Scimitar syndrome

11.4.2 Principles of Surgical Treatment

The key to surgical correction of pediatrics with SS is to dissect the anomalous pulmonary veins and reestablish the connection between the pulmonary veins and the left atrium. If necessary, the lung lobes involved should be removed. The success rate of surgery performed within 1 year of age is over 80%, especially for those children with SS who do not have other intracardiac malformations. Several factors can affect the incidence of postoperative adverse events in children with SS, which mainly include the age of onset of symptoms and signs, single ventricle physiology, and main pulmonary artery collateral formation.

11.5 Discussion

11.5.1 Preoperative Assessment and Preparation

The clinical manifestations of children with SS mainly depend on the changes in hemodynamics, right heart volume load, the degree of secondary pulmonary vein stenosis, the severity of other cardiovascular malformations, and lung development. Children with simple SS may have no clinical symptoms. At the same time, those with severe intracardiac malformations, pulmonary vein stenosis, poor development of the right lung, vascular disease, or systemic circulation artery (such as the aorta or bronchial artery) collateral supply may present with symptoms of pulmonary hypertension and heart failure.

Once children with SS develop heart and lung failure, they should be actively treated. Conservative treatment includes anti-infection treatment, enhancement of heart function, and pulmonary hypertension reduction. When conservative treatments cannot improve the functions of the heart and lungs and persistent acidosis occurs, emergency surgery is needed to save lives. In this case, the child was given active anti-infection treatment, heart function support (epinephrine and norepinephrine), and CPAP ventilation treatment before surgery. However, hemodynamics was still unstable. Therefore, emergency surgery was needed to correct the anatomical abnormalities.

11.5.2 Anesthetic Management During Surgery

Most SS patients have good cardiac reserve and can tolerate the inhalational induction of anesthesia well. Large doses of opioids such as fentanyl or sufentanil, with less suppression on hemodynamics, should be chosen for induction of anesthesia combined with hypnotic and muscle relaxants in those patients with mechanical ventilation and positive inotropic agents support before surgery. For those patients with pulmonary vein obstruction who usually have high pulmonary vascular reactivity, large doses of fentanyl or sufentanil can be used to reduce the increase in pulmonary vascular resistance caused by surgical stress stimuli.

Intraoperative anesthetic management aims to maintain age-matched heart rate, myocardial contractility, and preload. For patients who already have heart failure before surgery, positive inotropic agents and vasoactive drugs should be actively used to maintain cardiac output and systemic circulation perfusion.

A decreased PVR: SVR ratio should be avoided for patients with increased pulmonary blood flow and right ventricular volume overload. A decreased PVR: SVR ratio will increase left-to-right shunting and result in insufficient systemic circulation perfusion. Hyperventilation can cause the reduction of PVR and improve pulmonary blood flow. Therefore, hyperventilation should be avoided for such patients. It is better to maintain $PaCO_2$ at 40–50 mm Hg. For SS patients with pulmonary vein obstruction, hyperventilation or the use of pulmonary vasodilators will exacerbate pulmonary edema. However, appropriate PEEP can improve lung compliance, alleviate pulmonary edema, and thus improve oxygenation.

The DHCA technique reduces tissue oxygen demand and protects the brain during cardiac surgery. There are still some controversies about the impact of DHCA on the neurodevelopmental outcome of children with congenital heart disease. Some studies have shown that brain oxygen saturation monitoring can identify the risk of ischemic hypoxic brain injury in patients. The DHCA technique and cerebral oxygen saturation monitoring were simultaneously used during the operation. The lowest brain oxygen saturation during DHCA was 52%, within 15% of the baseline value.

11.5.3 Postoperative Anesthetic Management

The anesthetic management after CPB should focus on regulating cardiac insufficiency and pulmonary hypertension. Postoperative transesophageal echocardiography greatly helps to evaluate the anastomosis of pulmonary veins, the left atrium, and ventricular function. After ruling out the residual pulmonary vein obstruction, PVR can be reduced by adjusting mechanical ventilation. In addition, some selective pulmonary vasodilators, such as inhaling nitric oxide, can also be used. If blood pressure can be maintained, prostacyclin agents like remodulin can also be used. The positive inotropic agents should also be actively given to support right ventricular function while PVR is reduced. Dopamine (5.0–10 μg/(kg·min)) does not increase PVR but increases myocardial contractility. In SS patients, left-to-right shunting may lead to long-term preload insufficiency of the left ventricle, which may lead to poor development of the left heart. Thus, these patients may present with biventricular heart failure postoperatively. For patients with biventricular heart failure, small doses of epinephrine can be used. Postoperative fluid infusion in SS patients should be cautious. Excessive fluid may cause acute left heart failure.

11.6 Shortcomings and Limitations

During the surgery, the placement of pulmonary artery or left atrial pressure tubes can greatly help assess pulmonary artery pressure and identify the causes of pulmonary hypertension. However, due to a lack of relevant materials, pulmonary artery pressure and left atrial pressure were not monitored, which had some impact on the timely detection and treatment of postoperative pulmonary hypertension.

11.7 Conclusion

Children with Scimitar syndrome may need urgent anomalous pulmonary vein drainage correction surgery due to cardiopulmonary insufficiency. Anatomical correction can effectively improve the outcome of children with SS. Similarly, precise respiratory and circulatory management during the perioperative period is also essential (Yong Bian).

12 Anesthetic Management for Surgical Correction of Neonatal Obstructive Total Anomalous Pulmonary Venous Connection

Jingjing Lv

Abstract

A 1-day-old infant was found to have congenital heart disease during prenatal examination. Symptoms of cyanosis, difficulty in breathing, and low pulse oxygen saturation (SpO_2) appeared immediately after birth. He was then transferred to our hospital for further treatment in an emergency. Echocardiography demonstrated obstructed total anomalous pulmonary venous connection (TAPVC), and emergency corrective surgery of TAPVC was scheduled. Severe preoperative hypoxemia, acidosis, and circulatory failure significantly increase the risk of anesthesia in this infant. In perioperative comprehensive anesthetic management, the key points include the regulation of mechanical ventilation, application of vasoactive drugs, regulation of acid–base balance, and blood protection, which can help such infants safely pass through the perioperative period.

Total anomalous pulmonary venous connection (TAPVC) refers to the condition that the four pulmonary veins do not directly connect to the left atrium but anomalously connect to the right atrium or a branch of the systemic veins. Therefore, the oxygenated blood from the lungs is delivered to the right atrium instead of the left atrium, which only receives the mixed blood from the right atrium. The clinical symptoms and signs of TAPVC depend on the size of the atrial septal defect (ASD) and whether the pulmonary vein stenosis exists. For an obstructive TAPVC, pulmonary edema, pulmonary arterial hypertension, and poor systemic circulation can occur in the early postnatal period due to the increase of pressure at the venous end of the pulmonary circulation, which quickly leads to progressive hypoxemia, acidosis, and hemodynamic failure, etc. Once this situation happens, emergency surgery to relieve the anatomical obstruction is often required to save a life. This chapter reports the perioperative anesthetic management of emergency corrective surgery for supracardiac obstructive TAPVC.

12.1 Case Presentation

A 1-day-old boy with 3.5 kg in weight and 50 cm in length was born full-term without asphyxia by cesarean section. The boy was diagnosed with congenital heart disease during prenatal examination. After birth, the patient had cyanosis, difficulty in breathing, and 50% pulse oxygen saturation (SpO_2). Immediate endotracheal intubation, mechanical ventilation, and prostaglandin

J. Lv (✉)
The National Children's Medical Center (Shanghai), Department of Anesthesiology of Shanghai Children's Medical Center, Shanghai Jiao Tong University School of Medicine, Shanghai, China
e-mail: lvjingjing@scmc.com.cn

J. Zheng et al. (eds.), *Selected Pediatric Cardiovascular Surgery Anesthesia Cases*,
https://doi.org/10.1007/978-981-96-5614-1_12

Table 12.1 Results of blood gas analysis

Blood gas analysis	pH	$PaCO_2$ (mm Hg)	PaO_2 (mm Hg)	Na^+ (mmol/L)	K^+ (mmol/L)	CL^- (mmol/L)	HCO_3^- (mmol/L)	BE (mmol/L)	HCT (%)	Lac (mmol/L)
Preoperation	6.9	125.0	27.2	140	3.4	101	28.5	−10.9	51	1.6
Enter OR	7.1	101.6	27.3	139	3.6	108	28.7	−4.2	41	2
Exit OR	7.3	57.2	150	145	3.9	105	27	−2.6	34	3.1

infusion to maintain patent ductus arteriosus (PDA) were initiated, and the boy was then admitted to the Cardiac Surgery Intensive Care Unit (CICU).

Physical examination: The boy was mechanically ventilated, had normal physical development, gray complexion, SpO_2 50–70%, axillary temperature 36 °C, heart rate (HR) 134 beats/min, respiratory rate (RR) 45 breaths/min, blood pressure (BP) 75/48 mmHg.

Laboratory tests: Routine blood test: HCT 53.5%, platelets 323 × 10^9/L. Liver and kidney function: AST 54 U/L, ALB 29.8 g/L, TP 48.9 g/L, UREA 1.8 mmol/L. Coagulation function: APTT 80.3 s, PT 17 s, INR 1.7%, fibrinogen 1.27 g/L, D-dimer 0.38 mg/L.

Blood gas analysis: progressive increase in lactate and carbon dioxide partial pressure ($PaCO_2$) and decrease in pH (Table 12.1).

Emergency echocardiography: Supracardiac type TAPVC (obstructive), ASD (type II), patent ductus arteriosus (PDA), pulmonary arterial hypertension (PAH).

Preoperative diagnosis: Supracardiac type TAPVC (obstructive), ASD (type II), PDA, PAH, heart failure. Emergency surgical correction of TAPVC was scheduled.

12.2 Anesthetic Management

The boy was transferred to the operating room (OR) under mechanical ventilation and with epinephrine intravenous infusion at 0.1 μg/(kg·min). After entering OR, the pressure-controlled ventilation-volume guaranteed (PCV-VG) mode was used with respiratory parameters setting as: oxygen flow rate 1 L/min, fraction of inspired oxygen (FiO_2) 70%, tidal volume (VT) 30 mL, RR 40 times/min, inspiratory to expiratory (I:E) ratio 1:1.5, and positive end-expiratory pressure (PEEP) 3.0 cm H_2O. Invasive blood pressure (ABP) from the left radial artery and central venous pressure (CVP) from the right internal jugular vein were continuously monitored. SpO_2, electrocardiogram (ECG), and cerebral oxygen saturation (SrO_2) were also monitored. Baseline values: ABP 70/42 mm Hg, HR 160 times/min, SpO_2 70%, CVP 5.0 cm H_2O, SrO_2 40%. Midazolam 0.5 mg, rocuronium 2.0 mg, and sufentanil 5.0 μg were intravenously administered for anesthesia induction. Anesthesia was maintained by propofol 2.0 mg/(kg·h), sufentanil 1.0 μg/(kg·h), rocuronium 0.6 mg/(kg·h). The surgery was performed under cardiopulmonary bypass (CPB) support and deep hypothermic circulatory arrest. Before CPB was established, blood gas analysis showed a significant increase of $PaCO_2$ (101.6 mm Hg), and the respiratory parameters were adjusted to facilitate carbon dioxide elimination with intermittent manual lung recruitment.

Supracardiac TAPVC was found after the establishment of CPB and hypothermic circulatory arrest. The common confluence of the left and right pulmonary veins was very narrow. The openings of the pulmonary vein branches were also very narrow. The left and right pulmonary veins were cut open to the branches, and sutureless suturing was performed. After aortic cross-clamp release, the heart automatically resumed beating and sinus rhythm with HR 110–120 times/min, BP 55–60/35–40 mmHg. Through adjusting the dose of vasoactive drugs, BP was maintained at 60–70/40–45 mmHg, HR at 135–145 times/min with dopamine infusion at 7.5 μg/(kg·min), epinephrine at 0.2 μg/(kg·min), and isoprenaline at 0.05 μg/(kg·min). After removing the vena cava clamp, mechanical ventilation was resumed, and manual lung recruitment was performed simultaneously to maintain normal $ETCO_2$. The blood gas analysis results are shown in Table 12.1. Based on these results, 7 mL of sodium bicarbonate was given to correct acidosis, the respiratory parameters were adjusted to reduce $ETCO_2$, and 100 mg calcium was supplemented to correct hypocalcemia. Coagulation monitoring by Sonoclot suggested prolonged activated clotting time (ACT) and clot rate (CR) times, cryoprecipitate 1 U, and prothrombin complex 50 IU was given to supplement fibrinogen and coagulation factors.

The operation lasted 180 min, including 115 min for CPB, 66 min for aortic occlusion, and 39 min for circulatory arrest. During the operation, 40 mL of acetic acid Ringer's solution and 20 mL of plasma were transfused, and 35 mL of urine was output.

12.3 Postoperative Outcome

Delayed sternal closure (DSC) was conducted with a temporary pacemaker implanted. The patient was intubated and transferred to the CICU with continuous vasoactive drug infusion and constant monitoring of ABP, EKG, and SpO_2. Red blood cells and fresh frozen plasma were transfused postoperatively to improve anemia and coagulation status. The sternum chest was closed 3 days later. The tracheal tube was successfully removed on postoperative day 6, and the boy was discharged from the hospital on postoperative day 20.

12.4 Review of Knowledge Points

12.4.1 Anatomic Characteristics and Classification

TAPVC refers to a cyanotic congenital defect in which the four pulmonary veins fail to connect to the left atrium directly but connect to the right atrium or the systemic venous system. Therefore, the oxygenated pulmonary venous return was directly drained into the systemic venous circulation. The incidence of TAPVC is relatively low, ranging from 0.06% to 0.12%, less than 3% of congenital heart defects. TAPVC is commonly classified into four types: supracardiac, intracardiac, subcardiac, and mixed types. The supracardiac TAPVC is the most common type, accounting for about 46%, in which the pulmonary veins from each lung join to form a confluence posterior to the left atrium and connect with the right superior vena cava or right azygous vein or the left innominate vein through the vertical vein, then the blood flows back to the right atrium (Fig. 12.1a). The intracardiac type TAPVC accounts for about 24%, where the pulmonary veins from each lung join to form a confluence and drain to the coronary sinus or directly into the right atrium (Fig. 12.1b); the subcardiac type TAPVC accounts for about 22%, where the pulmonary veins from each lung join to form a confluence and connect with the inferior vena cava, portal vein or hepatic vein, etc. through the vertical vein passing the esophageal hiatus on the diaphragm, and then the blood returns to the right heart system (Fig. 12.1c); the mixed type accounts for about 8%, and may have the above two or three types of characteristics at the same time.

According to whether pulmonary venous obstruction presents, TAPVC can be classified into obstructive and nonobstructive types. Generally speaking, the longer the course of the vertical vein is, the greater the probability of pulmonary vein obstruction will be due to narrowing or compression of this pulmonary vein drainage pathway. Therefore, it is generally believed that pulmonary vein obstruction is most likely to occur in subcardiac TAPVC due to the long path of the vertical vein and passing the esophageal hiatus. In supracardiac patients, the vertical vein runs between the left main bronchus and the pulmonary artery, which may be easily compressed to cause pulmonary vein obstruction, increase the pulmonary artery pressure, further expand the pulmonary artery, and compress the vertical vein. This leads to almost complete obstruction of the vertical vein and a vicious cycle. Children with obstructed TAPVC often need emergency surgery to relieve the obstruction to save lives.

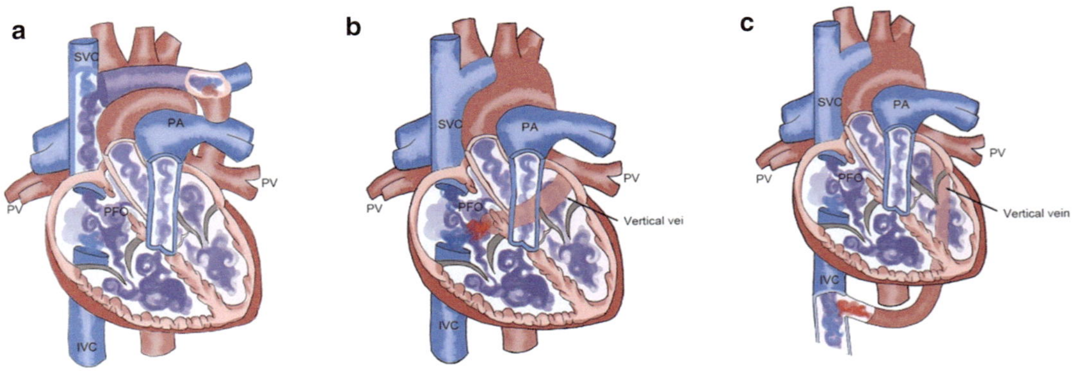

Fig. 12.1 Anatomical typing of TAPVC. (**a**) supracardiac; (**b**) intracardiac; (**c**) subcardiac. *PA* pulmonary artery, *PV* pulmonary vein, *SVC* superior vena cava, *IVC* inferior vena cava, *PFO* patent foramen ovale

12.4.2 Pathophysiological Characteristics

Due to the return of pulmonary venous blood to the right atrium, a large amount of the physiological left-to-right shunting in TAPVC children is significantly increased because both the systemic venous return and pulmonary venous return blood drains to the right atrium and cause overload in the right atrium volume. To keep surviving after birth, the TAPVC patients must have an anatomical mandatory right-to-left shunt, either through atrial septal defects or patent foramen ovale. During the intrauterine period, less blood flow to the left heart usually causes underdevelopment of the left heart with low compliance, which may limit the shunt at the level of the atrial septum.

Compression or obstruction of the vertical vein can cause increased pulmonary venous pressure and pulmonary vascular resistance, resulting in pulmonary hypertension and pulmonary edema. At this time, any factors to increase pulmonary blood flow will exacerbate pulmonary edema. Those drugs with direct dilation of the pulmonary vessels, such as NO, are definitely contraindicated. The cardiac output in children with obstructed TAPVC will be significantly reduced. As the obstruction worsens, the right ventricular pressure can approach or exceed the systemic circulation pressure, and the interventricular septum shifts to the left, further reducing compliance with the already underdeveloped left ventricle. These children's systemic circulation cardiac output largely depends on the right-to-left shunt provided by the exhausted right ventricle through the PDA.

12.5 Discussion

12.5.1 Preoperative Assessment and Preparation

Active preoperative preparation is essential for improving the tolerance of pediatric patients to surgical trauma. Children with obstructed TAPVC often have a certain degree of pulmonary arterial hypertension, hypoxemia, acidosis, low perfusion of the systemic circulation, and organ dysfunction before surgery, manifesting as tachycardia, hypotension, pulmonary edema, etc. Therefore, it is necessary to timely administer positive inotropic drugs, correct acidosis, and perform endotracheal intubation and mechanical ventilation to support heart and lung function and increase oxygenation. This patient showed systemic cyanosis immediately after birth, progressive hypoxemia, and acidosis. Therefore, this patient was immediately intubated and mechanically ventilated after admission. Epinephrine was continuously infused to increase cardiac output and maintain the perfusion of the systemic circulation. Acidosis was also corrected while preoperative assessment and preparation were actively optimized.

12.5.2 Anesthetic Management During Surgery

Compared to unobstructed TAPVC, children with obstructed TAPVC often experience quick hemodynamic failure due to pulmonary circulation congestion, pulmonary arterial hypertension, and poor systemic circulation perfusion, which poses great challenges to anesthetic management, especially during the anesthesia induction period. It is important to reduce the hemodynamic changes caused by various stressful stimulations, prevent the increase of pulmonary circulation resistance, and avoid hypoxia and excessive suppression of the cardiovascular system. The following points should be noted for maintaining circulatory system stability.

1. To maintain a certain depth of anesthesia and analgesia: Anesthesia is mainly maintained by muscle relaxants and opioid analgesics. Large doses of opioid analgesics can suppress the surgical stimulation-related increase of pulmonary vascular resistance and provide relatively stable hemodynamics.
2. To maintain the heart rate within the age-related normal ranges: For the obstructed TAPVC, many clinical symptoms often appear in the early neonatal period. However, the ability to increase cardiac output for these infants is limited, mainly relying on increasing heart rate. The reasons are that the myocardium of newborns and infants is immature, the myocardial cells are small, the myofibrils are few and disordered, and the reserve of myocardial contractility is limited. Therefore, maintaining a relatively fast heart rate is very important for these patients. In the present case, the heart rate was slow after the aorta cross-clamp was released. Isoproterenol was continuously infused at 0.05 μg/(kg·min) to maintain an appropriate heart rate, and temporary cardiac pacing leads were placed.
3. To timely use positive inotropic drugs: After the aorta cross-clamp was released, it is beneficial for the patient to be weaned off CPB smoothly by using positive inotropic drugs to enhance the function of the left ventricle and make the smaller volume left ventricle more adaptable to the sudden increase of preload.
4. To correct acid–base balance and electrolyte disorders: In the first few months after birth, the sarcoplasmic reticulum volume in neonates is smaller, and the calcium reserves are also less. However, the demand for exogenous calcium is relatively larger, which easily causes neonates to develop hypocalcemia and reduce myocardial contractility. Therefore, calcium gluconate should be routinely administered in these neonatal patients.

Postoperative metabolic acidosis is often related to tissue hypoxia and ischemia. Severe acidosis can cause cardiac pump dysfunction, coagulation dysfunction, and low or no response to catecholamines. Therefore, it is necessary to correct metabolic acidosis in time. Improving systemic circulation perfusion is the most effective way to prevent or treat metabolic acidosis.

5. Perioperative blood management is critical during neonatal anesthesia because the coagulation function of neonates, especially preterm neonates, is often abnormal, such as coagulation function reduction and hyperfibrinolysis. The acute hemodilution and the activation and consumption of coagulation factors and platelets caused by CPB further reduce neonates' coagulation function, making the hemostasis difficult during surgery. Low doses of lysine analogs, tranexamic acid (total dose 20 mg/kg), can effectively reduce the amount of bleeding and transfusion of allogeneic blood products during the perioperative period of cardiovascular surgery without increasing the incidence of postoperative seizures. Perioperative bedside coagulation function monitoring helps to observe the full picture of coagulation, guide component transfusion, and evaluate heparin residue. The coagulation and platelet function analyzer (Sonoclot) can predict abnormal bleeding after cardiac surgery and assess whether the platelet function is normal through the PF value, which helps to identify the cause of postoperative bleeding.

6. For obstructed TAPVC, overventilation should be avoided before CPB and obstruction relief because overventilation can reduce pulmonary vascular resistance, increase pulmonary blood flow, and thus aggravate pulmonary edema. In addition, any risk factors to reduce pulmonary vascular resistance will reduce the right-to-left shunt and exacerbate poor perfusion of the systemic circulation. After CPB, moderate overventilation and a higher inhaled oxygen concentration are needed to reduce pulmonary vascular resistance and alleviate the preload on the right ventricle.

12.6 Conclusion

In summary, proactive preoperative preparation, reasonable ventilation strategies, maintaining circulation, and homeostasis were the keys for children with obstructed TAPVC to safely pass through the perioperative period (Jingjing Lv).

13 Anesthetic Management of Surgical Repair of Obstructive Cor Triatriatum Sinister in a 3-Month-Old Female Infant

Yue Huang

Abstract

A 3-month-old female infant was brought to our hospital due to a heart murmur noted on a physical examination. The diagnosis of cor triatriatum sinister (obstruction), atrial septal defect (secundum), and pulmonary hypertension was made by transthoracic echocardiography, and surgery was proposed. In patients with obstructive cor triatriatum sinister, the return flow of blood from the pulmonary vein to the left heart was obstructed, which resulted in mild pulmonary hypertension (PH), and early surgery was required to relieve the obstruction. Physiologically, this condition is similar to mitral stenosis. The anesthetic strategies include avoiding tachycardia, ensuring myocardial contractility, maintaining blood volume, and avoiding hypotension. At the same time, it should also be noted to prevent an increase in pulmonary vascular resistance secondary to hypoxia and hypercapnia.

Cor triatriatum (CT) is a rare cardiac anomaly resulting from dividing the atrium into two chambers by a perforated fibromuscular septum. If the left atrium is involved, then the CT is also known as cor triatriatum sinister (CTS). If the right atrium is involved, it is called cor triatriatum dexter (CTD), with the latter being extremely rare and simple to treat surgically. CTS is reported to account for only 0.1–0.4% of all congenital heart malformations. In this case, we reported the anesthetic management of surgical repair of obstructive CTS in a 3-month-old female infant.

13.1 Case Presentation

A 3-month and 2-day-old term female infant (G1P1) with a weight of 6.0 kg and a height of 77 cm was brought to our hospital because of a heart murmur noted on a physical examination. There was no history of cyanosis, growth retardation, feeding difficulties, and recurrent respiratory infections, but there was a slight decrease in activity.

Physical examination: The baby presented with an axillary temperature of 36.8 °C, pulse rate at 136 beats per minute (bpm), respiratory rate at 32 bpm, and arm blood pressure at 86/52 mm Hg. She was conscious, had normal development, and had no obvious cyanosis. Clear breath sounds were heard in both lungs without any obvious dry or wet rales. There was no tremor in the precordial region and no sensation of elevation. The heart sounds were strong and rhythmic. Class III systolic murmur could be heard in

Y. Huang (✉)
The National Children's Medical Center (Shanghai), Department of Anesthesiology of Shanghai Children's Medical Center, Shanghai Jiao Tong University School of Medicine, Shanghai, China
e-mail: huangyue@scmc.com.cn

J. Zheng et al. (eds.), *Selected Pediatric Cardiovascular Surgery Anesthesia Cases*,
https://doi.org/10.1007/978-981-96-5614-1_13

the third to fourth intercostal space at the upper left sternal border and accentuated the pulmonary component of the second heart sound. The abdomen was flat and soft, and the liver and spleen were not palpable. The extremities were warm with no edema and clubbing.

Laboratory tests: Hb 104 g/L, TBIL 38.3 μmol/L, AST 66 U/L, NT-proBNP 1042 pg/mL, no apparent abnormalities in coagulation function.

Electrocardiogram (ECG): Sinus rhythm, right ventricular hypertrophy, left atrial hypertrophy, and I° atrioventricular block.

Chest radiograph: Cardiac chamber enlargement and increase of bilateral lung markings.

Transthoracic echocardiography (TTE): The left atrium was divided into proximal and distal atria by a horizontal membrane with an orifice of 0.31 cm, and the blood flow velocity through the orifice was 3.36 m/s, the pressure gradient was 45 mm Hg. All four pulmonary veins drain into the superior or proximal chamber. The atrial septal defect (ASD) was 1.33 cm (secundum) and located at the proximal chamber near the inferior vena cava with left-to-right shunting at the atrial level. The left ventricle was small, with acceptable contraction. The tricuspid annulus was measured at 2.0 cm with mild to moderate regurgitation; the regurgitant bundle width was 0.3 cm with a flow velocity of 3.27 m/s and a pressure gradient of 42.7 mm Hg. The interventricular septum was intact. All of which indicated Cor triatriatum (obstructive), Atrial septal defect (secundum), and Pulmonary hypertension (mild).

Chest CT: Double chambers in the left atrium with a horizontal membrane, normal pulmonary venous return. The atrial septal defect (secundum) was 15.1 × 15.9 mm. The right atrium and the right ventricle were enlarged. No significant stenosis exists in the outflow tracts of the left and right ventricles. Suggestions: ASD (II), CTS.

Preoperative diagnosis: CTS, ASD, PH.

13.2 Anesthetic Management

Upon entering the operating room, the basic vital signs included SpO_2 97%, HR (ECG) 132 bpm, and non-invasive blood pressure (NIBP) 78/52 mm Hg. Peripheral intravenous access was established for the induction by intravenous administration of midazolam 0.6 mg, etomidate 1.5 mg, sufentanil 12 μg, and rocuronium 3.6 mg. After the loss of eyelash reflex, the child was intubated with a cuffed ID 3.5 mm endotracheal tube under visual laryngoscopy, and mechanical ventilation was initiated. The depth of intubation was 11 cm. The left radial artery and right internal jugular vein were catheterization under ultrasound guidance for continuous monitoring of arterial blood pressure (ABP) and central venous pressure (CVP), respectively, and for periodic monitoring of arterial blood gases and electrolytes (Table 13.1). ABP and CVP were obtained after ultrasound-guided catheterization of the radial artery and right internal jugular vein, respectively. During the operation, pressure control ventilation (PCV) was applied with oxygen flow 2 L/min, a fraction of inspired oxygen (FiO_2) of 30–50%, Inspiratory time to expiratory time (I:E) of 1:2, Tidal Volume (VT) 45 mL. The end-tidal carbon dioxide partial pressure ($EtCO_2$) was maintained at 35–40 mm Hg by adjustment of the ventilation frequency and inspiratory pressure. Sufentanil 2.5 μg/(kg·h), propofol 4–5 mg/(kg·h), and rocuronium 0.6 mg/(kg·h) were continuously infused via a peripheral vein combined with sevoflurane intermittent inhalation at 1.0–2.5% to maintain the depth of anesthesia. The bispectral index (BIS) was maintained at 40–60.

After sternotomy, heparin sodium 18 mg was injected via the internal jugular vein. When activated clotting time (ACT) >480 s, surgery for CTS correction and ASD (secundum) repair was performed under cardiopulmonary bypass (CPB) with mild hypothermia. During the operation, it was found that the ASD was Type II with a diameter of 15 mm and close to the inferior vena cava. The left atrium was divided into an accessory chamber and a true chamber by a fibromuscular septum with a 3 mm orifice on the membrane. All four pulmonary veins drained into the accessory chamber. The membrane was completely excised, and the ASD was closed with continuous sutures using an autologous pericardial patch. There was no significant stenosis in the pulmonary veins. The heart resumed spontaneous sinus rhythm

Table 13.1 Intraoperative arterial blood gas and electrolyte analysis result

	pH	PaO_2 (mm Hg)	$PaCO_2$ (mm Hg)	Lac (mmol/L)	HCT (%)	ABE (mmol/L)	Na^+ (mmol/L)	K^+ (mmol/L)	Ca^{2+} (mmol/L)	Cl^- (mmol/L)
Post-induction	7.41	535	34.5	1.7	35.9	−1.8	147	4.07	1.07	110
Post-CPB	7.33	324	38.5	2.0	26.6	−5.2	141	5.0	0.86	103

after the release of the aortic cross-clamp. Dopamine at 5.0 μg/(kg·min) and epinephrine at 0.03 μg/(kg·min) were intravenously administered to maintain ABP around 70/40 mm Hg, HR of around 130 bpm. Pressure control ventilation was resumed with moderate hyperventilation to maintain an $EtCO_2$ level between 30 and 40 mm Hg. Transesophageal echocardiography (TEE) showed no residual membrane in the left atrium and unobstructed pulmonary venous return. After modified ultrafiltration, protamine sulfate was infused at a ratio of 1.2:1 to reverse the effects of heparin, and thrombin was administered to improve coagulation function. Arterial blood gases and electrolytes were rechecked with BE of 5.2 mmol/L and Ca^{2+} of 0.86 mmol/L. Metabolic acidosis was corrected with intravenous administration of 5% sodium bicarbonate 9 mL. Hypocalcemia was treated with a slow infusion of calcium gluconate 200 mg. The dosage of vasoactive drugs was adjusted based on blood pressure. Autologous blood 60 mL was infused to maintain ABP around 80/45 mm Hg and HR around 130–160 bpm. The sternum was closed after satisfactory hemostasis.

13.3 Postoperative Outcome

The operation lasted 120 min, with a CPB time of 59 min and an aortic cross-clamp time of 20 min. The estimated blood loss was about 200 mL. The total urine output was 70 mL. A total of 60 mL of sodium acetate Ringer's solution and 60 mL of autologous blood were transfused. Blood lactate levels remained within the normal range throughout the surgery. At the end of the procedure, the patient presented with ABP 82/45 mm Hg, HR 145 bpm, SpO_2 100%, CVP 14 cm H_2O, and rectal temperature 36.5 °C. She was transferred to the Cardiac Intensive Care Unit (CICU) with manual ventilation assistance under the monitoring of ABP, ECG, and SpO_2. The patient was extubated on the second postoperative day, discharged from the CICU on the third postoperative day, and discharged from the hospital on the fifth postoperative day.

13.4 Review of Knowledge Points

13.4.1 Pathophysiology

In CTS, the pulmonary venous blood generally enters the proximal or superior chamber, which is then drained into the distal or inferior chamber (true atrium) by a single orifice or multiple orifices. There is a fibromuscular septum between the accessory atrium and the true atrium. Most cases have an orifice on the septum. Blood flow from the proximal to the distal chamber depends on the size and number of fenestrations in the fibromuscular membrane. If the blood flow from the accessory atrium to the true atrium is significantly restricted by the orifice size, a pressure gradient within the atria is produced, and the patients can develop some clinical features similar to mitral stenosis, exertional dyspnea, telangiectasia, pulmonary edema, and pulmonary hypertension. If the communication between the proximal chamber and the right atrium causes significant right-to-left shunting, the pathophysiological changes resemble total anomalous pulmonary venous return.

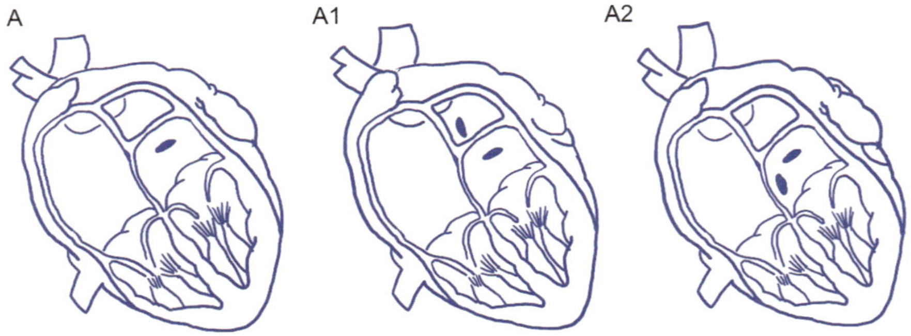

Fig. 13.1 Classification of cor triatriatum according to Lam et al. (type A, A1, and A2)

13.4.2 Anatomical Features and Classification

Several classification schemes have been reported to describe CTS. Lam's typing is the most commonly used. In type A, a proximal chamber receives all pulmonary venous blood flows, and a distal chamber contains the left atrial appendage and the mitral valve. There is communication through one or more fenestrations in the membrane between a proximal chamber and a distal chamber. According to the presence and location of an ASD, type A can be further subdivided. The ASD is located between the right atrium and the proximal chamber in subtype A1, whereas it is between the right atrium and distal chamber in type A2 (Fig. 13.1). In type B, all pulmonary venous blood returns to an enlarged coronary sinus, which is a form of TAPVC. In type C, there is no connection between the pulmonary veins and the proximal chamber. Type A is the most common form (64%), followed by subtype A1 (18%).

13.4.3 Surgical Management

Surgical resection of the fibromuscular septum is the definitive treatment and can generally be performed as an elective surgery. However, in infants and children with symptoms of heart failure or pulmonary congestion due to obstructive CTS, corrective surgery should be performed urgently. Surgery usually involves the removal of the fibromuscular membrane to allow unobstructed blood flow from the pulmonary veins to the mitral valve through median sternotomy with CPB support under normothermia or mild hypothermia. Treatment with balloon catheter dilatation has also been reported.

13.5 Discussion

13.5.1 Preoperative Assessment and Preparation

Children with CTS have many different clinical manifestations and pathophysiological characteristics depending on the anatomical subtype. Preoperative echocardiography can confirm the diagnosis and subtype. In children with a small orifice(s) in the membrane between the accessory and true chamber accompanied by an obstruction, pulmonary venous return is obstructed. Attention should be paid to the symptoms of PH or pulmonary congestion preoperatively. Tachycardia and increased PVR should be avoided during the perioperative period. Children with obstructive CTS may also have varying degrees of left ventricular hypoplasia and affect left heart function, which should be carefully evaluated during preoperative visits. In addition, 12–50% of children with CTS have other cardiac anomalies requiring targeted management based on the comorbidities. In this case, preoperative echocardiography revealed an orifice of 0.31 cm in the membrane with a perforated blood flow velocity at 3.36 m/s and a pressure gradient of 45 mm Hg, suggesting that the blood flow into the true chamber was restricted, and there was an obstruction. However, due to the relatively short duration of the disease, the child had not yet shown the symptoms of pulmonary congestion or PH. Echocardiography also indicated a smaller left ventricle but adequate contraction activity. Therefore, perioperative myocardial protection and support of cardiac function after weaning off CPB are important considerations.

13.5.2 Anesthetic Management Before CPB

1. Maintaining normal sinus rhythm
   Maintaining a normal sinus rhythm is better, allowing maximum blood flow across the intra-atrial membrane and facilitating ventricular filling. In this case, the preoperative ECG showed sinus rhythm. During surgery, arterial blood samples were periodically drawn for blood gas analysis to help promptly correct fluid, electrolyte, and acid–base imbalance, which can help prevent arrhythmias. All patients with CTS and symptoms should be medically managed, and the fast ventricular rate should also be controlled. Conversely, severe bradycardia can be equally detrimental.
2. Maintaining moderate preload
   Moderate preload before CPB is beneficial to increase the blood flow through the orifice in the membrane. However, excessive fluid loading due to an insufficient number or a limited size of orifice(s) can lead to cardiac decompensation. The margin between fluid underloading and overloading is narrow, thus posing a challenge in perioperative fluid management. After the relief of the obstruction, preload can be appropriately increased to ensure cardiac output.
3. Regulation of pulmonary vascular resistance
   The common cause of PH in children with CTS is usually due to obstruction of pulmonary venous blood to the left atrium, known as postcapillary PH. The preoperative echocardiography indicated that the blood flow into the true atrium was restricted, potentially resulting in pulmonary venous return obstruction, pulmonary congestion, and pulmonary edema, and PVR and pulmonary artery pressure increase because of the elevated pressure at the venous end of the pulmonary circulation. In addition, increased right ventricular pressure causes leftward deviation of the interventricular septum and further reduction of left ventricular volume, which can result in severe impairment of cardiac output and organ perfusion. Restriction of left atrial outflow also increases left-to-right shunting and right ventricular dilation. Children with pulmonary venous return obstruction usually have higher PVR. The use of larger doses of fentanyl or sufentanil is beneficial to reduce the increase in PVR caused by surgical stress. Before CPB, attempts to increase pulmonary blood flow by hyperventilation or using pulmonary vasodilators should be avoided because they can aggravate the pulmonary edema.

13.5.3 Anesthetic Management After CPB

Surgery for CTS, especially when combined with other cardiac anomalies, is complex and involves multiple intracardiac operations. These operations can easily damage the cardiac conduction bundle and lead to an atrioventricular (AV) block. The suture site's traction on the conduction bundle can also cause tissue injury and edema, which can also cause a conduction block. Myocardial ischemia, hypoxia, and reperfusion injury are likely to cause postoperative malignant arrhythmias, even cardiac arrest. Early detection and intervention are crucial.

1. Regulation of right ventricular function and pulmonary vascular resistance
   Preoperative pulmonary vein return obstruction can cause PH in children with CTS, pul-

monary vein congestion, and pulmonary artery pressure may be reduced after CPB, which can be confirmed by echocardiography. However, some children may still show postoperative high PVR due to irreversible changes in the pulmonary vascular bed from long-term pulmonary congestion. Adjusting mechanical ventilation parameters for moderate hyperventilation and avoiding hypercapnia and acidosis can help lower PVR as much as possible. Selective pulmonary vasodilators, such as inhaled nitric oxide, may be needed if pulmonary hypertension persists.

2. Low cardiac output syndrome
Low cardiac output syndrome (LCOS) is a major and quite severe complication following corrective surgery for infants with CTS. It is often related to varying degrees of left ventricular hypoplasia in these patients. This case had potential left ventricular hypoplasia before surgery and required intravenously infusing dopamine at 5.0 μg/(kg·min) and epinephrine at 0.03 μg/(kg·min) to increase myocardial contractility after the release of aortic cross-clamp, while closely monitoring circulatory function. Given the child's age or disease-specific challenges, preoperative placement of a pulmonary artery catheter to monitor cardiac output may be difficult. Therefore, transesophageal echocardiography would be the most appropriate monitoring technique to assess cardiac performance. The ventricular function can be evaluated by short-axis views of the left ventricle and the mid-esophageal four-chamber view, especially the myocardial contractility and volume status.

13.6 Conclusion

Although obstruction occurred in this case, the child tolerated the surgery and anesthesia well due to the relatively short course of the disease, which had not yet shown significant symptoms. However, suppose the child develops symptoms of pulmonary congestion or clinical manifestations similar to mitral stenosis.

In that case, the principles of anesthetic management for such cardiac lesions can be referred to, which need to monitor the cardiac function and the volume status closely. In addition, timely intervention is also required (Yue Huang).

14 Anesthetic Management of PDA Ligation in Extremely Low Birth Weight Infants

Ying Sun

Abstract

The patient, one of the twins, presented with respiratory distress immediately after birth. Post-admission echocardiography indicated: ventricular septal defect (VSD), atrial septal defect (ASD), and patent ductus arteriosus (PDA). After conservative treatment with ibuprofen to promote arterial duct closure combined with cardiac function support and mechanical ventilation, the arterial duct did not close. The respiratory and circulatory functions were not improved either. Multidisciplinary consultation suggested: PDA ligation under non-extracorporeal circulation first, and then VSD and ASD repair should be done when right. The anesthetic management of PDA ligation in these infants should be based on the physiological characteristics of extremely low birth weight infants and the pathophysiology of patent ductus arteriosus, maintaining age-appropriate heart rate and blood pressure during surgery to ensure perfusion of vital organs. Strengthen ventilation management to avoid hypoxia and acidosis and pay attention to perioperative temperature management.

Y. Sun (✉)
The National Children's Medical Center (Shanghai), Department of Anesthesiology of Shanghai Children's Medical Center, Shanghai Jiao Tong University School of Medicine, Shanghai, China
e-mail: sunying@scmc.com.cn

The ductus arteriosus is a physiological connection between the pulmonary artery and the descending aorta in the neonatal period. In normal newborns, the ductus arteriosus naturally closes within a few days after birth as arterial oxygen levels increase. In this special group of preterm infants, the probability of natural closure of the ductus arteriosus is inversely proportional to the gestational week. The patent ductus arteriosus (PDA) incidence can be as high as 60%. If the ductus arteriosus remains open, persistent ductal shunting can lead to over-circulation in the lungs, increasing the risk of pulmonary hemorrhage, pulmonary hypertension, and bronchopulmonary dysplasia. Meanwhile, shunting can lead to systemic perfusion insufficiency and increase the risk of necrotizing enterocolitis, intraventricular hemorrhage, renal failure, and death. Extremely low birth weight infants refer to preterm infants with a birth weight of <1500 g. The special pathophysiology of PDA challenges anesthetic management because the development of various aspects of extremely low birth weight infants is not perfected.

14.1 Case Presentation

The male patient (one of the twins), weighing 1.4 kg, was 31 weeks and 6 days gestation. He was delivered by cesarean section due to twin pregnancy, selective intrauterine growth restric-

J. Zheng et al. (eds.), *Selected Pediatric Cardiovascular Surgery Anesthesia Cases*,
https://doi.org/10.1007/978-981-96-5614-1_14

tion, and advanced maternal age. His birth weight was 1320 g with an Apgar score of 9, clear amniotic fluid, normal placenta, and normal umbilical cord. He was intravenously given 10% dextrose 2.5 mL in the maternity hospital due to postnatal hypoglycemia (2.2 mmol/L). Pulmonary surfactant (Curosurf) 120 mg was intratracheally given due to preterm birth and neonatal respiratory distress. He was then transferred to our hospital by ambulance. The admission diagnosis was preterm infant, extremely low birth weight infant, neonatal respiratory distress syndrome, and neonatal hypoglycemia. After admission, echocardiography showed ventricular septal defect (VSD), atrial septal defect (ASD), and PDA. He was given digoxin and spironolactone to improve myocardial contractility and increase urine output. Noninvasive continuous positive airway pressure (NCPAP) was given for ventilation support. Ibuprofen was given orally to promote PDA closure. After two courses of treatment, echocardiography showed that PDA was still not closed yet. The circulatory and respiratory function was not improved. It was difficult to maintain normal oxygenation by N-CPAP. Endotracheal intubation was then performed, and invasive ventilation was conducted with a ventilator. Both cardiologists and cardiac surgeons thought that it was an extremely high risk to perform VSD and ASD repair + PDA ligation under cardiopulmonary bypass (CPB) at this time. In order to improve the respiratory and circulatory function, protect the pulmonary vascular bed, and improve the perfusion of the systemic circulation, PDA ligation could be performed under non-CPB support VSD and ASD could be repaired when the timing was appropriate.

Physical examination: The patient was placed in an incubator with mechanical ventilation with PC-AC + VG mode (parameters: Fraction of inspired Oxygen (FiO_2) 25%, tidal volume (VT) 6 mL/time, time of inspiration (Ti) 0.34 s, respiration rate (RR) 50 times/min, positive end-expiratory pressure (PEEP) 5 cm H_2O, pulse oxygen saturation (SpO_2) 89–92%, heart rate (HR) 165–170 beats/min, noninvasive blood pressure (BP) was 69/31 mm Hg with dopamine 5.0 μg/(kg·min) and dobutamine 5.0 μg/(kg·min) maintenance. The patient was conscious, responsive, regular heart rhythm, strong heart sounds, and grade III cardiac murmur. Coarse breath sounds were heard in both lungs without rales. The liver was 2–3 cm below the ribs, slightly tough. The skin all over the body was slightly edematous. The extremities were somewhat cold.

Laboratory test: Routine blood tests, liver and kidney function, coagulation function, and blood gas were almost normal.

Echocardiography: Patent ductus arteriosus 0.35 cm, bidirectional shunt, mainly left to right shunt, flow rate 1.5 m/s. Perimembranous fusion type VSD 0.39 cm, left to right shunt 1.5 m/s, ASD (II) with two parts (0.78 cm and 0.22 cm, respectively), left to right shunt. The right atrium and right ventricle were slightly enlarged, and the left ventricular systolic activity was normal without pericardial effusion. The ratio for the left atrium to the aortic root (La/Ao) was 1.63, which was greater than the normal value of 1.4.

Preoperative diagnosis: Preterm birth, VSD, ASD, PDA, heart failure. Elective PDA ligation surgery was planned.

14.2 Anesthetic Management

The patient was transported to the operating room without preoperative medication. He was intubated with respiratory bag-assisted ventilation (spontaneous breathing retained). On admission, electrocardiogram, noninvasive BP, and SpO_2 were monitored. The right upper limb blood pressure was 80/39 mm Hg, HR 168 beats/min, and SpO_2 90%. The right elbow vein (24 G) catheterization was already performed. Dopamine 5.0 μg/(kg·min) and dobutamine 5.0 μg/(kg·min) were maintained by continuous intravenous infusion. Anesthesia was induced with intravenous bolus doses of etomidate 0.3 mg, sufentanil 1.0 μg, and rocuronium bromide 1.0 mg. Pressure control ventilation was used with respiratory parameters set as oxygen flow rate 1 L/min, FiO_2 30%, VT 4–6 mL, RR 50 beats/min, inspiratory time to expiratory time (I:E) ratio 1:2, and PEEP 5 cm H_2O. The respiratory parameters were adjusted during surgery to maintain end-tidal carbon dioxide ($ETCO_2$) at 35–45 mmHg.

After induction of anesthesia, the right femoral artery and right internal jugular vein were catheterized under ultrasound guidance for continuously monitoring invasive blood pressure (ABP) and central venous pressure (CVP).Sevoflurane intermittent inhalation was used to maintain anesthesia. Intraoperative temperature was observed, and active insulation measures such as warm air blankets and fluid warming were given. The total operative time was 50 min with estimated bleeding of about 5 mL, urine output of 2 mL, and infusion of Ringer's acetate solution of 10 mL.

No significant hemodynamic changes were seen after PDA ligation. At the end of the operation, invasive femoral arterial blood pressure was 45/31 mm Hg, the noninvasive blood pressure in the right upper extremity was 66/40 mm Hg, HR 163 beats/min, SpO_2 90%, CVP 8 cm H_2O, and anal temperature 36.5 °C.

14.3 Postoperative Outcome

After surgery, he was transferred to the Neonatal Intensive Care Unit with endotracheal intubation under invasive blood pressure and SpO_2 monitoring. Cardiac function improved on the seventh postoperative day, and then the mechanical ventilation was replaced by the noninvasive ventilation support after endotracheal tube removal. Two weeks later, high-flow nasal cannula oxygen therapy (HFNC) replaced the noninvasive ventilation support. Three weeks later, the noninvasive ventilation support was then replaced by nasal cannula oxygen therapy. The patient was discharged from hospital on the 38th day postoperatively.

14.4 Review of Knowledge Points

14.4.1 The Harm of PDA in Premature Infants

The incidence of PDA in preterm infants is inversely proportional to gestational age. Persistent opening of the PDA in preterm infants is due to the low oxygen sensitivity of immature ductus arteriosus and the lack of middle-layer muscle in the ductus arteriosus. The possibility of natural closure of PDA in preterm infants is small. The shunt between the systemic circulation and pulmonary circulation can cause some serious complications, such as pulmonary hemorrhage, bronchopulmonary dysplasia (BPD), intraventricular hemorrhage (IVH), and necrotizing enterocolitis (NEC), which can significantly increase the mortality rate of the patient.

14.4.2 Advancements in Drug Treatment for PDA in Preterm Infants

The treatments of PDA mainly include pharmacological or surgical treatment. Nonsteroidal anti-inflammatory drugs (NSAIDs) are usually used for pharmacological closure of PDA, with ibuprofen being the current first-line drug. The levels of blood prostaglandins in patients with persistent opening of the ductus arteriosus are usually high. Therefore, NSAIDs can be used to facilitate the closure of PDA due to the inhibition of prostaglandin production. Prostaglandins are produced from the conversion of arachidonic acid by prostaglandin-H synthase, which has two distinct catalytic activities, including cyclooxygenase activity and peroxidase activity. Indomethacin and ibuprofen inhibit the conversion of arachidonic acid to prostaglandins by inhibiting cyclooxygenase and are the two most commonly used drugs for PDA closure. Acetaminophen reduces the production of prostaglandins by inhibiting peroxidase. Indomethacin can cause more side effects than ibuprofen, which has now been largely replaced by ibuprofen. Ibuprofen is contraindicated in those patients with renal failure, severe hyperbilirubinemia, sepsis, necrotizing enterocolitis, gastrointestinal perforation, active bleeding at any site, severe thrombocytopenia, and hypersensitivity to ibuprofen. When ibuprofen is contraindicated, acetaminophen is the only treatment option.

14.4.3 Indications for Surgical Correction of PDA in Preterm Infants

Early intervention treatment is recommended for PDA with hemodynamically significant PDA (hsPDA) and/or clinically significant PDA. hsPDA is determined by the size of the shunt bundle of the arterial catheter, the degree of volume overload of the pulmonary circulation, the volume of pulmonary blood perfusion, and the systemic risk. The degree of pulmonary blood perfusion and the degree of systemic hypoperfusion are the main criteria for hsPDA. The current surgical indications in our hospital are as follows: For infants with a PDA diameter of more than 1. 5 mm and a ratio of 1.4 or greater for left atrium to aortic root, weighing less than 1500 g, regardless of whether it is hsPDA, ibuprofen is used for two courses first, and then the cardiac ultrasound is reperformed. If PDA is still >0.15 cm, La/Ao >1.4, surgery is required.

Clinically, arterial duct ligation is usually performed through a left posterior lateral incision for infants weighing less than 3 kg. This incision is larger and more traumatic than the axillary straight incision but has a clearer field of vision and ensures a safe surgical operation. PDA ligation in preterm infants significantly reduces mortality without increasing the risk of adverse complications such as chronic lung disease, retinopathy of prematurity, and neurodevelopmental disorders.

14.5 Discussion

The anesthetic management of extremely low birth weight infants undergoing PDA ligation should be based on their physiological characteristics and the pathophysiology of patent ductus arteriosus, emphasizing refined management to reduce anesthesia-related complications.

14.5.1 Preoperative Assessment and Preparation

During the preoperative visit, attention should be paid to the infant's gestational age, weight, birth conditions, lung development status, intubated or not, ventilator parameter settings, and the use of vasoactive drugs. Review the medical history, imaging data, and laboratory test results to assess the overall condition and heart and lung function. Prepare anesthesia machines and monitoring equipment suitable for extremely low birth weight infants, increase the operating room's temperature, equip them with corresponding warming blankets, etc. Some centers choose to complete this kind of surgery in the NICU to avoid a drop in body temperature during transport. Therefore, temperature management during transport is particularly important.

14.5.2 Intraoperative Anesthetic Management

Issues related to arterial and venous puncture: The extremely low weight of the infant poses a great challenge to arterial and venous catheterization, which can cause a relatively high incidence of complications related to arterial and venous catheterization. How can we increase the success rate of catheterization? How can we reduce the incidence of complications? How to evaluate the benefits and risks of catheterization? These are all difficult problems in the anesthesia of extremely low birth weight infants. Invasive arterial pressure monitoring may benefit major surgery or critically ill patients, facilitating real-time invasive blood pressure monitoring and arterial blood gas sampling. However, when arterial catheterization faces a high failure rate and incidence of complications, we may use noninvasive blood pressure monitoring and oxygen saturation waveform analysis to replace invasive blood pressure monitoring. For this patient, establishing invasive blood pressure monitoring of the lower limb artery was to enable the surgeon to detect in time if the descending aorta was mistakenly ligated. In addition, simultaneous monitoring of upper and lower limb oxygen saturation or blood pressure can also detect this mistake.

Performing arterial catheterization and central venous catheterization under ultrasound guidance is better. Ultrasound-guided arterial and venous catheterization can significantly increase the success rate and reduce the incidence of complications, especially in newborns and premature infants. The depth of internal jugular vein catheterization in extremely low birth weight infants is sometimes difficult to control. The internal jugular vein in newborns, premature infants, and extremely low birth weight infants is thinner, the subcutaneous tissue is thinner, and the superior vena cava is even shorter, which makes it easy to place it too deeply but also easy to slip it out if it is too shallow. Research has found that the correlation between the depth of central venous catheterization and weight is the best, with the depth of catheterization = 0.7 × weight (kg) + 2.6 ($R^2 = 0.723$, weight 580–3980 g). In this case, the patient's weight was 1.4 kg, and the depth of placement in the right neck was 3.5 cm, which was basically consistent with the above formula.

Selection of anesthetic induction and maintenance drugs: The fetal heart has more connective tissue and less contractile tissue than the infant heart and is more dependent on extracellular calcium ion concentration. The fetal heart's compliance is poorer, the Frank–Starling curve is flatter, and it is less sensitive to catecholamines. The heart rate is faster at rest, the cardiac output is mainly dependent on the heart rate, and the cardiac functional reserve is lower.

Anesthetic induction for immature infants undergoing PDA ligation is mainly based on a large dose of opioids and muscle relaxants. Of those opioids, fentanyl or sufentanil is usually chosen to ensure minimal suppression of myocardial contractility and sufficient HR. It is recommended to use atracurium as a muscle relaxant. For extremely low birth weight infants, 30–50 μg/kg of fentanyl and atracurium show stable hemodynamic performance with blood pressure fluctuations within 5% and no fluctuations in blood pressure and heart rate during skin incision. Studies have shown that plasma concentrations did not change for 120 min after 30 μg/kg of fentanyl was administered intravenously. The half-life of fentanyl in extremely low birth weight infants is as long as 6–32 h, compared to approximately 2–3 h in children and adults. The lower clearance and metabolism rates of opioids and such a long half-life indicate that almost no additional opioids or maintenance are needed during the operation. The longer mechanical ventilation time after surgery in such patients is also related to the pharmacokinetics and pharmacodynamics of opioids.

Perioperative blood pressure control and monitoring: Regarding blood pressure control before PDA ligation, extremely low birth weight infants generally do not need to achieve controlled hypotension through antihypertensive drugs. In this case, the child was maintained with sevoflurane inhalation anesthesia during the operation. The systolic pressure was controlled at 40–50 mm Hg during PDA ligation. It should be noted that the total blood volume of extremely low birth weight infants is very low, about 140 mL for a 1.4 kg patient. Therefore, small bleeding will account for a larger percentage of the total blood volume. Communication between the anesthesiologist and the surgeon can decide whether the red blood cells are needed to apply for standby before surgery.

Unexpectedly, the lower limb arterial blood pressure (ABP 45/31 mmHg) of the child in this case was significantly lower than the upper limb blood pressure (BP 66/40 mmHg) after the operation. Bedside transthoracic echocardiography confirmed that the child also had aortic arch stenosis.

Ventilation management and monitoring of end-tidal carbon dioxide: Severe hypoxemia and hypercapnia may occur in children during the operation due to the lateral position, plus the pulling and compression of lung tissues by surgical operation. Therefore, the respiratory function must be carefully assessed in patients with preoperative ventilation or oxygenation difficulties in case of surgical intolerance. Theoretically, a normal or slightly elevated carbon dioxide level should be maintained prior to PDA ligation. The concentration of inhalation oxygen should also be controlled in order to reduce the left-to-right shunt and control the pulmonary blood flow. However, hypoxia and severe acidosis should also be avoided to avoid exacerbating pulmonary hypertension. In neonates and preterm infants with rapid respiratory rate and small tidal volume, percutaneous carbon dioxide monitoring may be more accurate than side stream $ETCO_2$. Therefore, percutaneous carbon dioxide monitoring is recommended in these patients. Because extremely low birth weight infants have a low absolute blood volume, frequent blood sampling for blood gas analysis during surgery is not recommended.

Temperature management: Raising room temperature and using warm air blankets are very effective insulation measures. Attention should also be paid to insulation during transportation to prevent rapid heat loss.

14.6 Shortcomings and Limitations

Due to the lack of percutaneous carbon dioxide monitors, we still used side-stream $ETCO_2$ monitoring during surgery, which may have masked the increase of $ETCO_2$ to a certain extent due to its limited accuracy.

14.7 Conclusion

In conclusion, PDA ligation surgery in extremely low birth weight infants poses great challenges for both surgeons and anesthesiologists. A well-coordinated team with qualified neonatal specialists, including medical, surgical, and anesthetic members, is a guarantee of successful surgery (Ying Sun).

Anesthetic Management of Neonatal Ductus Arteriosus Aneurysm Resection

15

Ying Sun

Abstract

A 2-day-old male infant was referred to our hospital due to shortness of breath. Echocardiography indicated an arteriovenous duct aneurysm and severe left pulmonary artery compression. An emergency arteriovenous duct aneurysm resection under general anesthesia was planned. Preoperative transfer and anesthesia induction risks in such patients are very high. Therefore, the surgeon team should be present during the transfer and anesthesia induction process. Adequate sedation and analgesia, immobilization, and sufficient depth of anesthesia are required during the perioperative period. In addition, the site of arterial catheterization must be matched with the surgical plan, so that the surgical efficacy can be timely and effectively assessed.

Ductus arteriosus aneurysm (DAA) is an aneurysmal expansion of the arteriovenous duct, which is incidentally detected by echocardiography in most patients. Although fetal DAA is usually not associated with adverse consequences, adverse events such as rupture, infection, and compression of adjacent tissue structures can occur in infant or adult patients, requiring emergency surgery to remove the DAA. In this case, a 2-day-old neonate was diagnosed with DAA complicated by severe compression of the left pulmonary artery. Therefore, it was necessary to perform DAA resection to relieve the compression on the left pulmonary artery. It is not common to perform emergency DAA resection under general anesthesia in neonates, and we hope to gain further experience by using this case as an example.

15.1 Case Presentation

A 2-day-old male neonate was born full term (38 weeks gestation) by cesarean section due to gestational diabetes mellitus in the mother. He was 3.8 kg in weight and was admitted to the emergency room due to two episodes of cyanosis after choking on milk and shortness of breath for half a day. After admission, the patient was seen to have shortness of breath, moaning, and respiratory distress with suprasternal retraction. Then, he was urgently intubated in the emergency room. After intubation, the patient was transferred to the Neonatal Intensive Care Unit (NICU) for continued mechanical ventilation and anti-inflammatory treatment. The patient's vital signs were stable. Due to severe compression of the left pulmonary artery, it was decided to perform emergency exploratory surgery under general anesthesia. The echocardiography from the

Y. Sun (✉)
The National Children's Medical Center (Shanghai), Department of Anesthesiology of Shanghai Children's Medical Center, Shanghai Jiao Tong University School of Medicine, Shanghai, China
e-mail: sunying@scmc.com.cn

J. Zheng et al. (eds.), *Selected Pediatric Cardiovascular Surgery Anesthesia Cases*,
https://doi.org/10.1007/978-981-96-5614-1_15

local hospital showed an atrial septal defect (ASD, II) and pulmonary artery embolism.

Laboratory tests: The preoperative blood routine, liver and kidney function, coagulation function, and blood gas analysis showed no obvious abnormalities.

Echocardiography: ASD (septum secundum), bidirectional shunt at the atrial level, with a predominantly left-to-right shunt. A saclike cavity was seen at the distal end of the aortic arch, communicating with the descending aorta with back-and-forth blood flow. Two medium sizes of echo masses were seen inside, measuring 0.9 cm × 0.99 cm and 0.23 cm × 0.25 cm, respectively. The pulmonary artery trunk and the left pulmonary artery were compressed before the bifurcation. The flow speed of the pulmonary artery trunk before the bifurcation was 1.1 m/s. The flow bundle at the left pulmonary artery opening was about 0.19 cm in width; the flow rate was 3.0 m/s, and the pressure difference was 36 mm Hg (Fig. 15.1).

Chest CT showed concordant ventricular-aortic connection, left arch, no obvious aortic stenosis, arteriovenous duct aneurysmal expansion with a diameter of about 8.8 mm, and possible closure near the pulmonary artery end. Abnormal density shadow around the arteriovenous duct with enhanced CT value 86–110 HU protruded to the main pulmonary artery and compressed the origin of the left pulmonary artery; the origin of the left pulmonary artery was almost obstructed by severe stenosis. The distal end of the left pulmonary was about 2.4 mm. The right pulmonary artery was well developed, with the origin and distal end both about 6.7 mm (Fig. 15.2).

Cranial and abdominal ultrasound: No obvious abnormalities were observed.

Preoperative diagnosis: Neonatal pneumonia, respiratory failure, ASD, and pulmonary artery embolism.

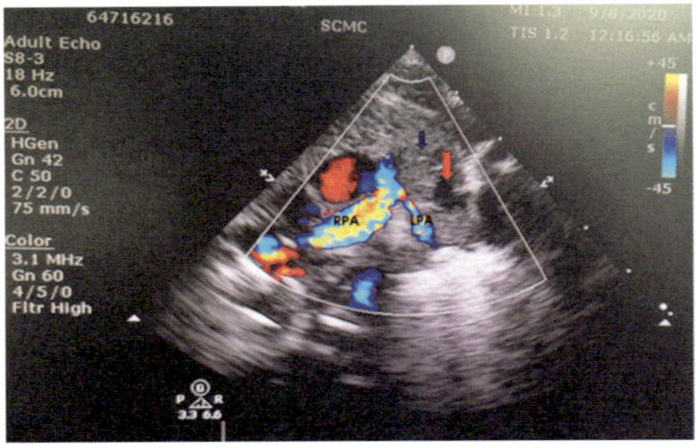

Fig. 15.1 Echocardiography of DAA compressing the left pulmonary artery. *RPA* right pulmonary artery, *LPA* left pulmonary artery. Blue arrow indicates thrombus, red arrow indicates tumor cavity

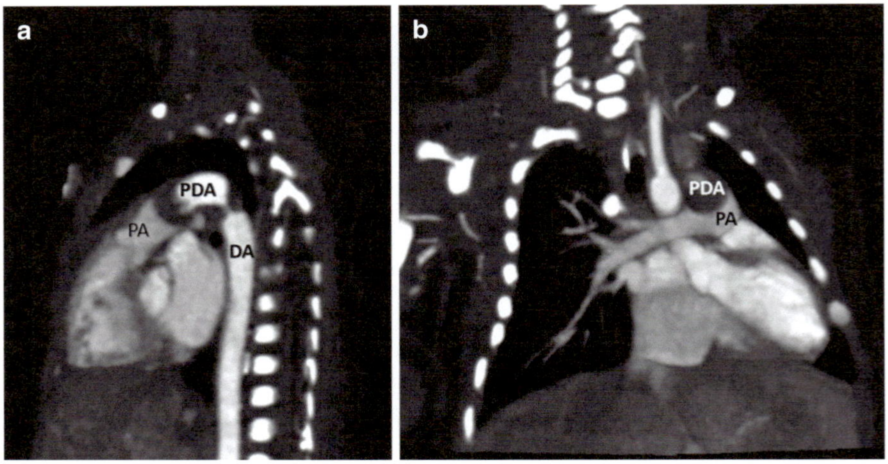

Fig. 15.2 CT image of DAA. (**a**) abnormally large PDA; (**b**) thrombus formation around PDA, compressing the pulmonary artery

15.2 Anesthetic Management

The patient was on mechanical ventilation in the NICU with normal-frequency ventilator PC-AC mode before the operation. The ventilation parameters were set as a fraction of inspired oxygen fraction (FiO_2) 30%, peak inspiratory pressure (PIP) 13 cm H_2O, positive end-expiratory pressure (PEEP)5 cm H_2O, inspiratory time (Ti) 0.42 s, and respiratory rate (RR) of 45 breaths/min. Midazolam 0.5 μg/(kg·min) was used for sedation, cefotaxime, and penicillin sodium for anti-inflammatory treatment, fasting, and fluid replacement were implemented. The patient's oxygenation was good, and hemodynamics was stable. Midazolam 0.3 mg and rocuronium bromide 2.0 mg were intravenously given for adequate sedation and muscle relaxation before transfer. The patient was smoothly transferred to the operating room under electrocardiogram (ECG) and pulse oxygen saturation (SpO_2) monitoring. The heart rate (HR) was 145–156 beats/min, blood pressure (BP) was around 65/42 mm Hg, and SpO_2 was 95%.

After entering the operating room, the patient was ventilated with pressure-controlled ventilation (PCV) mode with the following ventilator parameter settings: FiO_2 30%, PIP 20 cm H_2O, RR 28 breaths/min, tidal volume (VT) 35 mL, and kept warm by a warm air blanket. Anesthesia was first induced by intravenous injection of sufentanil 7.0 μg and etomidate 1.2 mg, then maintained by intravenous infusion of propofol 4.0 mg/(kg·h), sufentanil 2.0 μg/(kg·h), and rocuronium bromide 0.5 mg/(kg·h). Considering that the child was undergoing surgery at the PDA site, the right radial artery and right femoral artery were catheterized with ultrasound guidance for invasive artery blood pressure monitoring since the surgical operation might involve the descending part of the aortic arch. The right internal jugular vein was catheterization for central venous pressure (CVP) measurement, transfusion of blood and fluids, and administration of medications. The results of Preoperative blood gas analysis were: pH 7.42, PO_2 59.9 mm Hg, PCO_2 29 mm Hg, K^+ 3.61 mmol/L, Ca^{2+} 1.10 mmol/L, BE −4.5 mmol/L, Lac 1.5 mmol/L. The process of thoracotomy and establishing cardiopulmonary bypass (CPB) was smooth. After cardiac arrest, the PDA was found to be abnormally large with plaques inside. After opening the main trunk of the pulmonary artery longitudinally (Fig. 15.3), two large intercalated aneurysms were found inside. The aneurysm at the proximal end of the pulmonary artery was removed smoothly. The anatomical relationship between the aneurysm at the distal end and the descending aorta was unclear. Therefore, the aneurysm was isolated from the aorta by deep hypothermia circulatory arrest, and the aortic end of the PDA was sutured closed, and then the circulation was restored, the ASD was closed, and the pericardial patch was used to repair the pulmonary artery. After the aorta cross-clamp was released, the heart resumed beating automatically. Dopamine 5.0 μg/(kg·min) was intravenously administered. There was no pressure difference between the upper and lower limbs blood pressure. CPB was weaned off after suction 10 minutes of parallel circulation assis-

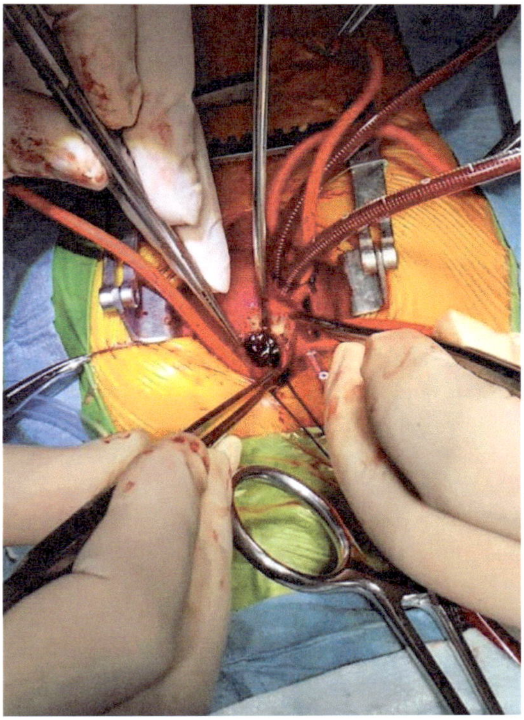

Fig. 15.3 Tumor body of the arterial duct tumor in the pulmonary artery

tance. Modified ultrafiltration took about 10 minutes. Blood gas analysis results: pH 7.39, PO_2 60 mm Hg, PCO_2 36 mm Hg, K^+ 3. 6 mmol/L, Ca^{2+} 1.16 mmol/L, BE −3.0 mmol/L, Lac 2.7 mmol/L. Prothrombin complex 80 IU was intravenously given to reduce bleeding.

The process of hemostasis and sternum closure went smoothly. After the operation, the patient's BP was 65–70/38–42 mm Hg (upper and lower limbs), HR was around 160 beats/min, and SpO_2 was 96%. Dopamine 5.0 μg/(kg·min) was intravenously infused.

15.3 Postoperative Outcome

The patient was transferred to the cardiac care unit with an endotracheal intubation and continued mechanical ventilation support. The endotracheal tube was removed on the postoperative day 2 with non-invasive ventilation support. The patient was transferred to the general ward on postoperative day 4 and discharged from the hospital on postoperative day 14.

Discharge diagnosis: Arterial duct aneurysm, PDA, ASD, neonatal pneumonia, respiratory failure.

15.4 Review of Knowledge Points

15.4.1 Anatomy of the Arterial Duct Aneurysm

DAA is characterized by a saccular or fusiform dilation and extension with a diameter ranging from 6.5 to 11.2 mm. Although DAA can be detected in prenatal ultrasound examinations, most DAAs are detected in the first 2 months after birth. The formation of DAA may be due to abnormal intimal cushion formation or defective elastin in the ductus, or it may be related to PDA ligation or infection. Most DAAs can heal alone without surgical treatment, which may be related to the progressive contraction of PDA and thrombosis.

15.4.2 Common Complications and Outcomes of Arterial Duct Aneurysm

According to a literature review by Lund et al., the incidence of complications in DAA patients under 2 months of age is about 30% and can be increased to 60% in patients over 2 months of age. These complications mainly include aneurysm dilation to the pulmonary artery or aorta, spontaneous rupture, erosion or compression of adjacent structures, and infection. Most DAA patients are asymptomatic; mildly affected patients may have hoarseness or difficulty breathing due to compression of the recurrent laryngeal nerve or diaphragmatic nerve, which may also compress the left main bronchus to cause obstruction. Only a very small number of patients may have life-threatening complications. Echocardiography follow-up is an important means to assess the spontaneous regression of DAA. Chen reported a case of a 3-day-old DAA newborn with a maximum diameter of 1.5 cm, compressing the left pulmonary artery, but he was asymptomatic, had no significant murmur, and was discharged without any treatment. At 1 month old, the echocardiography review suggested PDA was closed, and at the age of 9 months old, the CT examination suggested the aneurysm was well thrombosed with rim calcification.

15.4.3 Surgical Indications for Arterial Duct Aneurysm

Surgery should be considered in the following situations: ① The ductus arteriosus with DAA remains patent beyond the neonatal period. ② Association with connective tissue disease. ③ Evidence of thrombus extension to adjacent vessels or thromboembolism. ④ Significant compression of adjacent vessels.

15.5 Discussion

DAA was once considered a rare disease, but recent echocardiographic screening of full-term newborns shows that the incidence of ductus arteriosus aneurysm is as high as 8.8%, which is not as rare as we believe. Although most DAA patients are asymptomatic or self-healing, spontaneous rupture does occur with severe compression or erosion of surrounding tissues, requiring emergency surgery with extremely high anesthesia risk. It is particularly important to maintain circulatory stability during anesthesia to avoid rupture of the aneurysm, which can lead to death.

15.5.1 Preoperative Assessment and Preparation

In this case, the child had shortness of breath as the main clinical manifestation. Both ultrasound and CT showed signs of pulmonary artery compression, which required emergency surgery to relieve the compression. In addition to following the principles of anesthetic management for neonatal congenital heart surgery, special attention should be paid to maintaining hemodynamic stability during preoperative transfer, avoiding coughing and significant blood pressure fluctuations to prevent aneurysm rupture and sudden death caused by hypertension and insufficient perfusion of important tissues and organs caused by hypotension. Adequate depth of sedation and analgesia should be maintained before any operations. Midazolam and muscle relaxants were given before transfer to maintain sufficient sedation and muscle relaxation, avoid coughing, and ensure a smooth transfer process. In addition, anesthesiologists, cardiac surgeons, and CICU doctors should all participate in the patient's transfer while closely monitoring ECG, BP, SpO_2, and $ETCO_2$.

15.5.2 Intraoperative Anesthetic Management

All kinds of rescue drugs should be prepared before anesthesia induction. The surgeon and CPB teams should be ready to operate to deal with emergency surgery in case of sudden deterioration. It is better to choose etomidate supplemented by a high dose of opioids for the induction of anesthesia since etomidate has a mild impact on hemodynamics, and high doses of opioids can significantly reduce stress response, control catecholamine levels, and help maintain hemodynamic stability. Fentanyl or sufentanil are ideal opioids. In this case, the long-acting sufentanil was used. The anesthesia was maintained by continuous intravenous infusion of sufentanil, propofol, and rocuronium bromide to achieve adequate sedation, analgesia, immobilization, and minimal hemodynamic inhibition.

The lower limb arterial catheterization for invasive blood pressure measurement is preferred in this case since the surgery was performed on the PDA site. However, considering that the ductus arteriosus aneurysm is located close to the descending aorta, aortic end suturing may cause narrowing of the descending aorta and cause a significant difference in blood pressure between the upper and lower limbs. To avoid the impact of surgical operations on the pressure measurement in the left radial artery, the femoral artery and the right radial artery were simultaneously catheterized for timely intraoperative and postoperative blood pressure comparative observation. Although PDA surgery is usually performed in the lateral position without CPB, the surgeon chose to operate under deep hypothermia cardiac arrest with a clear anatomical field due to the young age, lightweight, and unclear structure of the surgical site. The surgery went smoothly.

In this case, the child's DAA aneurysm compresses the pulmonary artery and increases the pulmonary artery pressure. Combined with the high pulmonary artery resistance in the neonatal period, bidirectional shunting occurred at the level of the child's atrium, which led to the child's hypoxia, acidosis, cyanosis, etc. Hypoxia and carbon dioxide accumulation should be avoided, which exacerbates pulmonary hypertension and right-to-left shunting at the atrial level and causes worsening cyanosis, hypoxia, and further deterioration of hemodynamics.

15.6 Conclusion

Although the incidence of DAA is not low, only very few infants need emergency surgery. Surgery should be performed immediately after completing preoperative examinations if the patients require surgical treatment. The whole process of transfer and anesthesia should be smooth to avoid serious adverse events such as rupture of the tumor, massive bleeding, and sudden death (Ying Sun).

Anesthetic Management of Aortopulmonary Window Corrective Surgery in a Child with Severe Pneumonia

16

Yong Bian

Abstract

A one-month-old male infant was admitted to our hospital due to dyspnea and difficulty breathing. Echocardiography indicated aortopulmonary window, atrial septal defect (Type II), moderate tricuspid regurgitation, pulmonary valve regurgitation, and mild to severe pulmonary hypertension (100 mm Hg). Chest radiograph suggested bilateral pulmonary infiltrates. He was diagnosed with an aortopulmonary window complicated with severe pneumonia. After admission, active anti-infection and optimization of cardiac function were conducted. After the infection was controlled, the aortopulmonary window radical surgery was performed under general anesthesia. Anesthetic management should focus on preventing infection while optimizing ventilation management, rational use of positive inotropic agents, and maintaining the balance of systemic and pulmonary circulation.

Aortopulmonary window (APW), also known as aortopulmonary fistula or aortopulmonary septal defect, is a rare congenital heart disease, which is caused by abnormal fusion or arrangement of the arterial trunk during embryonic development, accounting for about 0.1–0.6% of congenital heart diseases. If APW is not corrected in time, pulmonary hypertension will progress rapidly, and about 40% of cases will face the risk of death within 1 year after birth. Long-term complications in children include heart failure, insufficient coronary artery perfusion, and severe pulmonary hypertension. These children generally have pulmonary circulation overload, and the amount of pulmonary blood mainly depends on the size of the aortopulmonary septal defect and the pressure difference between the systematic and pulmonary arteries. Increased pulmonary blood can lead to irreversible pulmonary vascular disease, which is incredibly complicated with severe pneumonia. So, significant challenges were faced in anesthetic management. This article reports the experience of the anesthetic management of aortopulmonary window corrective surgery in a child with severe pneumonia.

16.1 Case Presentation

The patient was a one-month-old and 26-day-old boy with a weight of 4.0 kg. He was born full-term with no history of asphyxia. The child was admitted to our hospital due to shortness of breath and difficulty breathing. At the time of admission, the child was restless, moaning with dyspnea, pale complexion, and nodding-like

Y. Bian (✉)
The National Children's Medical Center (Shanghai), Department of Anesthesiology of Shanghai Children's Medical Center, Shanghai Jiao Tong University School of Medicine, Shanghai, China
e-mail: bianyong@scmc.com.cn

J. Zheng et al. (eds.), *Selected Pediatric Cardiovascular Surgery Anesthesia Cases*,
https://doi.org/10.1007/978-981-96-5614-1_16

breathing. Pulse oxygen saturation (SpO_2) was 80%, respiratory rate (RR) 70 times/min, and heart rate (HR) 180 times/min. CT examination showed congenital heart disease, right aortic arch, right descending aorta, aortopulmonary window, and atrial septal defect (ASD). Echocardiography suggested aortopulmonary window, ASD (Type II) 1.13 cm, moderate tricuspid regurgitation (TR), pulmonary valve regurgitation (PR), and moderate to severe pulmonary hypertension (100 mm Hg). The child was tentatively diagnosed with bronchopneumonia, respiratory distress, aortopulmonary window, ASD, and pulmonary hypertension and was admitted to our PICU.

Physical examination: Wet rales were heard at lung auscultation. II/VI systolic murmur was heard at 2–3 intercostal space. The second heart sound of the pulmonary valve was accentuated.

Chest radiograph: Cardiac silhouette enlargement and bilateral lung infiltrates. Electrocardiogram (ECG): Sinus rhythm, left atrial enlargement, possible right ventricular hypertrophy, and QT shortening.

After admission, cefoperazone and piperacillin sodium tazobactam sodium were used to treat infection, digoxin was used to treat cardiac dysfunction, and furosemide was used for diuresis. At the admission night, the shortness of breath became worse with SpO_2 at 80% under mask oxygen inhalation, RR at 80 times/min, HR at 180 times/min, and cyanosis. Blood gas analysis showed $PaCO_2$ was 62 mm Hg and PaO_2 was 42 mm Hg, indicating severe pneumonia and respiratory failure. Endotracheal intubation was performed for mechanical ventilation. Pressure control assisted ventilation (PC-AC) mode was used with the following parameters: fraction of inspired oxygen (FiO_2) 50%, end-expiratory positive pressure (PEEP) 5 cm H_2O, peak airway pressure (PIP) 23 cm H_2O, RR 30 times/min. Hydrocortisone was given to reduce lung inflammation. After 10 days of hospitalization treatment, the lung infection was controlled. It was decided to conduct radical surgery on the aortopulmonary window after consultation with the cardiothoracic surgery department.

16.2 Anesthetic Management

The patient was transferred to the operating room with endotracheal intubation. Dobutamine 5.0 μg/(kg·min) was intravenously infused. After entering the operating room, routine monitoring was conducted. Baseline values for vital signs were as follows: non-invasive blood pressure (NBP) 72/35 mm Hg, HR 150 times/min, and SpO_2 90%. Midazolam 0.4 mg, etomidate 1.2 mg, sufentanil 5.0 μg, and rocuronium 2.5 mg were given for intravenous induction of anesthesia. Anesthesia was maintained with propofol 4.0 mg/(kg·h), rocuronium 0.6 mg/(kg·h), and sufentanil 2.0 μg/(kg·h) infusion. During the operation, pressure-controlled ventilation-volume guaranteed (PCV-VG) mode was used for mechanical ventilation. The oxygen flow rate was 1.0 L/min, FiO_2 50%, tidal volume (VT) 40 mL, RR 24 times/min, inspiratory time to expiratory time (I:E) ratio 1:2, PEEP 4.0 cm H_2O. The partial pressure of end-tidal carbon dioxide ($ETCO_2$) was maintained at 40–45 mm Hg.

After the induction of anesthesia, the right internal jugular vein was catheterized for intraoperative central venous pressure (CVP) monitoring and vasoactive drug infusion. The left radial artery was catheterized for invasive arterial pressure (ABP) monitoring and blood gas analysis. Near-infrared regional cerebral oxygen saturation ($rScO_2$) monitoring was used during the operation with a baseline value of 68%. The changes in $rScO_2$ were maintained within 15% of the baseline value. Blood was drawn from the superior vena cava to determine the oxygen saturation of mixed venous blood (SvO_2). The baseline value of SvO_2 was 67%, and SpO_2 was 90%. Based on the above information, the pulmonary circulation blood volume (Qp): the systemic circulation blood volume (Qs) was calculated to be 2.3:1 (see the discussion section for the calculation method). FiO_2 and respiratory parameters were adjusted to maintain the balance of the patient's Qp/Qs. After the sternum was opened, 3.0 mg/kg of sodium heparin was intravenously injected, and cardiopulmonary bypass (CBP) was quickly established. After the aorta was cross-clamped, the APW repair surgery was finished within 52 min. After the aorta cross-clamp was

Table 16.1 Intraoperative blood gas test results

Time point	pH	Hb (g/dL)	HCT (%)	PaO_2 (mm Hg)	$PaCO_2$ (mm Hg)	BE (mmol/L)	Na^+ (mmol/L)	K^+ (mmol/L)	Cl^- (mmol/L)	Ca^{2+} (mmol/L)	Lac (mmol/L)
Admission	7.32	12.5	38.9	132	48	−3.1	135	3.2	108	1.16	1.3
Discharge	7.448	11.5	35.6	127	35.2	0.7	132	4.2	105	1.26	1.1

released, Remodulin was intravenously infused at 20 ng/(kg·min) to reduce pulmonary artery hypertension. The pulmonary artery pressure and ABP were measured at 35/17 (23) mm Hg and 92/55 (50) mm Hg, respectively. The patient was successfully separated from CBP. Protamine was given in a 1.2:1 ratio to neutralize heparin. Considering the longer CBP time, factor VII was intravenously injected to improve coagulation function. After hemostasis was satisfied, the sternum was closed. The patient's respiratory and circulatory functions were stable. The results of blood gas tests upon entering and leaving the operating room are shown in Table 16.1.

16.3 Postoperative Outcome

The operation lasted 3 h and 40 min, during which 60 mL of acetate Ringer's solution and 50 mL of red cell suspension were transfused. The urine output was 15 mL. The patient's ABP was 96/49 mm Hg, HR 113 beats/min, and SpO_2 100% at the end of the operation. The patient was transferred to the cardiac surgery intensive care unit with endotracheal intubation, ABP, ECG, and SpO_2 monitoring. Continued cardiac support, fluid and electrolyte balance maintenance, infection intervention, nutritional support, and active intervention for pulmonary hypertension were provided. The tracheal tube was removed on postoperative day 12, and the patient was discharged from the hospital on postoperative day 27.

16.4 Review of Knowledge Points

16.4.1 Aortopulmonary Window

APW is referred to as a large defect between the ascending aorta and the main pulmonary artery, which is caused by the failure of the spiral septum to separate the embryonic arterial trunk. APW accounts for 0.1–0.6% of congenital heart diseases. Among them, 50–80% of patients have patent ductus arteriosus (PDA), anomalous coronary artery origin from the right pulmonary artery, the right pulmonary artery origin from the aorta, and interruption or stenosis of the aortic arch. The pathophysiology of APW is similar to that of large PDA. Early surgical intervention is vital for preventing congestive heart failure (large left-to-right shunt) and the development of late pulmonary artery hypertension. APW is classified into three types based on the defect location of the disease itself: proximal defect (Type I), distal defect (Type II), and complete defect or transitional defect(Type III). However, the size of the APW defect significantly impacts the pathophysiology and prognosis of the disease. This type of disease rarely co-exists with DiGeorge syndrome, indicating that APW does not originate from conotruncal anomalies, which distinguishes it from other major arterial malformations, such as ventricular septal defect (VSD) with aortic interruption, Tetralogy of Fallot (TOF), and persistent truncus arteriosus. A few APW patients can develop severe lung infections, manifesting as extensive parenchymal and vascular lung changes. This situation can result in more complex pathophysiological changes in APW. A large amount of pulmonary blood flow exacerbates pulmonary exudation and vascular disease, while severe infection reduces lung compliance, increases pulmonary resistance, and mismatch of pulmonary ventilation–perfusion ratio. These two pathological states increase the risk of pulmonary hypertension and heart failure in APW patients. The pathophysiological mechanism of APW patients with pneumonia is shown in Fig. 16.1.

During the fetal period, the shunt between the two is not apparent due to the roughly equal pressure at the root of the ascending aorta and pulmo-

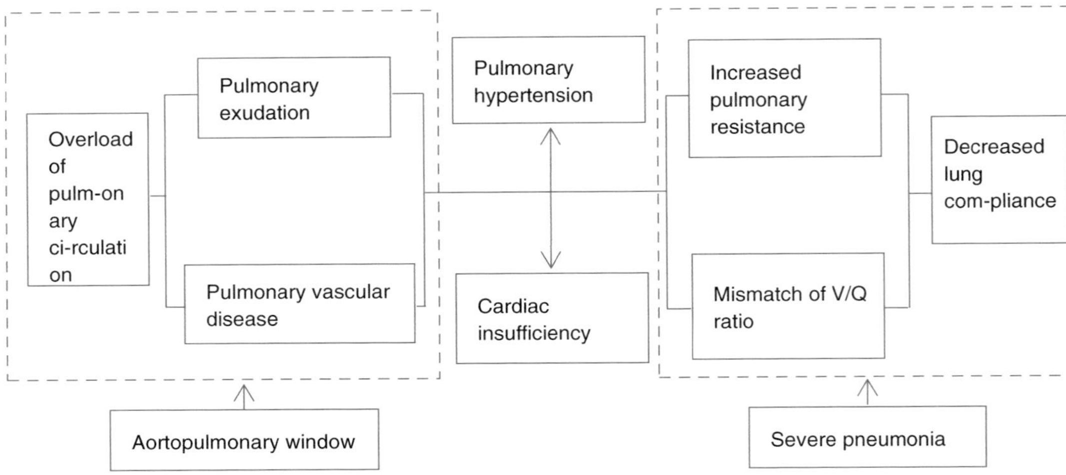

Fig. 16.1 Pathophysiological illustration of the aortopulmonary window with severe pneumonia

nary artery. Hence, the fetal ultrasound screening rate is very low. After birth, due to the rapid drop in pulmonary artery pressure, a significant defect may lead to early cardiac insufficiency or failure in patients. For large defects, early onset may exacerbate pulmonary hypertension, causing the shunt to change from the original left-to-right shunt to a bidirectional shunt, leading to cyanosis. The most common symptoms of APW include sweating, difficulty feeding, and unexplained non-gain in weight. Physical examination can reveal the patient's tachycardia, rapid breathing, and bounding pulse. Chest X-rays suggest an enlarged heart shadow and increased pulmonary perfusion.

Ultrasound diagnosis remains the golden standard for these types of diseases, and more attention should be paid to the size and location of the aortopulmonary defect during diagnosis.

16.4.2 Perioperative Management Principles

The focus of preoperative management for these children is to improve systemic circulation output by limiting pulmonary circulation blood flow. The management principles are similar to those with single ventricle physiology or persistent arterial trunk with non-obstructive pulmonary blood flow, that is, maintaining a physiological state of systemic to pulmonary circulation ratio of 1:1. Its hemodynamic changes are similar to persistent arterial trunk, but more severe than typical PDA. For cases with excessive pulmonary blood, mechanical ventilation, and positive inotropic agents can be used to regulate pulmonary blood flow and improve cardiac function. The ventilation strategies include higher $ETCO_2$, low FiO_2, and normal pH. CO_2 can be inhaled if necessary to increase pulmonary vascular resistance and improve the state of increased pulmonary blood flow. For children with chronic heart failure, small doses of positive inotropic agents and vasodilators can be used. It is worth noting that these children should avoid severe metabolic acidosis before surgery to improve the quality of survival after surgery.

The principle of surgery for children with simple APW is to repair the defect and protect the coronary arteries and large vessel valves. Milrinone is recommended during the off-pump process because it reduces cardiac and pulmonary vascular resistance. With the in-depth research on pulmonary hypertension, the use of prostacyclin analogs to reduce pulmonary hypertension has gradually increased, and the clinical application of prostacyclin analogs combined with other vasoactive drugs has also gradually increased.

Large doses of cardiotonic drugs should be avoided during postoperative care in these children. It also should be kept alert to the possibility of pulmonary hypertension crisis and low cardiac output caused by the increased pulmonary artery pressure in some children after surgery. This situation occurs more often in older children, which is related to the long-term existence of uncorrected APW, which leads to an overload of pulmonary circulation in these children. Therefore, perioperative monitoring of mixed venous oxygen saturation or near-infrared cerebral oxygen saturation can help understand the systematic pulmonary circulation blood volume and guide the adjustment of systematic pulmonary circulation balance, maintaining tissue oxygen delivery and oxygen supply balance.

16.5 Discussion

16.5.1 Preoperative Assessment and Preparation

The key to preoperative assessment for these children is to evaluate the pulmonary hypertension and the severity of pneumonia. The echocardiography revealed a significant APW defect and ASD. The child also had severe pulmonary hypertension before surgery, which could aggravate pulmonary hypertension. APW with severe pulmonary infection accelerated the progression of the disease because severe pneumonia might cause lung atelectasis, lung collapse, or pulmonary edema in the lungs with existing vascular disease (caused by APW), decreased lung function, pulmonary circulation overload caused by APW, which in turn might aggravate the degree of pulmonary infection. In addition, it is also very challenging to ameliorate pulmonary infection in children with congenital heart disease due to their low immunity.

16.5.2 Intraoperative Anesthetic Management

As previously mentioned, it is crucial to effectively control the balance of systemic-pulmonary circulation blood flow before CPB in such patients. According to the classic cardiac oxygen delivery mathematical model for children with systemic-pulmonary shunt diseases, tissue oxygen delivery is maximized when Qp/Qs is equal to or slightly less than 1. In clinical management of similar cases, such balance can be achieved by maintaining higher blood CO_2 levels, lower FiO_2, and normal pH through respiratory management. Appropriate positive inotropic agents can also be used if it is necessary. Evaluating the pulmonary blood flow when a pulmonary infection occurs may be difficult. Sometimes, the decrease in oxygenation is not necessarily caused by pulmonary blood changes but by pulmonary parenchymal diseases instead, which can also cause insufficient oxygenation. In this case, it may exacerbate the mismatch of the ventilation–perfusion ratio in lung tissue by regulating pulmonary blood flow, leading to hypoxia and heart failure. Therefore, effective perioperative monitoring and evaluation are of great significance for the outcome of such patients. It is essential to monitor cerebral tissue oxygen delivery since the cerebral tissue is the most vulnerable organ to oxygen delivery in the body. In this case, $rScO_2$ was maintained at about 68% during the operation, which effectively ensures brain tissue perfusion, reduces the occurrence of neurological complications, and indirectly reflects the balance of systemic-pulmonary circulation in the patient.

Some literature showed that the combination of $rScO_2$ and SvO_2 monitoring is more conducive to regulating the systemic-pulmonary circulation blood volume of children with shunt heart disease during the perioperative period and improving the outcome. According to the Fick principle, the ratio of systemic-pulmonary circulation blood flow is $(SaO_2\text{-}SvO_2)/(SpaO_2\text{-}SpvO_2)$, where SaO_2 is arterial oxygen saturation, SvO_2 is mixed venous oxygen saturation, $SpaO_2$ is pulmonary arterial oxygen saturation, and $SpvO_2$ is pulmonary venous oxygen saturation. Typically, the difference between $SpaO_2$ and $SpvO_2$ is tiny, around 10%, so after measuring SaO_2 and SvO_2, the systemic-pulmonary circulation blood flow ratio can be effectively evaluated to help manage and balance systemic-pulmonary arterial blood volume. The systemic-pulmonary circulation blood flow ratio can be estimated by drawing arterial and superior vena cava blood samples. In this case, the patient's baseline SaO_2 was 90%, SvO_2 was 67%, and the theoretical difference of $SpaO_2$–$SpvO_2$ was 10%. According to the calculation, Qp:Qs is 2.3:1, indicating a situation of excessive pulmonary blood flow. Therefore, it is not difficult to understand that the patient had symptoms of congestive heart failure at the early stage. The increased gradient between SaO_2 and SvO_2 may reflect the increase in pulmonary blood flow, which can be reduced by ventilation strategies, including reducing respiratory rate and VT. If the effective gradient of SaO_2 and SvO_2 cannot be maintained and continues to rise after the adjustment of respiratory parameters, possibly due to an insufficient oxygen uptake rate, heart failure should be considered. In this case, it is better to use vasoactive drugs to regulate arterial tension, which is beneficial in controlling the systemic-pulmonary circulation ratio and ensuring the stability of the aortopulmonary circulation. In addition to regulating the Qp/Qs balance through respiration and vasoactive drugs, anesthesiologists are more concerned about the impact of anesthetic drugs on systemic pulmonary circulation. Tracy et al. used the ultrasound velocity time integral method to calculate the systemic-pulmonary circulation ratio of children with left-to-right shunt heart disease. They found that 1–1.5 MAC sevoflurane, halothane, isoflurane, and fentanyl combined with midazolam did not change the systemic-pulmonary circulation ratio of this type of heart disease. The result suggests that the clinical routine dose of anesthetic drugs has a specific safety range for left-to-right shunt heart disease, and the basic pathophysiology of the aortopulmonary window also belongs to a large amount of left-to-right shunt, so it can be inferred that the routine dose of anesthetic drugs is also safe for these patients.

It is worth noting that the preoperative Qp/Qs of this patient were still high after preoperative respiratory management and the use of positive inotropic agents, which may be related to factors such as unrestricted shunting of the aortopulmonary window and pulmonary parenchymal disease, indicating the necessity of early surgery for these patients. Delaying the treatment of cardiac anatomical abnormalities may worsen the patient's condition. The surgery not only solved the shunt problem between the aorta and the pulmonary artery fundamentally, which effectively controlled the pulmonary blood flow on the one hand and alleviated the heart failure caused by the pulmonary blood flow increase on the other hand, but it also facilitated the control of pulmonary infections. This patient had uncorrectable hypoxia, hypotension, and severe signs of pulmonary infection before surgery, and the pulmonary infection was effectively controlled after surgery, all of which proved that early surgery was beneficial for this patient.

16.5.3 Postoperative Anesthetic Management

The key point of APW in postoperative management is to actively control pulmonary hypertension and prevent the occurrence of a pulmonary hypertension crisis. Other therapies include pain management, appropriate depth of sedation, effective ventilation management (such as appropriate PEEP, mild hyperventilation, etc.), and the use of drugs to alleviate pulmonary hypertension. If there is a severe lung infection, effective anti-infection, immune enhancement, and physical therapy are needed to help alleviate lung inflammation. After the above treatment, the lung inflammation of the child, in this case, was effectively controlled, and the cardiopulmonary function gradually recovered. The prognosis of this patient is good.

16.6 Shortcomings and Limitations

When conditions permit, the severity of pulmonary hypertension in such children can be assessed preoperatively through cardiac catheterization, which is of great significance for anesthesia and medication guidance as well as for the success of the surgery. In addition, catheter examination can also directly and effectively evaluate the blood flow of the systematic pulmonary circulation. Unfortunately, the disease progression of this child was rapid, and the comprehensive preoperative evaluation was not performed with a lack of objective indicators of preoperative pulmonary hypertension and Qp/Qs, which is a shortcoming in the treatment of this case.

16.7 Conclusion

In summary, this child had APW complicated with a severe lung infection, which made it difficult for the anesthesiologist to control the balance of the systematic -pulmonary circulation. The treatment principle is to prevent disease and maintain the balance of the systematic pulmonary circulation through ventilation management and positive inotropic agents. The combined use of near-infrared brain oxygen saturation and mixed venous oxygen saturation is of great importance for evaluating and managing the blood flow of the systematic pulmonary circulation (Yong Bian).

Anesthetic Management of Pediatric Isolated Coarctation of the Aorta Repair with End-to-End Anastomosis

17

Yanting Wang

Abstract

A one-year-old girl was found to have heart murmurs during a physical examination. Echocardiography showed coarctation of the aorta (CoA). She was scheduled to undergo an end-to-end anastomosis of the aorta under general anesthesia without cardiopulmonary bypass support. During the operation, controlled hypothermia, hypotension, and aortic cross-clamping were conducted to remove the narrowed segment and perform an end-to-end anastomosis to reconstruct the vascular structure. The blood pressure differences between the upper and lower limbs were significantly reduced, and the hemodynamics became stable after the circulation was resumed. After the operation, the patient was safely transferred to the Cardiac Intensive Care Unit (CICU). CoA may be relieved by resection and end-to-end anastomosis without cardiopulmonary bypass. The key point of anesthetic management is maintaining hemodynamic stability and protecting organ function.

Y. Wang (✉)
The National Children's Medical Center (Shanghai), Department of Anesthesiology of Shanghai Children's Medical Center, Shanghai Jiao Tong University School of Medicine, Shanghai, China
e-mail: wangyanting@scmc.com.cn

Aortic coarctation or coarctation of the aorta (CoA) is a relatively common congenital heart malformation with localized or non-continuous narrowing of the aorta. The narrowing segment is commonly located at the distal end of the left subclavian artery origin and the opposite side of the connection between the arterial duct and the aorta. Clinically, long-segment stenosis or abdominal aortic coarctation can also be found. The main clinical features of patients with CoA include Hypertension and strong pulse above the narrowed segment, hypotension, and weakened pulse below the narrowed segment, as well as left heart pressure overload and lower body hypoperfusion. The anatomical feature of CoA is characterized by the presence of convex or non-continuous fibrous ridges in the inner layer of the aorta. Still, its pathophysiological changes vary depending on the severity of stenosis, combined lesions, collateral circulation compensation, etc. Surgical options of CoA depend on whether there are other congenital heart defects. The isolated CoA in children without other congenital heart defects is usually corrected by surgery without the support of cardiopulmonary bypass (CBP). The key to anesthetic management is maintaining hemodynamic stability and protecting organ function. This article reports the anesthetic management of a case of isolated coarctation of the aorta repair with end-to-end anastomosis in a child.

J. Zheng et al. (eds.), *Selected Pediatric Cardiovascular Surgery Anesthesia Cases*,
https://doi.org/10.1007/978-981-96-5614-1_17

17.1 Case Presentation

The patient was a one-year and one-month-old girl with a height of 77 cm and a weight of 8.0 kg. She was born full-term without a history of asphyxia at birth. She was found to have heart murmurs during a physical examination. Echocardiography revealed CoA. She was scheduled to undergo isolated CoA repair with an end-to-end anastomosis under general anesthesia without CBP support.

Physical examination: She was consciousness with good mental response. No obvious cyanosis was found. The breathing sounds in both lungs are symmetric without obvious dry or wet rales. A II/VI-grade systolic murmur can be heard in the second to third intercostal space on the left side of the sternum. The pulse of the lower limb arteries is weakened.

Echocardiography: No obvious abnormalities were seen in the internal structure of the heart, CoA (pressure difference 58 mm Hg), and normal left heart systolic function.

Chest CT of the great vessels: CoA, the narrowed segment, has a diameter of 2.7 mm and is located at the beginning of the descending thoracic aorta. The distal descending aorta is dilated, with a diameter of 10.4 mm.

17.2 Anesthetic Management

Routine monitoring was conducted after the patient was transported to the operating room. The baseline non-invasive blood pressure (NBP) of the upper limb was 105/55 mm Hg, heart rate (HR) was 138 beats/min, and pulse oxygen saturation (SpO_2) was 100%. Anesthesia was induced by intravenous bolus injection of midazolam 1.0 mg, etomidate 2.5 mg, sufentanil 20 μg, and rocuronium 5.0 mg; mechanical ventilation with pressure-controlled ventilation-volume guaranteed (PCV-VG) mode was initiated after successful endotracheal intubation. The ventilation parameters were set as follows: oxygen flow rate 1 L/min, a fraction of inspired oxygen (FiO_2) 50%, tidal volume (VT) 80 mL, respiratory rate (RR) 24 times/min. The end-tidal carbon dioxide partial pressure ($ETCO_2$) was maintained at 30–40 mm Hg. After the induction of anesthesia, the right internal jugular vein was catheterized under ultrasound guidance for central venous pressure (CVP) monitoring and infusion of vasoactive agents. The right radial and femoral arteries were also catheterized under ultrasound guidance to continuously monitor the upper and lower limbs' invasive arterial pressure (ABP). The upper limb ABP was 112/65 mm Hg, and the lower limb ABP was 67/45 mm Hg. Anesthesia was maintained by continuous infusion of propofol 5.0 mg/(kg·h), sufentanil 2.5 μg/(kg·h), rocuronium 0.6 mg/(kg·h), and intermittent inhalation of 1–2% sevoflurane.

During the operation, the rectal temperature was reduced to 34 °C by a water blanket and an ice bag on her head. Before aortic cross-clamping, sodium nitroprusside 1.0 μg/(kg·min) was intravenously initiated to control the systolic pressure of the upper limb at 90–100 mm Hg. The surgery began with aortic cross-clamping, which lasted for about 15 minutes. The upper limb blood pressure was maintained at 90–100 mm Hg, and the lower limb blood pressure was maintained above 40 mm Hg. After the end-to-end anastomosis of the aorta was completed, the cross-clamping of the aorta was released, sodium nitroprusside was discontinued, and rewarming began. After the rectal temperature rose to above 36 °C, arterial blood gas was rechecked (Table 17.1). According to the arterial blood gas analysis results, 5% sodium bicarbonate 2 mL/kg was intravenously given to correct metabolic acidosis and maintain homeostasis. After the operation, the upper limb ABP was 99/61 mm Hg, the lower limb ABP was 88/56 mm Hg, and the pressure difference between the upper and lower limbs was significantly reduced. After sufficient hemostasis and closure of the sternum, the child was safely transferred to the Cardiac Intensive Care Unit (CICU).

Table 17.1 Intraoperative blood gas test results

Time point	pH	Hb (g/dL)	PaO_2 (mm Hg)	$PaCO_2$ (mm Hg)	BE (mmol/L)	HCT (%)	K^+ (mmol/L)	Ca^{2+} (mmol/L)	Cl^- (mmol/L)	Lac (mmol/L)	Na^+ (mmol/L)
Admission	7.39	11.9	275	33.7	−2.7	36.4	3.6	1.23	108	0.8	136
Discharge	7.31	11.5	299	34.9	−5.6	42.2	3.5	1.21	110	2.7	135

17.3 Postoperative Outcome

The operation lasted 90 minutes in total with aortic cross-clamping for 15 min. The estimated blood loss was approximately 10 mL. The urine output was 20 mL. 150 mL of Ringer's acetate solution was transfused. The patient was transferred to the CICU with endotracheal intubation after the operation. The endotracheal tube was removed 24 h after the operation. The patient was discharged from the CICU on postoperative day 2 and discharged from the hospital on postoperative day 7.

17.4 Review of Knowledge Points

17.4.1 CoA Classification

1. Depending on whether there are other intracardiac malformations, CoA can be divided into three categories:
   (a) Isolated CoA.
   (b) CoA combined with ventricular septal defect.
   (c) CoA combined with other intracardiac malformations.
2. Depending on the range and degree of narrowing, CoA can be divided into two categories:
   (a) Simple CoA.
   (b) Aortic arch hypoplasia (referring to a certain degree of narrowing in the aortic arch or isthmus).
   (c) Depending on the clinical manifestations, CoA can be divided into two categories:
      (i) Infantile type: Most of the patients with infantile type CoA manifest the symptoms of congestive heart failure, gallop rhythm and systolic murmur on cardiac auscultation, weakened or absent femoral artery pulsation, mild purplish skin on the lower limbs in some children.
      (ii) Adult type: Often no obvious symptoms. Physical examination reveals higher blood pressure in the upper limbs than in the lower limbs and weakened or absent femoral artery pulsation.

17.4.2 Surgical Indications for CoA

Suppose a child with CoA has symptoms of chronic heart failure, such as difficulty breathing, difficulty feeding, and delayed growth and development. In that case, surgery should be scheduled after adjusting heart function with medications. It is generally believed that surgery should be performed as early as possible, as the risk of hypertension, aneurysm, and sudden death increases with time. Although children with adult-type CoA have no obvious symptoms, surgery is still required in some specific situations. The surgical indications for CoA include:

1. Pressure gradient >20 mm Hg between the two ends of the aortic stenosis segment.
2. Even though the pressure gradient between the two ends of the aortic stenosis segment is ≤20 mm Hg and if there is clear anatomical narrowing evidence on imaging examination and there are abundant collaterals or existing systolic hypertension, surgery is indicated.

17.5 Discussion

17.5.1 Preoperative Assessment and Preparation

The pathophysiological changes in children with CoA mainly depend on the severity and location of aortic stenosis, the type and severity of other concurrent heart diseases, the blood flow that the patent ductus arteriosus (PDA) can provide to the aorta, and the status of collateral circulation formation at the distal side of the aorta. The preoperative assessment should focus on those factors which can cause the pathophysiological changes in children with CoA. In addition, aortic stenosis can increase left ventricular afterload, which makes children with CoA prone to congestive heart failure and pulmonary edema. Therefore, special attention should be paid to symptoms such as rapid breathing, cyanosis, and feeding difficulties. The cardiac function should be accurately assessed preoperatively. A significant increase in the pulse pressure difference between the upper and lower limbs and a decrease or disappearance of the pulse in the lower limb arteries are simple and feasible indicators reflecting the degree of aortic stenosis. The SpO_2 at the proximal side of stenosis is significantly higher than that at the distal side, which is an indicator of severe aortic stenosis, suggesting that the pulmonary artery provides blood perfusion to the distal side of the aortic stenosis through PDA, a situation also known as differential cyanosis. The vital organs in the lower body may be under perfused due to the blood pressure drop in the distal side of stenosis, so special attention should be paid to the functional assessment of the kidneys and spinal cord. For some children with severe CoA, especially those with underdeveloped left heart and aortic arch, the patient's survival depends on PDA, so the ductus arteriosus should be kept open preoperatively. The surgical procedures for different types of CoA are also different. CT and MRI can clearly define the location and length of the stenosis and whether there are other intracardiac malformations. Echocardiography can help to estimate the pressure gradient at both ends of the stenosis. Anesthesiologists must prepare in advance based on the results of these preoperative examinations and possible surgical procedures.

17.5.2 Intraoperative Anesthetic Management

Pediatric isolated aortic stenosis is usually corrected without CBP support, and the reconstruction of aortic vascular structure during surgery requires the interruption of aortic blood supply. Except for the heart and brain, all other important organs in the body may suffer from ischemia and hypoxia. Therefore, the key points of intraoperative anesthetic management should focus on:

1. Induction and maintenance of anesthesia. For older children with CoA who only have proximal hypertension or a small pulse pressure difference between the upper and lower limbs, whether it is inhalation general anesthesia or intravenous general anesthesia, the child can tolerate it quite well. For those newborns or infants who need to undergo CoA correction surgery, the CoA is usually more severe and more dependent on the patency of ductus arteriosus to provide forward blood flow to the distal side of the stenosis, often accompanied by insufficient distal perfusion, heart failure, and pulmonary edema. Prostaglandin is usually used to keep ductus arteriosus open before surgery. These children have poor tolerance to inhalation general anesthesia and better tolerance to intravenous general anesthesia with large doses of opioids.
2. Maintain intraoperative hemodynamic stability. Patients with CoA usually have a significant pressure difference between the upper and lower limbs, so it is recommended to simultaneously monitor the ABP of both the upper and lower limbs. Furthermore, it is necessary to establish ABP monitoring at the right upper limb because the cross-clamping of the aorta during surgery may cause the interruption of the left upper limb blood flow or affect the opening of the left subclavian artery. So, the ABP from the left radial artery cannot reliably reflect the overall blood pressure, while the ABP from the right radial artery is unaffected. The arterial pulsation of lower limbs in patients with CoA is usually weak or absent, which makes femoral artery catheterization difficult. Conducting the femoral artery catheterization under ultrasound guidance is recommended to increase the catheterization success rate. If femoral artery catheterization fails, a surgical incision of the femoral artery for catheterization or non-invasive pressure measurement at the lower

limb can be considered. In addition, it is better to simultaneously conduct SpO_2 monitoring at both the upper and lower limbs.

It is required to conduct the cross-clamping of the aorta during end-to-end anastomosis of the aorta, which can cause a sudden increase in proximal blood pressure and significantly increase the risks of cerebrovascular accidents and acute heart failure. Therefore, it is necessary to conduct controlled hypotension during the cross-clamping of the aorta, which can effectively reduce the risks of cerebrovascular accidents and acute heart failure. Before aortic cross-clamping, it is necessary to use antihypertensive drugs to lower the ABP of the upper limb to normal or slightly below normal levels. Still, the reduction of ABP should not exceed 20% of the baseline value. Controlled hypotension can significantly increase the risks of ischemia in important organs such as the spinal cord and kidneys due to lower body hypoperfusion, which can result in paraplegia and renal failure. Therefore, special attention should be paid to the degree and duration of hypotension during controlled hypotension. The ABP of the upper limb should be kept at normal or slightly below normal levels, and the duration should be as short as possible. To protect the spinal cord during aortic cross-clamping, permissive hypothermia should also be used with rectal and nasopharyngeal temperatures at 34–35 °C. However, excessive hypothermia should be avoided. In addition, intraoperative electrophysiological monitoring of the spinal cord is also very necessary for guiding controlled hypotension. In recent years, the use of controlled hypotension in CoA correction surgery has become less and less.

3. Organ function protection. After aortic cross-clamping during surgery, the decrease in distal blood pressure may lead to spinal cord injury and acute ischemic hypoxic injury to abdominal organs. These serious complications can be prevented by appropriate cooling and shortening the aortic cross-clamping time as much as possible. Hypothermia can reduce the oxygen demand of tissue cells and stabilize cell membranes by reducing the metabolic rate of tissues, thereby increasing the tolerance of tissues to ischemia and hypoxia. Furthermore, hypothermia can also indirectly protect the spinal cord by reducing excitatory neurotransmitters' release. Studies have shown that the safe time limit for aortic cross-clamping is 30 min. The incidence of paraplegia is as high as 25% or more if the cross-clamping of the aorta is released after 60 min. Therefore, special attention should be paid to protecting the function of important organs during CoA correction surgery. When the aortic arch is cross-clamped, at least one carotid artery must be kept open to ensure cerebral perfusion and prevent brain injury. Near-infrared spectroscopy (NIRS) can detect tissue oxygen saturation in the brain, kidneys, and intestinal areas, indirectly reflecting changes in blood flow in important organs, which is helpful in the early detection of organ damage.

17.5.3 Postoperative Anesthetic Management

Once the aortic vessel structure is reconstructed, the aorta's cross-clamping should be released immediately. Significant hemodynamic fluctuations can happen during this period due to the redistribution of blood flow and the entrance of anaerobic metabolites produced during the cross-clamping period into the blood circulation. The early complications that may occur after the cross-clamping of the aorta is released mainly include:

1. Transient hypotension. After the cross-clamping of the aorta is released, the patients may experience transient hypotension due to reactive congestion and vasodilation in the distal tissue. In addition, the blood lactic acid level and $PaCO_2$ will also be significantly increased. Transient hypotension can be reduced by replenishing blood volume before the release of aortic cross-clamping, increasing the minute ventilation, and giving sodium bicarbonate and vasoactive drugs when necessary.

2. Early postoperative hypertension. Early postoperative hypertension generally occurs immediately after surgery, which will subside in most of the patients with postoperative hypertension within 24 h after surgery. Still, some patients can last for about a week. This may be related to the severe hemodynamic fluctuations; the pressure receptors changes in the carotid sinus and aortic arch caused by the release of aortic cross-clamping, which further leads to the increase of catecholamines release and the activation of the renin–angiotensin–aldosterone system in the later time. β-Receptor blockers and/or vasodilators can be used to control this rebound hypertension in severe cases while maintaining adequate analgesia and sedation.
3. Low cardiac output syndrome. Newborns and small infants may develop low cardiac output syndrome after surgery, which may be related to preoperative left heart failure and longer cross-clamping time during surgery. Positive inotropic drugs can be used to enhance myocardial contractility and reduce left heart afterload. Severe cases can be supported by extracorporeal membrane oxygenation (ECMO).

17.6 Conclusion

In summary, the principles of anesthetic management for CoA repair surgery without CPB include Controlling blood pressure and maintaining heart function before aortic cross-clamping, protecting the function of vital organs during aortic cross-clamping, and replenishing blood volume, correcting acidosis, and supporting stable blood pressure after aortic cross-clamping. (Yanting Wang).

18 Anesthetic Management of Corrective Surgery in an Infant with Coarctation of the Aorta, Ventricular, and Atrial Septal Defects

Yanhui Huang

Abstract

A 2-month-old female infant with coarctation of the aorta (CoA) accompanied by ventricular septal defect (VSD) and atrial septal defect (ASD) was admitted to our hospital with pulse oxygen saturation (SpO_2) of 94% and liver 1.0 cm below the ribs. She was scheduled to undergo the corrective surgery of coarctation of the aorta and the repair of VSD and ASD under general anesthesia. The left ventricular pressure was overloaded, and the perfusion of the lower body was insufficient in this case. The left-to-right shunt of VSD and ASD further reduced the effective forward blood flow of the left ventricle and caused pulmonary arterial hypertension. Therefore, before cardiopulmonary bypass, it is necessary to maintain an appropriate systemic-pulmonary circulation resistance ratio and ensure tissue perfusion in the lower body by maintaining a higher preload. After cardiopulmonary bypass, it is necessary to reduce the afterload of the right ventricle through hyperventilation and use inotropic drugs to enhance myocardial contractility to maintain circulation stability and ensure systemic tissue perfusion.

Y. Huang (✉)
The National Children's Medical Center (Shanghai), Department of Anesthesiology of Shanghai Children's Medical Center, Shanghai Jiao Tong University School of Medicine, Shanghai, China
e-mail: huangyanhui@scmc.com.cn

Coarctation of the aorta (CoA) refers to narrowing the aorta near the ductus arteriosus or the ligamentum arteriosum. The pathophysiological changes of CoA are diverse and often combined with other congenital heart diseases. Therefore, the clinical manifestations of CoA vary dramatically. Mild cases may present as asymptomatic hypertension, while severe cases may present as acute congestive heart failure. The risk of organ ischemia distal to the stenosis is significantly increased in newborns and infants with CoA due to the insufficient establishment of collateral circulation, which can easily lead to renal failure and acidosis. Therefore, the risk of anesthetic management is relatively higher. This article reports the anesthetic management of an infant with CoA, VSD, and ASD for cardiac corrective surgery.

18.1 Case Presentation

The patient was 2 months and 9 days old girl with a weight of 4.7 kg. An abnormal fetal heart structure was found during prenatal screening. She was followed up at the outpatient clinic after birth. She was admitted to the hospital for further diagnosis and treatment at this time.

Physical examination: The patient's heart rate (HR) was 135 beats/min on cardiac auscultation, a III/VI systolic murmur was heard at the 3–4 intercostal space on the left edge of the sternum, the liver was 1.0 cm below the ribs, soft in texture,

J. Zheng et al. (eds.), *Selected Pediatric Cardiovascular Surgery Anesthesia Cases*,
https://doi.org/10.1007/978-981-96-5614-1_18

the pulse oxygen saturation (SpO_2) was 94% when breathing air.

Laboratory tests: Normal routine blood test, kidney, and coagulation functions. Liver function AST 77.

Chest X-ray: Enlarged heart shadow, multiple lung markings, blurred right lung markings.

Electrocardiogram (ECG): Sinus rhythm, left atrial enlargement, left anterior fascicular block (LAH), complete right bundle branch block (CRBBB) with right ventricular hypertrophy.

Echocardiography: Enlargement of the right atrium, left atrium, and left ventricle, aortic valve ring and ascending aorta hypoplasia, valve ring inner diameter 0.63 cm, ascending aorta inner diameter 0.64 cm, mild to moderate tricuspid regurgitation, regurgitation bundle width 0.35 cm, regurgitation speed 4.35 m/s, pressure difference 70 mm Hg. ASD (II) at the oval fossa position 0.4 cm, left to right shunting. Membranous VSD 0.86 cm, about 0.37 cm from the atrioventricular valve, bidirectional shunt. Left aortic arch, small arch development, arch transverse inner diameter 0.40 cm, isthmus inner diameter 0.4 cm, descending aorta distal inner diameter 0.48 cm, descending aorta flow speed 2.86 m/s, pressure difference 32 mm Hg.

Heart, thoracic major vessels, airway CT (plain scan + enhancement): Unobstructed trachea and bronchi, increased and blurred lung markings, patent oval foramen, left atrial and ventricular enlargement, VSD 7.1 mm × 8. 4 mm, slight right ventricular hypertrophy, the normal origin of the coronary arteries, and no patent ductus arteriosus. Left arch, aortic isthmus stenosis with a diameter of about 3.3 mm, distal ascending aorta about 7.2 mm, aortic arch about 5.7 mm, pulmonary artery trunk dilation, acceptable left and right pulmonary artery development.

Preoperative diagnosis: CoA, VSD, ASD. Elective CoA correction surgery and repair of VSD and ASD were planned.

18.2 Anesthetic Management

The infant did not receive any sedatives before surgery. Basic vital signs: HR 145 beats/min, blood pressure (BP) 75/38 mm Hg, SpO_2 94%. Anesthesia was induced with intravenous bolus doses of 1.0 mg midazolam, 8.0 μg sufentanil, and 3.0 mg rocuronium. Under the assistance of the visual laryngoscope, an ID 3.5 mm cuffed tracheal tube was orally intubated; the depth of the endotracheal tube was 10 cm. The pressure-controlled ventilation (PCV) mode was used with respiratory parameters set as 2 L/min oxygen flow rate, 50% fraction of inspired oxygen, and 1:2 inspiratory time to expiratory time (I:E) ratio. End-tidal carbon dioxide ($ETCO_2$) was maintained between 35 and 40 mm Hg through the adjustment of the peak inspiratory pressure (PIP) and respiratory rate (RR).

After anesthesia induction, the right radial artery, right femoral artery, and right internal jugular vein were catheterized under ultrasound guidance for continuously monitoring invasive blood pressure (ABP) and central venous pressure (CVP). The left femoral vein was also accessed for rapid intraoperative fluid infusion. Before the initiation of cardiopulmonary bypass (CBP), CVP was maintained at about 12 cm H_2O, and the regional cerebral tissue oxygen saturation ($rScO_2$) was monitored by near-infrared spectroscopy with a baseline value of 67% and dropped to a minimum value of 63% during CBP. General anesthesia was maintained by intravenous infusion of 4.0 mg/(kg·h) propofol, 2.0 μg/(kg·h) sufentanil, 0.5 mg/(kg·h) rocuronium combined with sevoflurane inhalation. Before the operation, tranexamic acid 10 mg/kg and ulinastatin 100,000 U were intravenously administered for anti-fibrinolysis and anti-inflammation. After thoracotomy, heparin 15 mg was infused via the right internal jugular vein, and CBP was started when the activated clotting time (ACT) reached more than 400 s. During the operation, the aortic coarctation was found to be pre-ductal, with the narrowest internal diameter of 2.0 mm. Therefore, under deep hypothermic selective cerebral perfusion, the descending aorta was cross-clamped, the coarctation segment was first removed, and then the descending aorta was anastomosed with the posterior wall of the aortic arch by end-to-side, and the anterior wall was enlarged with a pericardial patch. After the correction of aortic coarctation, the descending aorta was unclamped, and the temperature was warmed up. Under full bypass, a perimembranous VSD was found with a defect diameter of about 12 mm, which was closed with continuous suturing of a bovine pericardial patch. In addition, a PFO-type ASD was found with a diameter of about 4.0 mm, which was directly closed by suture. After the aortic cross-clamp was released, the heart automatically resumed beating with a 2:1 atrioventricular rhythm. The normal sinus rhythm was not restored even after the intravenous infusion of isoproterenol at 0.05 μg/(kg·min). So, an atrioventricular sequential pacemaker was implanted with DDD mode and a pacing rate of 140 beats/min. At the same time, dopamine 5.0 μg/(kg·min), epinephrine 0.05 μg/(kg·min), and norepinephrine 0.025 μg/(kg·min) were infused intravenously to maintain systolic blood pressure not less than 60 mm Hg. $ETCO_2$ was maintained at 32–35 mm Hg by adjusting PIP and RR. After weaning off CBP, protamine was infused intravenously to neutralize heparin (the ratio was 1.5:1), and red blood cell suspension was transfused to maintain CVP not less than 10 cm H_2O. The patient was sent back to the Cardiac Intensive Care Unit (CICU) with endotracheal intubation when the surgery was finished.

18.3 Postoperative Outcome

On postoperative day 7, the endotracheal tube was removed, and non-invasive ventilation was initiated, but SpO_2 continuously dropped. So, the endotracheal intubation was performed again for mechanical ventilation. On the postoperative day 13, the endotracheal tube was successfully removed. On the postoperative day 14, the patient was transferred to the general ward. The patient was discharged from the hospital on the postoperative day 21.

18.4 Review of Knowledge Points

CoA accounts for 6–8% of all congenital heart diseases, with an incidence of 3 to 4 cases per 10,000 live births; male to female ratio is approximately 2:1.

The pathological classification of CoA has not yet been unified. In clinical practice, it is often classified into preductal (infantile) and postductal (adult) types according to whether the narrowed segment is located at the proximal or distal end of the ductus arteriosus, which was proposed by Bonnet (Fig. 18.1). The narrowed segment of the preductal type is mainly located between the proximal end of the ductus arteriosus and the distal end of the left subclavian artery, and the aortic arch is often involved with diffuse stenosis. The ductus arteriosus usually remains open and the collateral circulation is less. The narrowed segment of postductal type CoA is frequently located at the distal end of the ductus arteriosus or the attachment of the arterial ligament. The narrowed segment is often more limited. Most of the ductus arteriosus has closed and the collateral circulation is usually abundant.

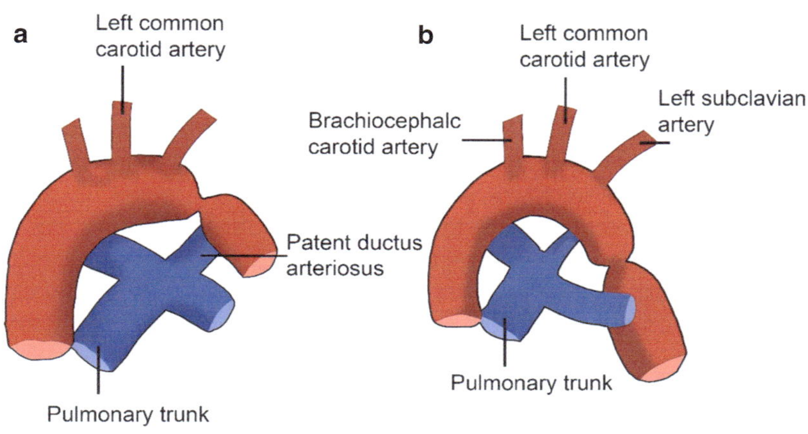

Fig. 18.1 Aortic stenosis classification. (**a**) preductal type; (**b**) postductal type

18.4.1 Clinical Manifestations of CoA

Infantile CoA often presents with symptoms of congestive heart failure, such as shortness of breath, excessive sweating, difficulty feeding, gallop rhythm, and systolic murmur on cardiac auscultation. The pulsation of the femoral artery is weak or disappears. The right-to-left shunting can occur in severe cases of infantile CoA with patent ductus arteriosus, that is to say, pulmonary artery blood flows into the descending aorta through the ductus arteriosus, which leads to differential cyanosis, i.e., cyanosis in the toes, but no cyanosis in the fingers and lips. In this situation, the lower limbs' arterial pulsation can be normal. Adult patients with CoA often have no obvious subjective symptoms but systemic arterial hypertension. The blood pressure in the upper limbs is higher than lower limbs. Weak or absent femoral artery pulsation can also be found during physical examination. Some patients may complain of headaches, palpitations after activities, shortness of breath, lower limb fatigue, etc. Regardless of the type of CoA, there is usually a significant difference in blood pressure between the upper and lower limbs. Suppose there is doubt about whether the formation of distal collateral circulation is sufficient. In that case, the blood pressure of the upper and lower limbs should be monitored perioperatively to clarify systemic blood flow perfusion status, and the pulse oxygen saturation of the lower limbs should be monitored.

18.4.2 Hemodynamic Changes in CoA

The hemodynamic changes of CoA mainly include increased blood pressure near the proximal end of the stenosis, which increases the afterload of the left ventricle, leading to hypertrophic damage of the left ventricle and resulting in congestive heart failure. The blood flow in the distal vessels decreases due to the stenosis; in severe cases, it can lead to reduced blood supply to the lower body and kidneys and decreased oxygen saturation in the lower limbs, resulting in hypoxia, oliguria, and acidosis. As the collateral circulation is established, symptoms can be improved. If CoA is combined with atrial septal defect, ventricular septal defect, and aortic valve stenosis, the aortic blood flow will decrease further.

18.4.3 Surgical Treatment of CoA

The timing of surgery for children with CoA is classified into emergency surgery, limited-time surgery, and elective surgery. For infantile CoA, acute heart failure and shock can easily occur as the arterial duct closes. Therefore, surgery should be performed in a timely manner while stabilizing the overall condition with medical treatment. Once the arterial duct shows a tendency to close, oliguria, and a progressive increase in lactic acid, emergency surgery is required. Suppose the child has symptoms of chronic heart failure such as difficulty breathing, difficulty feeding, delayed growth and development, etc. In that case, limited-time surgery should be performed after improving heart function with drug treatment. For children with adult-type CoA, although there are no obvious symptoms, if the pressure difference between the two ends of the stenosis is >20 mm Hg, or even if the pressure difference is ≤20 mm Hg but imaging shows clear anatomical stenosis evidence, and there is abundant collateral or existing systolic hypertension (greater than the 95th percentile of blood pressure in the same age and height population), children show an indication for surgical intervention and elective surgery is needed. When CoA is accompanied by other congenital heart defects that need to be corrected in one stage, surgery can be performed through a median sternotomy approach with the aid of CPB. During the aortic cross-clamp period, selective cerebral perfusion can be performed through the brachiocephalic artery to enhance brain protection and reduce postoperative neurological complications. Children who are planning for cerebral perfusion need to be monitored for right radial artery pressure to ensure the accuracy of invasive arterial blood pressure during cerebral perfusion.

18.4.4 Selective Cerebral Perfusion

Selective cerebral perfusion (SCP) refers to selective perfusion of the cerebral arteries by directly perfusing the right cerebral hemisphere and right upper limb. In contrast, the left cerebral hemisphere receives blood supply through the Willis circle. Because children's blood vessels are small and the diameter of the arterial cannulation is limited, continuous perfusion of the brain is usually performed by extending the cannula from the ascending aortic root into the brachiocephalic artery, maintaining the blood supply to the brain and right upper limb. At this time, invasive arterial blood pressure monitoring of the child's right radial artery needs to be established to obtain arterial blood pressure during cerebral perfusion. The purpose of SCP is to reduce the time of cerebral ischemia and hypoxia and reduce postoperative neurological complications. Typically, near-infrared spectroscopy (NIRS) is used to monitor $rScO_2$ in order to reflect the effect of SCP.

18.5 Discussion

18.5.1 Preoperative Assessment and Preparation

The preoperative chest X-ray did not show any signs of pulmonary edema or any symptoms of left heart congestive heart failure, such as rapid breathing and excessive sweating in this infant. However, the infant's liver was 1.0 cm below the ribs, indicating obvious symptoms of right heart failure. SpO_2 was 94% at room air, which was considered to be caused by preoperative pulmonary hypertension and bidirectional shunting at VSD. Therefore, during the perioperative period, it was necessary to avoid further increases in pulmonary artery pressure and prevent right heart failure. To prepare for the possible exacerbation of right heart failure during surgery, all kinds of cardiotonic drugs should be ready for use as needed.

18.5.2 Induction of Anesthesia

Considering the young age of this patient with CoA and insufficient collateral circulation, the fact that increased afterload of the left ventricle can easily lead to a decline in left ventricular function, and the patient also has bidirectional shunting, a project of induction and maintenance of anesthesia with benzodiazepines, opioids, rocuronium, and combined inhalation low concentration sevoflurane was performed in order to maintain circulation stability as much as possible.

18.5.3 Anesthetic Management Before CPB

During the perioperative period, special attention should be paid to the blood perfusion of the lower body in children with CoA. It is well-known that good blood perfusion is closely related to cardiac output, which depends on heart rate, myocardial contractility, and preload. So, if cardiotonic drugs are used before surgical correction of the narrowed segment, cardiotonic drugs not only increase heart rate and myocardial contractility but also increase systemic circulation resistance, which further exacerbates the pressure afterload of the left ventricle in children with CoA. Therefore, the use of cardiotonic drugs should be avoided as much as possible before surgical correction of the narrowed segment. In this case, the infant was given fluid supplementation to maintain CVP at around 12 cm H_2O. That is, cardiac output was increased by increasing cardiac preload to improve blood perfusion of the lower body.

The blood perfusion of the lower body in children with CoA is also affected by the increased left ventricular afterload caused by aortic stenosis, which depends on the severity of the stenosis, the presence of PDA, the degree of establishment of collateral circulation distal to the aorta, and other concurrent heart diseases. The PDA in this infant has already closed, so the blood perfusion of the lower body mainly comes from the blood flow through the aortic stenosis segment and collateral circulation. We cannot improve the blood perfusion of the lower body by altering the collateral circulation formation, but we can increase the blood flow through the aortic stenosis segment. In this case, at the ASD level, there exists a left-to-right shunting, which reduces the left heart output and the blood flow through the aortic stenosis segment. At the VSD level, a bidirectional shunting exists, which increases the left heart output and blood flow through the aortic stenosis segment through the right-to-left shunting. However, bidirectional shunting also indicates the presence of pulmonary hypertension. Considering that the preoperative physical examination found that the infant's liver was 1 cm below the ribs, which is one of the symptoms of right heart failure, we adopt hyperventilation to reduce pulmonary vascular resistance and relieve the right ventricular afterload. However, hyperventilation will cause an increase in pulmonary blood flow and a decrease in systemic blood flow and affect the blood perfusion of the lower body. Therefore, it is not appropriate to hyperventilate at this time but rather to maintain appropriate pulmonary vascular resistance to counteract the increased left-to-right shunting caused by increased aortic ejection impedance due to aortic stenosis. At the same time, we should avoid the increase of pulmonary vascular resistance and right ventricular afterload caused by excessive blood carbon dioxide accumulation. In short, the balance must be achieved between the right ventricular afterload reduction and the left-to-right shunting reduction. Therefore, $ETCO_2$ has maintained at 35–40 mm Hg by the adjustment of respiratory parameter settings in this case to avoid the increase of pulmonary blood flow and the further reduction of lower body blood perfusion caused by the reduction in pulmonary vascular resistance after hyperventilation and also avoid the increase of pulmonary vascular resistance and right ventricular afterload caused by carbon dioxide accumulation. CoA may involve the left subclavian artery. When the aorta is cross-clamped during surgery, the proximal aortic clamp may also block or affect the blood flow of the left subclavian artery and result in unreliable arterial pressure measurement in the left upper limb. In addition, the arterial pressure measurement in the left upper limb will be completely distorted during selective cerebral perfusion. Therefore, the invasive arterial pressure measurement was conducted on the right radial artery. The purpose of femoral artery pressure measurement is to compare the pressure difference between the upper and lower arteries to better understand the blood perfusion of the lower body and to evaluate the surgical effect simultaneously.

18.5.4 Anesthetic Management During CPB

Some children can develop neurological complications after surgery under CPB. A decrease in $rScO_2$ may be an important cause among various pathogenic factors. Near-infrared spectroscopy can continuously and reliably reflect the changes in cerebral blood flow by detecting the absorption and reflection of near-infrared light in brain tissue, which can provide useful information for timely intervention in brain tissue oxygenation. The value displayed by near-infrared spectroscopy is the regional tissue oxygenation index, the ratio of oxygenated hemoglobin to total hemoglobin in the near-infrared penetration area, which mainly reflects the venous blood oxygen content. The normal value of $rScO_2$ is about 68%. A decrease of more than 10% from the baseline value suggests insufficient cerebral perfusion, a decrease of 20% may be related to the occurrence of neurological symptoms. In this case, the maximum decrease of $rScO_2$ value was less than 6% during CPB, indicating that selective cerebral perfusion achieved a good effect.

18.5.5 Anesthetic Management After CPB

The one-stage repair surgery for CoA and other related heart abnormalities is very challenging due to the severe disease conditions, long time of aortic cross-clamp during the repair of aortic stenosis and intracardiac abnormalities, and low heart function commonly related to myocardial damage. Therefore, the inotropic drugs were given in this case to improve the heart function after the resuming of heart beating and the relief of the conduction block. Mild hyperventilation was conducted to reduce the afterload of the right ventricle to maintain circulation stability and systemic blood perfusion.

After surgery, the patient was transferred to the CICU. It was difficult to maintain oxygenation after the tracheal tube was removed. Hypoxia was subsequently resolved by tracheal intubation again. The longer postoperative mechanical ventilation time and the occurrence of postoperative respiratory failure may be related to the increase of airway mucoprotein caused by cardiopulmonary bypass.

18.6 Shortcomings and Limitations

Due to the limitations, the medical team did not monitor the tissue oxygen saturation of the lower half of the patient's body, especially the oxygen saturation in the kidney area, which is not conducive to the early detection of ischemic hypoxia events in important organs such as the kidneys, this may bring adverse consequences.

18.7 Conclusion

In summary, CoA is a type of obstructive disease of the left heart. Maintaining the cardiac output is the key point of anesthetic management. The reduction of systemic-pulmonary circulation resistance ratio should be avoided as much as possible before CPB if the patient with CoA is accompanied by ASD or VSD. In addition, the aggravation of pulmonary artery hypertension should also be avoided, and an appropriate pulmonary-systemic circulation resistance ratio should be maintained. Monitoring the changes in regional cerebral oxygen saturation during selective cerebral perfusion is necessary. Low cardiac output should also be corrected after CPB (Yanhui Huang).

19 Anesthetic Management of Aortic Supravalvular Stenosis Surgery in a Child with Williams Syndrome

Yanhui Huang

Abstract

A 5-year-old and 3-month-old child with Williams syndrome was found to have a heart murmur during a physical examination. An echocardiogram indicated supravalvular aortic stenosis. The child was scheduled to undergo corrective surgery for supravalvular aortic stenosis under general anesthesia. Children with Williams syndrome often have supravalvular aortic stenosis and coronary artery disease. Supravalvular aortic stenosis usually causes increased left ventricular afterload and left ventricular centripetal hypertrophy. Coronary artery disease causes poor myocardial perfusion and myocardial ischemia, which significantly increases the risk of arrhythmias and cardiac arrest. Anesthetic management for these children should maintain adequate circulatory volume and good coronary artery perfusion, avoid myocardial oxygen consumption increase, and prevent the occurrence of perioperative hypotension.

Y. Huang (✉)
The National Children's Medical Center (Shanghai), Department of Anesthesiology of Shanghai Children's Medical Center, Shanghai Jiao Tong University School of Medicine, Shanghai, China
e-mail: huangyanhui@scmc.com.cn

Williams syndrome is a relatively rare congenital multisystem disease that involves cardiovascular, connective tissue, and central nervous system disorders. Cardiovascular disorders include supravalvular aortic stenosis (SVAS), pulmonary artery stenosis, obstructive coronary artery disease, and diffuse aortic stenosis. The risk of sudden death in these patients during sedation or anesthesia is 25 to 100 times higher than that of the general patients. This article reports the anesthetic management of a child with Williams syndrome undergoing cardiac correction surgery.

19.1 Case Presentation

The patient was a 5-year-old and 3-month-old male with a weight of 19 kg. A heart murmur was found soon after birth during a physical examination at a local hospital. Still, no further diagnosis and treatment were conducted until he came to the hospital for further diagnosis and treatment.

Physical examination: Distinctive facial features, irregular teeth, regular heart rhythm, II/VI systolic murmur heard in the second to third intercostal space on the left sternal border, enhanced second heart sound in the pulmonary valve auscultation area, blood pressure (BP) 95/50 mm Hg, pulse oxygen saturation (SpO_2) 98%.

Laboratory tests: Normal blood routine test, normal coagulation, liver and kidney function.

J. Zheng et al. (eds.), *Selected Pediatric Cardiovascular Surgery Anesthesia Cases*,
https://doi.org/10.1007/978-981-96-5614-1_19

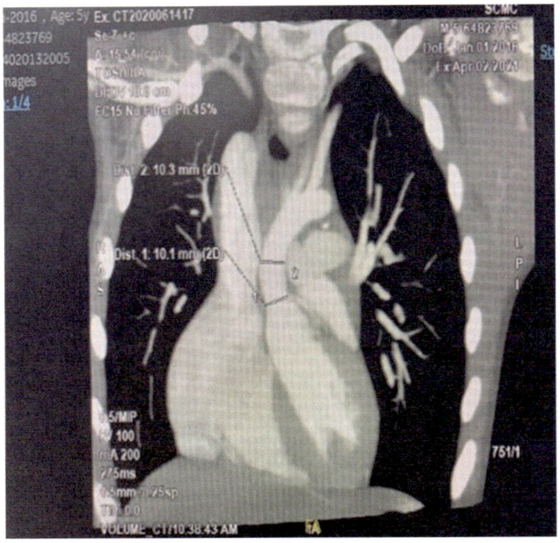

Fig. 19.1 Preoperative ascending aorta CT of the child

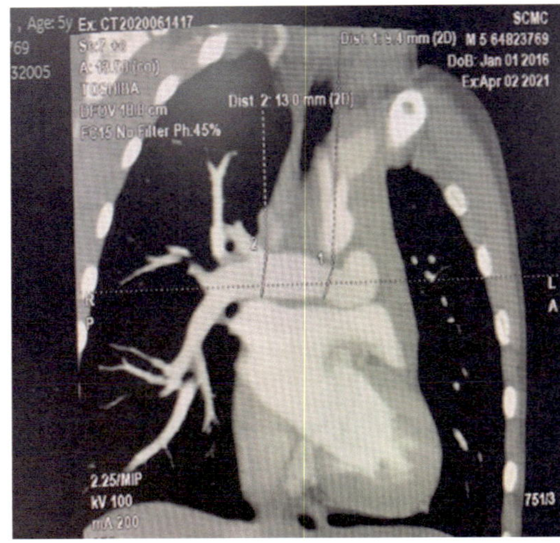

Fig. 19.2 Preoperative right pulmonary artery CT of the child

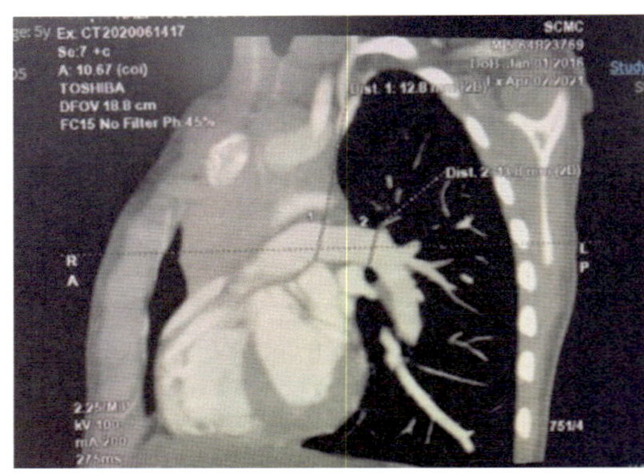

Fig. 19.3 Preoperative left pulmonary artery CT of the child

Chest X-ray: Heart shadow enlargement, multiple lung markings.

Electrocardiogram (ECG): Sinus tachycardia.

Echocardiography: Mild left ventricle enlargement and hypertrophy, acceptable tricuspid aortic valve mobility, valve ring 1.43 cm, transvalvular flow speed 1.5 m/s, sinutubular junction 0.96 cm, flow speed 3.9 m/s, pressure difference 61 mm Hg, ascending aorta diameter 1.23 cm. Left pulmonary artery flow speed 2.0 m/s, right pulmonary artery flow speed 2.06 m/s. Atrial septal defect (ASD, II) central part 0.71 cm, left aortic arch, acceptable arch transverse part morphology, isthmus part 0.71 cm, descending aorta flow speed 2.83 m/s.

Thoracic CT (plain scan + enhancement): Ventricular septal defect (VSD), right atrium and left ventricle enlargement (mild), myocardial hypertrophy (mild), left arch, aortic sinus enlargement, unclear display of the coronary arteries, SVAS with diameter 8.5 × 10.1 mm, ascending aorta 10.3 × 1.6 mm (Fig. 19.1), right pulmonary artery root 9.4 mm, slightly narrow, the distal portion 13.0 mm (Fig. 19.2), left pulmonary artery root 12.8 mm, the distal portion 13.8 mm (Fig. 19.3).

The diagnosis was Williams syndrome with stenosis above the aortic valve. He was scheduled to receive corrective surgery for stenosis above the aortic valve.

19.2 Anesthetic Management

The boy drank 100 mL of water 2 hours before surgery and took oral midazolam 0.5 mg/kg half an hour before surgery. He was separated from his parent after the Ramsay score reached 3. Routine ECG, BP, and SpO_2 were monitored after he was brought into the operating room.

Heart rate (HR) was 110 beats/min, BP was 117/65 mm Hg, and SpO_2 was 100%. Midazolam 1.5 mg, etomidate 5.0 mg, sufentanil 40 μg, and rocuronium 10 mg were intravenously injected for anesthesia induction. An ID 5.0 mm cuffed endotracheal tube was intubated orally with the assistance of visual laryngoscopy. The depth of the endotracheal tube was 15 cm. Pressure control ventilation (PCV) mode was used with respiratory parameters set as: 1.0 L/min oxygen flow rate, 50% fraction of inspired oxygen (FiO_2), 177 mL tidal volume (VT), 1:2 inspiratory time to expiratory time (I:E) ratio, end-tidal carbon dioxide ($ETCO_2$) was maintained between 35 and 40 mm Hg through adjustment of peak inspiratory pressure (PIP) and respiratory rate (RR).

After anesthesia induction, the left radial artery and right internal jugular vein were catheterized under ultrasound guidance to continuously monitor invasive blood pressure (ABP) and central venous pressure (CVP). The left femoral vein was catheterized for rapid fluid infusion to maintain CVP at 8–10 cm H_2O. General anesthesia was maintained by intravenous infusion of 4.0 mg/(kg·h) propofol, 2.0 μg/(kg·h) sufentanil, and 0.5 mg/(kg·h) rocuronium combined with sevoflurane intermittent inhalation. Before the aorta was cannulated after thoracotomy, heparin 60 mg was intravenously injected, and cardiopulmonary bypass (CPB) was initiated when the activated clotting time (ACT) was more than 400 seconds. The aortic wall at the oblique incision of the ascending aorta was found to be significantly thickened; the diameter of the sinutubular junction was about 5.0 mm, and the bovine pericardial patch was applied to enlarge the sinutubular junction. The diameter of secundum ASD was 10 mm, which was closed using the autologous pericardial patch. The heart automatically resumed beating and sinus rhythm soon after aortic cross-clamp was released, HR 115 beats/min, ABP 63/48 mm Hg, Dopamine 5.0 μg/(kg·min), epinephrine 0.05 μg/(kg·min), and norepinephrine 0.025 μg/(kg·min) were intravenously administered to maintain circulatory stability. After the boy was successfully separated from CPB, crystalloid fluids and blood products were supplemented to maintain HR around 120 beats/min, systolic blood pressure not less than 100 mm Hg, diastolic blood pressure not less than 65 mm Hg, and CVP kept at 9–13 cm H_2O. After ultrafiltration, protamine was given to neutralize heparin (the ratio of the two doses was 1.5:1), and 10% calcium gluconate 2.0 mL was supplemented according to the blood gas analysis results. 150 mL of autologous blood was infused during the hemostasis and chest closure period. The patient was transferred to the Cardiac Intensive Care Unit (CICU) with an endotracheal tube after surgery.

19.3 Postoperative Outcome

The child's hemodynamics were stable after surgery. No abnormalities were found during the follow-up examination of the chest radiograph and echocardiography. The endotracheal tube was removed on the second day after surgery. The child was transferred back to the general ward on the third day after surgery and discharged from the hospital on the sixth day after surgery.

19.4 Review of Knowledge Points

19.4.1 Genetic Basis of Williams Syndrome

Williams syndrome is caused by a deletion of 1.5–1.8 M base pairs on the long arm of chromosome 7q11.23, which encodes 27 genes, including the elastin gene. The deletion of the elastin gene results in the reduction of elastin formation. The lack of elastin formation is associated with a wide range of arterial diseases and abnormal cardiovascular development in children with Williams syndrome. The deletion of some other genes is related to hypertension, visual-spatial defects, and cognitive characteristics in children with Williams syndrome.

19.4.2 Pathological Anatomy and Pathophysiology of Williams Syndrome

In children with Williams syndrome, the lack of elastin in large blood vessels makes them become less elastic and more fragile, which leads the blood vessels to be exposed to higher stress than usual and progressive thickening and fibrosis of the smooth muscle and collagen layers in the middle of the blood vessels. As the vessels become narrowed, the blood flow speed will increase and cause more shear stress to vascular endothelium, leading to further thickening of the middle layer of the blood vessel wall. This vicious cycle repeats again and again. When elastin-related arterial disease occurs, the sinus tubular ridge at the top of the aortic valve junction often becomes thickened, which can lead to supravalvular aortic stenosis, left ventricular afterload increase, cardiac systolic work increase, and gradual left ventricular wall centripetal hypertrophy. Myocardial hypertrophy increases the demand for metabolic substrates and restricts the coronary blood flow supply. Due to the thickening of the Valsalva sinus wall in children with Williams syndrome, the coronary artery's openings may narrow. If the aortic valve leaf adheres to the sinus tubular ridge, it can also restrict blood flow to the sinus and reduce coronary perfusion. When the aortic valve is narrowed, the openings of the coronary artery are usually in the high-pressure chamber. Hence, the coronary artery is prone to expansion, twisting, thickening, hardening, and other degenerative changes. All these factors can contribute to the ventricular fibrillation and cardiac arrest.

19.4.3 Clinical Manifestations of Williams Syndrome

Williams syndrome involves multiple organ systems. 7% to 58% of children with Williams syndrome have renal artery stenosis. These children are usually hypersensitive to sound. They have elfin facies, small or irregularly shaped deciduous teeth, and malocclusion, which may lead to difficult airways and affect tracheal intubation. Hypercalcemia is common in newborns and infants with this syndrome, which leads to irritability, abdominal colic, difficulty feeding, and electrocardiogram abnormalities. Hypercalcemia usually disappears after 4 years old. In addition, low birth weight, developmental delay, and low muscle tone are also quite common. Pulmonary artery obstructive lesions can occur with SVAS.

19.5 Discussion

19.5.1 Preoperative Assessment and Preparation

As early as 1996, Bird and others identified the risk factors for sudden death in children with Williams syndrome, including young age, sedation or anesthesia, biventricular outflow tract obstruction, and coronary artery stenosis. For details, see Table 19.1. This case was classified as a high-risk patient based on the pressure difference at the sinutubular junction >40 mm Hg, left ventricular enlargement, and myocardial hypertrophy. Sinus tachycardia of preoperative ECG and unclear display of the coronary arteries on echocardiogram indicated the possibility of coronary artery disease. Therefore, it is important to control the fast heart rate to reduce myocardial oxygen consumption, avoid hypotension, and reduce the risk of sudden death during the perioperative period. It is also very important to maintain adequate blood volume before surgery, which can help to maintain the child's cardiac preload and myocardial contractility and ensure adequate cardiac output and coronary perfusion. To avoid preoperative fast-related dehydration and a reduction in circulating blood volume, the child, in this case, drank light fluids 2 h before surgery.

19.5.2 Preoperative Medication

Preoperative anxiety is very common in children with Williams syndrome, which can be exacerbated by hyperacusis. Children with Williams syndrome are very fond of music. Therefore, it is very useful to alleviate their anxiety through music. In this case, the child was given sedatives before surgery to relieve stress. Sedatives that do not cause tachycardia, hypotension, or respiratory depression were preferred to use, as these factors can cause or exacerbate myocardial ischemia and hypoxia, even leading to sudden cardiac arrest and death in this kind of child. In this case, the child was given oral midazolam 0.5 mg/kg before surgery, which achieved good anti-anxiety effects.

Table 19.1 Risk stratification in children with Williams syndrome

Low risk	Medium risk	High risk
Age > 20 years	Hypertension	Age < 3 years
Mild SVAS or PPS	Moderate SVAS or PPS	History of adverse cardiovascular events
Normal ECG	Moderate BVOTO	Arrhythmia
Renal artery not involved	Renal artery stenosis	Severe BVOTO
	Renal dysfunction	SVAS pressure difference > 40 mm hg and left ventricular hypertrophy
	ECG 450 ms < QTc < 500 ms	Significant involvement of the coronary arteries
	Airway abnormalities, lung disease or severe gastroesophageal reflux	Diffuse stenosis of the thoracic aorta
		Moderate left or right ventricular hypertrophy symptoms or ECG showing ischemic signs
		ECG: QTc >500 ms

SVAS supravalvular aortic stenosis, *PPS* peripheral pulmonary stenosis, *BVOTO* biventricular outflow tract obstruction, *QTc* corrected QT interval

19.5.3 Anesthesia Induction

Most intravenous anesthetics inhibit the sympathetic nervous system and cause varying degrees of peripheral vasodilation and systemic vascular resistance reduction, particularly propofol. Children with supravalvular aortic stenosis have reduced cardiac output and are prone to hypotension. Therefore, in this case, etomidate, which has a minimal impact on hemodynamics, was chosen instead of propofol for anesthesia induction to avoid excessive blood pressure drop, which could affect coronary perfusion. This child with Williams syndrome had misaligned teeth, which could indicate a difficult airway. A visual laryngoscope, which has advantages over a traditional laryngoscope in dealing with difficult airways, was chosen for endotracheal intubation. The entire anesthesia induction and intubation process went smoothly.

19.5.4 Perioperative Anesthetic Management

The pathophysiological mechanisms leading to death in children with Williams syndrome include reduced cardiac output, myocardial ischemia, and arrhythmias. Therefore, the overall goal of anesthetic management in children with Williams syndrome is to maintain adequate preload, appropriate myocardial contractility, and relatively high afterload, maintaining sufficient coronary perfusion while avoiding a sharp increase in heart rate, myocardial contractility, and myocardial oxygen consumption. Therefore, it is better to maintain a relatively sufficient circulating volume before CPB. After CPB, a small dose of epinephrine and norepinephrine can be infused intravenously to enhance myocardial contractility, increase cardiac output, and increase peripheral vascular resistance. In addition, it is also necessary to replenish the circulation volume after CPB. All of the above work is to maintain good coronary perfusion, ensure myocardial blood supply, avoid arrhythmias, and maintain hemodynamic stability.

19.6 Shortcomings and Limitations

Children with Williams syndrome are at a potential risk of severe hemodynamic fluctuations during anesthesia induction. Establishment of invasive arterial blood pressure monitoring before anesthesia induction can help avoid severe blood pressure fluctuations. However, due to the child's age of only 5 years and inability to cooperate, our team was unable to conduct arterial catheterization while the child was sedated. Therefore, our team adopted non-invasive blood pressure monitoring every 2 min to replace invasive arterial blood pressure monitoring during anesthesia induction. Additionally, the child's heart rate reached around 120 beats/min after CPB, faster than the normal physiological range for a 5-year-old child, which is not ideal for heart rate control.

19.7 Conclusion

Currently, there is no ideal anesthesia plan suitable for all children with Williams syndrome. However, it is well known that maintaining sufficient circulatory volume, appropriate myocardial contractility, higher diastolic pressure, adequate coronary blood supply, and avoiding increased myocardial oxygen consumption are key points of anesthetic management in children with Williams syndrome. To improve the perioperative safety of these children, emergency plans should be prepared for intraoperative crisis events, including standby surgical and CPB supporting teams` (Yanhui Huang).

20 Anesthetic Management of a Neonate with Persistent Fifth Aortic Arch Complicated by Distal Stenosis and an Interrupted Fourth Aortic Arch

Jie Hu

Abstract

A 6-day-old, 2.6 kg male neonate was admitted to the intensive care unit due to poor feeding and cyanosis after crying and was diagnosed with persistent fifth aortic arch (PFAA) complicated by distal stenosis and an interrupted fourth aortic arch. He manifested with progressive heart failure, shock, and acidosis. His clinical condition was progressively improved after endotracheal intubation and prostaglandin infusion was initiated. A surgical repair was performed through a standard median sternotomy.

Persistent fifth aortic arch (PFAA) is a rare congenital cardiac defect that was first described by Van Praagh R and Van Praagh S in 1969. Although PFAA can be an isolated disease, it is often associated with other cardiovascular anomalies, including aortic arch interruption, coarctation, transposition of the great arteries, pulmonary atresia, truncus arteriosus, and other complex congenital heart diseases. PFAA with severe distal stenosis and interrupted fourth aortic arch could cause shock in the neonatal period. This report describes the perioperative anesthetic management of a newborn with PFAA, distal stenosis, and interrupted fourth aortic arch.

20.1 Case Presentation

The patient was a 6-day-old male with a weight of 2.6 kg. He was born full-term via cesarean section. There was no history of asphyxia. On the day of admission, the patient refused to be fed, and cyanosis could be seen after crying. He was diagnosed with "coarctation of the aorta (CoA), neonatal acidosis, pneumonia" by another hospital. Oxygen was administered by a hood, but normal oxygen saturation could not be maintained. The patient was transferred to our hospital after endotracheal intubation for further treatment.

Physical examination: The newborn was sedated and gray under mechanical ventilation. When fraction of inspired oxygen (FiO_2) was 21%, pulse oxygen saturation (SpO_2) was 92%, heart rate (HR) was 146 beats/min, left upper limb blood pressure was 88/57 mm Hg, right upper limb blood pressure was 99/61 mm Hg, left lower limb blood pressure was 72/60 mm Hg, right lower limb blood pressure was 57/34 mm Hg, bilateral lung breathing sounds were clear, no rales were found, and II/VI systolic murmurs could be heard in the precordial region.

Routine blood test: WBC 21.97 × 10^9, RBC 4.15 × 10^{12}, HCT 43.1%, Hb 148 g/L, Plt

J. Hu (✉)
The National Children's Medical Center (Shanghai), Department of Anesthesiology of Shanghai Children's Medical Center, Shanghai Jiao Tong University School of Medicine, Shanghai, China
e-mail: hujie@scmc.com.cn

J. Zheng et al. (eds.), *Selected Pediatric Cardiovascular Surgery Anesthesia Cases*,
https://doi.org/10.1007/978-981-96-5614-1_20

304 × 10^9, N 59.8%. Liver and kidney function tests: AST 60 U/L, ALT 58 U/L, UREA 3.1 mmol/L, CREA 67 μmol/L. Coagulation routine: PT 15.2 s, APTT 44.4 s. Blood gas analysis: pH 7.21, PaO_2 87.3 mm Hg, $PaCO_2$ 36.9 mm Hg, BE 20.4 mmol/L, Na^+ 124 mmol/L, K^+ 4.8 mmol/L, Ca^{2+} 1.24 mmol/L, Cl^-10 6 mmol/L, Lac 10.3 mmol/L, Hb 18 g/L, HCT 55%.

Chest X-ray: Enlarged heart shadow, increased and blurred lung markings. Echocardiography: Type A interrupted aortic arch (IAA), residual fifth arch with stenosis, the narrowest inner diameter was 0.16 cm, flow speed 3.64 m/s, pressure difference 52.9 mm Hg, central atrial septal defect (ASD, II) 0.44 cm, bidirectional shunt, slightly enlarged left atrium and left ventricle, diffusely weakened left ventricular systolic activity, LVEF 29.4%.

Cardiac CT: IAA (Type A), residual fifth arch with distal stenosis, PDA, ASD.

After completing the relevant examinations, prostaglandin 5.0 ng/(kg·min) and dopamine 5.0 μg/(kg·min) were initiated to infuse intravenously. Furosemide 2.5 mg was administered intravenously q12h for diuresis. A surgical repair would be conducted when his clinical condition was stable.

20.2 Anesthetic Management

The patient was brought into the operating room with endotracheal intubation and intravenous infusion of prostaglandin 5.0 ng/(kg·min) and dopamine 5.0 μg/(kg·min). The ventilator parameters were adjusted after the endotracheal tube position was confirmed by bilateral auscultating the breath sounds. The pressure control ventilation mode was used, and end-tidal carbon dioxide ($ETCO_2$) was maintained at 35–45 mm Hg by peak inspiratory pressure (PIP) adjustment. The ventilation frequency was 30 times/min, the inspiratory time to expiratory time (I:E) ratio was 1:2, and a fraction of inspired oxygen (FiO_2) was 21%. In addition to routine monitoring, invasive arterial blood pressures (ABP) were measured from the right upper and right lower extremities, and central venous pressure (CVP) was measured from the right internal jugular vein catheterization. After induction of anesthesia, arterial blood was drawn for blood gas analysis (Table 20.1). General anesthesia was maintained by intravenous infusion of sufentanil, propofol, rocuronium, and sevoflurane intermittent inhalation during the operation.

Standard median sternotomy was conducted smoothly. ABP was 108/66 mm Hg, HR was 133 beats/min, SpO_2 was 97%, and CVP was 8 cm H_2O. After establishing cardiopulmonary bypass (CPB), the body temperature was reduced to 20 °C. Once the ascending aorta was cross-clamped, myocardial protective fluid was injected at the root of the aorta, which caused the heart to stop beating. An interrupted fourth aortic arch and residual fifth arch without development were found. The PDA connection was close to closing, ligated, and cut off. During the hypothermic circulatory arrest, the anterior wall of the fifth arch was cut open and enlarged by the pericardial patch. After CPB was restored, the temperature was gradually increased. Once the aortic cross-clamped was released, the spontaneous heartbeat automatically returned to sinus rhythm. The CPB time was 63 minutes. The hypothermic circulatory arrest time was 10 min. The withdrawal from CPB was smooth. Dopamine at 5.0 μg/(kg·min) and epinephrine at 0.2 μg/(kg·min) was continuously infused. ABP was 71/41 mm Hg, HR was 157 beats/min, SpO_2 was 98%, and CVP was 14 cm H_2O. Protamine was intravenously given to neutralize heparin after ultrafiltration. The blood gas analysis was then rechecked (Table 20.1). 5% sodium bicarbonate 2 mL/kg, calcium gluconate 20 mg/kg, and 10% KCl 1 mL were intravenously administrated based on the blood gas analysis results. After CPB, 30 mL concentrated autologous red blood cells, 200 μg VII factor, and 50 IU prothrombin complex were intravenously infused to assist hemostasis. Delayed sternal closure, in this case, was required after surgery. This neonate was transported to the CICU with endotracheal intubation.

Table 20.1 Intraoperative blood gas test results

Time point	pH	PaO_2 (mm Hg)	$PaCO_2$ (mm Hg)	BE (mmol/L)	HCT (%)	K^+ (mmol/L)	Ca^{2+} (mmol/L)	Cl^- (mmol/L)	Lac (mmol/L)	HCO^{3-} (mmol/L)
Before thoracotomy	7.37	72	45.5	0.5	46.7	2.63	1.068	109	1.3	21.5
After stopping ultrafiltration	7.29	111.8	44.7	−5.5	37.3	3.83	1.037	108.5	7.4	15.6

20.3 Postoperative Outcome

The sternum was successfully closed on the postoperative day 3. Non-invasive ventilation was initiated after the removal of endotracheal intubation on postoperative day 3. The non-invasive ventilation was switched to nasal cannula oxygenation 1 day later. The child recovered well and was discharged from the hospital 15 days after the surgery.

20.4 Review of Knowledge Points

20.4.1 Embryological Basis of PFAA

During embryological development of the great arteries, the bilateral fifth primitive arches usually do not form or degenerate early after formation at the 4th week of embryonic life. However, for some reason, the fifth arch may persist unilaterally or bilaterally and completely or partially, producing various appearances.

20.4.2 Pathological Anatomy of PFAA

PFAA is a rare congenital cardiovascular malformation that can occur alone or in combination with IAA, CoA, persistent arterial trunk, Tetralogy of Fallot, pulmonary artery atresia, and transposition of the great arteries. In 1969, Van Praagh R and Van Praagh S first reported PFAA cases or so-called double aortic arch. PFAA can be a right or left arch and be divided into two major categories. One type of PFAA is the connection between the systemic-systemic circulation (Type A and B), which is the most common type. The other is the connection between the systemic-pulmonary circulation (Type C). Type A is characterized by having upper and lower aortic arches. Both the upper arch (the fourth aortic arch) and the lower arch (the fifth aortic arch) on the same side are open, forming a parallel double-chamber aorta. Type B is based on Type A, with the fourth arch interrupted and the fifth arch open. Type C is the fifth arch open and connected to the pulmonary artery through the embryonic sixth arch, forming a systemic-pulmonary artery connection (Fig. 20.1).

20.4.3 Clinical Manifestations of PFAA

The clinical symptoms of PFAA vary greatly depending on the accompanied cardiovascular malformations. For simple Type A and B PFAA, the hemodynamic is usually normal when the blood flow in the fifth aortic arch is sufficient. As these children grow up, PFAA may be incidentally found due to hypertension, blood pressure differences between the upper and lower extremities, or systolic murmurs. If the patients with PFAA were accompanied by other complex cardiovascular malformations, the symptoms of cyanosis, tachypnea, or feeding problems usually occur in infancy or even the neonatal period. Echocardiography and cardiac catheterization are the most commonly used diagnostic methods. Still, CTA and MRI can provide more accurate information about the relationship between the fifth aortic arch and surrounding structures and vessels.

PFAA combined with CoA and Type A IAA is more common in clinics, of which the fourth aortic arch is interrupted distal to the left subclavian artery, and the fifth aortic arch originates from the ascending aorta opposite or adjacent to the brachiocephalic artery and ends

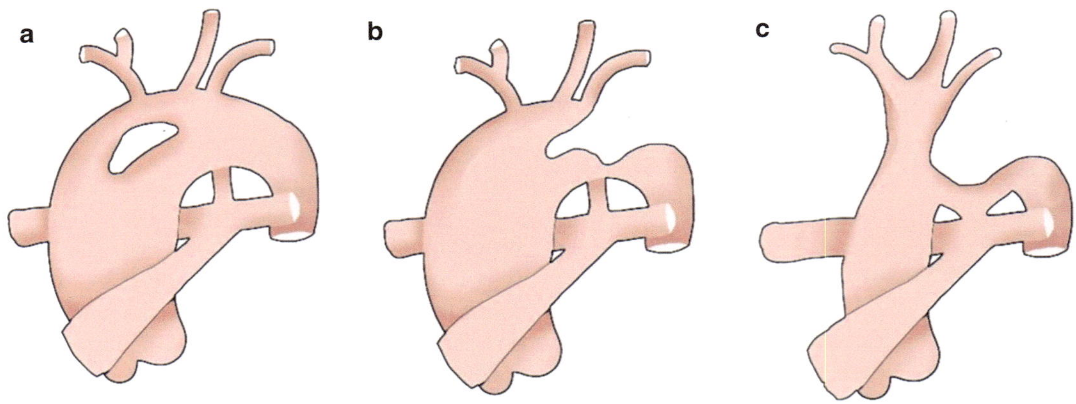

Fig. 20.1 Classification of persistent fifth aortic arch. (**a**) type A; (**b**) type B; (**c**) type C

at the descending aorta, where it narrows at the end. Because the fourth aortic arch is interrupted, the blood flow to the lower body is supplied by the fifth aortic arch, the unique channel connecting the ascending and descending aorta. It thus plays a crucial role in the survival of the child. However, the stenosis at the fifth aortic arch can severely affect hemodynamics. The child may show early clinical manifestations such as blood pressure differences between the upper and lower extremities, heart failure, etc., which require surgical treatment as soon as possible.

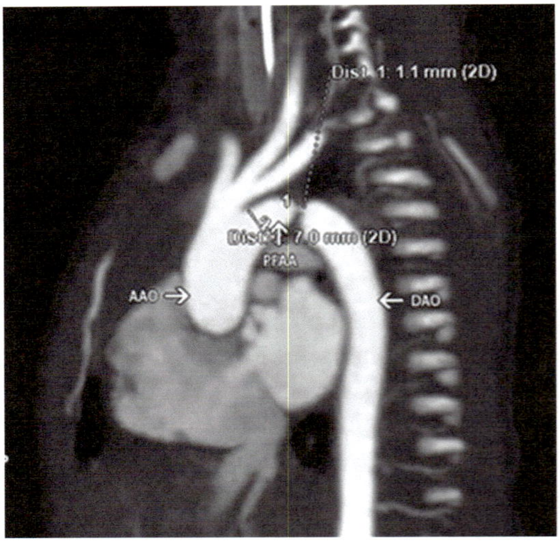

Fig. 20.2 Preoperative cardiac CT of the patient. *AAO* ascending aorta, *PFAA* persistent fifth aortic arch, *DAO* descending aorta

20.5 Discussion

We classified our case as PFAA type B with CoA according to the criteria. If the fourth arch is fully present, it is relatively simple to identify other arterial arches except this arch, namely the fifth arterial arch. Once the fourth arterial arch is interrupted, it is very challenging to make the diagnosis since the fifth arterial arch becomes the only arterial arch. Therefore, this case was initially diagnosed with CoA (Fig. 20.2). PFAA has been labeled as the great pretender in previous literature. PFAA is easily misdiagnosed as CoA because it is hard to identify, especially in the situation of PFAA combined with IAA. In fact, their hemodynamic changes are very similar.

20.5.1 Preoperative Assessment and Preparation

Patients with PFAA usually do not have significant symptoms. Many patients are diagnosed with PFAA due to the increased blood pressure in the upper extremities, and the systolic murmur is incidentally found during physical examination. Very few PFAA patients may be found due to shock caused by the closure of the patent ductus arteriosus in newborns or infants. Unlike CoA or IAA, the blood flow of the descending aorta in PFAA is supplied by both PDA and PFAA. The blood flow provided by PFAA is usually beneficial to maintain hemodynamic stability. There is enough time to develop collateral vessels unless the distal end of PFAA becomes severely narrow, which also explains why the clinical manifestations of PFAA are usually mild and the development is slow. However, once PFAA narrows, it can result in left ventricular pressure overload and lower body hypoperfusion. If the narrowing is very severe, the PDA must be kept open to provide blood flow to the distal aorta (right-to-left shunt from the pulmonary artery to the distal aorta through the PDA). The preoperative heart failure, in this case, was considered to be caused by severe CoA, acute increase in left ventricular afterload severely affected left ventricular systolic function, which manifested as low cardiac output and shock. Therefore, preoperative treatment focuses on using prostaglandin to keep the PDA open, mechanical ventilation, and cardiotonic and diuretic therapy. The preoperative increase in blood lactate indicates insufficient perfusion of important organs and requires emergency surgery to correct PFAA stenosis.

20.5.2 Anesthetic Management Before CPB

Anesthetic management before CPB should continue the treatment in the CICU. To ensure blood perfusion in the lower body, prostaglandin should be continuously infused to keep the PDA open. The left ventricular output is very sensitive to the decrease in myocardial contractility due to the relatively high left ventricle afterload. Therefore, positive inotropic drugs should be used to ensure myocardial contraction. SVR increase should also be avoided because the increase of SVR will increase the pressure load on the left ventricle, leading to a significant decrease in cardiac output. In addition to standard routine monitoring, invasive arterial pressure should be measured in the right upper limb as clamping of the proximal aorta can affect the blood flow in the subclavian artery, which makes the pressure in the left upper limb unreliable. The oxygen saturation probe should also be placed on the right hand. Furthermore, postoperatively, lower limb arterial pressure should be monitored to compare the pressure difference between the upper and lower limbs to evaluate the surgical outcome. If conditions permit, near-infrared spectroscopy (NIRS) should be used to monitor cerebral oxygen saturation to ensure cerebral perfusion. Renal NIRS should also be used to monitor lower body perfusion during surgery. Since this was an early case, we did not have the equipment to monitor cerebral oxygen saturation at the time.

20.5.3 Anesthetic Management After CPB

The common surgical approach for PFAA is lateral thoracotomy for arch reconstruction without CPB. However, considering the critical preoperative condition of this case, the neonate could not tolerate the surgical approach of aortic clamping after lateral thoracotomy, so a median sternotomy was chosen for surgery under CPB. Deep hypothermic circulatory arrest and selective antegrade cerebral perfusion are important measures for brain protection during aortic arch surgery. Some studies suggest that when the nasopharyngeal temperature drops to around 18 °C, the "safe" time limit for deep hypothermic circulatory arrest is 30–40 min. Prolonged circulatory arrest can cause ischemic effects on other organs, and many inflammatory factors and metabolic products will be released into the blood after reperfusion. In addition, it can cause myocardial edema, further damaging cardiac function. Newborns and small infants may develop acute low cardiac output postoperatively, which may be related to preoperative left heart dysfunction and prolonged cross-clamping time during surgery. The use of positive inotropic drugs such as dopamine and epinephrine in combination with afterload-reducing drugs can help improve left ventricular wall stress. Surgical bleeding and coagulation abnormalities after CPB are common complications after aortic arch surgery. Hypothermia is one of the factors affecting coagulation function. Therefore, postoperative supplementation of coagulation factors, fibrinogen, and platelets should be actively pursued.

20.6 Shortcomings and Limitations

This is an earlier case. Our team did not have the equipment to monitor cerebral and renal oxygen saturation. Therefore, we were unable to more accurately monitor the brain and lower body perfusion in this case during CPB, which was regrettable.

20.7 Conclusion

In summary, for those newborns with PFAA combined with IAA and severe CoA, it is crucial to use prostaglandin to maintain PDA open preoperatively. Intraoperatively, in addition to routine monitoring, attention should be paid to the perfusion of the brain and lower body organs. Coagulopathy and hemodynamic instability were the most common problems after surgery, which should be paid more attention (Jie Hu).

21 Anesthetic Management for the Surgical Correction of Tetralogy of Fallot in an Infant

Jing Jiang

Abstract

A 7-month-old male infant was diagnosed with Tetralogy of Fallot (TOF) shortly after birth. He was admitted to our hospital due to aggravated cyanosis after crying recently. He was scheduled to undergo TOF corrective surgery under general anesthesia. Children with TOF often have significant hypoxemia and cardiopulmonary dysfunction due to the obstruction of the right ventricular outflow tract and intracardiac right-to-left shunting, which reduces pulmonary blood flow. The right ventricular outflow tract spasm can also cause a sharp decrease in pulmonary blood flow and Tet spells, which can be life-threatening in severe cases. During the perioperative period, attention should be paid to managing systemic pulmonary vascular resistance to avoid further reduction of pulmonary blood flow. Proactive prevention and treatment of Tet spells should be conducted. After cardiopulmonary bypass, normal right heart and coagulation functions should be maintained.

J. Jiang (✉)
The National Children's Medical Center (Shanghai), Department of Anesthesiology of Shanghai Children's Medical Center, Shanghai Jiao Tong University School of Medicine, Shanghai, China
e-mail: jiangjing@scmc.com.cn

Tetralogy of Fallot (TOF) is the most common cyanotic congenital heart disease, with 3–6 cases per 10,000 births, accounting for 5–7% of congenital heart diseases. The basic pathological anatomical changes include right ventricular outflow tract (RVOT) obstruction, malpositioned ventricular septal defect (VSD), aortic override (override range ≤ 50%), and secondary right ventricular hypertrophy. Depending on the development of the pulmonary artery, TOF can be corrected in one stage or multistage. This article reports the anesthetic management of a one-stage correction surgery in a child with TOF.

21.1 Case Presentation

A 7-month-old boy of 66 cm in height and 8.5 kg in weight was born full-term by cesarean section. Auscultation detected a heart murmur at birth, and echocardiography suggested TOF, patent foramen ovale (PFO), and patent ductus arteriosus (PDA). In the past time, the child's face turned blue during crying, which has worsened recently. He was admitted to our hospital for further treatment.

Physical Examination: The infant was conscious without obvious abnormal mental reactions. His lips and extremities were cyanotic. No finger clubbing was observed. The lung sounds were slightly coarse without rales. The heart rhythm was regular. A coarse systolic murmur

J. Zheng et al. (eds.), *Selected Pediatric Cardiovascular Surgery Anesthesia Cases*,
https://doi.org/10.1007/978-981-96-5614-1_21

could be heard on the upper left edge of the sternum. The extremities were warm without edema. The pulse oxygen saturation (SpO_2) was 85% with air breathing.

Laboratory tests: Hemoglobin 137 g/L, hematocrit 43.2%, normal liver, kidney, and coagulation function.

Echocardiography: mild right atrium and right ventricle enlargement, mild right ventricular wall thickness, widened and straddled ventricular septum (straddle range = 50%), pulmonary valve and subvalvular stenosis, pulmonary artery flow velocity 4.3 m/s, transvalvular pressure difference 74 mm Hg. PFO, left-to-right shunt, malpositioned ventricular septal defect (VSD) 12.5 mm, bidirectional shunt, mainly right-to-left. Echocardiography indicated TOF, PFO, and small collateral vessel formation.

Cardiac CT: Malpositioned VSD about 12.3 mm, aorta straddling the ventricular septum, right ventricle and outflow tract muscle hypertrophy, pulmonary valve and subvalvular stenosis, nearly normal development of pulmonary artery trunk and the left and right pulmonary arteries, McGoon index 2.07.

Chest X-ray: Boot-shaped heart, normal lung imaging.

Electrocardiogram (ECG): Sinus rhythm, upright T wave in right precordial leads.

The preoperative diagnosis was TOF. Surgical correction of TOF under general anesthesia was scheduled.

21.2 Anesthetic Management

Carbohydrate drink (2.0 mL/kg) was orally administered 2 h before surgery. 0.5 mg/kg of midazolam was orally administered for preoperative sedation 30 min before surgery. After reaching a Ramsay sedation score of 4, the child was calmly separated from the parents and brought to the operating room. After entering the operating room, ECG, blood pressure (BP), and SpO_2 were routinely monitored. Basic vital signs: BP 80/45 mm Hg, heart rate (HR) 122 beats/min, SpO_2 75%. The induction of anesthesia was conducted with midazolam 0.5 mg, etomidate 1.5 mg, sufentanil 16 μg, and rocuronium 5.0 mg. After the eyelash reflex disappeared, an ID 4.0 mm cuffed endotracheal tube was intubated with a video laryngoscope's assistance; the intubation depth was 11 cm. Pressure-controlled ventilation-volume guaranteed (PCV-VG) mode was adopted with a 2 L/min oxygen flow rate, 50% fraction of inspired oxygen (FiO_2), 80 mL tidal volume (VT), 1:2 inspiratory time to expiratory time (I:E) ratio. Adjustment of respiratory rate to maintain end-tidal carbon dioxide ($ETCO_2$) between 35 and 40 mm Hg. After intubation, invasive arterial pressure (ABP) and central venous pressure (CVP) monitoring were quickly established. Bispectral index (BIS) and cerebral tissue oxygen saturation (rSO_2) monitoring were also applied. Vital signs after intubation: ABP 88/50 mm Hg, HR 133 beats/min, SpO_2 97%, CVP 10 cm H_2O, rSO_2 70%. During the operation, propofol 4.0 mg/(kg·h), sufentanil 2.0 μg/(kg·h), and rocuronium 0.5 mg/(kg·h) were intravenously infused for maintenance anesthesia, while 0.5–1.0 MAC sevoflurane was inhaled. BIS value was maintained at 40–60 during surgery. The intraoperative arterial blood gas analysis results are shown in Table 21.1: pH 7.32, BE −6.9 mmol/L and 5% $NaHCO_3$ 2 mL/kg were given to correct metabolic acidosis.

Before the operation, tranexamic acid 10 mg/kg and ulinastatin 100,000 U were intravenously administered. Heparin 3.0 mg/kg was intravenously administered after thoracotomy, and CPB

Table 21.1 Intraoperative blood gas test results

Condition	FiO_2 (%)	pH	PaO_2 (mm Hg)	$PaCO_2$ (mm Hg)	BE (mmol/L)	HCT (%)	K^+ (mmol/L)	Ca^{2+} (mmol/L)	Lac (mmol/L)	Cl^- (mmol/L)	Hb (g/dL)	HCO^3 (mmol/L)
Postintubation	30	7.32	47	35.5	−6.93	35.7	3.82	1.22	1.3	108	12.3	18.2
Post-ultrafiltration	50	7.44	185	28.6	−4.05	27.6	3.51	0.98	1.4	104.3	9.6	19.2

was initiated after activated clotting time (ACT) >480 s. The VSD was closed with a pericardial patch, RVOT was enlarged with a transvalvular patch, and the hypertrophic abnormal muscle bundle of the right ventricular outflow tract was removed. After the aortic cross-clamp was released, the heart automatically resumed beating and sinus rhythm. Dopamine 5.0 μg/(kg·min) and norepinephrine 0.03 μg/(kg·min) were intravenously infused to maintain ABP at 60/40 mm Hg and HR at 130 beats/min. After the vena cava cross-clamp was released, mechanical ventilation resumed, and the respiratory parameters were set as before. Transesophageal echocardiography showed a pulmonary artery flow rate of 0.8 m/s, no residual shunt around the VSD patch, and an ejection fraction of 65%. CPB flow was gradually reduced to prepare for weaning. During the weaning process, the patient's ABP and HR were stable. After modified ultrafiltration, protamine 55 mg (1.2:1) was intravenously dripped to neutralize heparin. 1 IU of thrombin was used to assist hemostasis. Recheck artery blood gas (Table 21.1), among which $PaCO_2$ was 28.6 mm Hg, BE was −4.05, and Ca^{2+} was 0.98 mmol/L. The respiratory rate was reduced to 16 breaths/min, 5% $NaHCO_3$ was infused at 2.0 mL/kg to correct metabolic acidosis and 150 mg of calcium gluconate was slowly infused. There was more bleeding in the operative field, then the coagulation function was measured: ACT 160 s (100–155), clotting rate (CR) 9.0 (9–35), and platelet function (PF) 1.7 (>1.5). Protamine 5.0 mg and prothrombin complex 20 IU/kg was infused. The dosage of vasoactive drugs and inhaled anesthetics was adjusted according to blood pressure, 100 mL of autologous blood was reinfused, ABP was maintained around 80/45 mm Hg, HR 130–160 beats/min.

21.3 Postoperative Outcome

The operation lasted a total of 125 min, with a mild hypothermia bypass time of 90 min and an aortic cross-clamping time of 60 min. Blood loss was estimated at around 100 mL. The urine output was 90 mL. During the surgery, 90 mL of Ringer's acetate solution and 100 mL of autologous blood were transfused; the lactate level remained within the normal range. At the end of the surgery, ABP was 82/45 mm Hg, HR was 155 beats/min, SpO_2 was 100%, CVP was 14 cm H_2O, rectal temperature was 36.5 °C, and rSO_2 was 65%. Under the monitoring of ABP, ECG, and SpO_2, the child was transferred to the Cardiac Intensive Care Unit (CICU). The child was extubated on the 6th day after surgery and discharged from CICU on the postoperative day 7. He was finally discharged from the hospital on postoperative day 19.

21.4 Review of Knowledge Points

21.4.1 TOF Anatomy

TOF is a type of congenital malformation disease. There is a spectrum of diseases in TOF, depending on the development of the pulmonary artery. In addition to classic TOF (TOF with varying degrees of pulmonary artery stenosis), it also includes TOF with absent pulmonary valve syndrome, TOF with pulmonary atresia, etc. In children with TOF combined with the absence of the pulmonary valve, poor development of the fetal pulmonary valve leads to significant pulmonary regurgitation, which in turn causes aneurysmal dilation of the developing main pulmonary artery and branch pulmonary arteries. These enlarged vessels may cause airway compression, with the potential for tracheobronchomalacia and severe neonatal respiratory compromise. TOF combined with pulmonary atresia is the most severe form of TOF, often classified separately as pulmonary atresia with VSD. Due to the lack of forward blood flow from the right ventricle to the pulmonary circulation, the main pulmonary artery is severely underdeveloped, and pulmonary blood flow depends upon a ductus arteriosus and/or major aortopulmonary collateral arteries.

21.4.2 TOF Surgical Procedures

Once a child is diagnosed with TOF, surgical treatment should be considered. The surgical procedures include one-stage radical surgery and staged correction. The selection of surgical procedures mainly depends on the development of the pulmonary artery. It is generally recognized that if the McGoon ratio > 1.2, and the pulmonary artery index (Nakata index) >150 mm^2/m^2, one-stage corrective surgery can be performed. Staged corrective surgery is performed for children who cannot meet the conditions for one-stage corrective surgery, mainly those with severe underdevelopment of the pulmonary artery branches (i.e., McGoon ratio < 1.2, Nakata index <150 mm^2/m^2). Common palliative surgical procedures in clinical practice include modified Blalock–Taussig shunt, central shunt, and RVOT patch widening. The child's McGoon index was 2.07 in this case, so one-stage corrective surgery was performed.

21.5 Discussion

21.5.1 Preoperative Assessment and Preparation

1. Degrees of pulmonary blood flow reduction. The pulmonary blood flow in children with TOF varies with the site and degree of obstruction, systemic-pulmonary vascular resistance ratio, and collateral circulation formation. Pulmonary blood flow plays a vital role in the anesthetic management of children with TOF. TOF with severe RVOT obstruction has reduced pulmonary blood flow, which is mainly manifested clinically as a decrease in SpO_2, severe cyanosis, polycythemia, and eventually digital clubbing. The choice of drugs aims to maintain or make the systemic vascular resistance higher than the pulmonary vascular resistance to reduce right-to-left shunting. TOF with less severe RVOT obstruction is manifested as left-to-right shunting through VSD, which can lead to increased pulmonary blood flow and symptoms of congestive heart failure. SpO_2 is basically normal. Anesthetic management must avoid interventions that reduce pulmonary vascular resistance and increase systemic vascular resistance. Therefore, preoperative assessment of pulmonary blood flow should be emphasized based on the patient's medical history, physical examination, and laboratory test results.

   Arterial blood oxygen saturation can reflect the pulmonary blood flow of children with TOF. The lower the arterial oxygen saturation, the less the pulmonary blood flow. In addition to the pulmonary valve and subvalvular stenosis, increased pressure difference across the pulmonary valve, and small collateral vessels formation to partly increase the pulmonary blood flow, this child's basic SpO_2 was low, the lips were cyanotic, the pulmonary blood flow was reduced, which was diagnosed as classic TOF.
2. Risk of Tet spells. For classic TOF patients, it is necessary to carefully verify the history of Tet spells before surgery, evaluate the potential possibility of Tet spells, and proactively prevent and treat Tet spells. Although this child has no history of Tet spells, the child's basic oxygenation is poor, and the possibility of perioperative Tet spells cannot be ruled out.
3. Pathophysiological changes affecting anesthetic management. Anatomical abnormalities such as abnormal coronary artery origin, large systemic pulmonary collateral branches, and long-term hypoxia-induced erythrocytosis will all affect anesthetic management. The child's preoperative hemoglobin and hematocrit were increased, which may be related to long-term hypoxia-induced erythrocytosis. When hemoglobin exceeds 20 g/dL, increased blood viscosity may affect important organ perfusion and coagulation function, dehydration should be avoided during the perioperative period, and anticoagulants may be used. Based on the above situations, the preoperative preparation for this child was: ① preoperative drink (≤5 mL/kg) was orally administrated 2 h before surgery to shorten the fasting drink time and avoid the decrease

in preload caused by long-term fasting food and drink, which can exacerbate the dynamic obstruction of the right ventricular outflow tract and further reduces pulmonary blood flow; ② Midazolam 0.5 mg/kg was orally administrated for preoperative sedation 20–30 min before surgery to reduce the child's anxiety due to unfamiliar environment and crying caused by venous access and avoid stress-induced Tet spells.

21.5.2 Intraoperative Anesthetic Management

1. Maintain HR, myocardial contractility, and preload to ensure sufficient cardiac output. Maintaining normal blood volume is also very important to prevent the reflexive acceleration of HR and the dynamic obstruction aggravation of RVOT caused by enhancement of myocardial contractility and hypovolemia. For children with TOF who have been fasting food and drink for a long time, venous access should be established immediately to give 10–15 mL/kg of crystalloid or 5% albumin.
2. The keys to induction of anesthesia should focus on preventing stressful stimuli and maintaining oxygenation and hemodynamic stability. The anesthetics with minimal effects on SVR, such as etomidate and ketamine, can be used for induction of anesthesia. To maintain hemodynamic stability, slow injection is also required. In this case, midazolam, etomidate, sufentanil, and rocuronium were intravenously administered for anesthesia induction. During the operation, propofol, sufentanil, rocuronium, and sevoflurane were used to maintain anesthesia. The speed of propofol was adjusted based on HR and ABP. The goal of anesthetic management was to maintain stable HR, blood pressure, and adequate anesthesia depth (BIS value 40–60).
3. Ventilation strategies that reduce pulmonary vascular resistance should be used before and after CPB, with moderate hyperventilation to maintain carbon dioxide levels at the lower normal range. At the same time, the mean airway pressure should be reduced as much as possible to avoid mechanical obstruction of pulmonary blood flow due to high mean airway pressure. Near-infrared cerebral oxygen monitors can be used to monitor cerebral tissue oxygenation (rSO_2) to avoid a reduction in cerebral oxygen supply caused by low carbon dioxide. It should be noted that in TOF patients, the difference between end-tidal carbon dioxide and $PaCO_2$ is large, which is related to their intracardiac shunt volume. In this case, we used PCV-VG mode ventilation to ensure VT while avoiding high airway pressure and maintained $PaCO_2$ at around 35 mm Hg. During the operation, the decrease in rSO_2 value did not exceed 15% of the baseline value.

21.5.3 Post-CPB Anesthetic Management

1. After CPB, cardiac output depends more on heart rate, and the heart rate should be maintained in accordance with age, preferably sinus rhythm.
2. Support right heart function. Using a patch across the right ventricular outflow tract can cause segmental motion impairment of the free wall of the right ventricle. After CPB, positive inotropic drugs such as dopamine or milrinone can be used to support right ventricular function. Dopamine has a strong positive inotropic effect and does not increase pulmonary vascular resistance. Therefore, in this case, dopamine was administered by infusion. Norepinephrine was also added to maintain blood pressure when the child's blood pressure was low.
3. In TOF surgery, exposure to VSD and RVOT can damage the atrioventricular node by pulling on the tricuspid valve, which results in about up to 20% junctional ectopic tachycardia (JET) after surgery. The use of dexmedetomidine during surgery can reduce the occurrence of JET.

4. Management of coagulation function. The long-term hypoxia in patients with TOF can cause an increase in red blood cells and blood viscosity, which finally impairs the coagulation function, including thrombocytopenia, disseminated intravascular coagulation, primary fibrinolysis, and coagulation factor production disorders. Therefore, the coagulation function should be closely monitored during the perioperative period. The blood product treatment should be guided according to the results of coagulation function monitoring after CPB. In this case, the preoperative hematocrit of the child was 43.2%, only slightly elevated, with normal platelet count and coagulation function. Tranexamic acid 10 mg/kg was intravenously administrated to inhibit fibrinolysis and reduce bleeding during the operation. The Sonoclot coagulation and platelet function monitor was used in this case to assess coagulation function at the end of CPB and guide the supplement of coagulation products.

21.6 Conclusion

In summary, accurate preoperative assessment of pulmonary blood flow, the proactive prevention and treatment of Tet spells, maintenance of appropriate systemic and pulmonary vascular resistance by optimization of ventilation management strategies and anesthetics, maintenance of cardiac coagulation function, and timely treatment of arrhythmia after CPB are the key points of perioperative anesthetic management in patients with TOF (Jing Jiang).

Anesthetic Management of Tet Spells During the Infant Tetralogy of Fallot Corrective Surgery

22

Jing Jiang

Abstract

A 5-month-old male infant was diagnosed with congenital heart disease after prenatal examination, which was confirmed as Tetralogy of Fallot (TOF) by echocardiography after birth. Recently, the infant experienced worsening cyanosis of the lips when he cried. The pulse oxygen saturation (SpO_2) was 77% with room air. He was scheduled for TOF corrective surgery under general anesthesia. During the surgery, the end-tidal carbon dioxide pressure ($ETCO_2$) quickly dropped when the pulmonary artery was exposed. SpO_2 also quickly dropped to 30%, indicating Tet spells. So, pure oxygen ventilation, rapid fluid replacement, correction of acidosis, and intravenous administration of phenylephrine were initiated quickly. Cardiopulmonary bypass (CPB) was also quickly established. After the above treatments, SpO_2 was gradually increased. The surgery went smoothly, and the outcome was good.

Tet spells are among the most common clinical emergencies in children with Tetralogy of Fallot (TOF). The increase of right-to-left shunting caused by right ventricular outflow tract (ROVT) spasm obstruction and the imbalance of systemic-pulmonary vascular resistance (PVR), etc. can lead to a sharp decrease in pulmonary blood flow, which may be the mechanism of Tet spells. The main clinical manifestations of Tet spells are dyspnea and worsening cyanosis, which can cause limb paralysis, convulsions, cerebrovascular accidents, and even sudden death in severe cases. This article reports a case of Tet spells during radical surgery in a child with TOF and discusses the mechanism, risk factors, and treatment of Tet spells.

22.1 Case Presentation

The patient was 5 months and 16 days old boy with a weight of 6.9 kg and a height of 68 cm. He was born full-term without asphyxia. Congenital heart disease was detected during a prenatal ultrasound examination. Local hospital echocardiography after birth indicated: TOF, patent foramen ovale (PFO). Recently, the cyanosis of the lips became worse during crying. The boy was brought to our hospital for further diagnosis and treatment.

Physical examination: The infant was conscious with a normal mental response. Cyanosis of lips became worse after crying. No obvious cyanosis of the limbs was found. Wet rales were heard in both lungs. The heart sounds were strong and regular, with a coarse systolic murmur in the

J. Jiang (✉)
The National Children's Medical Center (Shanghai), Department of Anesthesiology of Shanghai Children's Medical Center, Shanghai Jiao Tong University School of Medicine, Shanghai, China
e-mail: jiangjing@scmc.com.cn

J. Zheng et al. (eds.), *Selected Pediatric Cardiovascular Surgery Anesthesia Cases*,
https://doi.org/10.1007/978-981-96-5614-1_22

third intercostal space on the left side of the sternum. The abdomen was soft, and the extremities were warm. SpO_2 was 77% with room air.

Laboratory tests: Normal blood routine test, liver, kidney, and coagulation function. NT-proBNP 178 pg/mL (0–125).

Echocardiography: overriding aorta, pulmonary valve and subvalvular stenosis with transvalvular pressure gradient of 95 mm Hg. PFO with bidirectional shunting. Malalignment type ventricular septal defect (VSD) with bidirectional shunting, predominantly right-to-left shunting. The low position of the left innominate vein. Diagnosis: TOF, PFO, low position of innominate vein.

Cardiac CT: TOF, normal pulmonary artery development, low position of innominate vein.

Electrocardiogram (ECG): Sinus rhythm, right ventricular hypertrophy.

Chest X-ray: Boot-shaped heart, normal lung imaging.

Preoperative diagnosis: TOF, PFO. Surgical correction of TOF under general anesthesia was scheduled.

22.2 Anesthetic Management

After entering the operating room, ECG, blood pressure (BP), and SpO_2 were routinely monitored. Basic vital signs: SpO_2 90%, heart rate (HR) 151 beats/min, BP 80/52 mm Hg. The anesthesia was intravenously induced with midazolam 1.0 mg, etomidate 2.0 mg, sufentanil 10 μg, and rocuronium 5.0 mg. After the eyelash reflex disappeared, an ID 3.5 mm cuffed endotracheal tube was intubated with a video laryngoscope's assistance; the intubation depth was 12 cm. During surgery, propofol 4.0 mg/(kg·h), sufentanil 2.0 μg/(kg·h), and rocuronium 0.5 mg/(kg·h) were intravenously infused for the maintenance of anesthesia, while 0.5–1.0 MAC sevoflurane was intermittently inhaled. Bispectral index (BIS) was maintained at 40–60 during surgery. Pressure control ventilation (PCV) mode was adopted with 2 L/min oxygen flow rate, 50% fraction of inspired oxygen (FiO_2), 60 mL tidal volume (VT), and 1:2 inspiratory to expiratory (I:E) time ratio. The end-tidal carbon dioxide ($ETCO_2$) was maintained at 35–40 mm Hg by adjustment of ventilation frequency. After intubation, invasive arterial pressure (ABP) and central venous pressure (CVP) monitoring were quickly established. Cerebral tissue oxygen saturation (rSO_2) monitoring was also applied. Vital signs after intubation: SpO_2 93%, HR 133 beats/min, ABP 81/48 mm Hg, CVP 10 cm H_2O, BIS 55. The results of intraoperative arterial blood gas analysis at FiO_2 60%: pH 7.38, PaO_2 52 mm Hg, $PaCO_2$ 33.6 mm Hg, BE −4.9 mmol/L, HCT 38.6%, K^+3.4 mmol/L, Ca^{2+}1.23 mmol/L, Lac 1.0 mmol/L, Cl^- 108 mmol/L, Hb 12.8 g/dL, HCO_3^-19.4 mmol/L.

The surgery started at 9:00 am. The child's $ETCO_2$ suddenly dropped with a low and flat waveform at 9:25 am when the surgeon was exposing the pulmonary artery. The anesthesia machine works well without a respiratory circuit leak. Although VT was increased, SpO_2 still dropped to 40% rapidly. At the same time, ABP dropped to 50/30 mm Hg while HR was increased. It was suspected that Tet spells occurred. So, FiO_2 was immediately increased to 100%, Ringer's acetate solution 60 mL was quickly infused to increase blood volume, 5% $NaHCO_3$ 15 mL was slowly infused to correct acidosis, and phenylephrine 7.0 μg was intravenously injected to increase the systemic vascular resistance (SVR). Artery blood gas analysis was rechecked at the same time. After the above treatments, SpO_2 was increased to 75%, and ABP was gradually increased to 75/45 mm Hg. Then, the surgeon was informed to establish cardiopulmonary bypass (CPB) as soon as possible. The vital signs during Tet spells are shown in Table 22.1.

Surgical exploration confirmed the diagnosis of TOF (malalignment type VSD and right ventricular outflow tract hypertrophy). The VSD was closed with a pericardial patch. Patch augmentation and ablation of the abnormally hypertrophic muscle bundle of the RVOT was conducted. After the aortic cross-clamp was released, the heart automatically resumed beating and sinus rhythm. Dopamine 5.0 μg/(kg·min) and norepinephrine 0.02 μg/(kg·min) were intravenously infused. After the vena cava cross-clamp was released,

Table 22.1 Vital sign data during Tet spells

Time	9:25	9:30	9:35	9:40	9:45	9:50	9:55	10:00
SpO_2 (%)	40	40	38	40	65	76	76	86
HR (bpm)	140	117	112	111	105	120	126	145
ABP (mm Hg)	50/30	56/34	60/40	65/40	73/44	83/54	79/42	77/50

mechanical ventilation was resumed with the same ventilation parameter settings as before. Transesophageal echocardiography showed: a cardiac ejection fraction of 66%, pulmonary artery flow speed of 0.9 m/s, and no residual shunt around the VSD patch. The CPB was successfully weaned off after gradual adjustment of CPB flow. Protamine was intravenously dripped in to neutralize heparin after modified ultrafiltration. Thrombin was infused to assist hemostasis, and the sternum was closed.

22.3 Postoperative Outcome

The infant underwent TOF radical surgery, which lasted for 330 min in total, including a CPB time of 123 min and an aortic cross-clamping time of 87 min. The blood loss was estimated at around 200 mL. The urine output was 100 mL. 120 mL of Ringer's acetate solution, 100 mL of autologous salvaged blood, and 100 mL of fresh frozen plasma were transfused. At the end of the surgery, ABP was 80/48 mm Hg, HR was 148 beats/min, SpO_2 was 100%, CVP was 14 cm H_2O, and rectal temperature was 36.5 °C. Under ABP, ECG, and SpO_2 monitoring, the patient was transferred to the Cardiac Intensive Care Unit (CICU). The patient was extubated on postoperative day 3 and discharged from CICU on postoperative day 6. He was finally discharged from the hospital on postoperative day 12.

22.4 Review of Knowledge Points

22.4.1 Pathophysiology of TOF

TOF is anatomically characterized by aortic overriding, right ventricular hypertrophy, RVOT, and VSD. During ventricular contraction, the blood from the right ventricle enters the left ventricle through the VSD. It leads to a right-to-left shunt within the heart and reduced pulmonary circulation due to right ventricular hypertrophy and RVOT. The amount of shunting flow depends on the degree of RVOT obstruction and the ratio of SVR and PVR. In children with TOF, RVOT obstruction includes fixed and dynamic obstructions. Fixed RVOT obstruction is mainly caused by the narrowing of the infundibulum, pulmonary valve, and supravalvular regions. For those children with severe pulmonary valve stenosis, poor development of pulmonary artery branches, and severe infundibular muscle hypertrophy, the intracardiac shunting flow is relatively larger. In comparison, the pulmonary blood flow is relatively less. Chronic hypoxia can cause systemic-pulmonary collateral circulation formation, increasing the pulmonary blood flow and somewhat alleviating hypoxia. Dynamic RVOT obstruction (subpulmonary stenosis) is caused by functional changes in the right ventricular infundibulum diameter. The increased catecholamine release and low blood volume can increase the risk of dynamic RVOT obstruction occurrence.

22.4.2 Mechanism of Tet Spells

Tet or cyanotic spells are acute episodes characterized by a sudden worsening of cyanosis in patients with TOF, typically occurring during infancy and early childhood. However, they may persist into adulthood in some cases. It is generally believed that acute RVOT obstruction aggravation and SVR–PVR imbalance can lead to a significant increase in right-to-left shunting and a sharp decrease in pulmonary blood flow, which may contribute to the occurrence of Tet spells. Tet spells often occur in the awake state but can also happen during general anesthesia. Unlike SpO_2 decrease as the first sign of Tet spells in the awake state, Tet spells under general anesthesia

Table 22.2 Factors increasing right-to-left shunting

Pathophysiology	Pathogenesis
Increased PVR	Pain, light anesthesia, tachycardia, acidosis, hypoxemia, hypercapnia, hypothermia, and sympathetic stimulation caused by increased intrathoracic pressure
Dynamic outflow tract obstruction	Tachycardia, decreased blood volume, and increased myocardial contractility can cause infundibular spasm and dynamic outflow tract obstruction
Decreased systemic circulation resistance	Volatile anesthetics, drugs causing histamine release, α-adrenergic blockers

manifest as a progressive $ETCO_2$ decrease, followed by decreased SpO_2 and blood pressure. Several factors can trigger Tet spells during general anesthesia (Table 22.2).

22.5 Discussion

22.5.1 Preoperative Assessment and Preparation

It is very important to determine the possibility of Tet spells based on the patient's oxygenation status and the common factors related to Tet spells during the preoperative assessment and preparation. Those common factors related to Tet spells include:

1. Age. 2–3 months old is the peak period of Tet spells. As the age increases, more collateral circulation will be developed, and the risk of Tet spells will be reduced.
2. Cardiovascular development. Tet spells are more likely to occur in children with severe RVOT stenosis (fixed obstruction), fewer collateral circulations, and arterial duct closure.
3. Surgery. The surgical operation can cause reactive RVOT spasms.
4. Anemia. Anemia results in a hypoxic state in children, which can further trigger or exacerbate Tet spells.

In this case, although this patient was 5 months old and already passed the peak age of Tet spells, he was still at risk of Tet spells even without anemia since echocardiography showed that the pulmonary artery pressure difference had reached about 95 mm Hg, there existed bidirectional intracardiac shunting with right-to-left shunting predominately. The ductus arteriosus was patent without collateral vessel development.

Preoperative strategies to prevent Tet spells include:

1. Avoiding prolonged fasting time. Prolonged fasting time before surgery or sedation can reduce right ventricular preload, decrease RVOT diameter, and exacerbate dynamic RVOT obstruction, which is the major cause of Tet spells.
2. Preoperative sedation. Factors such as refusal to separate from parents before entering the room, refusal of mask touch, or intravenous puncture before anesthesia induction can all increase the release of endogenous catecholamine, which further causes the spasm of RVOT and triggers Tet spells.
3. Avoiding any factors that decrease SVR or increase PVR. High-concentration sevoflurane inhalation can dilate the systemic vessels and reduce SVR. Large doses of propofol can cause myocardial suppression and vasodilation. Inadequate ventilation can result in hypoxia and hypercapnia, which can further increase PVR. Therefore, anesthetics with minimal hemodynamic impact, such as etomidate and sufentanil, should be chosen for the induction and maintenance of general anesthesia. Also, the medications for treating Tet spells, such as phenylephrine, morphine, and sodium bicarbonate.

22.5.2 Intraoperative Anesthetic Management

The right-to-left intracardiac shunting can cause the reduction of pulmonary blood flow and hypoxemia in children with TOF. Therefore, anesthetic management focuses on reducing

PVR, increasing SVR, reducing right-to-left shunting, and maintaining effective pulmonary blood flow. In this case, anesthetics with minimal hemodynamic impact, such as etomidate and sufentanil, were chosen for slow induction to maintain hemodynamic stability and avoid hypotension. Intraoperatively, combined inhalation and intravenous anesthesia were used to maintain an appropriate depth of anesthesia based on BIS monitoring.

$ETCO_2$ waveform suddenly became low and flat, followed by a drop in SpO_2 during the exposure of the pulmonary artery by the cardiac surgeon. Although VT increased immediately, SpO_2 continued to drop rapidly, accompanied by an ABP decrease. After ruling out factors such as anesthesia machine breakdown, respiratory circuit leak, and allergic reactions, it was determined that Tet spells occurred due to the stimulation from pulmonary artery manipulation.

The treatments of intraoperative Tet spells are as follows:

1. Pure oxygen ventilation and moderate hyperventilation. Mechanical ventilation with 100% of oxygen can increase systemic oxygenation to the maximum. Although hyperventilation can decrease PVR and increase pulmonary blood flow to some extent, attention should be paid to the increase in mean airway pressure. Britta et al. show that reducing pulmonary perfusion during Tet spells can result in ventilation/perfusion mismatch, which can further reduce systemic arterial oxygen saturation. Higher mean airway pressure will reduce the right ventricular ejection, further reducing the pulmonary blood flow and exacerbating the ventilation/perfusion mismatch.
2. Manual compression of the aorta. During the surgery, manual compression of the ascending aorta can increase the left ventricular ejection resistance and pulmonary blood flow.
3. Blood Volume replenishment. 10–30 mL/kg of intravenous fluid supplementation can increase the ventricular preload and RVOT diameter, the pulmonary blood flow, and maintain blood pressure.
4. Correction of acidosis. Intravenous injection of sodium bicarbonate can treat severe metabolic acidosis. For children with acidosis, sodium bicarbonate has double the effects of volume expansion and acid correction, which can improve mean arterial pressure and cardiac output in the short term.
5. Medications for Tet spells therapy. Intravenous administration of phenylephrine at 5–10 μg/kg or 2–5 μg/(kg·min) can increase systemic blood pressure, reduce right-to-left shunting, and thus improve pulmonary blood flow. Intravenous administration of propranolol 0.1 mg/kg or esmolol 300–500 μg/kg can alleviate infundibular spasms by reducing myocardial contractility. In addition, they can also improve diastolic ventricular filling pressure through the reduction of HR to dilate RVOT diameter and alleviation of Tet spells.
6. For refractory Tet spells (hypoxic episodes that cannot be relieved by drug treatment), rapid establishment of cardiopulmonary bypass (CBP) can save the child's life. If emergency surgery cannot be performed, extracorporeal membrane oxygenation technology can be used to alleviate hypoxia.

In this case, after the above treatment, the child's $ETCO_2$ and SpO_2 gradually recovered, blood pressure rose, the Tet spells were relieved, and the surgery was continued. The key points of anesthetic management after CPB are maintaining a normal heart rate, using positive inotropic drugs to support right heart function, using ventilation strategies that reduce PVR, and treating arrhythmias, internal environment disorder, and coagulation dysfunction.

22.6 Shortcomings and Limitations

In this case, the preoperative sedation was not sufficient. The increase of right-to-left shunting induced by SVR after the induction of anesthesia was not corrected in time. In addition, blood volume supplementation might not be enough. Stimulation from strong surgical manipulation of the pulmonary vessels might cause the occurrence of Tet spells. All of these areas need to be improved in the future.

22.7 Conclusion

Severe Tet spells can lead to the death of the patient. All factors that can induce Tet spells should be avoided during the perioperative period. Early detection and rapid treatment of hypoxia, and ultimately, the use of CPB and surgery to relieve RVOT, can save lives (Jing Jiang).

Anesthetic Management of Emergency B-T Shunt Surgery in an Infant with Pulmonary Atresia and Intact Ventricular Septum

23

Lu Wang

Abstract

A 57-day-old boy, with prenatal echocardiography indicating pulmonary atresia with intact ventricular septum, developed cyanosis of the lips about 8 h after birth. The prenatal echocardiography indicated pulmonary atresia with intact ventricular septum (PA/IVS). He was admitted to our hospital because of acute exacerbation of cyanosis for 2 days. Wheezing respiration and severe cyanosis of the lips were observed. The blood pressure (BP) was 46/30 mm Hg, and the pulse oxygen saturation (SpO_2) was 45%. Immediate endotracheal intubation and mechanical ventilation were conducted. Dopamine at 5.0 μg/(kg·min) was intravenously administered to enhance cardiac function along with prostaglandin E_1 at 5.0 ng/(kg·min) to maintain the ductus arteriosus patency. However, the patient's BP and SpO_2 could not be maintained, and the lactate level continuously increased, which could not be alleviated by adjustment of drug dosages. Therefore, he was scheduled to undergo an emergency B-T shunt surgery under general anesthesia. This article introduced the key points of anesthetic management of emergency B-T shunt surgery in an infant with PA/IVS.

Pulmonary atresia with intact ventricular septum (PA/IVS) is a rare type of cyanotic congenital heart disease (CHD), which accounts for 1–3% of CHD. The pathological anatomy includes complete pulmonary valve obstruction, right ventricular hypoplasia, and tricuspid valve hypoplasia. Coronary artery malformations may coexist. The natural mortality rate of this disease is extremely high. Up to 50 percent of infants will die within 2 weeks without pharmacological and surgical intervention. The surgical approaches to PA/IVS vary depending on the development of the tricuspid valve, right ventricle, and right ventricle-dependent coronary circulation. This article reports the experience of anesthetic management of an emergency Blalock–Taussig (B-T) shunt surgery under general anesthesia in an infant with PA/IVS.

23.1 Case Presentation

The patient was a 57-day-old boy with 5.0 kg in weight and 50 cm in height. Prenatal ultrasound suggested PA/IVS, atrial septal defect (ASD), and patent ductus arteriosus (PDA). He was delivered by cesarean section at 38 weeks with an Apgar score of 9. He developed cyanosis in the lips about 8 h after birth. He was admitted to our

L. Wang (✉)
The National Children's Medical Center (Shanghai), Department of Anesthesiology of Shanghai Children's Medical Center, Shanghai Jiao Tong University School of Medicine, Shanghai, China
e-mail: wanglu@scmc.com.cn

J. Zheng et al. (eds.), *Selected Pediatric Cardiovascular Surgery Anesthesia Cases*,
https://doi.org/10.1007/978-981-96-5614-1_23

hospital due to tachypnea and acute exacerbation of cyanosis for 2 days.

Physical examination: The patient was on mechanical ventilation with a temperature of 36.8 °C, heart rate (HR) at 146 beats/min, and respiratory rate (RR) at 32 times/min. The respiratory sounds in bilateral lungs were symmetrical. The heart rhythm was regular with grade III/VI systolic murmur heard at the left sternal edge between the 2nd–3th ribs.

Laboratory tests: White blood cell 9.03×10^9/L, neutrophil 2.01×10^9/L, red blood cell 4.43×10^{12}/L, hemoglobin 151.0 g/L, hematocrit 45.6%, platelet 175×10^9/L, C-reactive protein 4.0 mg/L, normal liver and kidney function, PT 12.3 s, APTT 38.3 s, TT 20.7 s, INR 1.14.

Echocardiography: PA/IVS, ASD was 0.2 cm, predominantly right-to-left shunt, PDA 0.32 cm, and mild-to-moderate tricuspid regurgitation.

Wheezing respiration and severe cyanosis of the lips was observed while the patient was admitted. The blood pressure (BP) was as low as 46/30 mm Hg. The pulse oxygen saturation (SpO_2) was as low as 45%. He was immediately intubated for mechanical ventilation. The pressure-controlled ventilation (PCV) mode was used with the following parameter set: fraction of inspired oxygen (FiO_2) 21%, peak inspiratory pressure (PIP) 15.0 cm H_2O, RR 25 times/min, and positive end-expiratory pressure (PEEP) 5.0 cm H_2O. Then, the patient was transferred to the pediatric Cardiac Intensive Care Unit (CICU) with dopamine 5.0 μg/ (kg.min) and prostaglandin E_1 5.0 ng/(kg.min) infusion. Upon admission to CICU, the invasive arterial blood pressure (ABP) monitoring was rapidly established via the right brachial artery, and the arterial blood gas analysis was measured: pH 7.45, $PaCO_2$ 35.40 mm Hg, PaO_2 37.00 mm Hg, Ca^{2+} 1.04 mmol/L, and Lac 7.20 mmol/L. Calcium gluconate 100 mg was slowly dripped in. The dopamine dose was adjusted to 10 μg/(kg.min) due to ABP 52/31 mm Hg, HR 168 beats/min, and SpO_2 59%. Despite all of the above measures, it was difficult to maintain stable BP. Secondary blood gas analysis showed a persistent increase in lactate levels (8.2 mmol/L) and a decrease in PaO_2 (21.0 mm Hg). Therefore, an emergency modified B-T shunt, ASD enlargement, pulmonary atresia dilatation, and PDA ligation surgeries were planned to be conducted under general anesthesia.

Preoperative diagnosis: PA/IVS, ASD, PDA.

23.2 Anesthetic Management

A thermostatic incubator was used to transfer the patient to the operating room under mechanical ventilation with room air. The patient also received an intravenous infusion of midazolam, dopamine, and prostaglandin E_1. PCV mode was initiated with the following ventilation parameters: FiO_2 21%, PIP 20 cm H_2O, tidal volume (VT)30 mL, PEEP 2.0 cm H_2O, inspiratory to expiratory (I:E) time ratio 1:2. The partial pressure of end-tidal carbon dioxide ($ETCO_2$) was maintained at 35–45 mm Hg by RR adjustment. The right brachial artery was catheterized for continuous monitoring of artery blood pressure (ABP). Basic vital signs: SpO_2 53%, HR 153 times/min, ABP 58/42 mm Hg, and rectal temperature 36.7 °C. Sufentanil 5.0 μg and rocuronium 3 mg were given for intravenous induction of anesthesia. Anesthesia was maintained by continuous intravenous infusion of 4.0 mg/(kg·h) propofol, 2.0 μg/(kg·h)sufentanil, and 0.5 mg/(kg·h) rocuronium. In addition, sevoflurane 0.5–1.0 MAC was intermittently inhaled to maintain anesthesia. After the induction of anesthesia, the right internal jugular vein was successfully catheterized under ultrasound guidance for central venous pressure (CVP) monitoring and infusion of vasoactive drugs. The operating theatre temperature was 25 °C, and the warm air blanket temperature was set at 38 °C. After the sternum was opened, 3.0 mg/kg of sodium heparin was intravenously injected, and cardiopulmonary bypass (CBP) was quickly established after ACT >480 s. The warming air blanket was turned off after the initiation of CPB. RR was adjusted to 7 times/min, and PIP was adjusted to 7 cm H_2O. Modified B-T shunt surgery and atrial septal enlargement were conducted under CPB parallel circulation support. After the B-T anastomosis was finished, dopa-

Table 23.1 Blood gas analysis results

Time point	pH	PaO_2 (mm Hg)	$PaCO_2$ (mm Hg)	BE	HCT (%)	K^+ (mmol/L)	Ca^{2+} (mmol/L)	Lac (mmol/L)	FiO_2
Upon admission	7.376	47.7	44.2	0.8	43.9	5.3	1.14	1.6	21%
After CPB	7.404	38.4	46.5	3.5	44.2	4.6	1.1	2.5	45%
Upon discharge	7.41	41.9	44.8	3.1	39.5	4.5	1.0	2.4	60%

mine 7.5 μg/(kg·min), norepinephrine 0.1 μg/(kg·min), and epinephrine 0.1 μg/(kg·min) were initially infused to maintain ABP at 50–60/30–45 mm Hg, HR at 160–180 beats/min. Transesophageal echocardiography showed patent antegrade flow from the right ventricle to the pulmonary artery, visible blood flow in the B-T shunt conduit, and transvalvular pressure difference of the tricuspid valve 40 mm Hg. Respiratory parameters were adjusted: FiO_2 45%, PIP 15.0 cm H_2O, RR 25 times/min, SpO_2 89–95%. The CPB was successfully weaned off after rectal temperature was restored to 36 °C. Protamine was given in a 1.2:1 ratio to neutralize heparin after modified ultrafiltration. The results of intraoperative blood gas analysis results are shown in Table 23.1, among which PaO_2 after CPB was 38.4 mm Hg. After satisfied hemostasis, the sternum was closed. However, the HR was increased to about 190 beats/min, and ABP was stabilized with a slight drop in SpO_2 after the epinephrine dosage was reduced to 0.08 μg/(kg·min). SpO_2 was maintained at 85–90% after FiO_2 was increased to 60%. After stabilizing the hemodynamics, the patient was placed back into the thermostatic incubator and transferred to the Cardiac Intensive Care Unit (CICU) under close supervision.

23.3 Postoperative Outcome

The patient developed abdominal distension and anuria on the postoperative day 1, and peritoneal dialysis was not effective. Bedside ultrasonography showed slow blood flow in the B-T shunt conduit, enlarged right ventricle, ASD 0.5 cm with right-to-left shunt, and poor myocardial contractility. On postoperative day 2, the patient developed hypotension and hyperlactatemia, and bedside ultrasonography showed no blood flow in the B-T shunt conduit. It was suspected that the B-T shunt conduit was obstructed. Redo B-T shunt surgery was suggested, but the family members refused. On postoperative day 3, the patient suffered from recurrent ventricular fibrillation, which could not be corrected after cardiopulmonary resuscitation, and the family members decided to give up the treatment.

23.4 Review of Knowledge Points

23.4.1 Anatomical Features of PA/IVS

The anatomical characteristics of PA/IVS include the interrupted connection between the right ventricle and pulmonary artery and the intact ventricular septum. More than half of the cases have membranous pulmonary valvular atresia, separating the pulmonary trunk from the narrow right ventricular outflow tract. The pulmonary valve annulus is usually normal or slightly hypoplastic. The pulmonary valve leaflets are typically fused, but they are identifiable. The diameter of the pulmonary artery is generally normal. The tricuspid valve and right ventricle are hypoplastic. In children with severe hypoplasia of the tricuspid valve and right ventricle, the right ventricular pressure rises above systemic pressure, resulting in persistent sinus venosus patency. The foramen ovale is usually open, and 20% of patients may have a secondary ASD.

23.4.2 Pathophysiology of PA/IVS

In children with PA/IVS, venous return in the right ventricle cannot be pumped directly into the pulmonary artery during ventricular systole. Instead, it refluxes back into the right atrium through the tricuspid valve and then enters the left atrium through an ASD or patent foramen ovale, resulting in right-to-left shunting. After blood mixing in the left ventricle, the systemic and pulmonary venous blood in the left ventricle is parallelly distributed into the systemic and pulmonary circulation through the aorta and PDA. The pulmonary blood flow mainly depends on the opening of the ductus arteriosus, so prostaglandins should be used immediately after birth to maintain ductus arteriosus patency. Right ventricular pressure may be 2–3 times higher than the systemic pressure, which can cause fistula-like connections between the right ventricular cavity and the left and right coronary arteries. Retrograde blood flow from the ventricle to the coronary arteries can easily lead to fibromuscular intimal hyperplasia in the proximal coronary circulation and cause obstruction at the proximal end of the coronary arteries. The myocardium distal to the obstructed coronary artery will depend on retrograde perfusion from the high-pressure right ventricle to the coronary arteries, a physiological state known as right ventricular-dependent coronary circulation (RVDCC).

23.4.3 Surgical Treatment of PA/IVS

Children with RVDCC are contraindicated for right ventricular decompression because the forward blood flow of the coronary artery cannot meet the myocardial blood supply. These children can undergo single ventricle palliation surgery, such as modified B-T shunt (MBTS), followed by bidirectional Glenn shunt and Fontan surgery. The surgical method for non-RVDCC patients depends on developing the tricuspid valve and right ventricle. Patients with severe right ventricular and tricuspid valve dysplasia can undergo single ventricle palliation surgery. For those patients with moderate right ventricle and tricuspid valve dysplasia, 1¼ or 1½ ventricular repair can be conducted depending on the size of the right ventricle and the tricuspid valve. A biventricular repair can be performed for patients with a nearly normal right ventricle size and tricuspid valve size. Transthoracic echocardiography assesses the right ventricle and tricuspid valve size and function.

23.5 Discussion

The pathophysiology of PA/IVS is complex and variable. The more severe the heart malformation is, the earlier the onset of symptoms occurs. The younger the age at surgery, the higher the risk of perioperative anesthesia. These patients often undergo emergency surgery in the neonatal period, and their general preoperative conditions are relatively poor, especially for those combined with low body weight. Perioperative anesthetic management and organ function protection are more difficult.

23.5.1 Preoperative Assessment and Preparation

For those patients with PDA-dependent cardiac lesions, rapid infusion of prostaglandin is critical for the patient's survival. The newborns with suspected PA-IVS after birth should be given prostaglandin immediately after confirmation of the diagnosis. 15% to 20% of newborns treated with prostaglandin may experience apnea, which requires endotracheal intubation and mechanical ventilation. Supplemental oxygen may be required if cyanosis is severe. Preoperative management should focus on balancing the pulmonary and systemic blood flow (Qp/Qs), especially for those with mechanical ventilation. Excessive pulmonary blood flow may result from excessive blood flow through the PDA due to hyperoxemia and/or hypocapnia. In the absence of severe lung disease, severe hypoxemia or acidosis may indicate the closure of the arterial duct. Persistent hypoperfusion or acidosis after confirmation of the patency of the arterial duct may indicate an insufficient shunt at the atrial level, which requires urgent intervention. Prostaglandin infusion to maintain PDA open cannot improve the patient's internal environment and oxygenation situation. The general condition of the patient before surgery was poor, ASA grade IV(E), and emergency surgery was required.

23.5.2 Anesthetic Management Before CPB

1. Induction of anesthesia
   Anesthesia can be induced with intravenous and inhalation anesthetics, while the dosage and speed of administration should be adjusted. Hemodynamic management during the perioperative period should focus on maintaining proper Qp/Qs balance and appropriate cardiac output. Pay close attention to the diastolic blood pressure, and ECG changes to detect myocardial ischemia timely. In the case of severe right ventricular coronary artery fistula or RVDCC, right ventricular decompression caused by insufficient right ventricular volume load may cause fatal myocardial ischemia. Sevoflurane inhalation induction is most commonly used when venous access is lacking.
   For those patients with cardiac insufficiency and preoperative inotropic drug support, inhalational induction may not be tolerated. Ketamine or Esketamine can be chosen for the induction of anesthesia. The induction dosage of ketamine is usually 1.0–2.0 mg/kg. In this case, the patient was already in a state of basic sedation and mechanical ventilation preoperatively. Therefore, in order to minimize hemodynamic fluctuations, sufentanil was used for the induction of anesthesia, which has little effect on the hemodynamics.
2. Intraoperative monitoring
   In addition to routine monitoring, invasive monitoring (ABP, CVP) must be established according to the requirement of surgery. For example, the radial artery catheterization for invasive artery pressure measurement should be established on the contralateral side of the B-T shunt. The pulmonary blood flow in patients with PA/IVS mainly depends on the patency of ductus arteriosus, which may cause myocardial damage due to coronary steal. Therefore, it is very important to monitor the changes in diastolic blood pressure in patients with PA/IVS. Special attention should be paid to the preoperative ECG, which can be used as a reference for the changes in heart rate, arrhythmia, and ST segment caused by myocardial ischemia. Cerebral tissue oxygen saturation monitoring should also be conducted after B-T conduit construction due to blood supply from the systemic circulation to the pulmonary circulation, which may cause insufficient perfusion to the cerebral tissue.

23.5.3 Anesthetic Management After CPB

After the B-T shunt conduit is established, the anatomical issues, such as the proper size of the blood shunt and any twisting or narrowing of the B-T conduit, should be first ruled out if some issues occur. Once the anatomical problems are ruled out, physiological regulation should be considered. For the patients with single ventricle defects and fixed cardiac out, the systemic circulation oxygen supply (the product of systemic circulation oxygen content and systemic circulation blood flow) will be maximized when the Qp/Qs ratio is equal to or slightly less than 1. When Qp/Qs ratio is more than 1, the systemic circulation oxygen supply decreases progressively because the effect of increased systemic circulation oxygen content is offset by the progressive decrease in systemic circulation blood flow. When Qp/Qs ratio decreases below 1, the systemic circulation oxygen supply decreases precipitously because the precipitous decline in systemic circulation oxygen content offsets the increase in systemic circulation blood flow.

1. Hemodynamic management
   The hemodynamic fluctuations are very significant when the B-T shunt conduit is established. The arterial pulse pressure difference becomes wide because part of the systemic circulation blood enters the pulmonary circulation. To ensure normal coronary and cerebral blood supply, catecholamines such as dopamine and epinephrine can be used to elevate blood pressure. Maintaining the diastolic pressure above 40 mm Hg or 10–20 mm Hg higher than the normal value for the same age is better.

2. Ventilation management
   Changes in preload, sinus rhythm, myocardial contractility, SVR, shunt conduits, and changes in lung volume, alveolar oxygenation, pH, and carbon dioxide partial pressure all affect pulmonary vascular resistance. To maintain the balance of Qp/Qs, a FiO_2 of 40% is usually used to keep PaO_2 around 40 mm Hg.
3. Blood management
   Maintaining HCT at 38–45% is better by correcting anemia. The hemostatic drugs and coagulation factors should be used as little as possible. Anticoagulants should be used as early as possible after surgery to reduce the probability of conduit obstruction. Progressive hypoxemia after surgery may be due to the progressive conduit obstruction tendency.

23.6 Conclusion

In summary, PA-IVS is a rare ductal-dependent single ventricular physiological malformation. It is necessary to evaluate the size of the right ventricle and tricuspid valve annulus, the degree of the shunt at the atrial level, and the ductus arteriosus patency during the preoperative assessment. Cardiac catheterization is usually required to assess the coronary artery anatomy, right ventricular-coronary artery fistula, and RVDCC. Once the diagnosis of PA-IVS is confirmed in newborns, it is generally necessary to intravenously infuse prostaglandin to keep the ductus arteriosus patency before surgery. Surgical treatment options include biventricular repair, 1¼ or 1½ ventricular repair, or single ventricular palliation surgery. The goal of perioperative management is to balance Qp/Qs and maintain right ventricular filling pressure. (Lu Wang).

24 Anesthetic Management of Pediatric Pulmonary Artery Unifocalization Procedures for Pulmonary Artery Atresia with Ventricular Septal Defect

Bo Li

Abstract

A 4-year-old boy was diagnosed with pulmonary artery atresia accompanied by ventricular septal defect, branch pulmonary artery hypoplasia, and collateral vessel formation. He was scheduled to undergo pulmonary artery unifocalization procedures under general anesthesia. Refractory hypotension, hypoxemia, and metabolic acidosis occurred during the surgery, and cardiopulmonary bypass (CPB) support was needed to help finish unifocalization procedures. Pulmonary artery unifocalization procedures are often complex and very lengthy. Collateral vessel ligation may significantly reduce pulmonary blood flow and blood loss, leading to hemodynamic instability and arrhythmias. Anesthetic management poses a considerable challenge to anesthesiologists. The keys to anesthetic management during pulmonary artery unifocalization procedures include maintaining stable hemodynamics, ensuring sufficient organ perfusion, and keeping homeostasis.

B. Li (✉)
The National Children's Medical Center (Shanghai), Department of Anesthesiology of Shanghai Children's Medical Center, Shanghai Jiao Tong University School of Medicine, Shanghai, China
e-mail: libo@scmc.com.cn

Pulmonary artery atresia with ventricular septal defect (PA/VSD) is a relatively rare congenital disease with an incidence of approximately 7 per 100,000 live births. The pulmonary blood flow in a patient with pulmonary artery atresia is mainly supplied by major aortopulmonary collateral arteries (MAPCAs) instead of the main pulmonary artery. The clinical manifestations of patients with PA/VSD/MAPCAs vary greatly depending on the number and patency of collateral vessels and the ratio of pulmonary to systemic blood flow (Qp/Qs). The distal and branch vessels of the pulmonary artery in patients with PA/VSD/MAPCAs are often hypoplasia, which makes them unsuitable for radical surgery. Therefore, pulmonary artery unifocalization surgery is often required to consolidate the source of pulmonary blood flow, regulate pulmonary artery pressure, promote the development of pulmonary vessels, and facilitate subsequent radical surgery.

24.1 Case Presentation

A 4-year-old boy with 95 cm in height and 11.7 kg in weight has been found to have cyanosis since his birth. Echocardiography showed PA/VSD and collateral vessel formation. No history of convulsions, syncope, recurrent respiratory infections, edema, or oliguria in recent years, but with growth retardation. The preoperative diag-

J. Zheng et al. (eds.), *Selected Pediatric Cardiovascular Surgery Anesthesia Cases*,
https://doi.org/10.1007/978-981-96-5614-1_24

nosis was PA/VSD/MAPCAs. Pulmonary artery unifocalization surgery was planned to be performed under general anesthesia without CPB support.

Echocardiography showed PA/VSD, enlarged right atrium, and right ventricle hypertrophy.

Computerized tomography showed PA/VSD, a left pulmonary artery diameter of 1.3 mm, and a right pulmonary artery diameter of 1.2 mm. Multiple collateral vessels originated from the descending aorta.

Digital subtraction angiography indicated a poorly developed distal pulmonary artery. Five major collateral vessels originated from the aorta: (1) ascending aorta to left lung, with proximal and distal diameters of 4.3 mm and 3.3 mm, respectively; (2) descending aorta to left lung, with proximal and distal diameters of 3.2 mm and 2.6 mm, respectively; (3) descending aorta to left lung, with proximal and distal diameters of 2.5 mm and 2.9 mm, respectively; (4) descending aorta to right lung, with proximal and distal diameters of 1.8 mm and 3.0 mm, respectively; (5) descending aorta to right lung, with proximal and distal diameters of 2.2 mm and 2.4 mm, respectively.

Laboratory tests showed a hemoglobin level of 15.5 g/dL and hematocrit of 49.3%. No apparent abnormalities were found in liver, kidney, or coagulation function.

24.2 Anesthetic Management

Basic vital signs: heart rate (HR)152 beats/min, blood pressure (BP) 92/55 mmHg, pulse oxygen saturation (SpO_2) 71%.

Anesthesia was induced with intravenous bolus doses of 1.0 mg midazolam, 3.5 mg etomidate, 24 μg sufentanil, and 7.0 mg rocuronium. An ID 4.5 mm cuffed endotracheal tube was intubated under a visual laryngoscope, and the endotracheal tube was fixed after verification of the appropriate position by bilateral auscultation of the lungs. Pressure control ventilation (PCV) was initiated with the following respiratory parameters: 18 cm H_2O inspiratory pressure, 90–100 mL tidal volume (VT), 20 breaths/min respiratory rate (RR), and 1:2 I:E ratio. The fraction of inspired oxygen (FiO_2) was adjusted to maintain SpO_2 within 80–85%.

After anesthesia induction, arterial (right radial artery) and central venous (right internal jugular vein) catheterizations were performed under ultrasound guidance for continuous monitoring of invasive blood pressure (ABP) and central venous pressure (CVP). A right femoral vein access (20 G) was also established for blood transfusion. General anesthesia was maintained by continuous intravenous infusion of 4.0 mg/(kg·h) propofol, 2.0 μg/(kg·h)sufentanil, and 0.6 mg/(kg·h) rocuronium. Arterial blood gases were checked every 30 min to 1 h during surgery (Table 24.1).

About 3 h later, the patient's ABP suddenly dropped to approximately 50/30 mm Hg, and the SpO_2 dropped to 50–60%, but HR increased to approximately 160 beats/min upon ligation of a major collateral vessel. Despite the efforts to replenish blood volume, correct acidosis, and administer dopamine, no significant improvement in vital signs was observed. Arterial blood gas results indicated hypoxemia and metabolic acidosis (PaO_2 33.8 mmHg, pH 7.15, BE −6.2 mmol/L, Lac 4.5 mmol/L). Due to a significant reduction in pulmonary blood flow resulting from ligation of the major collateral artery, the surgeons opted to finish the pulmonary artery unifocalization procedures under CPB parallel circulation support. The respiratory parameters during parallel circulation were adjusted as follows: 12 cm H_2O inspiratory pressure, 50 mL VT, 10 breaths/min RR, 100% FiO_2. The surgery lasted for approximately 2 h under CPB parallel circulation support.

After completion of pulmonary artery unifocalization surgery, a flow-study test was conducted to assess pulmonary artery pressure. Despite the pulmonary artery perfusion flow had reached 2.5–3.0 L/(min·m^2), pulmonary artery pressure remained at approximately 30 mmHg, failing to meet the criteria for closing the VSD. Thus, the surgeons decided to retain the VSD.

The heart automatically resumed beating and sinus rhythm after aortic cross-clamp release. 5.0 μg/(kg·min) dopamine and 0.05 μg/(kg·min)

Table 24.1 Intraoperative blood gas test results

	30 min	90 min	150 min	180 min	240 min	300 min
Hb (g/dL)	14.9	14.0	13.2	9.2	11.7	11.6
HCT (%)	46.5	44	41.2	30.5	36.5	36.4
pH	7.27	7.34	7.37	7.15	7.41	7.33
PaO_2 (mmHg)	55.7	52.6	58.0	33.8	59.6	51.4
$PaCO_2$ (mmHg)	42.3	39.2	38.2	52.5	36.7	47.9
BE (mmol/L)	−3.9	−2.6	−1.2	−6.2	−1.5	−1.8
Na^+ (mmol/L)	141	138	140	142	139	141
K^+ (mmol/L)	3.9	4.1	3.8	3.9	4.0	3.8
Cl^- (mmol/L)	105	109	111	116	108	112
Ca^{2+} (mmol/L)	1.20	1.25	1.18	1.16	1.12	1.15
Lac (mmol/L)	0.6	0.6	0.7	4.5	2.6	1.9

epinephrine were continuously infused to maintain ABP within the range of 80–90/40–50 mmHg and HR 120–140 beats/min. FiO_2 was adjusted to maintain blood oxygen saturation, but SpO_2 remained around 70% even though FiO_2 was increased to 100%. Considering the possibility of lung reperfusion injury and atelectasis, the anesthesiologist first cleared airway secretions and applied 6 cm H_2O positive end-expiratory pressure (PEEP) and lung recruitment maneuvers. The patient's SpO_2 gradually rose to approximately 80%, and CPB was successfully weaned off.

24.3 Postoperative Outcome

The surgery lasted a total of 6.5 h. Ringer's acetate solution (400 mL) and 300 mL autologous blood were infused during surgery. The total urine output during surgery was 250 mL. The tracheal tube was successfully removed on the third postoperative day. The patient was discharged from the Cardiac Intensive Care Unit (CICU) on the seventh day and from the hospital on the fifteenth day.

24.4 Review of Knowledge Points

24.4.1 Pathophysiology of PA/VSD/MAPCAs

PA/VSD/MAPCAs is one of the functional single ventricle physiological diseases. Venous blood from the systemic circulation flows through the VSD into the left ventricle (right to left shunt), which mixes with the venous blood from the pulmonary circulation. The mixed venous blood is then ejected into the aorta, with a portion flowing to major organs and another portion entering the pulmonary circulation via the major aortopulmonary collateral arteries.

The clinical manifestations vary greatly depending on the number and patency of the collateral arteries. Patients with few or tortuous, blocked collateral arteries (Qp/Qs <1) may experience severe hypoxemia in the early stages of the disease. In contrast, those with many large or patent collateral arteries (Qp/Qs >1) may show signs and symptoms of congestive heart failure. Some patients with Qp/Qs ratios equal to or close to 1 may be asymptomatic.

24.4.2 Pulmonary Artery Unifocalization Procedures

Patients with PA/VSD/MAPCAs often present with poorly developed pulmonary arteries, which makes them unsuitable for one-stage radical surgery. Consequently, pulmonary artery unifocalization procedures are necessary for this population. The primary objective of this procedure is to consolidate the source of pulmonary blood flow, regulate pulmonary artery pressure and the Qp/Qs ratio, and facilitate and promote the development of pulmonary arteries and subsequent radical surgery.

24.4.3 Flow-Study Test

The flow-study test is a very important technique to help surgeons determine whether the VSD should be closed after pulmonary artery unifocalization procedures. The flow-study test works like an additional extracorporeal circulation connecting the pulmonary artery and left atrium, which measures pulmonary artery pressure under a perfusion flow of 2.5–3.0 L/(min·m^2). Generally, if the pulmonary artery pressure is <25 mmHg, VSD closure can be considered. Conversely, if the pulmonary artery pressure is >25 mmHg, VSD closure is not recommended.

24.5 Discussion

24.5.1 Preoperative Assessment and Preparation

The clinical manifestations of children with PA/VSD/MAPCAs vary greatly depending on different Qp/Qs ratios. For children without cyanosis before surgery, anesthesiologists should remain vigilant for potential signs and symptoms of congestive heart failure. Furthermore, 35% of 22q11 chromosomal deletion (DiGeorge syndrome) is reported with PA/VSD/MAPCAs, which may be associated with potential airway difficulties (such as a small mandible). Therefore, anesthesiologists should also be attentive to the possibility of a difficult airway.

24.5.2 Anesthetic Management Before CPB

The goal of anesthetic management is to balance blood flow between the systemic and pulmonary circulations and optimize systemic circulation perfusion. When the Qp/Qs ratio is equal to or slightly less than 1, systemic circulation oxygen supply is most optimized. Given the challenges in measuring the Qp/Qs ratio, arterial oxygen saturation (SaO_2) is a surrogate parameter. Studies indicate that systemic and pulmonary circulations reach equilibrium when SaO_2 is within the range of 75–80%. Therefore, the respiratory parameters setting during anesthesia should be adjusted to maintain SaO_2 within this range.

During anesthesia induction, propofol should be avoided or administered cautiously since propofol can cause significant vasodilation and blood pressure fluctuations. Etomidate combined with opioids is a relatively safer alternative. Additionally, due to the prolonged duration of pulmonary artery unifocalization surgery, anesthesiologists should reduce the maintenance dose of propofol to avoid acidosis. Inhaled anesthetics can dose-dependently reduce mean arterial pressure, systemic vascular resistance, and cardiac output. Therefore, the use of high doses or prolonged exposure to inhaled anesthetics should also be avoided.

Significant reduction in pulmonary blood flow may occur during the dissociation, ligation, and anastomosis of major collateral arteries, leading to severe hypoxia and metabolic acidosis. Although pulmonary artery unifocalization procedures are typically performed without CPB support, it is still necessary if intractable hypoxemia or metabolic acidosis occurs during the surgery.

24.5.3 Anesthetic Management After CPB

The patients undergoing pulmonary artery unifocalization procedures may develop intractable hypoxemia after CPB is weaned off. In addition to the surgery-induced reduction in pulmonary blood flow, other contributing factors may include (1) Ischemia-reperfusion injury of the lung; some lung segments in patients with PA/VSD/MAPCAs may be hypoperfused due to underdeveloped pulmonary vessels before surgery. However, the blood flow to these hypoperfused lung segments is increased after surgery and can lead to ischemia-reperfusion injury to the lung; (2) Reduced lung compliance after surgery, which can result in inadequate ventilation and oxygenation. Anesthesiologists should thoroughly clear airway secretions and manually perform lung recruitment following weaning from CPB.

24.6 Conclusion

In summary, the goal of anesthetic management for patients with PA/VSD/MAPCAs undergoing pulmonary artery unifocalization procedures is to maintain stable hemodynamics, ensure sufficient organ perfusion, and maintain homeostasis. If intractable hypoxemia and acidosis develop, CPB remains necessary. In this case, the patient experienced a significant reduction in pulmonary blood flow following ligating of major collateral arteries. Despite efforts to replenish blood volume, correct acidosis, and administer dopamine, no significant improvement was observed. Consequently, the procedure was conducted with CPB support (Bo Li).

25 Anesthetic Management of B-T Shunt Surgery in a Neonate with Pulmonary Atresia

Hongbin Gu

Abstract

The patient was a 7-day-old male neonate. He was diagnosed with pulmonary atresia (PA), ventricular septal defect (VSD), and patent ductus arteriosus (PDA) by echocardiography due to severe cyanosis after birth. The patient was admitted to our hospital after an emergency tracheal intubation, and an emergency PA correction surgery was subsequently carried out. During the operation, it was found that the patient had a small right ventricle, connections between the right ventricular myocardial sinusoids and intramural coronary artery branches, a lack of effective aorta-coronary communication, and an underdeveloped central confluence of the left and right pulmonary arteries. As a result, a modified systemic to pulmonary artery shunt surgery was performed, and the PDA was ligated. Delayed sternal closure was performed due to significant myocardial edema after the operation. He was then transferred to the cardiac intensive care unit (CICU) with mechanical ventilation and treatment of cardiovascular medications, creatine phosphate for myocardium nourishment, low-molecular-weight heparin calcium for anticoagulation, and antibiotics for infection prevention. The sternum and incision were closed 3 days later. Although the preoperative diagnosis was made by echocardiography in this case, intraoperative exploration showed abnormal coronary perfusion and significant myocardial edema, which led to palliative surgery. The medical team must focus on the cardiac anatomy and coronary development of children with PA.

The early mortality rate among children with PA is very high. Surgical treatment is the only curative option. If the proactive treatment of PA is adopted during infancy, there is a chance for the pulmonary vessels to develop normally. Most patients have a dual supply of blood vessels to the lung segments from collateral vessels and ductus arteriosus. However, the function of the collateral circulation will change with age and the development of the right heart system varies significantly among individuals. There are various purposes and methods for surgical treatment of such patients. This article reports a case of emergency surgery under general anesthesia to correct PA in a neonate. During intraoperative exploration, abnormal perfusion of the right ventricle, which was dependent on the connection of right ventricular myocardial sinusoids and the coronary artery, and poor development of the distal pulmonary arteries were found. Anesthesiologists should focus on preoperative assessment of cardiac func-

H. Gu (✉)
The National Children's Medical Center (Shanghai), Department of Anesthesiology of Shanghai Children's Medical Center, Shanghai Jiao Tong University School of Medicine, Shanghai, China
e-mail: guhongbin@scmc.com.cn

J. Zheng et al. (eds.), *Selected Pediatric Cardiovascular Surgery Anesthesia Cases*,
https://doi.org/10.1007/978-981-96-5614-1_25

tion and the presence of cardiac and major vascular anatomical abnormalities when administering anesthesia to children with PA. During perioperative, anesthesiologists must monitor cardiac function and maintain vital organ functions.

25.1 Case Presentation

A 7-day-old male presented with cyanotic lips, low responsiveness, difficulty feeding, and a weak cry. A two-dimensional multifunctional color ultrasound examination of the heart showed PA, VSD, and PDA. The patient was admitted to our hospital with endotracheal intubation for emergency surgery due to the diagnosis of PA, VSD, and PDA.

Physical examination:

At admission, the patient was 3.5 kg in weight and 51 cm in height. He did not experience asphyxia at birth, and his birth weight was 3.6 kg. He appeared sleepy, and the pulse oxygen saturation (SpO_2) in the left upper limb was 34%–40%. The infant's anterior fontanel was not closed yet. His limbs were in natural flexion. His breathing was rapid, with a respiratory rate (RR) of 35 times per minute. The heart rate (HR) was 149 beats per minute, and the non-invasive blood pressure was 55/32 mmHg in the left upper limb. The skin elasticity was good. The abdomen was soft with the liver 1.5 cm below the right rib. His extremities were warm without pallor, jaundice, bleeding points, or rash. He had no central cyanosis, eyelid edema, conjunctival congestion, or apparent scleral jaundice. Capillary refill time was 5 seconds. The eyes freely moved with both pupils' diameters of about 2.0 mm, and the light reflex was good. There were no tremors at the apex of the heart. The rhythm was regular, with strong heart sounds. An II–III/VI systolic murmur was heard with low P2 in the precordial area.

Laboratory examination:

The result of arterial blood gas analysis at a fraction of inspired oxygen (FiO_2) of 21% was as follows: pH 7.24, $PaCO_2$ 36.6 mmHg, PaO_2 14.8 mmHg, Na^+ 135 mmol/L, K^+ 3.2 mmol/L, Ca^{2+} 1.10 mmol/L, Cl^- 110 mmol/L, GLU 75.0 mg/dL, Lac 10.2 mmol/L, HCT 53.4%, HCO_3^- 14.2 mmol/L, ABE -11.2, SBE −10.6, Hb 17.5 g/dL.

Echocardiography:

The heart was in a regular position with the right atrium and right ventricle enlargement. The right ventricular wall was thickened. The aorta was widened and straddled 50% of the interventricular septum. The left ventricular contraction activity was regular. The left and right coronary arteries were not clearly visible. Forward blood flow wasn't detected because of pulmonary valve atresia. The diameter of the pulmonary valve ring was 0.56 cm. The diameter of the pulmonary artery's main trunk was 0.80 cm. The diameters of the left and right pulmonary arteries were 0.47 cm and 0.42 cm, respectively. The atrioventricular valve had normal activity. There was mild regurgitation of the tricuspid valve with a regurgitation bundle width of 0.23 cm and regurgitation speed of 3.70 m/s, and the pressure difference was 54.9 mmHg. Patent foramen ovale in the atrial septum with a diameter of 0.30 cm, right-to-left shunt. Malalignment type VSD and bidirectional shunt. The aortic arch was located on the left. PDA with a diameter of 0.20 cm (vertical type) and left-to-right shunt with a shunt speed of 3.44 m/s. Rich blood flow signals in the interventricular septum. Minor muscular VSD could not be ruled out.

25.1.1 Chest X-Ray

Thoracic skeleton or chest wall soft tissues were normal. The mediastinum and trachea were centrally located without any displacement. The cardiac silhouette was enlarged, and bilateral lung marking was increased. Diaphragms were smooth, and costophrenic angles were sharp.

The preoperative diagnosis was PA, VSD, PFO, and PDA. The modified B-T shunt surgery was scheduled.

25.2 Anesthetic Management

The patient was transferred to the operating room from the CICU with endotracheal intubation, invasive artery pressure (ABP) monitor, end-tidal carbon dioxide ($ETCO_2$) monitor, and mechanical ventilation. The pressure-controlled ventilation (PCV) mode was used with 24 times/min RR and peak inspiratory pressure (PIP) of approximately 20 cm H_2O. The tidal volume (VT) was maintained at about 8 mL/kg. In addition, epinephrine 0.05 μg/(kg·min), milrinone 0.5 μg/(kg·min), and $CaCl_2$ 10 mg/(kg·h)were continuously infused. Prostaglandin E_1 was intravenously infused at 0.2 μg/(kg·h) to keep the arterial duct open. It was important to regularly review and maintain fluid, electrolyte balance, and acid–base balance.

Anesthesia was induced by bolus injection of 0.1 mg/kg of midazolam and etomidate 0.2 mg/kg. Anesthesia was maintained by continuous infusion of propofol 3.0 mg/(kg·h), rocuronium 0.6 mg/(kg·h), and sufentanil 2.5 μg/(kg·h). The dosage of cardiovascular active drugs was adjusted according to the changes in ABP, HR, and SpO_2. Prostaglandin E_1 0.2 μg/(kg·h) was intravenously infused to maintain the arterial duct open until it was ligated and the new pulmonary blood flow pathway was established. The pressure-controlled ventilation-volume guaranteed (PCV-VG) mode with RR24 times/minute, VT approximately 8.0 mL/kg, and PIP below 20 cm H_2O was used for mechanical ventilation support during the operation. $ETCO_2$ at 30 mm Hg was maintained for appropriate hyperventilation. The synchronous trigger sensitivity was −2.0 cm H_2O. Following the induction of anesthesia, a 4F 5.0 cm double-lumen central venous catheter was inserted into the right internal jugular vein to monitor central venous pressure (CVP), and a 22 G 3.1 cm catheter was inserted into the femoral vein. The surgery was performed under the cardiopulmonary bypass (CPB) parallel circulation. During this process, FiO_2 was adjusted between 40% to 60%, RR 10 to 15 times/minute, and VT approximately 3 to 5 mL/kg. Following thoracotomy, it was found that the patient's right ventricle was less than one-third of the standard size. Segmental dilation and abnormal obstruction existed in both the left and right coronary arteries. The right ventricular myocardial sinusoids connected with intramural coronary artery branches didn't have effective aortic-coronary communication, indicating the possibility of the right ventricle-dependent coronary circulation. The distal branches of the pulmonary artery central confluence were poorly developed. To address this issue, a modified Blalock–Taussig shunt (mBTS) with a 4.0 mm balloon-expandable polytetrafluoroethylene tube was performed under parallel circulation to connect the right subclavian and the pulmonary arteries. Additionally, the arterial duct was ligated. After separation from CPB, dopamine 5 μg/(kg·min), milrinone 0.5 μg/(kg·min), and epinephrine 0.02–0.08 μg/(kg·min)was continuously infused to enhance the myocardial contractility. PCV-VG mode was continued with FiO_2 at 40–60%, RR at 24–30 times/min, VT at 6–8 mL/kg, PIP below 20 cm H_2O, end-expiratory positive pressure (PEEP) at 4.0 cm H_2O. $ETCO_2$ was maintained at about 35 mmHg. Due to the apparent myocardial edema and heart compression signs with one-stage sternum closure, delayed sternal closure was conducted, and the patient was then transferred to the CICU. In the process of transfer, the patient's HR, SpO_2, and ABP were maintained at 145 bpm, 80% (FiO_2 40%), and 65/40 mmHg, respectively. Upon admission to the CICU, the patient was placed on continuous mechanical ventilation using the intermittent positive pressure ventilation + synchronized intermittent mandatory ventilation (IPPV + SIMV) mode with PEEP of 4.0 cm H_2O. The cardiovascular active drugs were adjusted, which included intravenous infusion of dopamine 7.5 μg/(kg·min) and epinephrine 0.05 μg/(kg·min). $CaCl_2$ 10 mg/(kg·h) were also used. On the day of surgery, methylprednisolone was administered at a rate of 1.0 mg/(kg·48 h). In addition, creatine phosphate was used to nourish the myocardium. Low-molecular-weight heparin calcium injection was administered for anticoagulation, and antibiotics were given for anti-infection treatment.

25.3 Postoperative Outcome

The surgery proceeded without complications. The total CPB time lasted 55 min, with 35 min of parallel circulation time. The child's blood gas analysis results gradually returned to normal in the CICU. The sternum and skin were closed on the third postoperative day. The mechanical ventilation was withdrawn on the fifth postoperative day. The endotracheal intubation was also removed on the same day. The patient was discharged from the CICU on the seventh postoperative day and discharged from the hospital on the 15th postoperative day. The first follow-up color Doppler ultrasound assessment of pulmonary vascular development and cardiac function was scheduled 6 months later. The subsequent surgical plan would be determined based on the development of the pulmonary vessels.

25.4 Review of Knowledge Points

25.4.1 Pulmonary Atresia

PA can be divided into two types: PA/intact ventricular septum (IVS) and PA/VSD. Some scholars suggest that the term Tetralogy of Fallot (TOF) with pulmonary atresia may describe the pathology and treatment characteristics of PA/VSD more accurately. Anesthesiologists should pay special attention to several factors during anesthesia, which include the presence of multiple VSDs and atrial septal defects (ASDs), coronary artery abnormalities, and main pulmonary artery collaterals. Prostaglandin E_1 infusion may be necessary to maintain arterial duct patency. SpO_2 levels can be maintained at 80–90% if pulmonary blood flow is sufficient. It is also essential to consider the presence of other malformations, such as VACTERL syndrome, which involves congenital malformations of the spine, anus, heart, trachea, esophagus, kidney, and limbs. The signs and symptoms may not be apparent at birth if the patient presents with multiple main pulmonary artery collateral vessels formation. Hypoxic attacks may occasionally occur in children with TOF and PA. It is vital to maintain the balance of systemic-pulmonary circulation resistance during anesthesia to prevent the decrease of systemic circulation resistance and aggravation of cyanosis.

TOF with PA (Fig. 25.1) is characterized by the anterior malalignment of the outlet septum and blind pouch of the right ventricular outflow tract. The anatomy of the pulmonary artery varies greatly. The left and right pulmonary arteries can be either continuous or discontinuous, connected to the degenerated residual pulmonary trunk or

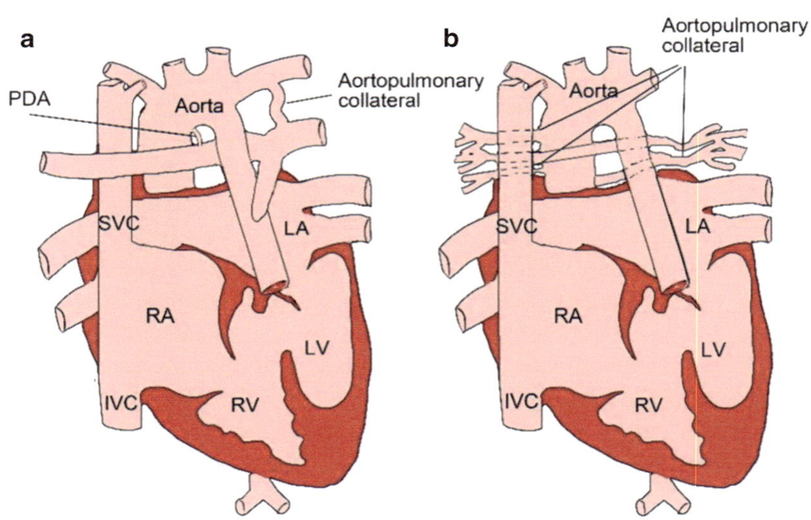

Fig. 25.1 The anatomy of TOF with pulmonary atresia. (**a**) type I of TOF/PA presents with short-segment pulmonary atresia, an average size of the pulmonary artery, continuous branch pulmonary arteries, a right aortic arch, and pulmonary blood flow provided by a sizeable systemic-pulmonary collateral from the left subclavian artery and a right PDA. (**b**) type III of TOF/PA is characterized by the absence of the pulmonary trunk, small branch pulmonary arteries that are continuous, and pulmonary blood flow provided by extensive systemic-pulmonary collaterals

supplied by PDA. In some patients, the collateral vessels between the aorta and the pulmonary artery can supply blood to the pulmonary circulation. Excessive blood flow from these collateral vessels can lead to congestive heart failure, the rapid formation of pulmonary vascular obstructive disease, and oxygen saturation reduction.

25.4.2 Treatment and Surgery

Drug and interventional treatment for PA: For those children dependent on PDA, intravenous infusion of prostaglandin E_1 is required to keep the ductus arteriosus open and provide sufficient pulmonary blood flow. It is not appropriate to use β-blockers for long-time prophylactic treatment of hypoxic episodes. The use of vasoconstrictors such as phenylephrine for the management of hypoxic episodes should be cautious to avoid immediate vasoconstriction before CPB. It is better to use digoxin and diuretics for children with congestive heart failure.

Prostaglandin E_1 can be used to keep the arterial arteriosus patency and maintain the continuity of the pulmonary artery. If SpO_2 can be maintained at 85% after prostaglandin E_1 infusion, then the children with PA can undergo one-stage radical surgery. Suppose there are other sources of pulmonary blood and SpO_2 can still be maintained at 70–75% during experimental occlusion. In that case, radical surgery can be performed after the collateral vessels for double pulmonary blood supply are occluded.

Palliative surgeries: Palliative surgeries typically include systemic-pulmonary shunt surgery and central aortopulmonary shunt procedure. Systemic-pulmonary shunt surgery can increase the pulmonary blood flow, expand the diameter of the pulmonary artery, and promote the development of some small pulmonary arteries. Elective radical surgery can be performed if the left-to-right shunting predominates 1–2 years after surgery. The cardiac catheterization examination can be performed 3–6 months after establishing the right ventricle and the pulmonary artery (central confluence) connection to assess the condition of pulmonary artery growth and occlude the aortopulmonary collateral vessels at an appropriate time. The unifocalization operation (UF) refers to directly connecting the large systemic-pulmonary collateral vessels to the main pulmonary artery and making the source of pulmonary blood single, meaning that the pulmonary blood flow is supplied by the central pulmonary artery.

25.5 Discussion

25.5.1 Preoperative Assessment and Preparation

The surgical procedures of children with TOF and PA vary depending on several factors, which include the development of the right ventricle (such as the Z value of the tricuspid valve), the development of the pulmonary vessels, and other accompanying malformations. These factors determine whether the radical or unifocalization surgery should be conducted. This is a rare complex PA case accompanied by coronary artery malformation and the poor development of pulmonary vessels and the right ventricle. Therefore, an mBTS shunt procedure was performed to increase pulmonary blood flow, improve hypoxemia, and promote the development of pulmonary vessels. During perioperative anesthetic management, it is essential to maintain the balance between pulmonary circulation resistance (Qp) and systemic circulation resistance (Qs), supplement appropriate fluid volume, and avoid excessive pulmonary congestion or reduced pulmonary artery blood flow.

25.5.2 Intraoperative Anesthetic Management

During the neonatal period, the pulmonary blood flow mainly depends on the PDA in patients with PA until an effective pulmonary blood flow source is established. Room air inhalation is recommended instead of pure oxygen inhalation to avoid accelerating PDA closure. Before surgery, preventing hyperventilation-induced pulmonary blood flow, left heart return blood volume increase, and left heart failure is better. During surgery, the arterial systolic pressure, SpO_2, and $ETCO_2$ should be maintained at around 80 mmHg, 75–85%, and 40 to 45 mmHg, respectively. Finally, 5% $CaCl_2$ can be appropriately used to enhance myocardial contractility and improve hypocalcemia after CPB.

25.5.3 Postoperative Anesthetic Management

(1) To maintain sufficient fluid volume, maintain appropriate arterial blood pressure, CVP 12–15 cm H_2O, left atrial pressure 10–12 mmHg, HCT about 40%, postoperative arterial systolic pressure maintained at 75–90 mmHg. (2) To maintain appropriate HR, better in the high range of the normal age group in younger children and synchronous atrial and ventricular rhythm. (3) 5% $CaCl_2$ 5–10 mg/(kg·h)and small doses of catecholamine drugs can be used together in infants under 3 months. (4) To maintain fluid, electrolytes, an acid–base balance, urine volume $\geq$ 2 mL/(kg·h), body temperature at 36–37 °C, and serum lactate change rate < 0.75 mmol/(L·h). (5) To apply the mechanical ventilation appropriately, SpO_2 and $ETCO_2$ should be maintained at 75–85% and 40–45 mmHg, respectively when FiO_2 is 0.4. The intrapleural pressure should be minimized to reduce the impedance to the venous return. Tidal volume should be maintained at 6–8 mL/kg, usually no or low level of PEEP, early withdrawal of mechanical ventilation, and active management atelectasis before the withdrawal of mechanical ventilation. (6) Generally, initiating heparin intravenous infusion at 5–10 U/(kg·h) 3 hours after non-CPB surgery or 6 h after CPB surgery is generally better. Avoiding or reducing the use of hemostatic agents and coagulation factors is better. (7) To check the artificial conduit's inner diameter and blood flow velocity by echocardiography.

25.6 Conclusion

The key points of anesthetic management of palliative surgeries in children with PA include: ① Anesthesiologists should carefully assess the function of coronary artery before anesthesia. ② It is appropriate to inhale 40% O_2 before surgery, and 100% O_2 inhalation should be avoided during surgery. ③ Excessive reduction in pulmonary artery pressure should be avoided in children with mBTS or central aortopulmonary shunting to prevent pulmonary congestion and heart failure. ④ To maintain sufficient fluid volume and relatively high arterial pressure after surgery to ensure adequate blood perfusion in the conduit. ⑤ It should be very cautious in using all kinds of hemostatic drugs, and a relatively low coagulation state should be maintained to avoid conduit occlusion.

The early mortality rate of PA is very high. These children often have severe coronary artery malformations (including proximal coronary artery stenosis and t coronary artery fistula supplied by the right ventricle to the distal coronary artery). Any measures to decompress the right ventricle pressure will cause large-area myocardial ischemia or even infarction in the left ventricle or death. The surgical treatment must follow the principle of diversified treatment plans due to dramatic differences in the size and morphological development of the right ventricle. The anesthesiologist needs to conduct an in-depth study of this situation and assist in formulating the best treatment principles (Hongbin Gu).

Anesthetic Management of Arterial Switch Operation in a Child with Taussig–Bing Anomaly

26

Yingzhi Dan

Abstract

A 4-month-old male infant was diagnosed with transposition of the great arteries and double outlet right ventricle (Taussig–Bing anomaly) due to cyanosis of the lips and fingertips. He was scheduled to undergo an arterial switch operation (ASO) under general anesthesia. After the aortic cross-clamp was released, the heart quickly resumed the sinus rhythm without defibrillation, but the electrocardiogram showed severe ST segment depression. The ST segment gradually returned to normal after treatment with dopamine, epinephrine, norepinephrine, and cardiopulmonary bypass support. The goals of perioperative management for such cases are to optimize cardiac output and balance myocardial oxygen supply and demand.

Taussig–Bing anomaly is a special type of congenital heart disease with a double outlet right ventricle (DORV), which includes transposition of the aorta to the right ventricle and malposition of the pulmonary artery with subpulmonary ventricular septal defect (VSD). There is no pulmonary stenosis. Clinically, it mainly manifests as cyanosis, developmental delay, and congestive heart failure. The natural course of the Taussig–Bing anomaly is similar to that of complete transposition of the great arteries combined with pulmonary hypertension, with early secondary pulmonary vascular obstructive disease. This article reports the anesthetic management of a Taussig–Bing anomaly undergoing ASO.

26.1 Case Presentation

A 4-months and 15-day-old male infant with 6.1 kg in weight and 52 cm in height. He was admitted to our hospital because of cyanosis in his lips and extremities over a month.

Physical examination: Body temperature 36.4 °C, heart rate (HR) 153 beats/min, respiratory rate (RR) 32 breaths/min, blood pressure (BP) 80/59 mm Hg, pulse oxygen saturation (SpO_2) 83% with air breathing. The patient was conscious and gave a normal response. Symmetrical chest without deformities and vein distention on the chest wall. There was no bulging in the precordial area and no thrill at the cardiac apex. The heart rhythm was regular with strong heart sounds. A coarse systolic murmur with thrill was heard in the third to fourth intercostal space on the left sternal border, the second sound of the pulmonary artery was weak.

Y. Dan (✉)
The National Children's Medical Center (Shanghai), Department of Anesthesiology of Shanghai Children's Medical Center, Shanghai Jiao Tong University School of Medicine, Shanghai, China
e-mail: danyingzhi@scmc.com.cn

J. Zheng et al. (eds.), *Selected Pediatric Cardiovascular Surgery Anesthesia Cases*,
https://doi.org/10.1007/978-981-96-5614-1_26

Bilateral respiratory movements were symmetrical. The breath sounds are clear without rales.

Echocardiography: DORV (Taussig–Bing anomaly), multiple VSD, atrial septal defect (ASD), pulmonary arterial hypertension (PAH), and slightly increased pulmonary artery flow speed. The heart, including the atrium and ventricles, is in a normal position with a concordant atrioventricular connection. The aorta originates from the right ventricle and is located at the left anterior. The pulmonary artery straddles the ventricular septum, mostly originating from the right ventricle, and is located at the right posterior. The aortic valve is functioning with an annulus of 1.27 cm with an ascending aorta diameter of 1.27 cm, mild aortic regurgitation, and a regurgitation jet width of 0.15 cm. The openings of the left and right coronary arteries are unclear. The pulmonary artery is widened, and the valve is functioning with an annulus of 1.22 cm, main trunk diameter of 1.84 cm, left pulmonary artery diameter of 0.69 cm, and right pulmonary artery diameter of 0.69 cm. The right atrium and right ventricle are enlarged. The right ventricular wall is thickened. The left ventricular contractibility is normal. The atrioventricular valve works well. The size of ASD is 0.26 cm. There are at least two VSDs. One VSD is 1.25 cm and located below the pulmonary artery; the other VSD is located at the muscular apex, with multiple jets, a range of 1.05 cm, a wider jet of 0.47 cm, and bidirectional shunting, predominantly left to right shunting. The aortic arch is on the left. No obvious shunting was observed at the level of the great arteries.

Cardiac and chest CT (plain scan + enhancement): DORV (S, D, L), VSD (below the pulmonary artery, muscular), ASD, lung infection. The mediastinum is basically in the midline of the thoracic cavity, the trachea with left and right bronchi are not compressed, and patchy exudation shadows are seen in both lungs. The atrium is in the normal position, the pulmonary vein return is normal, and the shunting at the atrial septal level is unclear. The right atrium is enlarged. The atrioventricular connection is concordant, there is a VSD below the pulmonary artery with a size of 12.3 mm and a muscular VSD with a size of 9.1 mm. Hypertrophic and enlarged right ventricle and well-developed left ventricle. The ventricular and great arterial connections are disconcordant. The origins of the left and right coronary arteries can be seen. The aorta is on the left and originates from the right ventricle. The pulmonary artery is on the right and mostly originates from the right ventricle, straddling the ventricular septum. No obvious aortic stenosis and patent ductus arteriosus are seen. The pulmonary artery main trunk is dilated with slightly widened left and right pulmonary arteries.

Preoperative diagnosis: DORV (Taussig–Bing anomaly), VSD (multiple), ASD, PAH.

26.2 Anesthetic Management

No preoperative medicines were given. Routine monitoring was initiated after entering the operating room with BP 85/50 mm Hg, HR 130 beats/min, and SpO_2 85%. After a peripheral venous cauterization was established, midazolam 0.6 mg, etomidate 1.8 mg, sufentanil 12 μg, and rocuronium 4.0 mg were intravenously administrated for induction of anesthesia. After the eyelash reflex disappeared, an ID 3.5 mm cuffed endotracheal tube was inserted with the assistance of video laryngoscopy. The depth of the tube was 11 cm. Pressure-controlled ventilation-volume guaranteed (PCV-VG) mode was used with oxygen flow rate 2.0 L/min, fraction of inspired oxygen fraction (FiO_2) 50%, tidal volume (VT) 50 mL, RR 24 times/min, inhalation time to exhalation time ratio (I:E) 1:2, positive end-expiratory pressure (PEEP) 4.0 cm H_2O, end-tidal carbon dioxide partial pressure ($EtCO_2$) about 38 mm Hg.

After induction of anesthesia, arterial (left femoral artery) and central venous (right internal jugular vein) were catheterized under ultrasound guidance for continuously monitoring invasive blood pressure (ABP) and central venous pressure (CVP). INVOS regional cerebral oxygen saturation ($rScO_2$) was continuously monitored.

Table 26.1 Blood gas test results before and after CPB

Time point	Hb (g/dL)	HCT (%)	pH	PaO_2 (mm Hg)	$PaCO_2$ (mm Hg)	BE (mmol/L)	Na^- (mmol/L)	K^+ (mmol/L)	Cl^- (mmol/L)	Ca^{2+} (mmol/L)	Lac (mmol/L)
Before CPB	10.8	32.4	7.46	58.0	33.6	−0.3	136.0	4.0	102.0	1.2	1.2
After stopping CPB	12.3	40.8	7.33	284.0	43.0	−3.7	133.0	4.1	94.0	1.1	2.1

The right femoral vein was also catheterized for rapid fluid replacement and blood transfusion. Tranexamic acid 10 mg/kg was intravenously administrated. General anesthesia was maintained by intravenous infusion of propofol 4.0 mg/(kg·h), sufentanil 2.5 μg/(kg·h), and rocuronium 0.6 mg/(kg·h) combined with sevoflurane intermittent inhalation. Before the operation, BP was 80/52 mm Hg, HR was 108 beats/min, SpO_2 was 95%, CVP was 12 cm H_2O, and $rScO_2$ was 75%. After cardiopulmonary bypass (CPB) was successfully established, a bovine pericardial patch was used to create an intracardiac tunnel connecting the left ventricle to the pulmonary artery. The aorta and pulmonary artery were transected, and an arterial switch operation was performed. The freed coronary artery openings were transplanted to the new aorta. The ASD was directly closed with a suture. The aortic cross-clamp was released after cardiac de-airing. The heartbeat spontaneously resumed to sinus rhythm without defibrillation, but the ECG showed severe ST segment depression. Dopamine 5.0 μg/(kg·min), epinephrine 0.02 μg/(kg·min), and norepinephrine 0.02 μg/(kg·min) were initiated immediately. Postoperative transesophageal echocardiography showed no residual shunting around the membranous VSD, two muscular shunts of 4.0 mm and 2.0 mm were still visible at the cardiac apex. There was no obstruction at the anastomosis of the two large arteries, mild to moderate mitral regurgitation, and no aortic valve insufficiency was found. After CPB, the aortic pressure was 80/47 mm Hg, and the pulmonary artery pressure was 31/15 mm Hg. Then, the epinephrine was increased to 0.1 μg/(kg·min), and CPB support was initiated until the ECG showed that the ST segment had returned to baseline. After the blood pressure was stabilized around 90/50 mm Hg, CPB was gradually weaned off. After ultrafiltration was completed, protamine was intravenously infused to neutralize heparin. Blood gas analysis was rechecked and electrolytes were supplemented according to the blood gas analysis results (Table 26.1). In addition, 120 IU of prothrombin complex were supplemented. Intraoperative body temperature was monitored, and active warming measures such as warm air blankets and fluid warming were also provided.

26.3 Postoperative Outcome

The operation lasted 345 min. The time of mildly hypothermic CPB support was 175 min. The aortic cross-clamping time was 127 min. The urine output was 10 mL. Approximately 150 mL of Ringer's acetate was infused. The $rScO_2$ was maintained at 73–80%. The lactate level remained within the normal range. After the operation, the BP was 90/50 mm Hg, HR was 140 beats/min, SpO_2 was 100%, CVP was 13 cm H_2O, and the rectal temperature was 36.5 °C. After the operation, dopamine was continuously infused at 5.0 μg/(kg·min), epinephrine at 0.1 μg/(kg·min), and norepinephrine at 0.02 μg/(kg·min). The patient was transferred to the Cardiac Intensive Care Unit (CICU) with an endotracheal tube and monitored by invasive blood pressure, ECG, and SpO_2. The tracheal tube was removed on the 5th day after surgery. The patient was discharged from the CICU on the 6th day after surgery and discharged from the hospital on the 10th day after surgery.

26.4 Review of Knowledge Points

26.4.1 Definition and Classification of DORV

The definition of DORV is still controversial in academia. The classic definition of double outlet right ventricle is ①The aorta and pulmonary artery both originate from the morphological right ventricle; ② The ventricular septal defect is the only outlet for the left ventricle; ③ There is no fibrous continuity between the semilunar valve and the atrioventricular valve due to the separation of the conus tissue. The widely accepted definition is that one major artery and most of the opening of the other major artery (>50%) originate from the morphological right ventricle, and there may or may not be a fibrous continuity between the aortic valve and the mitral valve.

In 2000, the Society of Thoracic Surgeons (STS) and the European Association for Cardio-Thoracic Surgery (EACTS) proposed a new classification: ① VSD type: VSD is located under the aortic valve, prone to pulmonary hypertension, and is the most common type; ② Tetralogy of Fallot (TOF) type: The ventricular septal defect is located under the aorta or the openings of the two major arteries, combined with right ventricular outflow tract stenosis; ③ Transposition of the great arteries (TGA) type: The ventricular septal defect is located under the pulmonary valve, this physiological type is seen in Taussig–Bing malformation, with or without infundibular and pulmonary stenosis; ④ VSD far from the great arteries type: The minimum distance between the VSD margin and the annulus of the two semilunar valves is greater than the diameter of the aortic valve ring. VSD is far from the great arteries, often combined with atrioventricular canal defect and/or heterotaxy syndrome. The new classification has good clinical practicality and is widely accepted by surgeons.

26.4.2 Anatomical Features of Children with DORV-TGA Type

This type of DORV is characterized by a subpulmonary VSD with or without PS. These patients usually have a conal septum that is displaced posteriorly and rightwardly, causing the VSD to be located near the pulmonary valve. Taussig–Bing anomaly is a subtype of DORV-TGA type, and typical Taussig–Bing anomaly includes atrial situs solitus and right ventricular loop, and both the aortic and pulmonary conus separate the aortic and pulmonary valves from the atrioventricular valve. The two semilunar valves are parallel at the same height. The position of the great vessels is lateral. The aorta originates entirely from the right ventricle, while the pulmonary valve straddles the ventricular septum, the septum is under the pulmonary artery, and there is no pulmonary stenosis. Taussig–Bing anomaly is often accompanied by other related cardiac anatomical abnormalities, commonly coronary artery anatomical abnormalities. It has been reported that 51% and 16% of patients were found to have aortic arch obstruction and coarctation of the aorta, respectively. The DORV with subpulmonary VSD is distinguished from TGA with VSD by lack of fibrous continuity between the pulmonary and mitral valves and both great arteries being primarily related to the right ventricle

26.4.3 Pathophysiology of DORV-TGA Type

Those children with DORV-TGA are similar to those with TGA /VSD in pathophysiology, which is characterized by the parallel circulation between systemic circulation and pulmonary circulation. The blood from the left ventricle is ejected primarily into the pulmonary artery through VSD, and the blood from the right ventricle mainly enters the aorta, which causes obvious hypoxemia and pulmonary hypertension. In addition, the risks of congestive heart failure and pulmonary vascular obstructive diseases are significantly increased due to the increased pulmonary blood flow. The blood oxygen saturation in the pulmonary artery is usually higher than that in the aorta, so these children present cyanosis, recurrent respiratory infections, and congestive heart failure in the neonatal period. When combined with pulmonary valve stenosis, cyanosis is more obvious, but the symptoms of heart failure may be alleviated. The development of these children is severely delayed. Physical examination shows bulging in the precordial area, third to fourth intercostal space on the left edge of the sternum with grade 3 or above systolic murmur and tremor, the second sound in the pulmonary valve area is enhanced or weakened, and most of these children die in the neonatal period.

26.4.4 Surgical Management

The "Congenital Heart Disease Surgery Chinese Expert Consensus (Seven): Double Outlet Right Ventricle" released by the National Cardiovascular Disease Expert Committee Congenital Heart Disease Professional Committee in 2020 considers that children with Taussig–Bing anomaly or combined with mild pulmonary valve stenosis (transvalvular pressure gradient<35 mm Hg), or good pulmonary valve function are recommended to undergo biventricular correction surgery as early as possible before the age of 6 months. First, to establish a baffle from the VSD to the pulmonary artery, then perform an arterial switch operation (ASO) or establish a baffle from the VSD to the aorta through the Kawashima procedure after removing the conus muscle.

The aorta and pulmonary artery are cut at the distal end of their respective valve membranes. The coronary artery with 3–4 mm aortic wall tissue is cut from the ascending aorta, and the gap is repaired with autologous pericardial tissue or artificial materials. Finally, the two major arteries are switched. Therefore, whether the coronary artery transplantation is successful has a decisive effect on whether the myocardial oxygen supply is sufficient after resuscitation. To make translocation of the coronary arteries successfully is very important for the sufficient myocardial oxygen supply after resuscitation.

26.5 Discussion

The goals of perioperative anesthetic management for children with Taussig–Bing anomaly are to optimize cardiac output and maintain a balance between oxygen supply and demand.

26.5.1 Preoperative Assessment and Preparation

During preoperative assessment, it is required to comprehensively understand the medical history, correctly assess the risks of surgery and anesthesia, and appropriately adjust the functions of important organs. We should focus on echocardiography, cardiac and large blood vessel CT, electrocardiogram, and laboratory tests related to cardiac function. It is better to confirm the diagnosis of Taussig–Bing anomaly before surgery. Our team assessed the child's cardiac function status and anesthesia risk. The child's current heart function belonged to grade IV (NAHA and modified Ross heart function grading). We fully communicated with the parents before surgery and fully informed them of the anesthesia risks.

26.5.2 Induction and Maintenance of Anesthesia

In this case, we used a high-dose opioid anesthesia technique due to the minimal suppression of cardiac function. We can effectively reduce the increase of pulmonary artery resistance caused by stress stimuli. The induction of anesthesia was conducted by intravenous injection of midazolam, etomidate, sufentanil, and rocuronium. General anesthesia was maintained with intravenous infusion of propofol, sufentanil, and rocuronium and combined with sevoflurane intermittent inhalation to keep the heart rate and blood pressure stable. Hypercapnia, acidosis, and hypoxemia can further increase pulmonary vascular resistance, which should be avoided in newborns and infants with limited myocardial reserve capacity. On the contrary, higher concentrations of inhaled oxygen and or mild hyperventilation can reduce PVR. In addition, the pulmonary vascular reactivity is typically higher in an immature pulmonary vascular bed, which can seriously affect pulmonary blood flow. According to these principles, the Qp/Qs ratio during surgery could be regulated by adjusting the inhaled oxygen concentration and ventilator parameters.

26.5.3 Hemodynamic Maintenance

The anesthetic management should focus on keeping heart rate in age-related normal range (preferably sinus rhythm), sufficient myocardial contractility, and suitable preload to maintain cardiac output.

In children with Taussig–Bing anomaly, VSD is close to the pulmonary valve. Most oxygenated blood from the left ventricular is ejected into the pulmonary artery, while most deoxygenated blood from the right ventricularis ejected into the aorta. When cardiac output decreases, the mixing between systemic and pulmonary circulation decreases, leading to a decrease in the oxygen saturation of deoxygenated blood in the systemic circulation, ultimately decreasing the oxygen saturation of oxygenated blood. At the same time, to avoid an increase in PVR, ventilatory interventions are needed for patients with concomitant pulmonary hypertension. After weaning off CPB, it is important to reduce aortic pressure and pulmonary artery pressure, which is beneficial to reduce bleeding at the suture site after ASO surgery.

26.5.4 If There Is Difficulty in Weaning Off CPB and Low Cardiac Output Syndrome, Coronary Ischemia Should Be First Considered

1. ASO surgery includes reimplantation of the coronary arteries. The first step is to investigate whether there is any twisting, pulling, or compression by a blood clot, surgical hemostatic material, or pulmonary artery in the coronary arteries. If these situations do occur, CPB should be restarted decisively, and conduct the corresponding surgical treatment.
2. Monitor the ST segment with multi-lead ECG, actively treat myocardial ischemia after coronary reimplantation, and use drugs such as nitroglycerin and β-blockers to improve the balance of myocardial oxygen supply and demand, but this is not a long-term solution.
3. Sometimes, there is transient myocardial ischemia secondary to coronary air embolism. Maintaining high perfusion pressure of CPB after releasing the aorta cross-clamp will help the coronary air embolism to migrate distally.
4. A temporary pacemaker is routinely placed during surgery to avoid excessive cardiac filling and compression of the coronary arteries when the heart rate slows down.
5. Transesophageal echocardiography (TEE) is very helpful in ensuring the complete removal of air embolism from the left atrium and left ventricle before weaning from cardiopulmonary bypass (CPB). It is also very useful to assess the patency of coronary artery reimplantation.
6. Enhancing the myocardial contractility of the left ventricle and reducing afterload are also necessary for separating from CPB support. Dopamine is the first choice of positive inotropic drugs. Epinephrine can be used for severe left ventricular dysfunction.

The child showed a transient significant decrease in the ST segment after CPB. Under the guidance of TEE, de-airing in the left ventricle by the cardiac surgeon was conducted combined with lung inflation. Then the child was reconfirmed that there was no twisting or opening damage to the coronary artery. The doses of positive inotropic drugs dopamine and, epinephrine, and norepinephrine were gradually increased to enhance the myocardial contractility of the left ventricle increase myocardial perfusion pressure. The parallel circulation was supported after the release of the aorta cross-clamp until the ST segment gradually returned to baseline.

26.5.5 Monitoring of Local Tissue Oxygen Saturation

Although supplement oxygen may lead to an increase in arterial oxygen saturation in the child with transposition physiology, it is important to recognize that there is a significant pulmonary overcirculation. While regulating the fraction of inspired oxygen before CPB can reduce pulmonary blood flow, it is necessary to closely monitor the systemic oxygen supply. During anesthesia, especially deep hypothermic circulatory arrest for VSD repair during CPB, frequent analysis of lactate levels and the use of non-invasive monitoring of $rScO_2$ can help to detect early alterations in systemic cardiac output induced by mechanical ventilation, anesthesia, and surgery. Several prospective observational studies have shown that non-invasive systemic oxygen balance indicators derived from near-infrared spectroscopy (NIRS) can effectively detect circulatory insufficiency in specific organ systems (such as the brain, kidneys, and intestines). NIRS has been widely used for $rScO_2$ monitoring, significantly reducing postoperative neurological complications in children with congenital heart disease. In this case, the child's $rScO_2$ was maintained at about 80% throughout the anesthesia and only decreased to about 73% during deep hypothermic circulatory arrest; it remained within the normal range.

26.6 Conclusion

The keys to anesthetic management in children with Taussig–Bing anomaly are to optimize cardiac output and maintain a balance between oxygen supply and demand. Monitoring cerebral oxygen saturation plays a crucial role in reducing postoperative central nervous system damage in these patients. By adjusting the parameters of mechanical ventilation, the balance between systemic and pulmonary vascular resistance can be regulated to ensure circulatory stability. The rational use of positive inotropic drugs can increase myocardial perfusion and improve cardiac contractility. Additionally, transfusion of red blood cells can increase oxygen-carrying capacity (Yingzhi Dan).

27 Anesthetic Management of Rastelli Surgery in a Child with Complete Transposition of the Great Arteries

Chi Wu

Abstract

A 6-month-old female infant was found with a heart murmur during physical examination, and cardiac ultrasound showed complete transposition of the great arteries (TGA) with ventricular septal defect (VSD) and left ventricular outflow tract (LVOT) obstruction. She was scheduled to undergo the Rastelli procedure under general anesthesia. The preoperative examination indicated a relative decrease in pulmonary blood flow. Before cardiopulmonary bypass (CPB), it is better to moderately reduce the pulmonary vascular resistance (PVR) and maintain the systemic vascular resistance (SVR) to increase the pulmonary blood flow and the blood mix of systemic and pulmonary circulation. After CPB, it is better to maintain a preload slightly below the normal range, increase the myocardial contractility, and decrease the afterload to maintain hemodynamic stability. The key point of anesthetic management in these children with TGA before CPB is adjusting the pulmonary-to-systemic pressure ratio (SVR/PVR) to balance the pulmonary cardiac output to the systemic cardiac output (Qp/Qs ratio). After CPB, the focus is on the smooth transition of the circulatory system after surgical operation.

The incidence of complete transposition of the great arteries (TGA) with VSD and LVOT obstruction is about 1/4500–1/2100, accounting for 7–9% of congenital heart diseases. The basic patho-anatomical changes include concordant atrioventricular connections together with discordant ventricular–arterial connections, ventricular septal defect (VSD), and left ventricular outflow tract stenosis (pulmonary and/or subvalvular stenosis). The systemic and pulmonary circulations rely on the VSD for oxygenated blood exchange. If the patients were left untreated, 90% of the patients with TGA would die within 1 year. The prognosis of children undergoing the Rastelli procedure is relatively good, and it is currently the preferred treatment option for complete TGA with VSD and LVOT stenosis. Due to the complexity of the procedure and the long duration of CBP, hemodynamics support in the early postoperative period is needed. This case report focuses on the anesthetic management of a child with TGA with VSD and LVOT obstruction who underwent the Rastelli procedure.

C. Wu (✉)
The National Children's Medical Center (Shanghai), Department of Anesthesiology of Shanghai Children's Medical Center, Shanghai Jiao Tong University School of Medicine, Shanghai, China
e-mail: wuchi@scmc.com.cn

J. Zheng et al. (eds.), *Selected Pediatric Cardiovascular Surgery Anesthesia Cases*,
https://doi.org/10.1007/978-981-96-5614-1_27

27.1 Case Presentation

A 6-month-old boy was 63 cm in height and 8.1 kg in weight. He was born by cesarean section at full term. Physical examination found a heart murmur after birth. Cardiac ultrasound showed complete TGA, VSD, and pulmonary valve and subvalvular stenosis. The patient was admitted to our hospital to seek surgical treatment.

Physical examination: The boy's consciousness was clear. The mental reaction was not obviously abnormal. The lips and extremity endings were cyanosed. Bilateral lung breath sounds were slightly coarse without rales. Arrhythmia occurred occasionally. Grade II/VI systolic murmur was heard at the left border of the sternum. The extremity endings were warm without edema. The pulse oxygen saturation (SpO_2) under room air was 89%.

Laboratory tests: hemoglobin 211 g/L, hematocrit 64.5%; no apparent abnormalities in the liver, kidney, or coagulation function.

Echocardiography: Right atrium and right ventricle enlargement, mild right ventricular wall hypertrophy; atrium orthotopic, ventricle orthotopic, atrioventricular concordance, ventriculoarterial discordance, aorta originates from the right ventricle, pulmonary artery arises from the left ventricle; VSD 0.66 cm, bidirectional shunt; pulmonary valve and subvalvular stenosis, pulmonary artery flow velocity 4.19 m/s, transvalvular pressure difference 70.3 mm Hg. Diagnosis: complete TGA, VSD, pulmonary valve and subvalvular stenosis.

Cardiac CT: Ventriculoarterial discordance with the aorta originating from the right ventricle and the pulmonary artery originating from the left ventricle; VSD approximately 6.9 mm; pulmonary valve and subvalvular stenosis; some small collateral vessels were seen.

Chest X-ray: Heart shadow enlargement, increased markings in both lungs, slightly blurred.

Electrocardiogram (ECG): Sinus rhythm, right ventricular hypertrophy.

The preoperative diagnosis: complete TGA, pulmonary valve and subvalvular stenosis, and VSD. Elective Rastelli surgery was scheduled under general anesthesia.

27.2 Anesthetic Management

Basic vital signs before anesthesia induction: heart rate (HR) 135 beats/min, blood pressure (BP) 82/45 mm Hg, SpO_2 86%. Anesthesia was induced by intravenous bolus injection of etomidate 1.5 mg, sufentanil 16 μg, rocuronium 5.0 mg. An ID 4.0 mm cuffed endotracheal tube was intubated under a visual laryngoscope and fixed after verification of the appropriate position by bilateral auscultation of the lungs. Pressure-controlled ventilation-volume guaranteed (PCV-VG) mode was used with respiratory parameters set as 50% fraction of inspired oxygen (FiO_2), 16 cm H_2O peak inspiratory pressure (PIP), 70–80 mL tidal volume (VT), 30 breaths/min respiratory rate (RR), and 1:2 inspiratory to expiratory time (I:E) ratio. The end-tidal carbon dioxide ($ETCO_2$) was maintained between 30 and 35 mm Hg by the adjustment of respiratory parameters.

After anesthesia induction, the left radial artery and right internal jugular vein were catheterized under ultrasound guidance for continuously monitoring invasive blood pressure (ABP) and central venous pressure (CVP). Bispectral index (BIS) and regional cereal oxygen saturation (rSO_2) monitoring were also conducted. The vital signs after endotracheal intubation: ABP 85/47 mm Hg, HR 128 beats/min, SpO_2 97%, CVP 13 cm H_2O, rSO_2 70%. General anesthesia was maintained by continuous intravenous infusion of propofol 5.0 mg/(kg·min), sufentanil 2.5 μg/(kg·min), 0.6 mg /(kg·min) rocuronium, and combined with 0.5–1.0 MAC sevoflurane inhalation. BIS value was maintained at 40–60. The artery blood gas (ABG) analysis results during operation were included in Table 27.1. The ABG result after intubation: pH 7.20, BE −12 mmol/L, HCO_3^-15.3 mmol/L. Five percent of sodium bicarbonate was intravenously infused for correction of metabolic acidosis.

Tranexamic acid 10 mg/kg and ulinastatin 100,000 U were intravenously administered before surgery. After thoracotomy, heparin

Table 27.1 Intraoperative blood gas results

	FiO_2 (%)	pH	PaO_2 (mm Hg)	$PaCO_2$ (mm Hg)	BE (mmol/L)	HCT (%)	K^+ (mmol/L)	Ca^{2+} (mmol/L)	Lac (mmol/L)	Cl^- (mmol/L)	Hb (g/dL)	HCO_3^- (mmol/L)
Post-intubation	60	7.20	33.6	40.4	−12.00	65.9	3.70	1.26	5.3	102	20.2	15.3
Ultrafiltration	60	7.38	122	37.0	−3.20	44.6	3.34	0.89	1.3	103	15.2	21.4

3.0 mg/kg was intravenously given. Once ACT was over 480 s, CPB was initiated. The surgery was performed under CPB support. Intraoperative exploration confirmed complete TGA accompanied by malalignment type VSD and hypertrophy of the right ventricular outflow tract. The VSD was closed with an autologous pericardial patch by consecutive sutures to form an intraventricular tunnel and baffle the aorta to the left ventricle. The root of the main pulmonary artery was transected, and an autologous pericardial patch sutured the proximal end of the main pulmonary artery. The abnormal hypertrophic muscle bundle of the right ventricular outflow tract was excised. The valved conduit was used to connect the right ventricular outflow tract with the main pulmonary artery and a probe strip was used to check for the patency of the outflow tract. The heart automatically resumed beating and sinus rhythm after the aortic cross-clamp release. Dopamine 5.0 μg/(kg·min) and epinephrine 0.1 μg/(kg·min) were intravenously infused. ABP 59/45 mm Hg, HR 152 beats/min. After the superior and inferior vena cava cross-clamp was released, mechanical ventilation with PCV-VG mode was resumed with similar respiratory parameters settings as before CPB.

Transesophageal echocardiography showed normal contractile activity in the left ventricular wall, cardiac ejection fraction of 62%, and no residual shunt around the intracardiac lateral tunnel patch. The flow rate of LVOT and right ventricular outflow tract was 0.9 m/s and 1.6 m/s, respectively. CBP was gradually weaned off after the adjustment of perfusion flow. After stopping the extracorporeal circulation, the ABP and HR were stable after CPB. After the modified ultrafiltration, protamine 90 mg (1.5:1) was intravenously infused to neutralize heparin, and hemocoagulase 1 U was used to facilitate hemostasis. ABG was rechecked (see Table 27.1), in which the Ca^{2+} level was 0.89 mmol/L; calcium gluconate 120 mg was then slowly infused. The dose of vasoactive drugs and the concentration of inhalational anesthetics were adjusted according to the blood pressure. Autologous salvaged blood 150 mL was transfused to maintain the blood pressure at around 75/42 mm Hg and the heart rate at 130–160 bpm. Delayed sternal closure was conducted due to the young age of this child and the adaption to the external ducts from the right ventricle to the pulmonary artery.

27.3 Postoperative Outcome

The total operation time was 230 min, the CBP time was 151 min, and the aortic cross-clamping time was 101 min. The estimated bleeding volume was about 250 mL. The urine volume was 120 mL. 150 mL of Ringer's acetate, 200 mL of erythrocyte suspension, and 100 mL of fresh frozen plasma were intravenously infused. At the end of the surgery, the ABP was 85/61 mm Hg; HR was 143 bpm, SpO_2 was 100%, CVP was 10 cm H_2O, rectal temperature was 36.3 °C, and rSO_2 was 65%. The child was transferred to the cardiac intensive care unit (CICU) under the monitoring of ABP, ECG, and SpO_2. The endotracheal tube was removed on the postoperative day 6. The child was discharged from CICU on the postoperative day nine and discharged from the hospital on the postoperative day 20.

27.4 Review of Knowledge Points

27.4.1 TGA/VSD/LVOT Obstruction

Complete TGA with VSD and LVOT obstruction is characterized by atrioventricular concordance and ventriculoarterial discordance. That means the morphological left ventricle connects with the pulmonary artery, and the morphological right ventricle connects with the aorta, creating the pathophysiological basis for separating the systemic and pulmonary circulations. The patient can only survive under the existence of a VSD shunt. The larger VSD can cause more oxygenated blood to mix at the defect and improve the oxygenation of the systemic circulation. However, if VSD is too large, too much blood flow will enter into the pulmonary circulation and cause pulmonary hypertension. The more severe the LVOT obstruction is, the less pulmonary blood flow is, and the lower the systemic blood oxygen saturation is.

27.4.2 Rastelli Surgery

The 20-year survival rate after arterial switch operation is approximately 90%, which is the preferred treatment option for TGA. However, in children with TGA accompanied by VSD and LVOT obstruction, sufficient left cardiac output cannot be maintained to achieve the goal of corrective treatment after the arterial switch operation due to the limitation of LVOT obstruction. For those children with TGA/VSD/LVOT obstruction, who have well-developed pulmonary arteries at the level of the left and right pulmonary arteries or bifurcation of the pulmonary arteries with fewer large aortic-pulmonary collateral branches but not high pulmonary artery pressures, the Rastelli procedure with intracardiac tunnel and external conduit can be performed. A pulmonary valve or subvalvular stenosis effectively protects the pulmonary vasculature, and the pulmonary vascular resistance is usually low. Furthermore, the large VSD usually causes the left ventricle to be hypertrophic enough to support the systemic circulation in this group of children, which is the physiological basis of the Rastelli procedure. The procedure includes VSD closure, a patch, and a baffle of the aorta into the left ventricle, which creates an intraventricular tunnel to establish access to the systemic circulation. The main pulmonary artery is transected at the root and closed proximally with a patch. The obvious hypertrophic muscle bundle of the right ventricular outflow tract is excised, and a valved conduit is used to connect the right ventricular outflow tract to the distal part of the main pulmonary artery to establish access to the pulmonary circulation.

27.5 Discussion

27.5.1 Preoperative Assessment and Preparation

SpO_2 89%, hemoglobin 211 g/L, hematocrit 64.5%, and collateral formation indicated that this patient experienced insufficient oxygenation in the systemic circulation, which could be improved by increasing the pulmonary blood flow and left ventricular output during surgery. This patient did not show any signs and symptoms of cardiac insufficiency before surgery, but postoperative low cardiac output syndrome is prone to occur. Therefore, conducting a detailed preoperative assessment and preparation and enhancing intraoperative monitoring is necessary. The left and right cardiac outflow tract obstruction after surgical reconstruction were common complications, which can be identified by intraoperative transesophageal echocardiography and hemodynamic manifestations.

27.5.2 Anesthetic Management Before CPB

Before CPB, anesthetic management aims to preserve cardiac output by maintaining HR, myocardial contractility, and preload. To avoid the relative increase in pulmonary vascular resistance (PVR) or relative decrease in systemic vascular resistance (SVR). Due to the pulmonary blood flow insufficiency before CPB, a higher FiO_2 and mild hyperventilation instead of PEEP were used to reduce pulmonary artery pressure before

CPB. A decrease in the systemic circulatory pressure was avoided by maintaining preload through volume supplementation, less myocardial contraction suppression by optimal selection of anesthetics, and timely adjustment of the depth of anesthesia.

27.5.3 Anesthetic Management After CPB

1. To maintain an age-appropriate HR and sinus rhythm since cardiac output after CPB is more dependent on HR. If it is necessary, a pacemaker should be installed in advance. A temporary pacemaker was routinely placed in this child for backup.
2. The preload should be appropriately reduced with the left atrial pressure at 6–9 mm Hg. After Rastelli surgery, the original morphological left ventricle becomes the real left ventricle to eject blood into the systemic circulation, which still needs some time to adapt. The blood volume changes very rapidly in young and low-body-weight children due to bleeding, diuretic drugs, ultrafiltration, and volume redistribution after CPB. Considering that these children cannot tolerate the higher preload at the early stage of the postoperative period, it is necessary to closely monitor the blood volume change at this stage, and the preload should be adjusted promptly. In addition to the changes in hemodynamic parameters and urine output, ultrasound assessment and direct observation of the degree of cardiac filling before chest closure can also provide a reference for blood and fluid infusion.
3. To Increase the left ventricle contractility and decrease the left ventricle afterload. Dopamine or dobutamine support may be required after separation from CPB. If SVR is higher, milrinone can be chosen since it can also directly reduce SVR in addition to the positive inotropic, myocardial diastolic, and PVR-reducing effects. There was no pulmonary hypertension in this patient due to the pulmonary valve and subvalvular stenosis. The large VSD (0.66 cm) exercised this patient's ability left ventricular to eject blood. Furthermore, the surgical correction and myocardial protection were satisfactory. All of these factors contributed to the smooth separation from CPB and more satisfactory hemodynamic status with a lower dose of vasoactive agents after surgery in this patient.
4. To maintain a relatively low right atrial pressure at 7–10 mm Hg. The right ventricular afterload can be appropriately reduced by lowering the pulmonary artery pressure. The strategies to lower pulmonary artery pressure and right ventricular afterload after CPB are similar to those before CPB.

27.6 Shortcomings and Limitations

There must be good matches between the systolic forces of the left and right ventricles and the aorta and pulmonary artery resistances after Rastelli surgery to facilitate the smooth conversion of the systemic and pulmonary circulatory functions. Due to the limitations of the monitoring equipment in children, we did not measure the aortic resistance, which makes it difficult to assess whether there was a good match between the left ventricular systolic force and the aortic resistance.

27.7 Conclusion

In conclusion, the anesthetic management of Rastelli surgery in a child with complete TGA should focus on the preoperative assessment of the severity of cyanosis, the optimal choice of ventilation management strategy and anesthetics, the maintenance of appropriate systemic-to-pulmonary circulatory resistance ratio before CPB, and the maintenance of cardiac function and the prevention and treatment of cardiac arrhythmias after CPB (Chi Wu).

28 Anesthetic Management of Nikaidoh Surgery in a Child with Complete Transposition of the Great Arteries

Chi Wu

Abstract

A 3-year-old boy was admitted to the hospital due to a recent exacerbation of cyanosis around the lips. Echocardiography showed complete transposition of the great arteries (TGA) with ventricular septal defect (VSD) and ventricular outflow tract obstruction (LVOTO). He was scheduled to undergo Nikaidoh under general anesthesia. The anatomical abnormalities related to coronary insufficiency and the mismatch of the ventricle and aortic resistance related to low cardiac output syndrome occurred after surgery. The boy's hemodynamics were stabilized after decompression of the coronary artery by reoperation and ECMO-assisted circulation. The anesthetic management before cardiopulmonary bypass (CPB) should focus on balancing the pulmonary-to-systemic flow ratio (Qp/Qs) by adjusting the systemic-to-pulmonary vascular resistance ratio (SVR/PVR). After CPB, the anesthetic management should focus on assessing and treating coronary perfusion and myocardial contractile function.

C. Wu (✉)
The National Children's Medical Center (Shanghai), Department of Anesthesiology of Shanghai Children's Medical Center, Shanghai Jiao Tong University School of Medicine, Shanghai, China
e-mail: wuchi@scmc.com.cn

The incidence of complete TGA with VSD and LVOTO is about 1/4500–1/2100, accounting for 7–9% of congenital heart diseases. The underlying pathoanatomic changes include transposition of the great arteries from left and right ventricles, ventricular septal defects, and pulmonary artery stenosis (PS) and/or subvalvular stenosis. The exchanges of oxygenated blood between the systemic and pulmonary circulations rely on VSD. Compared to the Rastelli procedure, the Nikaidoh procedure is more difficult to perform, but fewer long-term complications occur. Due to the complex adjustments in the cardiac anatomy, the Nikaidoh procedure usually takes a prolonged operative time, poses a greater impact on circulatory function, and results in more complex anesthetic management. This article described the anesthetic management of Nikaidoh surgery in a child with TGA accompanied by VSD and LVOTO.

28.1 Case Presentation

A 3-year-old boy with 96 cm in height and 12.3 kg in weight. The boy was delivered by cesarean section at full term. He was brought to the local hospital for a cold 2 years ago. A cardiac murmur was detected during a physical examination. Echocardiography indicated: TGA, VSD, and PS. During the follow-up period, recurrent pneumonia and cyanosis of the lips significantly

J. Zheng et al. (eds.), *Selected Pediatric Cardiovascular Surgery Anesthesia Cases*,
https://doi.org/10.1007/978-981-96-5614-1_28

deteriorated recently. The boy was admitted to our hospital for surgical treatment.

Physical examination: the boy was conscious with normal mental response. The lips were cyanotic, but no clubbing digits were found. Slight coarse respiratory sounds of both lungs were heard without rales. His heartbeat was regular with grade III–IV/VI systolic murmur heard at the third and fourth intercostal spaces on the left edge of the sternum and augmented second heart sound in the area of pulmonary valve auscultation. Warm extremities were found without edema. The pulse oximetry (SpO_2) was 82% with air breathing.

Laboratory tests: hemoglobin 145 g/L, hematocrit 48.4%, total protein 60.0 g/L, no apparent abnormalities in the liver, kidney, or coagulation function.

Echocardiography: Slight enlargement of the left atrium and left ventricle, concordant connection between atria and ventricles, concordant atrioventricular connection is consistent, discordant ventricle-aortic or pulmonary trunk connections, aorta originating from the right ventricle, pulmonary artery trunk originating from the left ventricle, VSD about 0.91 cm, bi-directional shunts, pulmonary artery valve and subvalvular stenosis, pulmonary flow velocity 3.91 m/s, transvalvular pressure gradient 61.2 mm Hg. The primary diagnosis was TGA, VSD, and PS.

Angiography: Discordant ventricle—aortic or pulmonary trunk connections, aorta originating from the right ventricle, pulmonary artery originating from the left ventricle, VSD approximately 10.8 mm.

Chest X-ray: heart shadow enlargement, increased markings in both lungs.

Electrocardiogram (ECG): Sinus rhythm, right ventricle enlargement, prolonged QT interval.

The preoperative diagnosis was TGA, VSD, and PS. Nikaidoh's surgical procedure was proposed to be conducted under general anesthesia.

28.2 Anesthetic Management

Basic vital signs: heart rate (HR) 112 beats/min, blood pressure (BP) 86/52 mm Hg, SpO_2 78%. Anesthesia was induced with intravenous bolus doses of 2.5 mg etomidate, 25 μg sufentanil, and 10.0 mg rocuronium. An ID 4.5 mm cuffed endotracheal tube was intubated under a visual laryngoscope and fixed after verification of the appropriate position by bilateral auscultation of the lungs. Pressure control ventilation was used with respiratory parameters set as fraction of inspiration oxygen (FiO_2) 60%, inspiratory pressure 16 cm H_2O, tidal volume (VT) 110–120 mL, respiratory rate (RR) 30 breaths/min, and inspiratory time: expiratory time (I:E) ratio 1:2. General anesthesia was maintained by continuous intravenous infusion of 5.0 mg/(kg·h) propofol, 2.5 μg/(kg·h) sufentanil, and 0.6 mg/(kg·h) rocuronium combined with 1–2% sevoflurane intermittent inhalation, end-tidal carbon dioxide ($ETCO_2$) was maintained between 30 and 35 mm Hg.

Invasive arterial pressure (ABP) from the left radial artery, central venous pressure (CVP) from the right internal jugular vein, bispectral index (BIS), and regional cerebral oxygen saturation (rSO_2) monitoring was rapidly set up after endotracheal intubation. Vital signs after intubation: ABP 89/46 mm Hg, HR 117 beats/min, SpO_2 95%, CVP 15 cm H_2O, rSO_2 78%. Anesthesia was maintained by intravenous infusion of propofol 4.0 mg/(kg·h), sufentanil 2.0 μg/(kg·h), rocuronium 0.5 mg/(kg·h), and combined with intermittent inhalation of sevoflurane 0.5–1.0 MAC. The BIS value was maintained between 40 and 60. Arterial blood gas analysis was shown in Table 28.1 with pH 7.28, BE −9.6 mmol/L, and 35 mL of 5% sodium bicarbonate was given to correct metabolic acidosis.

After anesthesia induction, left radial artery and right internal jugular vein catheterization were conducted under ultrasound guidance for continuously monitoring ABP and CVP. The surgery was performed under CPB support.

Table 28.1 Intraoperative blood gas results

	FiO_2 (%)	pH	PaO_2 (mm Hg)	$PaCO_2$ (mm Hg)	BE (mmol/L)	HCT (%)	K^+ (mmol/L)	Ca^{2+} (mmol/L)	Lac (mmol/L)	Cl^- (mmol/L)	Hb (g/dL)	HCO_3^- (mmol/L)
Post-intubation	60	7.28	67	35.3	−9.6	49.2	3.54	1.18	1.1	98	15.3	20.1
Ultrafiltration	60	7.39	260	37.9	−1.7	44.4	3.60	0.91	3.1	102	14.7	23.5

Intraoperative exploration showed that the two great arteries were in an anteroposterior relationship. The pericardial patch was used to repair the ventricular septal defect and reconstruct the left ventricular outflow tract. The aorta, combined with the coronary artery, was transplanted to the original position of the pulmonary artery. The pulmonary artery was enlarged by a patch and sutured to the anterior wall of the aorta. The right ventricular outflow tract was reconstructed. After aortic cross-clamp release, the heart resumed beating automatically. The rhythm was sinus rhythm with ST-segment elevation on ECG. Dopamine 5.0 μg/(kg·min) and epinephrine 0.02 μg/(kg·min) were infused. The blood pressure was 52/40 mm Hg, and HR was 113 bpm. Ventricular fibrillation occurred 2 minutes later. Open chest defibrillation was conducted with 6 joules and 3 times, then the sinus rhythm was restored with a heart rate of 72 beats/min and a blood pressure of 55/42 mm Hg. The dose of epinephrine was adjusted, and nitroglycerin 0.5 μg/(kg·min) was intravenously supplemented by an intravenous infusion pump. After the vena cava cross-clamp was released, pressure control ventilation was resumed with respiratory parameters set as inspiratory pressure 18 cm H_2O, VT 110–120 mL, RR 24 times/min. Transesophageal echocardiography (TEE) showed left ventricle enlargement with reduced wall motion. No residual shunt was detected around the VSD patch. Thereafter, the dose of epinephrine was gradually increased to 0.1 μg/(kg·min) according to blood pressure level. Before separation from CPB support, ABP was 62/36 mm Hg, HR was 165 bpm, and CVP was 13 cm H_2O. The CPB was gradually weaned off by decreasing the perfusion flow. BP and HR were stable after separation from CPB. At the end of the modified ultrafiltration, protamine 95 mg was intravenously dripped to neutralize heparin. Hemocoagulase 1 U was used to assist hemostasis. The blood gases were retested (see Table 28.1), in which Ca^{2+} was measured at 0.91 mmol/l, and then 150 mg of calcium gluconate was slowly injected. After that, 100 mL of autologous blood was transfused, and ABP was maintained around 85/42 mm Hg, HR at 130–160 beats/min. The sternum was closed after careful hemostasis.

28.3 Postoperative Outcome

The total operation time was 445 min, the CPB time was 231 min, and the aortic cross-clamp time was 108 min. The estimated blood loss and urine output were about 300 mL and 200 mL, respectively. 200 mL of Ringer's acetate and 100 mL of autologous blood were intravenously infused. The intraoperative lactate value remained in the normal range. At the end of the operation, ABP 90/45 mm Hg, HR 140 beats/min, SpO_2 100%, CVP 11 cm H_2O, rectal temperature 36.5 °C, rSO_2 65%. ST-segment depression on ECG was significantly improved compared to that at the time of CPB separation. The boy was intubated and transferred to the cardiac intensive care unit (CICU) with ABP, ECG, and SpO_2 monitoring.

On the postoperative day 1, blood pressure fluctuated with significant ST-segment depression on EEG. Emergency thoracotomy was performed, and the right pulmonary artery was found to be dilated at the patch enlargement, which compressed the coronary artery. Then, decompression of the coronary artery was performed. On postoperative day 3, ECMO was urgently instituted at the bedside to assist circulation due to the occurrence of low cardiac output syndrome. ECMO was withdrawn on the postoperative day 7. The endotracheal tube was removed on the postoperative day 20 and transferred from CICU to the general ward on the postoperative day 24. The boy was discharged from the hospital on postoperative day 40.

28.4 Review of Knowledge Points

28.4.1 TGA/VSD/LVOTO

The physiology, anatomy, and pathophysiology of TGA with VSD and LVOTO were described in Chap. 27.

28.4.2 Nikaidoh Procedure

The Rastelli procedure has been the most common technique used for the surgical treatment of TGA with VSD and LVOTO, which mainly includes the baffling of the VSD to the aorta and the reconstruction of the right ventricle outflow tract (RVOT). Although the early morbidity and mortality are relatively low, substantial late morbidity and mortality have been reported due to left and right-sided obstruction with a late survival of 52–59% at 20 years follow-up. The angular internal tunnel and external conduit constructed in the Rastelli procedure are susceptible to compression, which may contribute to the high incidence of late left and right ventricle outflow obstruction. The Nikaidoh procedure can reach the anatomical correction of TGA with VSD and LVOTO, and the reconstructed biventricular outflow tract is physiologically functional and hemodynamically stable. Furthermore, the energy consumption is relatively low, and the right ventricular volume is preserved. Therefore, the late incidence of obstruction and severe side events are significantly reduced. More and more children with TGA/VSD/LVOTO are now treated with Nikaidoh procedure, which involves: the two great arteries, and the right and left coronary arteries are first freed and transected, then the aortic root is grafted together with the coronary arteries to the original pulmonary artery, VSD is repaired with a patch continued to the aorta, the left ventricular outflow tract is reconstructed, the distal part of the pulmonary artery is enlarged with a patch and sutured to the anterior wall of the aorta to reconstruct the right ventricular outflow tract.

28.5 Discussion

28.5.1 Preoperative Assessment and Preparation

The SpO_2 was 82%, hemoglobin was 145 g/L, and hematocrit was 48.4% in this case, indicating that the systemic circulation's oxygen supply was insufficient. Although the boy did not show any signs and symptoms of cardiac insufficiency before the operation, postoperative low cardiac output syndrome is prone to occur after the Nikaidoh procedure. Reinforced monitoring and preparation of inotropic and vasoactive drugs in advance are required. If it is possible, mechanical circulatory assist devices should also be prepared in advance. Due to the stretching of the coronary arteries during surgery, the coronary artery can easily produce obstruction during the postoperative period. Therefore, dynamically monitoring and preparation of coronary vasodilators are needed. The obstruction of the right and left ventricular outflow tract after surgical reconstruction is another common complication, which should be identified by intraoperative TEE and hemodynamic manifestations.

28.5.2 Anesthetic Management Before CPB

1. Maintaining HR, myocardial contractility, and preload to maintain cardiac output.
2. Avoiding relative increase in PVR and relative decrease in SVR. In this child, pulmonary blood flow was reduced, so higher oxygen concentration and mild hyperventilation were given before CPB in order to reduce PVR and increase the pulmonary blood flow and the blood flow mixing between the systemic-

pulmonary circulations. On the other hand, blood volume should be adequately supplemented, and the depth of anesthesia should be well controlled in order to avoid a relative decrease in SVR, which could result in the increase in recirculation of venous blood and the decrease of arterial oxygen saturation level.

28.5.3 Anesthetic Management After CPB

1. Assessment and treatment of coronary perfusion insufficiency

   ECG monitoring and TEE provide insight into coronary artery damage. The air in the left atrium and left ventricle before separation from CPB can be adequately assessed to avoid coronary gas embolism. After the aortic cross-clamp is released, it is useful to maintain a high perfusion pressure by CPB to facilitate the distal migration of coronary gas embolism. After CPB separation, nitroglycerin and β-blockers should be used along with the enhancement of blood pressure if the ECG shows ST-segment depression and ruling out electrolyte disturbances, hypothermia, and other risk factors. Left ventricular enlargement can also lead to increased tension or distortion of the coronary anastomosis. TEE can be helpful in aiding in making a diagnosis. If all the above-mentioned measures fail to work, surgical problems should be considered, and the coronary artery obstruction should be surgically released. In this boy, ST depression on ECG after separation from CPB occurred, which indicated that the coronary arteries had not yet returned to their normal state. Nitroglycerin was given to dilate the coronary arteries, while epinephrine increased blood pressure and improved coronary perfusion. However, because the anatomical factors of coronary artery compression had not been relieved, the child experienced hemodynamic fluctuations on the same day of surgery, indicating that more precise monitoring techniques are required to enhance the assessment of the coronary arteries.

2. Assessment and treatment of ventricular function insufficiency

   Before surgery, the left ventricle mainly provides blood flow into the pulmonary circulation. However, after surgery, the left ventricle is changed to provide blood flow to the systemic circulation. It takes some time for myocardial contractility and ventricular volume to adapt to this change. The left ventricle cannot tolerate excessive volume loading. It is necessary to control the amount and rate of fluid input and maintain the left atrial pressure around 6–9 mm Hg. In the early postoperative period, positive inotropic drugs, such as dopamine, epinephrine, milrinone, etc., are usually required to support cardiovascular function. In addition to the positive inotropic action, milrinone can also enhance the ventricular diastolic function and reduce PVR. In addition, milrinone can also reduce SVR and the left ventricular afterload. In this case, ventricular fibrillation occurred after separation from CPB, to which the prolonged duration of CPB, myocardial edema, myocardial damage, and insufficient coronary perfusion (the postoperative finding) might contribute. CPB was successfully weaned off after the use of inotropic drugs to increase myocardial contractility and coronary perfusion. Low cardiac output syndrome happened on postoperative day 3, and the hemodynamics were stabilized after 1 week of bedside ECMO support. The low cardiac output syndrome may be related to the mismatch between ventricular contractility and aortic resistance after surgery, which takes time to establish a good match. One-year follow-up echocardiography showed that the left ventricular contractility was still inadequate. Therefore, the use of positive inotropic drugs or cardiac assist devices to improve ventricular function during the perioperative period can have a positive effect on those children who rely on self-regulation to adapt to the new anatomic changes.

28.6 Conclusion

Reviewing the intraoperative and postoperative course of this boy, we recognized that intraoperative positive inotropic and vasoactive drugs may mask the potential problems in coronary artery and myocardial systolic function. On the other hand, the postoperative cardiac function in children can be dynamically changed, which requires continuous monitoring and dynamic adjustment of positive inotropic and vasoactive drugs. The goal of anesthetic management in children with TGA/VSD/LVOTO before CPB is to balance the Qp/Qs by adjustment of the SVR/PVR ratio. After CPB, assessing and treating coronary artery perfusion and myocardial contractile function should be the key to anesthetic management (Chi Wu).

Anesthetic Management of Senning + Rastelli Procedure in a Child with Corrected Transposition of the Great Arteries

29

Chi Wu

Abstract

A 15-year-old male child was found to have exacerbation of end extremity bruising and decreased mobility recently. Echocardiography showed corrected transposition of the great arteries (C-TGA) with ventricular septal defect (VSD) and ventricular outflow tract (LVOT) obstruction. He was scheduled to undergo the Senning + Rastelli procedure under general anesthesia. The preoperative examination indicated a relative decrease in pulmonary blood flow. Before cardiopulmonary bypass (CPB), it is better to adjust the systemic-pulmonary vascular resistance ratio (SVR/PVR) to balance the systemic-pulmonary circulation blood flow (Qp/Qs ratio). The increase of Qp and mixing blood mix between the systemic-pulmonary circulation can be achieved by moderate reduction of PVR while maintaining the SVR. After CPB, it is better to maintain the smooth transition of myocardial systolic function, actively manage the cardiac arrhythmia, maintain a slightly lower-than-normal range of preload, and increase the myocardial contractility while decreasing the ventricular afterload.

C-TGA with VSD and LVOT obstruction accounts for 0.7% of all congenital heart malformations. The basic patho-anatomical changes include atrial-ventricular disconcordance and ventricular aortic disconcordance. To be more specific, the right atrium is connected to the left ventricle via the mitral valve and then to the pulmonary artery. The left atrium is connected to the right ventricle via the tricuspid valve and then to the aorta. In addition, there exists VSD and pulmonary and subvalvular stenosis. Such patients may be asymptomatic early because the circulation is adequate for physiological exchanges. However, since the anatomical right ventricle carries the function of systemic circulation for a long time, severe tricuspid regurgitation and right heart failure often occur in the long term. The anatomical left ventricle carries the function of pulmonary circulation. Therefore, it is possible that degeneration can occur. Therefore, surgical intervention should be performed at the optimal time after diagnosis. Senning + Rastelli is the most widely used corrective surgery. The procedure is highly complex, usually takes a long time, and significantly impacts the circulatory function. This article describes the anesthetic management of a patient with C-TGA, VSD, and

C. Wu (✉)
The National Children's Medical Center (Shanghai), Department of Anesthesiology of Shanghai Children's Medical Center, Shanghai Jiao Tong University School of Medicine, Shanghai, China
e-mail: wuchi@scmc.com.cn

J. Zheng et al. (eds.), *Selected Pediatric Cardiovascular Surgery Anesthesia Cases*,
https://doi.org/10.1007/978-981-96-5614-1_29

LVOT stenosis who underwent the Senning + Rastelli procedure.

29.1 Case Presentation

A 15-year-old boy was 155 cm in height and 32.5 kg in weight. He was born by cesarean section at full term. Physical examination found a heart murmur after birth when he was treated at a local hospital for "neonatal asphyxia." Cardiac ultrasound showed C-TGA, VSD, pulmonary stenosis (PS), and patent ductus arteriosus (PDA). The patient suffered from growth retardation, bruising at the end of the extremities, cyanosis, and decreased mobility, which became significantly worse recently. The patient was admitted to our hospital to seek surgical treatment.

Physical examination: The boy was conscious. The mental reaction was not obviously abnormal. The lips and extremity endings were bruising. Bilateral lung breath sounds were slightly coarse without rales. Grade III/VI systolic murmur was heard between two and four ribs at the left edge of the sternum. The extremity endings were warm without edema. The pulse oximetry (SpO_2) with room air was 81%.

Laboratory tests: hemoglobin 163 g/L, hematocrit 46.3%, no apparent abnormalities in the liver, kidney, or coagulation function.

Echocardiography: right atrium enlargement, anatomical right ventricular wall hypertrophy. The left atrium was connected to the anatomical right ventricle, and the right atrium was connected to the anatomical left ventricle. The aorta originates from the right ventricle, and the pulmonary artery arises from the left ventricle. VSD 1.6 cm, bidirectional shunt. Pulmonary valve and subvalvular stenosis. The pulmonary artery flow velocity was 4.7 m/s. The transvalvular pressure difference was 87.3 mm Hg. Tricuspid regurgitation with regurgitation bundle width 0.29 cm. Collateral vessel formation. Diagnosis: C-TGA, VSD, pulmonary valve and subvalvular stenosis, mild tricuspid regurgitation, collateral vessel formation.

Cardiac CT: atrial-ventricular disconcordance; ventricular-arterial disconcordance, VSD 16.8 mm, Coarctation, and PDA was not found.

Angiography: atriums are orthotropic, and ventricles are inverted. The anatomical right ventricle is located on the left, and the anatomical left ventricle is located on the right. The anatomical left ventricle connects with the pulmonary artery, which is located on the right, and the anatomical right ventricle connects with the aorta, which is located on the left. The origins of the coronary arteries are normal.

Chest X-ray: No obvious abnormalities in the cardiac shadow, increased lung markings.

Electrocardiogram (ECG): Sinus rhythm, high voltage in limb leads.

The preoperative diagnosis: C-TGA, pulmonary valve and subvalvular stenosis, and VSD. Elective Senning + Rastelli surgery was scheduled under general anesthesia.

29.2 Anesthetic Management

The patient drank 2 mL/kg of Outfast® 2 h before the operation, and he also orally took 10.0 mg midazolam syrup 30 min before the operation. After Ramsay sedation score reached 4, the patient was calmly separated from his parents and transported to the operating room. ECG, blood pressure (BP), and SpO_2 were routinely monitored: BP 113/65 mm Hg, heart rate (HR) 85 beats per minute (bpm), and SpO_2 82%. After the peripheral vein catheterization was established, general anesthesia was induced by intravenous bolus injection of midazolam 1.5 mg, etomidate 6.5 mg, sufentanil 30 μg, and rocuronium 25.0 mg. After the lash reflex disappeared, an ID 6.5 mm cuffed endotracheal tube was intubated with the assistance of visual laryngoscopy. The depth of intubation was 17 cm. Pressure-controlled ventilation-volume guaranteed (PCV-VG) mode was used with the following ventilation parameters: oxygen flow rate 2 L/min, fraction of inspired oxygen (FiO_2) 60%, tidal volume (VT) 300 mL, the inspiratory/expiratory (I:E) time ratio was 1:2, and the respiratory parameters were adjusted to maintain the partial

Table 29.1 Intraoperative blood gas results

	FiO_2 (%)	pH	PaO_2 (mm Hg)	$PaCO_2$ (mm Hg)	BE (mmol/L)	HCT (%)	K^+ (mmol/L)	Ca^{2+} (mmol/L)	Lac (mmol/L)	Cl^- (mmol/L)	Hb (g/dL)	HCO_3^- (mmol/L)
Post-intubation	60	7.31	65	33.0	−9.26	44.9	3.62	1.23	1.6	108	16.1	15.9
Ultrafiltration	60	7.42	140	32.4	−3.3	39.6	2.90	0.95	2.0	106	12.9	22.4

pressure of end-expiratory carbon dioxide ($ETCO_2$) between 35 and 40 mm Hg.

Invasive arterial pressure (ABP) from the left radial artery, central venous pressure (CVP) from the right jugular vein, frequency index (BIS), and regional cerebral tissue oxygen saturation (rSO_2) monitoring were rapidly established after endotracheal intubation. Post-intubation vital signs: ABP 105/58 mm Hg, HR 88 bpm, SpO_2 97%, CVP 10 cm H_2O, rSO_2 68%. Propofol 4.0 mg/(kg·h), sufentanil 2.0 μg/(kg·h), and rocuronium 0.5 mg/(kg·h) were intravenously infused with 0.5–1.0 MAC sevoflurane intermittent inhalation to maintain the depth of anesthesia. The BIS value was maintained between 40 and 60. Arterial blood gas analysis results were shown in Table 29.1, in which pH 7.20, BE −9.26 mmol/L, HCO_3^- 15.9 mmol/L, and 5% sodium bicarbonate 80 mL was intravenously given to correct metabolic acidosis.

Tranexamic acid 10 mg/kg and ulinastatin 100,000 U were intravenously given before the start of surgery. Heparin 3.0 mg/kg was intravenously given after the sternotomy. CPB was started after ACT >480 s. Intraoperative exploration confirmed the diagnosis of C-TGA combined with VSD and PS. A patch was used to segregate the vena cava into the tricuspid valve and the pulmonary venous cavity into the mitral valve to complete the Senning procedure. A pericardial patch suture was used to close VSD and segregate the aorta into the left ventricle creating an intraventricular tunnel. A polyester tube connected the right ventricular outflow tract to the principal pulmonary artery. The heart automatically resumed beating after aortic cross-clamping release, and the cardiac rhythm was sinus rhythm. Dopamine 5.0 μg/(kg·min) and epinephrine 0.05 μg/(kg·min) were intravenously infused, ABP 55/40 mm Hg, HR 155 bpm, and mechanical ventilation with the same parameters as before was resumed after vena cava cross-clamping was released. Transesophageal echocardiography showed that no significant residual shunt was detected in the septal patch. The aorta was connected to the left ventricle with an anterior blood flow of 1.2 m/s. The anastomosis between the valved conduit and the right ventricle was smooth. The pulmonary vein flowed back into the right atrium with a flow of 0.48 m/s. The vena cava flowed back into the left atrium with a flow of 0.40 m/s. Mild tricuspid valve regurgitation. CBP was gradually weaned off after the adjustment of perfusion flow. The ABP was 75/42 mm Hg, and HR was about 150 bpm. After the modified ultrafiltration ended, protamine 210 mg (1.2:1) was intravenously given to neutralize heparin. Hemagglutinin 1 U was used to assist in hemostasis. Blood gas analysis was rechecked (see Table 29.1), in which Ca^{2+} was 0.95 mmol/L. Calcium gluconate (300 mg) was slowly injected to correct the low Ca^{2+} level. The dosage of vasoactive drugs and the concentration of inhalational anesthetics were adjusted according to the blood pressure. The sternum was closed after the transfusion of 300 mL of erythrocyte suspension and 50 mL of plasma adequate hemostasis.

29.3 Postoperative Outcome

The operation lasted for 360 min in total, which included the CPB time of 200 min and the aortic cross-clamping time of 153 min. The temperature was lowered to 28 °C during the aortic cross-clamping. A total of 200 mL of Ringer's acetate, 300 mL of erythrocyte suspension, and 50 mL of plasma were infused intraoperatively (none of the volumes replenished and lost during CPB were calculated). At the end of the operation, ABP 82/45 mm Hg, HR 93 bpm, SpO_2 99%, CVP 8 cm H_2O, anal temperature 36.5 °C. The child was transferred to the Cardiac Intensive Care

Unit (CICU) with endotracheal intubation under ABP, ECG, and SpO_2 monitoring. The endotracheal tube was removed on the postoperative day 5. The patient was discharged from CICU on postoperative day 7 and discharged from the hospital on postoperative day 12.

29.4 Review of Knowledge Points

29.4.1 C-TGA/VSD/LVOT Obstruction

C-TGA alone is rare; more than 80% of cases are accompanied by other malformations, including VSDs, LVOT obstruction, and tricuspid valve malformation. Sixty percent to eighty percent of C-TGA patients are accompanied by VSD, and about 50% of patients are accompanied by LVOT obstruction (pulmonary and/or subvalvular stenosis). VSDs can increase the pulmonary artery blood flow, but the LVOT can limit the pulmonary artery blood flow. The ratio between them determines whether pulmonary congestion or cyanosis occurs. Although the majority of C-TGA patients present with cyanosis, 1–2% of patients are asymptomatic. Thirty percent of patients will produce tricuspid valve insufficiency with the increase of age and can even progress to severe tricuspid regurgitation and anatomic right ventricular dysfunction. Tricuspid regurgitation is an independent risk factor for death. The 20-year survival rate in C-TGA patients without significant tricuspid regurgitation is 93%, but only 49% in the patients with tricuspid regurgitation. Conduction system disorders occur in 15–50% of patients. The complete atrioventricular block is common due to atrioventricular disconcordance, the abnormal pathway of the atrioventricular bundle, and fibrosis of some atrioventricular bundles with the increase of age.

29.4.2 Senning + Rastelli Surgery

Senning (or Mustard) + ASO (aortic switching) does not resolve the inadequate left ventricular output due to LVOT obstruction. Therefore, the patients with LVOT obstruction are generally treated with the Senning (or Mustard) + Rastelli procedure. The Senning or Mustard procedure uses a patch or pericardium to make a plate barrier to segregate the non-oxygenated blood from the superior and inferior vena cava to the right atrium and the oxygenated blood from the pulmonary veins to the left atrium. Then the blood reversal is achieved at the atrial level. The Rastelli procedure creates a left ventricular outflow tunnel from the left ventricle to the aorta after the closure of VSD and a right ventricular outflow tunnel with an artificial conduit connecting the right ventricle to the pulmonary artery. Then, the blood reversal is achieved at the ventricular level.

29.5 Discussion

29.5.1 Preoperative Assessment and Preparation

In this case, SpO_2 was 81%, hemoglobin was 163 g/L, hematocrit was 46.3%, and systemic-pulmonary collateral branch formation indicated that the patient's pulmonary blood flow was insufficient. It is necessary to adjust the intraoperative ventilation parameters to regulate the pulmonary blood flow and increase oxygenation. A cardiac ultrasound showed anatomical right ventricle hypertrophy and dysfunction. So, special attention should be paid to controlling the preload and afterload of the right heart system and increasing the myocardial contractility after surgery. Although cardiac ultrasound did not report the size of the anatomical left ventricle and the ejection fraction, the decreased mobility indicated the anatomical left ventricular insufficiency. So, the preload and afterload of the left heart system should be reduced, and the contractility should also be increased. Such patients are at a high risk of intraoperative arrhythmias. The defibrillator and pacemaker should be prepared in advance.

29.5.2 Anesthetic Management Before CPB

As mentioned above, the patient's pulmonary blood was reduced, so measures to reduce pulmonary circulatory resistance, such as increasing FiO_2 and mild hyperventilation without PEEP, should be used before CPB to increase pulmonary blood flow and maintain normal left ventricular output. Furthermore, vigilance is required for the occurrence of cardiac arrhythmias.

29.5.3 Anesthetic Management After CPB

1. Smooth transition of the ventricular function. Cardiac dysfunction and cardiac output reduction are prone to occur during the postoperative period due to the gigantic changes in cardiac anatomy and myocardial edema caused by CPB. After aortic cross-clamping release, positive inotropic drugs should be actively used to support ventricular contractility. Small doses of dopamine and epinephrine can be intravenously infused. After separation from CPB, fluid supplementation should be appropriately controlled to maintain central venous pressure at 7–9 cm H_2O. It is better to control the arterial blood pressure in a lower range on the basis of sufficient systemic circulation perfusion to reduce the afterload of the left and right ventricles. The heart rate can be maintained in a higher range of 120–160 bpm to compensate for the low arterial blood pressure and maintain sufficient cardiac output to guarantee organ perfusion. After the above treatment, the patient's hemodynamics were stable, and the perfusion of the systemic circulation was satisfactory (blood lactate value 2.0 mmol/L).
2. Arrhythmia. Because of the abnormal pathways of the atrioventricular bundle, these patients are more prone to atrioventricular block and atrial arrhythmias after surgery. Although no conduction block occurred in this patient, a temporary pacemaker was routinely placed to prevent early postoperative arrhythmias.

29.6 Conclusion

In conclusion, despite the complexity and long duration of the procedure in this patient, no significant intraoperative hemodynamic fluctuations were observed. Before CPB, the key to anesthetic management is to adjust the SVR/PVR ratio to balance the Qp/Qs ratio. After CPB, the focus is to maintain the smooth transition of circulatory function (Chi Wu).

30 Anesthetic Management for the Single-Ventricle Palliation in a Small Infant with Ebstein's Anomaly

Jie Hu

Abstract

A 4-month-old male infant was found to have Ebstein's anomaly with moderate to severe tricuspid valve insufficiency immediately after birth. His symptoms, such as cyanosis and difficulty feeding, gradually worsened recently. He was admitted to our hospital for elective single-ventricle palliation. The patient had frequent attacks of tachyarrhythmia and heart failure before surgery. Tachyarrhythmia occurred repeatedly after thoracotomy. In this case, the key points of anesthetic management include perioperative tachyarrhythmia management, maintenance of preoperative forward blood flow in the pulmonary artery, and optimization of systemic circulation oxygen supply and perfusion pressure based on single-ventricle physiology after palliative surgery.

Children with Ebstein's anomaly (EA) who exhibit significant symptoms in the newborn or early infant are a subgroup with a high mortality rate in the EA spectrum. This article reports a case of a severe EA infant who showed early signs of cyanosis, severe arrhythmia, and heart failure and underwent single-ventricle palliation under general anesthesia.

J. Hu (✉)
The National Children's Medical Center (Shanghai), Department of Anesthesiology of Shanghai Children's Medical Center, Shanghai Jiao Tong University School of Medicine, Shanghai, China
e-mail: hujie@scmc.com.cn

30.1 Case Presentation

The patient was a 4-month-old boy with a weight of 5.7 kg. He was born full-term without asphyxia. After birth, he was hospitalized for newborn ABO hemolytic disease. During this period, a heart murmur was detected by auscultation, and echocardiography indicated apically displaced tricuspid valve anomaly with moderate to severe tricuspid valve closure insufficiency. Recently, the child gradually showed cyanosis after crying, milk intake reduction, obvious sweating, and pauses during feeding. Shortly after admission, the child was restless and crying with a cyanotic complexion. The heart rate (HR) monitored by electrocardiogram (ECG) was 220 beats/min, showing paroxysmal supraventricular tachycardia. Immediate oxygen inhalation through a mask, intranasal dexmedetomidine, and intramuscular phenobarbital was administered for sedation, followed by a slow intravenous propofol injection. The child's HR dropped and maintained around 190 beats/min. After administering 3 joules of synchronized electrical cardioversion to the child, the rhythm turned into sinus rhythm, the HR was maintained at around 140 beats/min, and the crying was relieved. Subsequently, oral

J. Zheng et al. (eds.), *Selected Pediatric Cardiovascular Surgery Anesthesia Cases*,
https://doi.org/10.1007/978-981-96-5614-1_30

propafenone, furosemide, spironolactone, and intravenous vitamin C were administered. The child was transferred to the Department of Cardiothoracic Surgery for surgical treatment 4 days later.

Physical examination: The child was conscious, lethargic, with a cyanotic complexion, cyanotic lips, SpO_2 85%, HR fluctuating between 140 and 220 beats/min, irregular rhythm, and continuous murmur of II/VI level in the precordial area.

Laboratory tests: Normal routine blood test, normal liver and kidney function. CK-MB 7.8 μg/L, cTnI 0.137 μg/L, NT-pro BNP 10,030 pg/mL.

Chest X-ray: Enlarged heart shadow, mild blurred lung markings.

Chest CT: Apical displacement of the tricuspid valve leaflets, no obvious abnormal changes in the aortic arch.

Echocardiography: Apical displacement of the tricuspid valve leaflets, patent foramen ovale (PFO), patent ductus arteriosus (PDA), severe tricuspid regurgitation (TR), mild left ventricular systolic function reduction, (RA + aRV) area/(LA + LV + RV) (RA, right atrial; aRV, atrialized right ventricle; RV, right ventricle; LA, left atrium; LV, left ventricle)area ratio = 1.15, LVEF (left ventricular ejection fraction) 50.89%.

Cardiac MRI: Apical displacement of the tricuspid valve leaflets, significant right atrium enlargement, LVEF 39.3%, RVEF 41%, atrialized right ventricular chamber EDV 20.14 mL (65.07 mL/m^2).

ECG: Ectopic rhythm, paroxysmal supraventricular tachycardia, incomplete right bundle branch block (IRBBB), right ventricular hypertrophy (possible?), secondary ST-T changes.

Preoperative diagnosis: Apical displacement of the tricuspid valve leaflet deformity, TR, PFO, PDA, paroxysmal supraventricular tachycardia, heart failure. Elective functional single-ventricle correction surgery was scheduled.

30.2 Anesthetic Management

The child did not take any oral premedication. After entering the operating room, routine ECG, blood pressure (BP), pulse oxygen saturation (SpO_2), and end-tidal carbon dioxide ($ETCO_2$) monitoring were conducted. Self-adhesive disposable external defibrillation pads were set up in advance. Anesthesia was induced by peripheral intravenous administration of midazolam 0.5 mg, sufentanil 10 μg, etomidate 1.5 mg, and rocuronium 3.0 mg. An ID 3.5 mm cuffed endotracheal tube was orally inserted with the assistance of video laryngoscopy. Pressure-controlled ventilation mode was used with the following ventilation parameter setting: fraction of inspired oxygen (FiO_2) 60%, ventilation frequency 30 times/min, the inspiratory time to expiratory time (I:E) 1:2. $ETCO_2$ was maintained at 35–40 mm Hg through the adjustment of the peak inspiratory pressure. After endotracheal intubation, the right radial artery and right internal jugular vein were quickly catheterized under ultrasound guidance for invasive artery pressure (ABP) and central venous pressure (CVP) monitor, respectively. A 4 F double-lumen catheter was chosen as a CVP catheter and placed at a depth of 5 cm. Vasoactive drugs were also infused through the internal jugular vein. The left femoral vein was accessed for rapid fluid replacement. After the induction of anesthesia, ABP was 82/44 mm Hg, HR was 127 beats/min, SpO_2 was 92%, and CVP was 12 cm H_2O. Anesthesia was maintained with intravenous infusion of sufentanil, propofol, rocuronium, and intermittent inhalation of sevoflurane. The artery blood gas analysis results before skin incision are shown in Table 30.1. Recurrent paroxysmal supraventricular tachycardia (PSVT) occurred after thoracotomy with HR 220 beats/min, BP 55/32 mm Hg, which rapidly progressed to ventricular fibrillation. Immediate defibrillation was conducted with 10 joules through the external defibrillation pads; the ventricular fibrillation was quickly converted to sinus rhythm. Epinephrine was intravenously adminis-

Table 30.1 Intraoperative blood gas test results

Time point	pH	PaO_2 (mm Hg)	$PaCO_2$ (mm Hg)	BE (mmol/L)	HCT (%)	K^+ (mmol/L)	Ca^{2+} (mmol/L)	Cl^- (mmol/L)	Lac (mmol/L)	HCO_3^- (mmol/L)
After chest opening	7.33	180	40.4	−4.36	37.7	3.83	1.194	109	1.2	21.2
Before cardiopulmonary bypass	7.22	111.2	38.5	−1.19	38.1	3.6	1.212	108.5	5.1	15.7
After stopping ultrafiltration	7.34	27.6	42.2	−3.37	32.5	4.05	0.731	109	2.5	22.3

tered to improve the blood pressure. The blood gas analysis results before the start of cardiopulmonary bypass (CPB) are shown in Table 30.1.

Pulmonary artery pressure and aortic pressure were simultaneously measured at 36/23(27) mm Hg and 99/66(83) mm Hg, respectively. Mild hypothermic CPB was used. A small PDA was found and ligated during surgery. The right ventricular cavity was small, with the septal leaflet of the tricuspid valve apical displacement. The right atrial tissue was partially excised and sutured to the tricuspid valve annulus. The tricuspid valve was closed with a 4 mm hole left. The atrial septal defect (ASD) was enlarged to about 1.0 cm. After intracardiac deaeration, the aortic cross-clamp was released, and the heart automatically resumed sinus rhythmic beating. Under parallel circulation, the right brachiocephalic and right pulmonary arteries were separated and connected with a 4 mm Goretex conduit for mBTS shunting. Transesophageal echocardiography (TEE) assessment indicated right unobstructed Blalock–Taussig (B-T) shunting and bidirectional shunting with dominant right-to-left shunting. CBP was successfully weaned off. Dopamine 5.0 μg/(kg·min) and norepinephrine 0.08 μg/(kg·min) were respectively infused to maintain blood pressure. After modified ultrafiltration, blood gas analysis was rechecked (Table 30.1). The ventilator parameters were adjusted based on the blood gas test results.

30.3 Postoperative Outcome

The operation lasted 2 h and 30 min, including CPB, which was 65 min, and aortic cross-clamp, which was 22 min. Before leaving the operating room, dopamine and norepinephrine were infused at 5.0 μg/(kg·min) and 0.08 μg/(kg·min), respectively. ABP was 74/38 mm Hg, HR was 142 beats/min, CVP was 9 cm H_2O, and SpO_2 was 84%. Delayed sternal closure was performed. The patient was transferred to the cardiac intensive care unit (CICU) with endotracheal intubation and mechanical ventilation support. The sternum was closed on the postoperative day 3. PSVT with HR 220 beats/min and BP 60/30 mm Hg occurred again in the CICU. The child's HR gradually decreased to 170 beats/min, and ABP increased to 80/50 mm Hg after cooling, intravenous administration of digoxin, and synchronized defibrillation. The child was successfully extubated on the third day after sternal closure. The child recovered well and was discharged from the hospital.

30.4 Review of Knowledge Points

30.4.1 Pathological Anatomy and Clinical Manifestations of EA

The main pathological changes of EA are apical displacement of the septal and posterior leaflets of the tricuspid valve, which results in valve insufficiency and the right ventricular effective chamber volume reduction. The clinical manifestations and pathophysiology of EA vary dramatically depending on EA anatomy and physiology heterogeneity. The severity of EA mainly depends on the degree of apical displacement of the tricuspid valve and the development of the right ventricle. Those with mild anatomical anomalies may have no symptoms or only mild cyanosis, fatigue, shortness of breath, and palpitations; they can grow into adults without EA diagnosis. However, those EA patients diagnosed by fetal echocardiography are often severe. They can have enlarged hearts, arrhythmia, edema, underdeveloped lungs, and even fetal distress. The intrauterine mortality rate is usually high. For those who are fortunate enough to survive to live birth, severe symptoms such as cyanosis and acidosis can be found within a few hours after birth and even threaten life safety. Celermajer and others proposed to evaluate the EA outcome by the Glasgow Outcome Score Extended Score (GOSE). The severity of EA in newborns is assessed by the ratio of the sum of the areas of the right atrium and atrialized right ventricle to the sum of the areas of the functional right ventricle, left atrium, and left ventricle on the four-chamber view of the Echocardiography. Grade 1 is <0.5, grade 2 is 0.5–0.99, grade 3 is 1–1.49, and grade 4 is ≥1.5. The higher the grade is, the more severe the condition is.

30.4.2 Pathophysiology of Critical EA

Neonates with EA present with circulatory shock or profound cyanosis represent a subgroup of patients with severe disease and increased morbidity and mortality. For these infants, severe tricuspid valve malformation can lead to severe regurgitation, and the capacity and contract function of the functional right ventricle is significantly reduced. Furthermore, the pulmonary artery pressure has not yet dropped to normal levels in the newborn period. All of the above factors result in no forward blood flow into the pulmonary artery during right ventricular systole. Restricted right ventricular outflow is similar to pulmonary artery atresia in pathophysiology. Pulmonary circulation is completely dependent on left-to-right shunting through the arterial duct or collateral circulation. The right-to-left shunting through ASD is an important source of preload for the left ventricle. Therefore, it is necessary to infuse prostaglandin intravenously to ensure the PDA supplies pulmonary blood flow. In some cases, a large PDA may cause circular shunting, i.e., blood flow from the aorta flows to the pulmonary artery through the PDA, then regurgitates into the right ventricle due to pulmonary artery regurgitation, regurgitates into the right atrium through the tricuspid valve, and then returns to the systemic circulation through the ASD, ultimately leading to volume overload, cardiac dilation, increased filling pressure, decreased cardiac output, and cyanosis. If this circular shunt occurs, prostaglandin should be discontinued, and the arterial duct should be closed. The risk of death is significantly increased in patients with pulmonary dysfunction and circular shunt physiology. In addition to severe impairment of the right heart function, the left heart function of the patient can also be severely affected. The left ventricle is flattened by the vast right heart. It appears "pancake-like" and abnormal movement of the interventricular septum towards the left ventricle will cause the left ventricle to be unable to fill effectively and severely affect cardiac output, requiring emergency surgical intervention or ECMO support. If the infant can survive in this critical period, as the pulmonary artery pressure gradually decreases, symptoms of cyanosis and heart failure will be relieved.

30.4.3 Surgical Treatments of Critical EA

Tricuspid valve repair with ASD closure is the preferred intervention for severely affected small infants and neonates who have adequate RV size and function to support a two-ventricle circulation. However, for newborns or infants with severe tricuspid valve malformations, poor right ventricular development, and symptoms of right ventricular outflow tract obstruction, they can be performed with univentricular palliation (i.e., right ventricular exclusion or Starnes procedure). In 1991, Starnes and others introduced an innovative surgical treatment for severe EA newborns known as the Starnes procedure. This procedure involved the univentricularization of the heart by TV closure using a fenestrated patch and a modified Blalock–Taussig shunt (B-T shunt). EA patients who undergo the Starnes procedure will usually undergo bidirectional cavopulmonary anastomosis in the future, followed by the Fontan procedure. Heart transplantation is also an option for severe EA newborns or infants, but it is usually only suitable for patients with poor biventricular function.

30.5 Discussion

30.5.1 Preoperative Assessment and Treatment

The child, in this case, showed obvious symptoms such as cyanosis, milk intake reduction, obvious sweating during feeding, and pauses in early infancy. Before the operation, he was treated for paroxysmal supraventricular tachycardia. The echocardiogram showed severe TR, GOSE ratio of 3, and mild left heart systolic function reduction. Laboratory test results showed that CK-MB 7.8 μg/L, cTnI 0.137 μg/L, and NT-proBNP 10,030 pg/mL, all indicating that the EA child was in a critical situation. He not only had right heart failure, but the vast right heart also had affected the left heart function, posing an extremely high anesthetic risk.

Another main problem before the operation for this child was that he was accompanied by paroxysmal supraventricular tachycardia, which further worsened the already unbearable heart function, reduced the forward blood flow of the pulmonary artery, aggravated cardiac output reduction, and cyanosis, and threatened life safety. Arrhythmias are very common in patients with EA, especially supraventricular arrhythmias, which mainly include paroxysmal supraventricular tachycardia and atrial fibrillation or flutter. Ten percent to Twenty percent of patients with EA may also have pre-excitation syndrome (Wolf–Parkinson–White). Frequent ventricular premature beats or ventricular tachycardia can also occur. Therefore, the child should be fully sedated before the operation to prevent arrhythmias caused by crying and anxiety. The vital signs should be closely monitored. Once arrhythmias occur, oxygen therapy, myocardial nutritional support, and anti-arrhythmic treatment should be initiated. Furthermore, surgical treatment of EA should be started as soon as possible after drug treatment.

30.5.2 Intraoperative Anesthetic Management

It is very important to paste disposable external defibrillation pads before the induction of anesthesia and closely monitor the ECG changes during the induction of anesthesia in case of arrhythmia occurrence. Every precaution, including the depth of the wire, should be taken to avoid the occurrence of arrhythmia during the internal jugular catheterization. Since the child was scheduled to undergo right-side B-T shunt surgery, the shunt side upper limb artery catheterization should be avoided, and the left radial artery was chosen for invasive artery blood pressure measurement. Before CPB, anesthetic management focuses on optimizing pulmonary forward blood flow and providing sufficient cardiac support. During mechanical ventilation, the average airway pressure should be reduced as much as possible to reduce pulmonary forward blood flow resistance. Avoid hypoxia and hypercapnia, which can increase pulmonary vascular resistance (PVR) and reduce pulmonary forward blood flow. For newborns with PDA-dependent pulmonary blood flow, prostaglandin must be used to open the PDA. In this case, the child had heart failure before surgery and repeated arrhythmias during the thoracotomy process. Although electrical defibrillation quickly restored sinus rhythm, it significantly impacted cardiac function, so epinephrine was used to enhance myocardial contraction and maintain cardiac output.

This case is not appropriate to conduct biventricular repair due to the displacement of the septal valve to the apex, the small undeveloped right ventricular cavity, and the unfavorable function of the right ventricle. Therefore, the tricuspid valve was closed, leaving a hole facilitating right ventricular decompression. The ASD was enlarged, which allowed systemic venous blood to reach the left ventricle, and then provided pulmonary arterial blood flow through the B-T shunt. After weaning off CPB, the anesthetic management should follow the post-B-T shunt management principles. After the B-T shunt is established, part of the aortic blood is shunted to the pulmonary circulation, similar to the "stealing blood" phenomenon, which will cause a decrease in systemic perfusion, an increase in pulmonary perfusion, and a reduction in coronary perfusion. Therefore, first, it is necessary to properly increase the blood volume to ensure that there is enough capacity to meet the increased pulmonary blood flow. Secondly, it is necessary to maintain a diastolic pressure not lower than 30 mm Hg to ensure sufficient coronary perfusion. In addition, regulating systemic-pulmonary blood flow distribution is the key to postoperative management since the shunt volume depends on the resistance between systemic and pulmonary circulation. When the resistance of the pulmonary circulation decreases, blood will enter the pulmonary circulation more and cause a decrease in coronary blood flow and even cardiac arrest in severe cases. The regulation of respiratory parameters is crucial to regulating pulmonary resistance. Both high oxygen concentration and hyperventilation can cause a decrease. Theoretically, when the inhaled oxygen concentration is controlled at 21%, PaO_2 is maintained at 45 mm Hg, $PaCO_2$ is maintained at 40–45 mm Hg, the distribution ratio of systemic-pulmonary blood flow is more appropriate, so SpO_2 should be controlled between 75% and 80%. Finally, sufficient diastolic pressure is needed after the B-T shunt surgery to ensure coronary perfusion. The left-to-right shunt increases the cardiac volume load and significantly impacts cardiac function. Considering the poor preoperative cardiac function, a large dose of positive inotropic drugs and vasoactive drugs are given to maintain stable blood pressure after weaning off CBP.

30.6 Conclusion

For severe newborns or infants with EA who undergo single-ventricular function correction surgery, attention should be paid to maintaining pulmonary forward blood flow before CPB and following the principles of post-B-T shunt management after CPB (Jie Hu).

Anesthetic Management of One-and-a-Half Ventricle Repair in a Child with Ebstein's Anomaly

31

Jie Hu

Abstract

A 10-year-old girl was diagnosed with Ebstein's anomaly at 11 months of age. As she grew older, exercise tolerance was gradually reduced, and she was scheduled for tricuspid valve repair surgery. After the completion of the conical reconstruction of the tricuspid valve and the folding of the atrialized ventricle, it was found that it was very difficult to maintain cardiac output and separate from cardiopulmonary bypass. So, the Glenn procedure was further performed. The anesthetic management of this patient should focus on the hemodynamic changes caused by tricuspid regurgitation and right ventricular dysfunction and the characteristics of Glenn circulation.

Ebstein's anomaly (EA), also known as tricuspid valve displacement malformation, is a relatively rare, complex congenital heart disease. The severity of the disease depends on the degree of tricuspid valve displacement and the development of the right ventricle. Due to the variety of EA severity and complexity, the choice of surgical methods varies dramatically. This article reports the anesthetic management of one-and-a-half ventricle repair in a child with EA.

J. Hu (✉)
The National Children's Medical Center (Shanghai), Department of Anesthesiology of Shanghai Children's Medical Center, Shanghai Jiao Tong University School of Medicine, Shanghai, China
e-mail: hujie@scmc.com.cn

31.1 Case Presentation

The patient was 10 years and 9 months old girl with a weight of 35 kg. She was diagnosed with tricuspid valve displacement malformation at 11 months of age due to cyanosis and fatigue at a local hospital. No treatment was given at that time. Since the onset of the disease, the patient's exercise tolerance has gradually decreased with occasional palpitations and fatigue, which are getting worse. Recently, she visited a local hospital, and a 24-h dynamic electrocardiogram showed "premature ventricular contractions 22731 times, short-term supraventricular tachycardia 18 times."

Physical examination: The patient was conscious without cyanosis. The lung sounds were clear without rales. The heart rhythm was regular, with no obvious murmurs. The liver was 2 cm below the ribs, not palpable below the xiphoid process, and the spleen was not palpable below the ribs.

Laboratory tests: The routine blood tests, the functions of the liver and kidney, and coagulation were all normal.

Echocardiography: tricuspid valve displacement, moderate tricuspid regurgitation, bidirec-

J. Zheng et al. (eds.), *Selected Pediatric Cardiovascular Surgery Anesthesia Cases*,
https://doi.org/10.1007/978-981-96-5614-1_31

tional shunting due to an unclosed oval foramen, normal left ventricular systolic activity. The ratio of (RA + aRV) area to (RV + LA + LV) area was 0.81 (RA, right atrium; aRV, atrialized right ventricle; RV, functional right ventricle; LA, left atrium; LV, left ventricle).

Cardiac MRI: the septal and posterior leaflets of the tricuspid valve displacement, with the septal leaflet displaced by 34.8 mm and the posterior leaflet by 38.9 mm. The interventricular septum at the atrialized right ventricle bulges into the left ventricle. The end-diastolic volume of the left ventricle was 72 mL (57 mL/m^2 body surface area), LVEF 62%, and the end-diastolic volume of the right ventricle was 78 mL (61 mL/m^2 body surface area), RVEF 59%.

Electrocardiogram (ECG): Sinus arrhythmia.

Preoperative diagnosis: the tricuspid valve displacement, patent foramen ovale, arrhythmia. Elective tricuspid valve plasty was scheduled.

31.2 Anesthetic Management

The child did not take any preoperative medications. After entering the operating room, routine ECG, blood pressure (BP), and pulse oxygen saturation (SpO_2) monitoring was performed. BP was 110/50 mm Hg, HR was 110 beats/min, and SpO_2 was 94%. A disposable external defibrillation electrode pad was pre-set under conscious state. After intravenous induction with midazolam 2.0 mg, sufentanil 70 μg, etomidate 10 mg, and rocuronium 20 mg, endotracheal intubation was conducted. A 6.0 ID cuffed tube was inserted orally. Pressure control ventilation mode was used with initial ventilator parameter settings as tidal volume (Vt) of about 280 mL by adjustment of peak inspiratory pressure (PIP), ventilation frequency 16 times/min, inspiratory to expiratory time (I:E) ratio 1:2, and fraction of inspired oxygen (FiO_2) 60%. The PIP and ventilation frequency was adjusted to maintain end-tidal carbon dioxide ($ETCO_2$) at 35–40 mm Hg. Then, the right radial artery was catheterized for invasive arterial pressure (ABP) monitoring, and a 5F double-lumen central venous catheter was successfully placed under ultrasound guidance to measure central venous pressure (CVP) and administer vasoactive drugs. The catheter was inserted to a depth of 9 cm. The left femoral vein was accessed for rapid fluid replacement. After anesthesia induction, arterial blood was drawn for blood gas analysis (Table 31.1). Anesthesia was maintained with sevoflurane inhalation combined with intravenous infusion of sufentanil, propofol, and rocuronium.

The thoracotomy process went smoothly, ABP was 94/55 mm Hg, HR was 80 beats/min, SpO_2 was 98%, CVP was 12 cm H_2O, and pulmonary artery pressure was measured directly as 18/13(15) mm Hg. Normothermic cardiopulmonary bypass (CBP) was used. After the aorta was cross-clamped, the septal and posterior leaflets of the tricuspid valve were significantly displaced (about 4–5 cm). Tricuspid valve conical reconstruction and the atrialized ventricle folding surgery were performed. After the aortic cross-clamping was released, the heart automatically resumed beating with a sinus rhythm. Dopamine 5.0 μg/(kg·min), epinephrine 0.05 μg/(kg·min), and norepinephrine 0.05 μg/(kg·min) were intravenously infused. However, at this time, the ABP was 71/41 mm Hg, HR 124 beats/min, SpO_2 89%, CVP 27 cm H_2O, the right atrium was significantly filled, and the right heart function was poor. It was difficult to maintain a stable BP. The dose of epinephrine and norepinephrine was increased to 0.1 μg/(kg·min), and there was no significant hemodynamic improvement, and it was difficult to separate from CBP. The surgeon team decided to perform a right-sided Glenn procedure which included the transection of the superior vena cava, the suture of the proximal end suture, the anastomosis of the distal end with the right pulmonary artery, and then enlargement of the oval foramen (1.5 cm). Postoperative transesophageal echocardiography (TEE) showed mild tricuspid regurgitation and bidirectional shunting at the atrial level. ABP was 90/38 mm Hg, HR was 116 beats/min, SpO_2 was 75%, and CVP was 23 cm H_2O. CBP was successfully weaned off at the end. After ultrafiltration, protamine was given to neutralize heparin. Blood gas analysis (Table 31.1) was performed. Internal environment adjustments were made according

Table 31.1 Intraoperative blood gas test results

Time point	pH	PaO_2 (mm Hg)	$PaCO_2$ (mm Hg)	BE (mmol/L)	HCT (%)	K^+ (mmol/L)	Ca^{2+} (mmol/L)	Cl^- mmol/L)	Lac (mmol/L)	HCO_3^- mmol/L)
After chest opening	7.42	167	33.1	−2.32	39.8	4	1.12	106	2.4	21.2
After stopping ultrafiltration	7.35	42	39.2	−3.94	31.2	3.24	0.94	106.7	5.6	21.3
Before leaving the room	7.35	39	38	−4.46	34.1	3.7	0.96	107	7.2	20.6

to the blood gas results. After separating from CBP, 200 mL of plasma, 1 U of concentrated red blood cells, and 600 U of prothrombin complex were intravenously transfused. Blood gas was rechecked before leaving the operating room (Table 31.1), and ACT was measured to be 122 s.

31.3 Postoperative Outcome

The operation lasted a total of 4 h, including 136 min of CBP and 101 min of aortic cross-clamp. At the time of leaving the operating room, dopamine was infused at 5.0 μg/(kg·min), epinephrine at 0.1 μg/(kg·min), norepinephrine at 0.1 μg/(kg·min), ABP 105/54 mm Hg, HR 122 beats/min, SpO_2 80%, CVP 23 cm H_2O. The patient was transferred to the Cardiac Intensive Care Unit (CICU) with endotracheal intubation, which was removed on postoperative day 2. The patient was transferred to the general ward on the postoperative day 4 and discharged on the postoperative day 14.

31.4 Review of Knowledge Points

31.4.1 Pathological Anatomy of EA

EA is a rare congenital heart disease with an incidence of about 1/200,000 in live births, accounting for less than 1% of congenital heart diseases. EA anatomical deformities are caused by the failure of the tricuspid valve leaflets to detach normally and free to the atrioventricular valve ring during embryonic development, which includes: ① The tricuspid valve leaflets are adhered to their below myocardium and cannot be lifted. ② The tricuspid valve ring is displaced towards the apex (the degree of downward displacement is septal valve > posterior valve > anterior valve). ③ The atrialized part of the right ventricle is dilated, combined with varying degrees of hypertrophy and thinning of the right ventricular wall. ④ The anterior valve is long and changes like a sail with openings and thrombosis. ⑤ The right atrioventricular junction (the real tricuspid valve ring) is dilated.

The key feature distinguishing EA from other congenital regurgitation diseases is that the displacement of the tricuspid septal valve is ≥8 mm/m^2 body surface area compared to the anterior mitral valve. Carpentier and others divided EA into four types: Type A has a sufficiently large functional right ventricular capacity; Type B has a larger atrialized right ventricle, and the anterior tricuspid valve activity is still acceptable; Type C has severely limited anterior valve activity, leading to right ventricular outflow tract obstruction; Type D has almost completely atrialized, except for a small part of the remaining right ventricular infundibulum.

31.4.2 Clinical Manifestations of EA

The severity of anatomical deformities in this disease forms the EA disease spectrum. At the lighter end of the disease spectrum, the degree of tricuspid valve displacement and the condition of right ventricular dysplasia in children are lighter. In infancy, there may be no obvious symptoms until children, adolescents, or adults show a series of symptoms caused by tricuspid regurgitation, such as arrhythmia and clinical manifestations of right heart failure. Tricuspid valve displacement and regurgitation causing right atrial enlargement is the anatomical basis for EA children to develop atrial fibrillation and flutter. In addition, abnormalities in the structure of the tricuspid valve ring and perivalvular tissue can lead to the formation of conduction bypasses, and the partial atrialization of the right ventricle often causes children to develop pre-excitation or ventricular/supraventricular arrhythmias. As age increases, children also show progressive cyanosis, reduced exercise tolerance, fatigue, or right heart failure.

31.4.3 Surgical Treatment of EA

For children and adolescents with NYHA heart function levels III to IV, progressive cyanosis, and fatigue combined with other malformations or arrhythmias, surgery can be considered. As the right heart function of children with EA progressively deteriorates, the worsening of heart function is inevitable, and early surgery can better protect the right heart function. Therefore, some studies suggest that severe tricuspid regurgitation shown by echocardiography indicates the need for surgery. The surgical methods vary depending on the degree of tricuspid valve and right ventricular cavity lesion, which include three types: ① For those with acceptable development of the effective cavity of the right ventricle, i.e., the ratio of the area measured by cardiac ultrasound (RA + aRV) to the area of (RV + LA + LV) is less than 1.0, only tricuspid valvuloplasty is performed, preserving all functions of the left and right ventricles. Currently, the most commonly used tricuspid valvuloplasty technique is conical reconstruction, which starts from the anterior leaflet, successively freeing the leaflet tissue and part of the chordae tendineae of the posterior and septal leaflets, rotating clockwise, and suturing in a ring to the normal atrioventricular connection of the tricuspid valve ring; near the atrioventricular junction of the septal leaflet, interrupted sutures are used. This makes the three leaflets form a sufficient and nearly normal tricuspid leaflet coaptation relationship, effectively reducing regurgitation, making the shape and function of the tricuspid valve after repair closer to normal, and reducing the possibility of postoperative tricuspid regurgitation recurrence and aggravation. ② For those with significant downward displacement of the tricuspid valve leading to poor development of the right ventricle (i.e., the above area ratio is 1.0–1.5) because the effective contraction chamber of the right ventricle cannot bear all the blood returning from the systemic circulation, a partial cavity pulmonary shunt is added, allowing the blood flow from the superior vena cava to directly enter the pulmonary artery, allowing the right ventricle to function as half a ventricle. ③ For those with stiff, curled, perforated development of the anterior leaflet of the tricuspid valve and significant downward displacement of the septal and posterior leaflets (ratio $\geq$ 1.5), the tricuspid valve cannot be shaped, and the function of the right ventricle should be abandoned, choosing single-ventricle palliation.

31.5 Discussion

The surgical treatment of children and adolescents with EA often chooses cone reconstruction. The main issues of the anesthetic management in these patients are tricuspid regurgitation, right ventricular dysfunction, possible right-to-left shunting at the atrial level, and potential arrhythmias. In addition, some patients' left ventricles can be squeezed by the enormous right heart, causing geometric abnormalities and resulting in left heart dysfunction.

31.5.1 Preoperative Assessment and Management

During the preoperative visit, it is essential to inquire about the child's exercise tolerance and whether there are fatigue, palpitations, and syncope symptoms. Physical examination should pay attention to whether there is liver enlargement, cyanosis, and abnormal heart sounds. Children with EA have enlarged right atrium and atrialized right ventricle with good compliance, so although there may be signs of right heart failure, jugular vein distension is not common. Echocardiography is the crucial method to make a diagnosis of children with EA, but cardiac catheterization can easily induce arrhythmia. Unless there are serious coronary artery problems, it should not be used as a routine preoperative examination for such patients. Although the child, in this case, does not have obvious cyanosis, his exercise endurance has gradually decreased since the onset of the disease, indicating that the deformity has significantly affected heart function and he also has arrhythmia, so caution should be maintained during anesthesia.

31.5.2 Induction of Anesthesia

Intravenous anesthetics are routinely used during the induction of anesthesia for pediatric cardiac surgery. Still, the vast right atrium of children with EA can cause convergence of intravenous anesthetics. A large amount of blood stays in the right atrium due to the tricuspid regurgitation, which causes the blood circulation to be slower and the onset time of the drug is prolonged. Therefore, special attention should be paid to the onset time of the drug during the induction of anesthesia to avoid serious hemodynamic fluctuations caused by the too short induction time and drug overdose. During the induction, it is also necessary to closely observe changes in the electrocardiogram. Up to 20% of children with EA have pre-excitation syndrome, which can easily cause supraventricular tachycardia during the placement of central venous catheters and thoracotomy. Therefore, a disposable external defibrillation electrode plate was pre-set before the induction of anesthesia in this case, and the guide wire should not be inserted too deep to induce arrhythmia. Placement of a pulmonary artery catheter in children with EA is challenging; the catheter can cause rupture of the reconstructed tricuspid valve, and the measurement of cardiac output using the thermodilution method is unreliable in the case of tricuspid regurgitation, so it is generally not recommended.

31.5.3 Anesthetic Management Before CBP

The goal of anesthetic management before CBP is to maintain the sinus rhythm as much as possible and maintain a slightly faster heart rate to alleviate the tricuspid regurgitation. Children with EA usually have right heart dysfunction, so it is necessary to ensure myocardial contractility, maintain appropriate right heart preload, and avoid hypercapnia, hypoxia, acidosis, etc., which can increase the pulmonary artery pressure and the right heart afterload. The Reduction of right heart afterload is also beneficial to alleviate the tricuspid regurgitation. Through these measures, the ultimate goal is to improve right heart output and subsequent left heart output. Suppose the patient has little forward blood flow in the pulmonary artery before surgery (right heart dysfunction or high PVR). In that case, it is very important to maintain right-to-left shunting at the atrial level. At this time, cardiac output can be maintained by sacrificing some oxygen saturation.

31.5.4 Anesthetic Management After CBP

Although the ratio of the area of the child in this case (RA + aRV) to the area of (LA + LV + RV) was less than 1.0, the CVP was greater than 24 cm H_2O, the arterial systolic pressure was less than 65 mm Hg. There was no significant effect after the increase of positive inotropic drug doses. It was difficult to wean off CBP after cone reconstruction surgery, and the effect significantly improved after the surgeon performed Glenn surgery and atrial septal enlargement. At this time, Glenn surgery can divert about half of the venous return blood, reduce the preload of the right ventricle to protect the right heart function, and reduce the inferior vena cava pressure under the premise of ensuring the forward pulsatile blood flow of the pulmonary artery, and reduce the tricuspid regurgitation. Atrial septal enlargement can partially reduce the preload of the right heart, reduce tricuspid regurgitation, and effectively reduce the occurrence of low cardiac output syndrome in the early postoperative period in children.

After the cone reconstruction, the underdeveloped right ventricle cannot adapt to the changes in hemodynamics. Furthermore, the contractility is impaired. Positive inotropic drugs can be used to maintain the contractility of the right ventricle. Glenn circulation was also established in this case. Therefore, it was necessary to maintain a lower pulmonary vascular resistance and appropriate right atrial pressure to ensure sufficient pulmonary blood flow and cardiac output. Regarding respiratory management, inhaling high oxygen concentrations and appropriate hyperventilation can reduce pulmonary vascular resistance. Positive pressure ventilation reduces venous return and increases pulmonary vascular resistance, so intraoperative airway peak pressure should be maintained at the lowest level. Weaning off mechanical ventilation as soon as possible after surgery is better if the child's heart function can tolerate it. Regarding volume management, it is better to maintain CVP at 20–26 cm H_2O and LAP at 10–15 mm Hg through appropriate blood volume expansion. The preferred route for fluid replacement is the inferior vena cava (femoral vein) to minimize the impact on the cavopulmonary anastomosis and avoid thrombosis in the superior vena cava.

31.6 Conclusion

In summary, EA is a complex and variable congenital heart disease. The severity and complexity of the malformation determine the method of anesthetic management and surgery. The critical points of anesthetic management in older children with EA should focus on right heart function protection, pulmonary vascular resistance reduction, avoidance of arrhythmias, and hemodynamic stability (Jie Hu).

Anesthetic Management of Central Shunt Procedure for an Infant with Tricuspid Atresia

32

Ruidong Zhang

Abstract

A one-month-old male infant was diagnosed with tricuspid atresia due to cyanosis of the lips. He was scheduled to undergo a central shunt procedure under general anesthesia. Tricuspid atresia is one of the single-ventricle physiological disorders. Central shunt procedure is referred to as systemic-pulmonary artery shunt between the ascending aorta and the pulmonary artery by a Gore-Tex artificial blood vessel, which is aimed to relieve hypoxia, promote the development of pulmonary artery, and prepare for staged Fontan surgery in the future. The key to anesthesia during the central shunt procedure includes optimizing systemic oxygen supply and maintaining a balance between systemic and pulmonary circulation as much as possible.

Tricuspid atresia (TA) ranks as the third most common cyanotic congenital heart disease. The incidence of patients with TA is estimated as 0.5–1.2 cases per 10,000 live births without significant gender difference. TA is a complex single-ventricle disorder with complete right ventricular inflow obstruction and varying degrees of right ventricular outflow obstruction. More than 70 percent of TA patients depend on the patent ductus arteriosus (PDA) for pulmonary blood flow. Therefore, it is necessary to establish a shunt between the systemic artery and the pulmonary artery in the neonatal period. This article reports the anesthetic management of a one-month-old TA patient undergoing a central shunt procedure.

32.1 Case Presentation

A 1-month-old male infant with 4.5 kg in weight and 54 cm in length was admitted to the hospital for treatment due to cyanosis after birth.

Physical examination: The patient was conscious and cyanotic. Peripheral oxygen saturation (SpO_2) was 71% with air breathing. The heart rhythm is regular. III/VI-grade systolic murmur can be heard at the second to fourth intercostal spaces on the left side of the sternum.

Laboratory tests: Hemoglobin 155 g/L, hematocrit 46.9%, no significant abnormalities in liver, kidney, and coagulation function.

Electrocardiogram (ECG): Sinus tachycardia, slight left axis deviation, T wave peak flat trajectory, IRBBB type.

Echocardiography: TA, right ventricular hypoplasia, right ventricular outflow tract

R. Zhang (✉)
The National Children's Medical Center (Shanghai), Department of Anesthesiology of Shanghai Children's Medical Center, Shanghai Jiao Tong University School of Medicine, Shanghai, China
e-mail: zhangruidong@scmc.com.cn

J. Zheng et al. (eds.), *Selected Pediatric Cardiovascular Surgery Anesthesia Cases*,
https://doi.org/10.1007/978-981-96-5614-1_32

obstruction (pressure difference 61 mm Hg), ventricular septal defect (VSD, bidirectional shunt), patent foramen ovale (right to left shunt), and collateral vessel formation.

Cardiac CT: The diameter of the left pulmonary artery opening was 4.7 mm, the diameter of the distal bifurcation was 4.1 mm, the diameter of the right pulmonary artery opening was 4.4 mm, the diameter of the distal bifurcation was 4.3 mm, and the diameter of the descending aorta at the level of the diaphragm was 6.8 mm.

Preoperative diagnosis: TA, VSD, atrial septal defect (ASD), right ventricular outflow tract obstruction, pulmonary artery stenosis with right ventricular hypoplasia.

32.2 Anesthetic Management

No preoperative medications were administrated. Routine monitoring was performed to monitor ECG, SpO_2, and non-invasive arterial blood pressure after admission to the operating room. The patient was given 6% sevoflurane inhalation to facilitate venous catheterization. After the peripheral vein was accessed, midazolam 0.1 mg/kg, etomidate 0.3 mg/kg, sufentanil 2.0 μg/kg, and rocuronium 0.6 mg/kg were intravenously administered for the induction of anesthesia. An ID 3.5 mm cuffed endotracheal tube was intubated orally under direct laryngoscopy. Mechanical ventilation was conducted in PCV-VG mode. The respiratory parameters were set as 2 L/min gas flow, 50% fraction of inspired oxygen (FiO_2), 6–8 mL/kg tidal volume (VT), 18 breaths/min respiratory rate (RR),1:2 inspiratory time to expiratory time (I:E) ratio. The end-tidal carbon dioxide ($ETCO_2$) was maintained at 35–40 mm Hg. General anesthesia was maintained by continuous intravenous infusion of 2.0 μg/(kg·h) sufentanil, 6.0 mg/(kg·h)propofol, and 0.6 mg/(kg·h) rocuronium combined with 1–2% sevoflurane intermittent inhalation. The left radial artery, left femoral vein, and right internal jugular vein were catheterized under ultrasound guidance to continuously monitor invasive arterial blood pressure (ABP) and central venous pressure (CVP). The results of arterial blood gas analysis after induction showed pH 7.27, PaO_2 25.2 mm Hg, $PaCO_2$ 46 mm Hg, BE −5.3 mmol/L, HCT 49%, serum potassium 4.6 mmol/L, serum calcium 1.27 mmol/L, lactate 1.4 mmol/L. Then 5% sodium bicarbonate 10 mL was injected intravenously to correct acidosis. The patient's body temperature was continuously monitored and maintained by warming blankets and fluid warming during the operation. Before thoracotomy, 10 mg/kg tranexamic acid and 10,000 U/kg ulinastatin were intravenously infused.

A median sternotomy was conducted on this patient. After heparinization, ascending aorta and right atrium cannulation was performed to establish cardiopulmonary bypass (CPB). The ductus arteriosus ligament was severed under parallel circulation. After the aorta was cross-clamped, the right atrium was opened, and the atrial septum was cut and enlarged to 1.5 cm. After the aorta cross-clamp was released, the heart automatically resumed beating, and a 3.5 mm diameter Gore-Tex artificial conduit connected the left wall of the ascending aorta and the pulmonary artery. Dopamine at 5–7.5 μg/(kg·min), epinephrine at 0.03–0.05 μg/(kg·min), and norepinephrine at 0.08 μg/(kg·min) were intravenously infused, respectively. The hemodynamics of the patient was stable. The SpO_2 has been improved from 70% to 85%. Transesophageal echocardiography showed that the ASD had been expanded to 1.5 cm with bidirectional shunting, the blood flow velocity in the central shunt tube was 2.9 m/s, mild mitral valve regurgitation, and normal left ventricular wall movement. After weaning off CPB assistance and ultrafiltration, protamine is intravenously infused with a ratio of protamine to heparin 1:1. Arterial blood gas analysis showed pH 7.28, PaO_2 41 mm Hg, $PaCO_2$ 47 mm Hg, BE −3.2 mmol/L, HCT 31.3%, serum potassium 3.73 mmol/L, serum calcium 1.16 mmol/L, lactate 2.3 mmol/L, and ACT rechecked at 151 s. Acidosis was corrected by 5% sodium bicarbonate injection. After placing a mediastinal drainage tube and carefully checking that there was no significant bleeding from the incisions, the sternum was closed layer by layer, and the patient was transferred to the Cardiac Intensive Care Unit (CICU) with an endotracheal tube in place.

32.3 Postoperative Outcome

The surgery lasted 2.5 h, including 44 min of CPB and 6 min of aortic cross-clamp. A total of 150 mL packed red blood cells and 100 mL plasma were transfused. Due to oliguria, peritoneal dialysis was performed on the first postoperative day. The patient was extubated on the fourth postoperative day, discharged from the CICU on the 8th day, and discharged from the hospital on the 15th day.

32.4 Review of Knowledge Points

32.4.1 Systemic-Pulmonary Artery Shunt Procedure

Systemic-pulmonary artery shunt is a common palliative procedure for treating children with cyanotic congenital heart disease, which provides pulmonary blood flow to promote pulmonary artery growth in children with TA and other single-ventricle diseases and be prepared for later staged surgery. Blalock and Taussig first reported the subclavian-pulmonary artery shunt procedure in 1945, and then Potts reported the descending aorta to the left pulmonary artery shunt procedure in 1946. In 1962 and 1966, Waterson and Cooley reported the ascending aorta to right pulmonary artery shunt procedure, respectively. De Leval used polytetrafluoroethylene (PTFE) artificial material and improved the Blalock–Taussig (BT) shunt procedure in 1975. Using a Gore-Tex thin-walled artificial blood vessel, the central shunt procedure establishes a connection between the ascending aorta and the pulmonary artery.

The requirements for ideal shunt surgery include: the technical operation is simple and feasible, it can provide appropriate rather than excessive pulmonary blood flow to avoid congestive heart failure and pulmonary hypertension, it can maintain long-term patency of the conduit, it can easily close the shunt after radical surgery, and there are no residual cardiopulmonary abnormalities after closing the shunt.

32.4.2 Central Shunt Procedure

The advantages of central shunt procedure include: it can be applied to infants and young children with poorly developed pulmonary artery branches, it can prevent the pulmonary artery from twisting, it can provide equal amounts of pulmonary blood flow to both lungs, the incidence of conduit blockage after central shunt surgery is lower compared to the classic and improved BT shunt procedure, it can avoid subclavian artery steal, it is easy to close the shunt during radical surgery. The disadvantage of the central shunt procedure is that it requires operation within the pericardial cavity, which can cause postoperative adhesions. If the patient does not have an open arterial duct or other sources of pulmonary blood, a central shunt procedure cannot be performed.

32.5 Discussion

32.5.1 Preoperative Assessment and Preparation

The increased oxygen consumption caused by anxiety, fear, and crying in children with congenital heart disease may result in their cardiac work being intolerable due to limited cardiac reserve. To reduce the sympathetic stress, children (age $\geq$ 6 months) are usually given oral midazolam 0.5 mg/kg for sedation half an hour before surgery. If the child has already established venous access and has resolved airway safety and respiratory issues before anesthesia, the dose of midazolam can be further increased by 0.1–0.25 mg/kg.

A defibrillator should be prepared before anesthesia. If the conditions permit, CPB equipment should be on standby. For those re-operative cases, major bleeding can occur during the dissecting of the sternum. Therefore, it is necessary to prepare sufficient blood sources in advance.

32.5.2 Intraoperative Anesthetic Management

Whether patients can tolerate inhalational or intravenous anesthesia depends mainly on the dosage and speed of administration. Sevoflurane inhalation induction is the most commonly used approach when there is a lack of venous access. If the patient is maintained or treated by positive inotropic drugs due to heart failure, they may not tolerate inhalational induction of anesthesia. It is better to choose intravenous induction of anesthesia. If intravenous induction of anesthesia is selected, the balance between systemic and pulmonary vascular resistance must be considered.

Pay attention to the characteristics of preoperative electrocardiograms and comparatively analyze the heart rate (HR), arrhythmia, and ST segment changes caused by myocardial ischemia. The central shunting procedure does not require contralateral radial artery catheterization for continuous artery blood pressure monitoring. The femoral artery can also be used for constant artery blood pressure measurement. Myocardial damage may occur due to coronary steal if PDA exists. Therefore, accurate monitoring and measurement of diastolic pressure is essential. It is worth noting that $PaCO_2$ is underestimated by $ETCO_2$ if a right-to-left shunt exists. The difference between $PaCO_2$ and $ETCO_2$ will be more pronounced when hypoxemia occurs. Rechecking blood gas analysis during surgery should be compared with the preoperative arterial blood gas baseline value. The central venous pathway can be used for volume management and positive inotropic drug infusion. Patients with TA are more likely to have preoperative respiratory tract infections, which can result in increased airway pressure and decreased oxygen saturation due to bronchospasm. During the operation, it may be necessary to hyperventilate and increase FiO_2 to maintain an acceptable blood oxygen saturation.

Balanced anesthesia combined with hypnotics, analgesics, inhaled anesthetics, and muscle relaxants is usually used for anesthesia maintenance. One hundred percent oxygen inhalation, hyperventilation, and a high concentration of inhalational anesthetics all reduce pulmonary vascular resistance, increase Qp/Qs, reduce diastolic pressure and systemic circulation perfusion, and ultimately cause myocardial ischemia.

Before the aortic cross-clamp was released, positive inotropic drugs and sodium bicarbonate were preventively given to reduce hypoxia, and acidosis-related severe complications, which were caused by the increase of pulmonary vascular resistance (PVR), impaired hypoxic pulmonary vasoconstriction, atelectasis, and mismatched ventilation–perfusion ratio. Reducing FiO_2 with the gradual increases of blood oxygen saturation is recommended. $ETCO_2$ will increase after the central shunt is established. At this time, blood dilution should be avoided, arterial blood gas analysis should be rechecked, and sufficient diastolic pressure should be maintained to avoid myocardial ischemia. The utilization of positive inotropic drugs can improve hemodynamic stability and oxygen supply at the cost of oxygen consumption increase.

If hemodynamic problems occur after the establishment of the central shunt, anatomical problems such as unsuitable size or twisting of the shunt, twisting should be ruled out first; then, the issues will be further analyzed from a physiological perspective. In order to achieve a "balanced circulation," when the Qp:Qs is equal to or slightly less than 1:1 in the case of a fixed cardiac output in patients with single-ventricle physiology, the systemic circulation oxygen supply (the product of systemic circulation oxygen content and systemic circulation blood flow) is the largest. When Qp:Qs exceeds 1:1, the systemic circu-

Table 32.1 Management of single-ventricle physiology

Clinical manifestation	Physiology	Management plan
SaO_2 75–80% Sa-vO_2 25–30% BP > 60/30 mm hg	Balanced blood flow Qp:Qs = (0.7–1.5):1	No treatment required
SaO_2 > 85–90% Sa-vO_2 35–40% BP < 60/30	Excessive pulmonary blood flow Qp:Qs > 2:1–3:1 Cause: Low PVR Shunt tube too thick Residual obstruction of aortic arch High SVR	Increase PVR: Controlled hypoventilation Mild acidosis Lower FiO_2 (0.17–0.19) Brain oxygen supply may be affected Increase systemic oxygen supply: Reduce afterload Inotropic support Hematocrit >40% Surgical operation: Partial occlusion of shunt tube Corrective reconstruction of aortic arch
SaO_2 < 65–75% Sa-vO_2 25–30%; but SvO_2 may be <30% critical value	Insufficient pulmonary blood flow Qp:Qs < 0.7:1	Reduce PVR: Controlled hyperventilation
BP >70/40 mm Hg Diastolic pressure > 40 mm Hg	Cause: PVR too high Shunt tube too thin Pulmonary vein hypoxia and underestimation of real Qp:Qs	Alkalosis Sedation/muscle relaxation Active treatment of atelectasis (pulmonary vein hypoxia) Consider using NO Increase systemic oxygen supply: Cardiotonic drug support Surgery: Correct shunt tube
SaO_2 < 70–75% Sa-vO_2 35–40% and SvO_2 possible Possibly <30% critical value BP <60/30 mm Hg	Low cardiac output Cause: Ventricular dysfunction Myocardial ischemia Myocardial contraction inhibited Afterload mismatch (residual aortic arch obstruction) AV valve regurgitation	Reduce oxygen consumption: Sedation/muscle relaxation Cardiotonic drug support/reduce afterload Surgery: Repair AV valve Adjust aortic arch Consider mechanical support: Post-cardiotomy support Transition to heart transplant

AV atrioventricular, *BP* blood pressure, *PVR* pulmonary vascular resistance, *SVR* systemic vascular resistance

lation oxygen supply progressively decreases because the effect of increasing systemic circulation oxygen content is offset by the progressive decrease in systemic circulation blood flow. When Qp:Qs drops below 1:1, the systemic circulation oxygen supply drops sharply because the increase in systemic circulation blood flow is more offset by the sharp drop in systemic circulation oxygen content. The management measures after the shunt operation for single-ventricle physiology are summarized in Table 32.1.

32.5.3 Postoperative Anesthetic Management

Although heparin is always intravenously administered during the aortic cross-clamping period, heparin therapy should be given as soon as possible after surgery. If there are no significant severe bleeding risks 4 h after surgery, such as chest drainage <3 mL/(kg·h), aPTT <60 s, heparin therapy should be restarted. The incidence of shunt failure is also high during the early postoperative period, which can result in a sharp drop in blood oxygen saturation, possibly secondary to the blood clot formation or shunt tube twisting. Once it happens, it is an emergent situation and should be resolved immediately.

32.6 Conclusion

As a palliative operation, the central shunt procedure increases the pulmonary blood flow, promotes the development of pulmonary artery, and provides opportunities for children with single-ventricle congenital heart disease for subsequent treatment by establishing a shunt between the systemic and pulmonary circulation. During anesthetic management, the goal should always be to optimize the oxygen supply and perfusion pressure of the systemic circulation, and maintenance of the balanced systemic and pulmonary circulation is the key to successful anesthetic management of central shunt procedure in patients with single-ventricle physiological disorder (Ruidong Zhang).

33 Anesthetic Management of Glenn Procedure for Infant with Tricuspid Atresia

Yunan Song

Abstract

A 1-year-old male cyanotic infant was diagnosed with tricuspid atresia by cardiac ultrasound. In order to improve hypoxia, reduce cardiac volume loading, and prepare for the final surgical correction of a single ventricle, a right-sided bidirectional superior vena cava-pulmonary artery anastomosis under cardiopulmonary bypass support was performed. As a staged procedure in treating a single ventricle, the goal of anesthetic management is to improve the pulmonary blood flow status, maintain the balance of blood flow between systemic and pulmonary circulation, and optimize the oxygen supply and perfusion of the systemic circulation. In this regard, the effect of mechanical ventilation on the patient's systemic-pulmonary blood flow status is an aspect of anesthetic management that should be given special attention.

The incidence of tricuspid atresia (TA) is about 0.5–1.2/10,000 live births without sex difference. TA is usually characterized by tricuspid hypoplasia, right atrium and right ventricle hypoplasia, and blood flow interruption from the right atrium to the right ventricle. There are several different anatomical subtypes based on the presence of transposition of the great arteries (TGA), the degree of pulmonary atresia (PA) or stenosis (PS), and the size of the ventricular septal defect (VSD). The patients with TA are treated based on the principle of single-ventricle physiology, which typically involves multiple stages of staged surgery and establishes the single-ventricle physiological circulation in the end. Superior vena cava to pulmonary artery anastomosis (bidirectional cavopulmonary anastomosis, bi-directional Glenn procedure) is staged. This article described the anesthetic management for an infant with TA undergoing a bi-directional Glenn procedure. The anesthetic management for the Blalock–Taussig and Fontan procedures in single-ventricle patients will not be repeated here.

33.1 Case Presentation

The patient was a year and 27-day-old male with a weight of 9 kg and a height of 75 cm. He was delivered at full-term by cesarean section. There was no history of postnatal asphyxia. He was admitted to our hospital due to a heart murmur found during a physical examination. The child presented with cyanosis, which was aggravated by crying and noise. Growth and development

Y. Song (✉)
The National Children's Medical Center (Shanghai), Department of Anesthesiology of Shanghai Children's Medical Center, Shanghai Jiao Tong University School of Medicine, Shanghai, China
e-mail: songyunan@scmc.com.cn

J. Zheng et al. (eds.), *Selected Pediatric Cardiovascular Surgery Anesthesia Cases*,
https://doi.org/10.1007/978-981-96-5614-1_33

were slightly delayed, but normal feeding and acceptable mobility were.

Laboratory tests: Hemoglobin 145 g/L, hematocrit 42.3%, no significant abnormalities in liver, kidney, and coagulation function.

Electrocardiogram (ECG): Sinus tachycardia, mild left axis deviation, ST-T changes.

Physical examination: Pulse rate 120 beats/min, respiratory rate (RR) 30 breaths/min, blood pressure (BP) 85/43 mm Hg, pulse oxygen saturation (SpO_2) 78%, cardiac dullness boundary enlargement, strong heart sounds, regular rhythm was, and grade III murmur in the precordial area, cyanotic lips, coarse breath sounds in both lungs, no rales. No significant liver and spleen enlargement, soft abdomen, shifting dullness, or edema in the whole body or limbs.

Cardiac ultrasound: TA, atrial septal defect (ASD II), VSD, right ventricular outflow tract obstruction (pressure gradient 67 mm Hg), fast flow velocity in the common pulmonary artery trunk and right pulmonary artery, mild pulmonary regurgitation. Pulmonary artery pressure could not be evaluated.

Cardiac CT: TA, ASD, VSD, mild narrowed right ventricular outflow tract.

Preoperative diagnosis: TA, VSD, ASD, right ventricular outflow tract obstruction. A bidirectional Glenn procedure was proposed.

33.2 Anesthetic Management

The child was brought into the operating room with basal heart rate (HR) at 125 bpm, BP at 82/43 mm Hg, and SpO_2 at 77%. Midazolam 0.1 mg/kg, sufentanil 2.0 μg/kg, etomidate 0.2 mg/kg, and rocuronium 0.6 mg/kg were intravenously injected for the induction of anesthesia. The endotracheal tube (ID 4.0 with cuff) was orally inserted into the trachea with a depth of 11 cm. Bilateral respiratory sounds were symmetrical. Anesthesia was maintained with sufentanil 2.5 μg/(kg·h), propofol 4.0 mg/(kg·h), rocuronium 0.6 mg/(kg·h). Pressure-controlled ventilation-volume guaranteed (PCV-VG) mode was used for intraoperative mechanical ventilation. The ventilator parameters were set as tidal volume (VT) 6–8 mL/kg, RR 20–24 beats/min, and the peak of inspiratory pressure P_{peak} 20 cm H_2O. The radial artery was catheterized to monitor the invasive arterial blood pressure (ABP), which fluctuated at 75–85/40–45 mm Hg before the operation. A double-lumen catheter was placed into the right internal jugular vein for the central venous pressure (CVP) monitor; the basal CVP was 8–10 cm H_2O. Intraoperative regional oxygen saturation (rSO_2) of the left brain tissue was monitored at 50–65. Arterial blood gas analysis was performed after intubation with a fraction of inspired oxygen (FiO_2) 40%: pH 7.33, PaO_2 42.6 mm Hg, $PaCO_2$ 30 mm Hg, HCT 25%, BE −10.1 mmol/L, and Lac 1.2 mmol/L. The ventilator parameters were adjusted to maintain an $ETCO_2$ at 35–40 mm Hg. The mean pulmonary artery pressure was 15 mm Hg after chest opening. After cardiopulmonary bypass (CPB) was established, the right-sided bidirectional Glenn procedure was performed under normothermic parallel circulation.

After most of Glenn's procedure was completed, mechanical ventilation was resumed, PCV-VG mode, VT 6–7 mL/kg, P_{peak} 16–18 cm H_2O, RR 20–22 times/min. Dopamine 5.0 μg/(kg·min) and milrinone 0.5 μg/(kg·min) were given for hemodynamic maintenance, ABP was 80–85/40 mm Hg, HR was 130–140 beats/min, CVP was 16–18 cm H_2O, and SpO_2 was 82%. CPB was successfully weaned off. Blood gas analysis (FiO_2 40%): pH 7.43, PaO_2 47.7 mm Hg, $PaCO_2$ 31 mm Hg, HCT 30%, BE −3.4 mmol/L, Lac 1.7 mmol/L. The RR was reduced to 15 times/min, and $ETCO_2$ was maintained around 45 mm Hg. Rocuronium was discontinued at the time of sternal closure. The dose of sufentanil was halved for early extubation. After the operation, the child was transferred to the Cardiac Intensive Care Unit (CICU). PCA analgesia (controlled by the ICU nurse) was given within the first 2 days after the operation. The background and bonus dose of sufentanil were 0.05 μg/(kg·h) and 0.01 μg/kg, respectively. The lockout time was 15 minutes.

33.3 Postoperative Outcome

The total surgical duration was 150 min, with 21 min of CPB time. The estimated blood loss was 20 mL, and urine output was 100 mL. Ringer's acetate solution of 150 mL, packed red blood cells of 150 mL, and plasma of 100 mL were intravenously infused. After returning to the CICU, the child was placed in a 30-degree head-up position, and the tracheal tube was removed 4 h later.

33.4 Review of Knowledge Points

33.4.1 Pathophysiology of TA

TA is a complex cyanotic congenital heart disease belonging to the category of single-ventricle diseases with right ventricular hypoplasia. Patients with complete right ventricular inflow tract obstruction may also have varying degrees of outflow tract obstruction. In patients with a nonrestrictive shunt at the atrial level, such as an ASD or PFO, the obligatory right-to-left shunt can lead to the complete mixing of systemic venous blood with oxygenated blood from the pulmonary veins in the left atrium. When shunting is restricted at ASD or PFO, a large right-to-left pressure gradient will result in poor right atrial decompression and systemic venous stasis.

Partially oxygenated blood mixed in the left atrium produces a left-to-right shunt through the septal defect into the right ventricular outflow tract. There may be stenosis at the entrance to the common pulmonary artery or overall dysplasia of the pulmonary arteries. Some cases of TA without VSD or with pulmonary vascular dysplasia rely on patent ductus arteriosus to introduce blood flow into the pulmonary circulation. Although the left ventricular output of patients with TA is mixed, if it contains sufficient oxygenated blood from the pulmonary venous return, it provides adequate oxygenation to alleviate cyanosis. Thus, insufficient pulmonary blood flow is the main cause of cyanosis in children, which depends on the degree of pulmonary vascular development, the presence and size of VSD, the location of the great arteries, and the status of the arterial conduit.

33.4.2 Glenn Procedure

Children with functional single ventricle may have various intracardiac malformations. In order to ultimately achieve physiological correction, a complete surgical strategy should be formulated in the neonatal period. The overall principle is to maintain the balance between systemic and pulmonary circulation. It is very important to protect the pulmonary vasculature from excessive pulmonary congestion and pulmonary hypertension and ensure the pulmonary vasculature development to prevent severe hypoxemia. Therefore, the child can survive and ultimately complete the physiological correction. If the pulmonary artery pressure is satisfactorily decreased, a bidirectional Glenn procedure should be performed over 6 months old.

The bidirectional Glenn procedure is generally known as a transitional procedure of a series of palliative operations for functional single-ventricular treatment. The major purpose is to improve the cyanosis and reduce the cardiac volume load, which further reduces the risk of total cavopulmonary connection (TCPC) surgery in the future. In order to get a better surgical outcome, Glenn's procedure should be performed under lower pulmonary vascular resistance. Therefore, the Glenn procedure is generally performed over 3–6 months old. It is not recommended to perform the Glenn procedure before 2–3 months old. The Glenn procedure requires a certain degree of pulmonary artery development. It is recommended that the McGoon ratio is beyond 1.5 (in patients with bilateral pulmonary arteries). Bidirectional Glenn surgery is also recommended in older children with risk factors for total cavopulmonary surgery, such as mean pulmonary artery pressure > 15 mm Hg, critical ventricular function, and malformations requiring concomitant management, such as atrioventricular valve regurgitation, restrictive pulmonary artery stenosis of the, and anomalous pulmonary venous drainage.

Although the bidirectional Glenn procedure is generally considered as a transitional operation, it may be the final palliative operation for some high-risk patients with multiple risk factors. Risk factors for the Glenn procedure include pulmonary artery resistance >4 WU and/or pulmonary artery torsion caused by previous systemic-pulmonary shunt surgery, concurrent anomalous pulmonary venous connection, preoperative moderate to severe atrioventricular valve regurgitation, age under 4 months, and long hospital stay after previous palliative surgery, etc.

33.5 Discussion

33.5.1 Preoperative Assessment and Preparation

Before surgery, children with TA should have a clear anatomical classification with a focus on the assessment of pulmonary blood flow (less, more, balanced) and cardiac function. The degree of cyanosis in children with TA depends on the pulmonary cardiac output (Qp) to the systemic cardiac output (Qs) (Qp:Qs) ratio. Pulmonary artery outflow tract stenosis or atresia and restrictive VSD can cause (Qp:Qs) <1. The cyanosis in patients with (Qp:Qs) <1 is more pronounced than in those with increased or normal pulmonary blood flow. However, patients with TA and increased pulmonary blood flow may show signs of preoperative congestive heart failure.

It is not easy to measure (Qp:Qs) clinically. SaO_2 instead of (Qp:Qs) ratio is often used to assess the degree of systemic and pulmonary circulatory balance. When the arterial blood oxygen saturation reaches 75–80%, it indicates that the systemic and pulmonary circulation has reached a balance. This patient's preoperative SpO_2 was 77%, indicating the systemic and pulmonary circulatory balance has reached. This may benefit from the mild preoperative right ventricular outflow tract obstruction.

These patients may have experienced surgeries or long-term hospitalization. Therefore, it is very important to provide preoperative sedation to relieve anxiety and stress, which further makes the subsequent anesthesia induction smoother. Midazolam and dexmedetomidine are the ideal sedatives for preoperative sedation. S-ketamine can increase peripheral vascular resistance, reduce right-to-left shunting, maintain pulmonary blood flow, alleviate hypoxia symptoms, and can also be used for preoperative sedation in children. In this case, the patient was given oral midazolam 0.5 mg/kg preoperatively. The patient was successfully separated from the parents with a Ramsay score of 4 after 30 min and entered the room calmly.

Due to the high hematocrit in cyanotic patients, long-term preoperative fasting, venous and arterial puncture-related fluid loss, etc., they often experience volume deficiency, hemoconcentration, metabolic acidosis, etc., so it is necessary to replenish the volume appropriately. In this case, sufficient volume was given immediately after intravenous cannulation and 150 mL of fluid was transfused before bypass.

33.5.2 Intraoperative Anesthetic Management

1. Maintain appropriate pulmonary vascular resistance before the Glenn surgery. For patients who have undergone B-T shunt or central shunt, it is important to maintain a balance between appropriate pulmonary vascular resistance and systemic vascular resistance to prevent systemic blood stealing. Excessive reduction of pulmonary vascular resistance can lead to excessive left-to-right shunt at the level of the great vessels, leading to excessive pulmonary blood flow or even pulmonary edema. For patients after systemic-pulmonary shunt surgery, the significant decreases in diastolic pressure can significantly affect coronary artery blood supply, which further causes circulatory instability, arrhythmia, and serious adverse consequences.

   Before the establishment of Glenn circulation, the key point of anesthetic management is to maintain a balance between pulmonary vascular resistance (PVR) and systemic vascular resistance (SVR) with the goal of optimizing systemic circulation oxygen supply and perfusion pressure. Maintaining PaO_2 at 40–45 mm Hg and SaO_2 at 70–80% is reasonable, which can achieve an appropriate systemic circulation oxygen supply.

2. Ventilation management after Glenn procedure. After the establishment of Glenn circulation, pulmonary vascular resistance should be appropriately reduced to increase pulmonary blood flow, which can be achieved by increasing FiO_2), reducing peak inspiratory pressure, etc. Tracheal intubation with positive pressure ventilation can reduce the return of venous blood and increase pulmonary vascular resistance. The pulmonary blood flow in children undergoing bidirectional Glenn surgery is passive and is dominated by the expiratory phase of positive pressure ventilation. The platform pressure of respiration is reduced by adjusting the I:E ratio, extending the expiratory time, and shortening the inspiratory time. Excessive positive end-expiratory pressure (PEEP) would increase intrapleural pressure and reduce pulmonary blood flow. So, PEEP pressure should be cautiously chosen for children undergoing bidirectional Glenn surgery.

   Although hyperventilation can significantly reduce pulmonary artery resistance and blood carbon dioxide partial pressure, low carbon dioxide partial pressure will cause a significant reduction of cerebral blood flow, superior vena cava return, and pulmonary blood flow, which is not conducive to maintaining effective pulmonary circulation. Therefore, for such patients, normal carbon dioxide levels or mild hypercapnia should be maintained. In this case, the PCV-VG mode was used with VT 6–7 mL/kg, P_{peak} 16 cm H_2O, RR 15–20 times/minute, and respiratory parameters were adjusted according to blood gas analysis to maintain $PaCO_2$ at 40–45 mm Hg.

   For patients with insufficient pulmonary blood flow, inhaling nitric oxide (NO) or prostacyclin can reduce pulmonary vascular resistance and increase pulmonary blood flow.

33.6 Conclusion

The Glenn procedure as a staged surgical palliative treatment for various complex congenital heart diseases can improve the postoperative pulmonary blood flow status and reduce the volume load of the systemic circulatory ventricle. The appropriate development and hemodynamic conditions are required for patients to undergo the Glenn procedure. The key point of anesthetic management for these patients is to reasonably regulate the mechanical ventilation and maintain a good balance between systemic and pulmonary vascular resistance (Yunan Song).

Anesthetic Management for Fontan Surgery in Pediatric Patients with Tricuspid Atresia

34

Ruidong Zhang

Abstract

A 10-year-old girl, who was diagnosed with tricuspid atresia (TA) due to cyanosis after birth, had undergone superior vena cava-pulmonary artery anastomosis surgery 7 years ago. She is now scheduled to undergo Fontan surgery under general anesthesia. After the initial surgery, the ventricular function of children with TA was partially preserved, but eventually, the Fontan surgery needs to be performed to bypass the obstructed tricuspid valve and right ventricle and introduce the venous blood completely into the pulmonary artery to establish the Fontan circulation. In addition to assessing the condition of the child after palliative surgery, both ventricular function and pulmonary blood flow are key points of concern for anesthesia during Fontan surgery.

Tricuspid atresia (TA) is one of the cyanotic congenital heart diseases characterized by tricuspid valve undevelopment, accounting for about 1% of all congenital heart diseases. In children with TA, the tricuspid valve is underdeveloped, and there is no communication between the right atrium and the underdeveloped right ventricle. TA is a single ventricle physiological lesion, which usually needs to undergo staged Fontan surgery. This article reports the anesthetic management of a 10-year-old girl with TA who underwent Fontan surgery again after superior vena cava (SVC)-pulmonary artery anastomosis surgery.

34.1 Case Presentation

The patient was a 10-year-old girl with 26 kg in weight and 125 cm in height. She was admitted to the hospital for Fontan surgery 7 years after SVC-pulmonary artery anastomosis surgery (bidirectional Glenn procedure) for TA.

Physical examination: The patient was conscious with central cyanosis. Her pulse oxygen saturation (SpO_2) was 72% in breathing air. She had clubbed fingers.

Laboratory tests: The red blood cell count is 6.53×10^{12}/L, hemoglobin 197 g/L, and hematocrit 60.4%. No significant abnormalities were found in liver, kidney, and coagulation functions.

Electrocardiogram (ECG): Ectopic rhythm (junctional rhythm) with irregular rhythm, left axis deviation, possible left anterior hemiblock (LAH), and ST segment changes.

R. Zhang (✉)
The National Children's Medical Center (Shanghai), Department of Anesthesiology of Shanghai Children's Medical Center, Shanghai Jiao Tong University School of Medicine, Shanghai, China
e-mail: zhangruidong@scmc.com.cn

J. Zheng et al. (eds.), *Selected Pediatric Cardiovascular Surgery Anesthesia Cases*,
https://doi.org/10.1007/978-981-96-5614-1_34

Echocardiography (local hospital): Single ventricle (one set of atrioventricular valves) after right Glenn procedure, anastomotic blood flow is smooth, bidirectional shunt at the atrial level.

Cardiac catheterization: After right cavity pulmonary shunt surgery, the anastomosis between the right superior vena cava and the right pulmonary artery was unobstructed. Rich collateral vessels were visible, including a large collateral vessel supplying the right lung, which had been obstructed by the coil.

Preoperative diagnosis: Tricuspid atresia/ after a bi-directional Glenn procedure.

34.2 Anesthetic Management

No preoperative medications were administered. After entering the operating room, the patient was connected to an anesthesia monitor device. ECG showed sinus rhythm, heart rate (HR) 102 beats/min, SpO_2 73%, non-invasive blood pressure (NIBP) 96/55 mm Hg. The peripheral venous catheter was placed, and midazolam 0.1 mg/kg, etomidate 0.3 mg/kg, sufentanil 2.0 μg/kg, and rocuronium 0.6 mg/kg were administered intravenously for induction. An ID 6.0 mm cuffed tube was inserted orally under direct laryngoscopy and mechanical ventilation was performed in PCV-VG mode with the following parameters: gas flow rate 2 L/min, fraction of inspired oxygen (FiO_2) 50%, tidal volume (VT) 6–8 mL/kg, respiration rate (RR) 16–18 times/ min, inspiratory time to expiratory time (I:E) ratio 1:2. End-tidal carbon dioxide ($ETCO_2$) was maintained at 35–40 mm Hg by adjustment of RR. Sufentanil 2.0 μg/(kg·h), propofol 6.0 mg/(kg·h), and rocuronium 0.6 mg/(kg·h) were continuously infused intravenously combined with 1–2% sevoflurane intermittent inhalation to maintain anesthesia. The left radial artery and right internal jugular vein were catheterized for monitoring invasive arterial blood pressure (ABP) and central venous pressure (CVP). The body temperature was also monitored. The left femoral vein was accessed for fluid replacement. The preoperative CVP was 14–16 cm H_2O. Warming blankets were used during the perioperative period. After intubation, arterial blood gas analysis showed pH 7.353, PaO_2 51.8 mm Hg, $PaCO_2$ 38.6 mm Hg, BE-4.0 mmol/L, HCT 51.6%, serum potassium 3.5 mmol/L, serum calcium 1.15 mmol/L, and lactate 1.2 mmol/L. Tranexamic acid 10 mg/kg was intravenously administered before thoracotomy.

The operation was performed under mild hypothermia and cardiopulmonary bypass (CPB) support via median sternotomy. During the operation, it was found that there existed subvalvular pulmonary, but the anastomosis between the right superior vena cava and the right pulmonary artery was patent. After cross-clamping the aorta, the right atrium was cut open, and the atrial septal defect (ASD) was enlarged. The lower end of the $19^{\#}$ GORE-TEX conduit was connected to the inferior vena cava, and the other end was connected to the lower edge of the pulmonary artery through the right atrium. A 5 mm hole was made on the conduit to establish a fenestrated intracardiac tunnel Fontan circulation, and a patch enlarged the anterior wall of the pulmonary artery. After the aorta cross-clamp was released, the heart automatically resumed sinus rhythm on ECG. After restarting mechanical ventilation, dopamine 5.0 μg/(kg·min), epinephrine 0.03 μg/(kg·min), norepinephrine 0.05 μg/(kg·min), and treprostinil 10–40 ng/(kg·min) were initiated to intravenously infused. The perfusion flow rate was gradually reduced until CPB was weaned off. After separating from CPB, the dose of vasoactive drugs was adjusted according to the hemodynamics. Dopamine and epinephrine were increased to 7.5 μg/(kg·min) and 0.1 μg/(kg·min), respectively. The blood pressure was maintained at 96/55 mm Hg, heart rate at 89 beats/min, SpO_2 at 80–85%, $ETCO_2$ at 30–35 mm Hg, and CVP at 19–22 cm H_2O. Postoperative transesophageal echocardiography showed the baffle opening was 0.56 cm, with a right-to-left shunt and flow velocity of 2.24 m/s. The arterial blood gas analysis was reviewed and showed pH 7.439, PaO_2 33.5 mm Hg, $PaCO_2$ 34.6 mm Hg, BE −0.56 mmol/L, HCT 44.3%, serum potassium 3.4 mmol/L, serum calcium 1.15 mmol/L, and lactate 2.3 mmol/L. The ventilator parameters were adjusted as FiO_2 100%, VT 10 mL/kg, RR 12 times/min, I:E ratio 1:3, and positive end-expiratory pressure (PEEP) 4 cm H_2O. After modified ultrafiltration, protamine was intravenously injected to neutralize heparin at a 1:1 ratio. A total of 150 mL of packed red blood cells, 400 mL of plasma, and 300 IU of prothrombin complex were intravenously transfused. After satisfied hemostasis, the sternum was closed, and the patient was sent to the Cardiac Intensive Care Unit (CICU) with endotracheal intubation under ABP, ECG, and SpO_2 monitoring. The operation lasted 5 h, including 100 min of CPB and 53 min of aortic cross-clamping. The total urine output during the operation was 1000 mL.

34.3 Postoperative Outcome

The patient underwent peritoneal dialysis on the postoperative day 1. The endotracheal tube was removed on the postoperative day 2. The patient left CICU on postoperative day 5 and was successfully discharged on postoperative day 11.

34.4 Review of Knowledge Points

34.4.1 Tricuspid Atresia

In children with TA, the right atrium is separated from the underdeveloped right ventricle, and the venous blood from the systemic circulation mixes with the oxygenated blood returning from the lungs in the left atrium through the patent foramen ovale or ASD. Therefore, part of the oxygenated blood is ejected into the aorta by the left ventricle, and another part of the oxygenated blood enters the right ventricular outflow tract through the ventricular septal defect (VSD) (Fig. 34.1). The entrance of the pulmonary artery trunk may be stenotic, or the pulmonary artery may be underdeveloped. Some cases of TA without VSD or with underdeveloped pulmonary vessels rely on the patent ductus arteriosus (PDA) to direct blood flow into the pulmonary circulation. Although the cardiac output in TA cases is mixed blood, if it contains a sufficient amount of oxygenated blood returning from the pulmonary veins, it can provide sufficient oxygenation to alleviate cyanosis. Therefore, pulmonary blood flow is the main factor determining the cyanosis of the child, and the pulmonary blood flow itself depends on the degree of pulmonary vessel development, the presence and size of the VSD, the relationship of the position of the great arteries, and whether there is PDA. Tricuspid atresia with increased pulmonary blood flow may pose a risk of congestive heart failure and pulmonary hypertension.

34.4.2 Fontan Procedure

In 1971, Fontan and Baudet first reported the surgical treatment of TA in children. The purpose was to bypass the right ventricle through surgery and directly introduce systemic venous blood

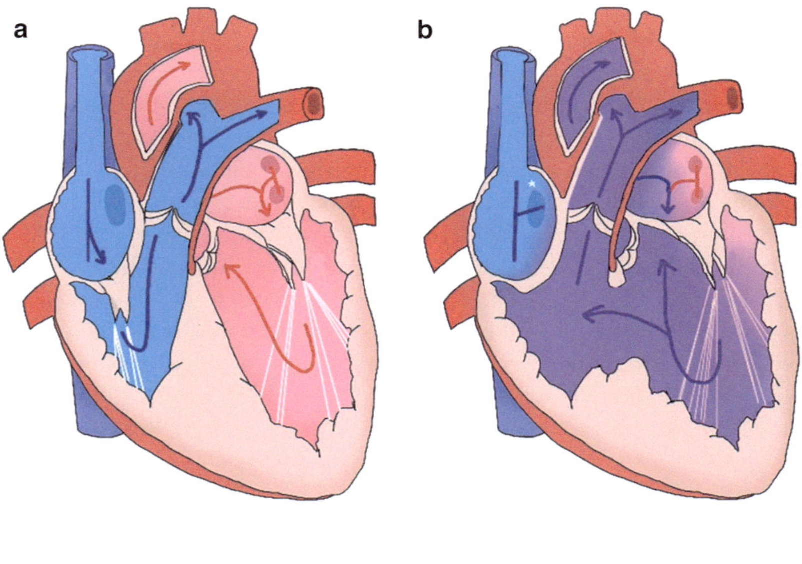

Fig. 34.1 Blood flow in normal heart (**a**) and tricuspid atresia (**b**)

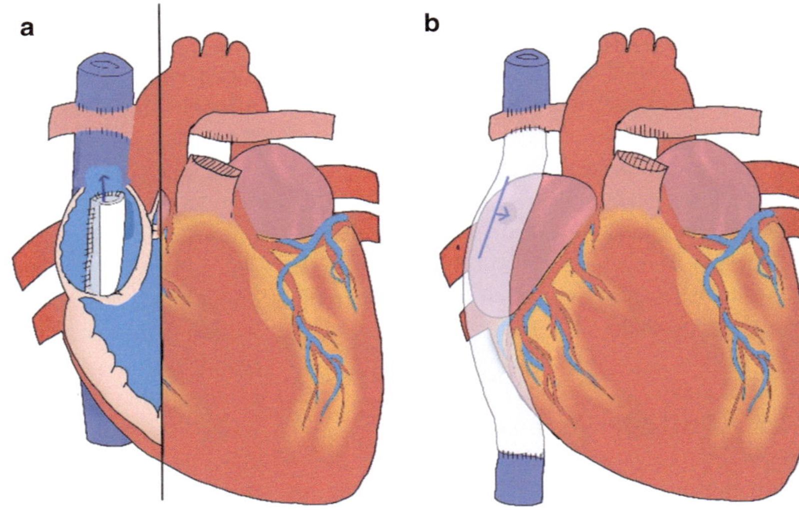

Fig. 34.2 Surgical repair of tricuspid atresia. (**a**) intra-atrial lateral tunnel Fontan technique. (**b**) extracardiac conduit Fontan technique with fenestration

into the pulmonary circulation, which was driven sequentially by a single ventricle for systemic and pulmonary circulation. The surgical steps include connecting the SVC and the right pulmonary artery, severing the connection between the SVC and the atrium, using an aortic valve homograft to establish a valved conduit connection between the right atrium or right atrial appendage and the left pulmonary artery, closing the ASD, inserting a homograft pulmonary valve at the inferior vena cava (IVC), ligating the pulmonary trunk. After the operation, the SVC blood flow enters the right pulmonary artery, and the IVC blood flow enters the left pulmonary artery. Establishing the Fontan circulation can reduce volume load, preserve ventricular function, and reduce atrial dilation. Since then, the Fontan procedure has been greatly improved. Currently, there are two main surgical methods. The intracardiac tunnel Fontan procedure uses an artificial patch to construct a tunnel connecting the IVC and the right pulmonary artery inside the right atrium. In contrast, the extracardiac conduit Fontan procedure uses a conduit to directly connect the IVC and the right pulmonary artery outside the heart (Fig. 34.2). The Fontan procedure is usually performed in children aged 2–4 years old. Preoperative evaluation of pulmonary artery anatomy and pressure, transpulmonary pressure, pulmonary vascular resistance, and left ventricular end-diastolic pressure is required by cardiac catheterization. Complications after the Fontan procedure include arrhythmias (commonly atrial arrhythmias, such as atrial flutter, atrial fibrillation, and supraventricular tachycardia), Fontan pathway obstruction, cyanosis and paradoxical embolism, thrombosis, collateral vessel formation, and protein-losing enteropathy. Risk factors include elevated pulmonary artery pressure, left/right pulmonary artery anatomical malformations, atrioventricular valve regurgitation, and ventricular dysfunction.

34.5 Discussion

34.5.1 Preoperative Assessment and Preparation

In the past, contraindications for Fontan surgery included early infancy, pulmonary vascular resistance (PVR) higher than 4 WU, severe pulmonary artery stenosis, ventricular ejection fraction lower than 25–30%, and ventricular diastolic pressure higher than 25 mm Hg. With the development of surgical techniques, atrioventricular valve regurgitation, localized pulmonary artery stenosis, or twisting, which were previously considered relative contraindications, can all be corrected through Fontan surgery. The patient had been evaluated preoperatively through echocardiography, electrocardiogram, and cardiac catheterization to assess the condition after the bidirectional Glenn procedure and the collateral vessels were occluded by cardiac catheterization, all of which were prepared for the subsequent Fontan surgery.

34.5.2 Anesthetic Management

1. Before CPB. Anesthesia induction in the patient can be achieved through mask inhalation of anesthetic gas or the use of intravenous anesthetics. Ketamine does not increase PVR in children and can be used if necessary. Invasive arterial pressure monitoring is usually established after anesthesia induction in pediatric patients. Re-opening the sternum in patients who have undergone multiple surgeries may lead to massive bleeding, so sufficient blood products must be prepared in advance. To facilitate the volume resuscitation, sufficient venous accesses must be established in the patient. Although CVP monitoring is required, there is still controversy over the placement of the catheter. If the central venous catheter is placed in the right internal jugular vein, it will interfere with the construction of the Glenn anastomosis and may cause thrombosis. Femoral vein catheterization can be used to monitor CVP, but it may also cause thrombosis. The patient may have scars at the femoral vein site due to previous cardiac catheterization. Surgeons may perform femoral artery and vein cannulation before splitting the sternum to quickly establish femoral artery-femoral vein CPB in case of massive bleeding during thoracotomy. In the past, large doses of analgesics were used during anesthesia. Still, now small doses of fentanyl-like drugs combined with inhaled anesthetics and nerve block are used to provide postoperative analgesia and extubate as early as possible. Patients with bidirectional Glenn shunts can be treated for hypoxia by increasing pulmonary blood flow through fluid replacement.
2. After CPB. The focus of postoperative anesthetic management is to reduce pulmonary vascular resistance and increase pulmonary blood flow. Inhalation of 100% pure oxygen, maintaining moderate hypocapnia and alkalosis, and reducing inspiratory pressure can lower PVR. If necessary, inhaled nitric oxide, prostacyclin, and treprostinil infusion can lower PVR and increase pulmonary blood flow. Maintaining sinus rhythm helps to maintain ventricular preload and cardiac output. Monitoring of CVP and atrial pressure (through a chest atrial pressure tube placed by the surgeon) in the early stages of weaning off CPB is used to calculate transpulmonary pressure (CVP-atrial pressure) and estimate PVR. The ideal transpulmonary pressure value is 7–8 mm Hg. An increase in atrial pressure indicates ventricular dysfunction or valve problems. Positive inotropic drugs can treat ventricular dysfunction and decrease the afterload of the systemic circulation, while atrioventricular valve regurgitation needs to be corrected surgically. If the atrial pressure is normal and the transpulmonary pressure is high, PVR is considered high, and pulmonary resistance needs to be reduced. A CVP above 27 cm H_2O reflects an increase in PVR and/or ventricular dysfunction, and the patient's related mortality rate will increase.

Positive pressure mechanical ventilation reduces venous return and increases PVR. In Fontan patients, pulmonary blood flow is passive and mainly occurs during the exhalation phase of positive-pressure mechanical ventilation. Measures such as shortening the inhalation time, extending the exhalation time, increasing tidal volume, and reducing respiratory rate can increase pulmonary blood flow. Minimizing plateau pressure, PEEP, and increasing the inspiratory pressure rising rate can improve pulmonary blood flow. Although PEEP is beneficial for accelerating alveolar re-expansion, it can potentially increase intrathoracic pressure and reduce pulmonary blood flow, so it needs to be balanced when used. Using PEEP after Fontan surgery can retain functional residual capacity and increase

PaO_2. Maintaining functional residual capacity reduces pulmonary vascular resistance by avoiding atelectasis and hypoxic pulmonary vasoconstriction. However, the level of PEEP suitable for Fontan patients is still unknown. Because negative intrapleural pressure increases pulmonary blood flow and cardiac output, it is recommended that Fontan the endotracheal intubation should be removed and resume spontaneous breathing as soon as possible after surgery. If the patients with the Fontan procedure cannot maintain sufficient spontaneous breathing, a negative pressure thoracic device can be used for ventilation assistance.

34.6 Shortcomings and Limitations

The patient underwent a second-stage thoracotomy, which may induce ventricular fibrillation due to the use of an electrocautery during the thoracotomy. Due to the limitations at the time, the placement of external defibrillation electrodes was not considered before anesthesia for automatic external defibrillation during surgery. In addition, the diameter of the patient's femoral vein should be measured in advance to assist femoral vein cannulation to establish CPB in case of major bleeding during thoracotomy.

34.7 Conclusion

Anesthetic management for Fontan surgery in children with TA poses a great challenge to anesthesiologists. The patient's existing disease pathology and post-palliative status should be comprehensively considered during preoperative assessment. Protecting ventricular function and promoting pulmonary blood flow are the main goals of anesthetic management for Fontan surgery. Improving the quality of perioperative anesthetic management can improve the prognosis of surgical patients and help avoid complications related to Fontan circulation (Ruidong Zhang).

35 Anesthetic Management of Valve Replacement Surgery in a Child with Mitral Regurgitation

Bo Li

Abstract

A 13-year-old girl underwent pulmonary artery plasty and mitral valvuloplasty 7 years ago due to pulmonary artery stenosis (PS) and mitral regurgitation (MR). She recently experienced aggravated shortness of breath after exercises. The echocardiography showed severe MR 1 month ago. She was consequently admitted to our hospital for mitral valve replacement under general anesthesia. During the operation, the patient experienced left heart failure while being weaned from cardiopulmonary bypass (CPB). Following the optimal adjustment of positive inotropic drugs, the left ventricular function was improved, and the patient was successfully weaned from CPB. The key points of anesthetic management during valve replacement surgery in a child with MR were to ensure adequate preload, avoid excessive afterload on the left heart, and maintain a relatively rapid heart rate. Given the increased pressure and volume load on the left ventricle, attention should be paid to potential occurrences of left ventricular failure.

B. Li (✉)
The National Children's Medical Center (Shanghai), Department of Anesthesiology of Shanghai Children's Medical Center, Shanghai Jiao Tong University School of Medicine, Shanghai, China
e-mail: libo@scmc.com.cn

Mitral regurgitation (MR) is the incomplete closure of the valves between the left atrium and ventricle and causes retrograde blood flow from the left ventricle to the left atrium. Valve replacement surgery is usually not considered as the primary option for pediatric patients with MR. According to the European Cardiothoracic Surgery Guidelines, valvuloplasty surgery is prioritized whenever possible for infants and children with MR. However, in cases where irreversible valve lesions such as calcification of the valve annulus or severe mitral valve prolapse are present in infants and children, valve replacement surgery remains an effective intervention. This case report focuses on the anesthetic management of elective mitral valve replacement surgery in a child with severe MR.

35.1 Case Presentation

A 13-year-old girl with 147 cm in height and 35 kg in weight was diagnosed with severe MR by echocardiographic examination. She had a history of pulmonary artery plasty and mitral valvuloplasty 7 years ago but no other systemic disease history. She complained of decreased exercise tolerance recently.

Preoperative diagnosis: Severe MR. She was scheduled to undergo mitral valve replacement surgery under general anesthesia.

J. Zheng et al. (eds.), *Selected Pediatric Cardiovascular Surgery Anesthesia Cases*,
https://doi.org/10.1007/978-981-96-5614-1_35

Echocardiography: Left atrium (LA) and left ventricle (LV) enlargement, LV hypertrophy, MR jet width 1.2 cm, MR jet area to LA area ratio (MR/LA ratio) 45%, and left ventricular ejection fraction (LVEF) 42%.

Laboratory tests: No apparent abnormalities in the liver, kidney, or coagulation function.

35.2 Anesthetic Management

Basic vital signs: Heart rate (HR) 108 beats/min, blood pressure (BP) 106/62 mmHg, pulse oxygen saturation (SpO_2) 98%. Anesthesia was induced with an intravenous bolus dose of 2.0 mg midazolam, 10.5 mg etomidate, 70 μg sufentanil, and 21 mg rocuronium. Volume control ventilation mode was used with respiratory parameters set as 60% fraction of inspired oxygen (FiO_2), 300 mL tidal volume (VT), 16 breaths/min respiratory rate (RR), and 1:2I:E (inspiratory to expiratory time) ratio. General anesthesia was maintained by intravenous infusion of 5.0 mg/(kg·h) of propofol, 2.5 μg/(kg·h) of sufentanil, and 0.6 mg/(kg·h) of rocuronium. End-tidal carbon dioxide ($ETCO_2$) was maintained at around 35 mmHg.

After anesthesia induction, the left radial artery and right internal jugular vein were catheterized under ultrasound guidance to continuously monitor invasive blood pressure (ABP) and central venous pressure (CVP). Arterial blood gas analysis after anesthesia induction revealed no significant abnormalities. The right great saphenous vein (20 G) was also accessed for fluid replacement and blood transfusion.

The valve replacement surgery was performed under cardiopulmonary bypass (CPB) support. After the aorta cross-clamp was released, the heart automatically resumed beating and sinus rhythm. After the vena cava cross-clamp was released, dopamine, epinephrine, and norepinephrine were infused at 5.0 μg/(kg·min),0.05 μg/(kg·min), and 0.02 μg/(kg·min), respectively. ABP was maintained at 80–100/50–60 mmHg, HR at 80–100 beats/min, and CVP at 10–12 cm H_2O. Transesophageal ultrasonography showed that the artificial mitral valve worked properly without perivalvular leakage.

CPB flow was gradually reduced to prepare for weaning. During the weaning process, the patient's ABP gradually dropped to 50–60/30–40 mmHg, and HR increased to 160 beats/min, indicating the occurrence of left heart failure. CPB perfusion flow rose again for assistance, and the dose of dopamine, epinephrine, and norepinephrine was increased to 10 μg/(kg·min), 0.1 μg/(kg·min), and 0.1 μg/(kg·min), respectively.

The patient's ABP was gradually increased to 90/50 mmHg, and the HR was decreased to 140 beats/min. Thirty minutes later, another attempt was made to wean off CBP. The CPB perfusion flow was gradually reduced with stable hemodynamics. Finally, the patient was successfully weaned from CPB.

35.3 Postoperative Outcome

The operation lasted approximately 6 h with an estimated blood loss of 500 mL and urine output of 800 mL. During the operation, 500 mL of Ringer's acetate solution, 350 mL of red blood cells, and 200 mL of plasma were intravenously transfused. The tracheal tube was successfully removed on the postoperative day 3. The patient was discharged from the Cardiac Intensive Care Unit on postoperative day 5 and discharged from the hospital on postoperative day 14.

35.4 Review of Knowledge Points

35.4.1 Pathophysiology of MR

MR can be divided into three levels according to the MR/LA ratio: mild (<20%), moderate (20–40%), and severe (>40%). The presence of Mild MR is typically asymptomatic; however, the regurgitation volume will progressively increase over time without treatment. Consequently, the patient may exhibit symptoms such as decreased exercise tolerance, chest tightness, and dyspnea.

In cases of severe MR, the patient's growth and development may be negatively impacted. The regurgitation volume of MR depends on the MR orifice area, MR duration, and the pressure gradient between the left atrium and ventricle. Anesthesiologists can indirectly regulate the regurgitation volume by controlling the heart rate and systemic vascular resistance. Specific measures include the following: ① Keeping the heart rate around the upper limit of the normal range for the patient's age. Both tachycardia and bradycardia increased the regurgitation volume. ② Controlling blood pressure to reduce the ejection resistance of the left ventricle.

35.4.2 Indicators for Valve Replacement Surgery

Generally speaking, valvuloplasty, rather than valve replacement surgery, is the first choice for infants and children with MR. Valve replacement surgery was considered only if the following conditions occurred:

1. The valve is severely dysplastic and cannot be repaired.
2. Accompanied by outflow tract stenosis or vascular stenosis, valve repair surgery cannot solve all these issues.
3. The valve is affected by infections, rheumatic endocarditis, neoplasms, or severe lesions and cannot be repaired.
4. Postoperative calcification, or severe degenerative lesions, cause valve function loss.
5. Cardiac insufficiency before surgery and valvuloplasty cannot improve heart function.

35.5 Discussion

35.5.1 Preoperative Assessment and Preparation

Preoperative assessment should focus on the signs and symptoms of left heart failure in children with MR. Children with mild MR are usually asymptomatic, whereas severe cases often present the following symptoms and signs:

1. Physical examination: Infants and young children may show feeding difficulties and shortness of breath. Elderly children may show development delay and exercise tolerance decrease.
2. Chest radiography: Cardiothoracic ratio increase, left atrium and ventricle enlargement, and pulmonary congestion.
3. Echocardiography: Left atrium and ventricle enlargement, LVEF decrease.

In this case, the patient already experienced shortness of breath after exercises, and echocardiography showed left atrium and ventricle enlargement and LVEF decrease (42%), all of which indicate that the patient was at a high risk of left heart failure after surgery.

35.5.2 Anesthetic Management Before CPB

1. To avoid the increase of left heart afterload: Increased left ventricular afterload in children with MR can exacerbate regurgitation volume. An appropriate reduction in systemic vascular resistance is beneficial in mitigating the regurgitation volume. In the setting of elevated pulmonary vascular resistance or right ventricular systolic insufficiency, reducing right ventricular afterload can improve right ventricular function and subsequently enhance left ventricular function and cardiac output.
2. To maintain the age-related normal upper limit of HR: Tachycardia in children with MR can lead to left ventricular filling insufficiency, and bradycardia can prolong the regurgitation duration, increasing the regurgitation volume.

35.5.3 Anesthetic Management After CPB

After valve replacement in children with MR, the left heart function usually improves, and the cardiac output increases. However, some children may still experience the following problems after surgery:

1. Left ventricular insufficiency: The blood flow in the left ventricle can only be pumped into the high-resistant aorta instead of partial leak back to the left atrium after valve replacement, which results in a significant increase in the pressure and volume load on the left ventricle. If myocardial protection is insufficient during CPB, or if left heart function has been impaired before surgery, left ventricular insufficiency may occur after surgery.
2. Pulmonary hypertension: Preexisting pulmonary hypertension may persist after surgery. If pulmonary hypertension persists after excluding factors such as hypoxia, hypercapnia, and acidosis, it is necessary to use pulmonary vasodilators to control pulmonary artery pressure.

35.6 Shortcomings and Limitations

In this case, left heart failure occurred following the first attempt to wean off CPB, possibly due to inadequate duration of post-CPB support. The patient was successfully weaned from CPB by increasing the CPB perfusion flow again and adjusting the dosage of positive inotropic drugs.

35.7 Conclusion

In summary, the key points of anesthetic management during valve replacement surgery in a child with MR are to control blood pressure to reduce left heart afterload and keep the heart rate around age-related normal upper limit before surgery. After surgery, anesthesiologists should be vigilant of left ventricular insufficiency. In this case, the anesthesiologist successfully treated the left ventricular insufficiency using positive inotropic drugs (Bo Li).

36 Anesthetic Management of Valvuloplasty Surgery in a Child with Tricuspid Regurgitation

Bo Li

Abstract

A 9-month-old male infant with a heart murmur was diagnosed with moderate-to-severe tricuspid regurgitation (TR) and scheduled to undergo tricuspid valve plasty under general anesthesia. The patient experienced right heart failure during weaning from cardiopulmonary bypass (CPB). After an optimal adjustment of ventilation parameters and positive inotropic drugs, the right ventricle function was improved, and the infant was successfully weaned from CPB. The keys to anesthetic management during valvuloplasty surgery in a TR child include maintaining sufficient right ventricular preload before CPB, reducing pulmonary vascular resistance, and maintaining myocardial contractility. Due to the increased pressure and volume load on the right ventricle, attention should be paid to the possible occurrence of right heart failure.

Tricuspid regurgitation (TR) is a relatively common heart valve disease in which the valve between the right atrium and right ventricle does not close properly, and the right ventricular blood leaks back into the right atrium during cardiac contraction. The incidence of TR in the normal population is about 65–85%. Mild TR is usually benign, but structural abnormalities of valve leaflets and annular dilation often accompany moderate and severe TRs. This case report focuses on the anesthetic management of elective valvuloplasty surgery in an infant with moderate-to-severe TR.

36.1 Case Presentation

A 9-month-old boy with 68 cm in height and 9 kg in weight was diagnosed with moderate-to-severe tricuspid regurgitation and right atrial enlargement by echocardiographic examination. The infant was a full-term cesarean section with no history of asphyxia at birth. The patient has no apparent symptoms such as cyanosis, difficulty breathing, convulsions, fainting, history of respiratory tract infection, edema, or oliguria.

Preoperative diagnosis: Moderate-to-severe tricuspid regurgitation. Tricuspid valve plasty surgery was planned under general anesthesia.

Echocardiography demonstrated right atrial enlargement, tricuspid annulus widening, poor diaphragmatic valve activity, adhesion to the ventricular septum, and moderate-to-severe regurgitation with a regurgitation jet width of 6.6 mm.

B. Li (✉)
The National Children's Medical Center (Shanghai), Department of Anesthesiology of Shanghai Children's Medical Center, Shanghai Jiao Tong University School of Medicine, Shanghai, China
e-mail: libo@scmc.com.cn

J. Zheng et al. (eds.), *Selected Pediatric Cardiovascular Surgery Anesthesia Cases*,
https://doi.org/10.1007/978-981-96-5614-1_36

Laboratory examination: AST 52 U/L, no apparent abnormalities in the liver, kidney, or coagulation function.

36.2 Anesthetic Management

Basic vital signs: Heart rate 136 beats/min, blood pressure 85/55 mm Hg, pulse oxygen saturation (SpO_2) 98%. Anesthesia was induced with intravenous bolus doses of 3.0 mg etomidate, 20 μg sufentanil, and 6.0 mg rocuronium. An ID 4.0 mm cuffed endotracheal tube was intubated under a visual laryngoscope and fixed after verification of the appropriate position by bilateral auscultation of the lungs. Pressure control ventilation was used with respiratory parameters set as 50% inhaled oxygen concentration, 16 cm H_2O inspiratory pressure, 70–80 mL tidal volume (VT), 30 breaths/min respiratory rate (RR), and 1:2 I:E ratio. General anesthesia was maintained by continuous intravenous infusion of 5.0 mg/(kg·h) of propofol, 2.5 μg/(kg·h) of sufentanil, and 0.6 mg/(kg·h) of rocuronium combined with 1% sevoflurane inhalation, end-tidal carbon dioxide ($EtCO_2$) was maintained between 30 and 35 mm Hg.

After anesthesia induction, arterial (left radial artery) and central venous (right internal jugular vein) catheterization were performed under ultrasound guidance to continuously monitor invasive blood pressure (ABP) and central venous pressure (CVP).The valvuloplasty surgery was performed under CPB support. The heart automatically resumed beating and sinus rhythm. After vena cava cross-clamp release, dopamine was infused at 5.0 μg/(kg·min), and pressure control ventilation was resumed with respiratory parameters set as inspiratory pressure 18 cm H_2O, VT 70–80 mL, RR 24 times/min. ABP was maintained at 80–100/50–60 mmHg, HR at 140–160 beats/min, and CVP at 10–12 cm H_2O. Transesophageal echocardiography showed that the tricuspid valve worked properly with mild regurgitation.

CPB flow was gradually reduced to prepare for weaning. During the weaning process, the patient's ABP dropped to approximately 50/30 mmHg, and his CVP rose to 18–20 cm H_2O. Considering right heart failure, the CPB perfusion flow was increased again for assistance, the dose of dopamine was increased to 10 μg/(kg·min), and norepinephrine was added at 0.05 μg/(kg·min). The respiratory parameters were adjusted as follows: inspiratory pressure, 12 cm H_2O; VT 50–60 mL; RR, 30 times/min.

The infant's ABP increased to 80/50 mmHg, and the CVP gradually decreased to 12–14 cm H_2O. Thirty minutes later, CPB perfusion flow gradually reduced, and the infant's vital signs remained stable. Then, the infant was successfully weaned from CPB.

36.3 Postoperative Outcome

The surgery lasted approximately 3.5 hours in total, with an estimated blood loss of 200 mL and urine output of 150 mL. One hundred milliliter of sodium acetate Ringer's solution, 150 mL of red blood cells, and 50 mL of 5% albumin were transfused during the surgery. The tracheal tube was successfully removed the next day. The infant was discharged from the Cardiac Intensive Care Unit (CICU) on the third day and from the hospital 1 week later.

36.4 Review of Knowledge Points

36.4.1 Grading of TR Severity

The width of the regurgitation jet can grade TR severity. Regurgitation jet <3 mm, mild; 3–7 mm, moderate; and > 7 mm, severe. Mild TR is generally asymptomatic, moderate-to-severe TR can cause an increase in right atrium pressure, and severe TR cases can present with symptoms of right heart failure, such as ascites, edema, and hepatomegaly.

36.4.2 Determinants of TR Volume

The regurgitation volume of TR depends on the TR orifice area, TR duration, and the pressure gradient between the right atrium and right ventricle. It is difficult for an anesthesiologist to intervene TR orifice area. Still, TR duration and pressure gradient between the right atrium and right ventricle can be indirectly regulated to reduce TR volume by adjustment of heart rate and pulmonary vascular resistance. Specific measures include the following: ① To keep the heart rate around the upper limit of the normal range for the patient's age and ② to reduce pulmonary vascular resistance by mild hyperventilation.

36.5 Discussion

36.5.1 Preoperative Assessment and Preparation

During preoperative assessment, an anesthesiologist needs to find any possible signs and symptoms of right heart failure in children with TR. Patients with mild TR are often asymptomatic, whereas severe cases may present with jugular vein distension, ascites, hepatomegaly, or lower limb edema. Echocardiography can directly assess the tricuspid valve's morphology, activity status, and regurgitation. If a patient has symptoms of right heart failure before surgery, the anesthesiologist should be vigilant regarding the possibility of right heart failure after surgery.

36.5.2 Anesthetic Management Before CPB

Before CPB, anesthetic management should focus on:

1. Ensuring sufficient right heart preload, which includes replenishment of circulatory volume, avoiding PEEP, and reducing ventilation pressure to minimize the impact on venous return.
2. Maintaining mild hyperventilation to reduce pulmonary vascular resistance, which includes maintenance of PaO_2 above 60 mmHg, $PaCO_2$ between 30 and 35 mmHg, and pH between 7.50 and 7.60. In addition, hypoxia, hypercapnia, and acidosis should also be avoided.
3. Keeping the heart rate around age-related normal upper limit.
4. Using anesthetic drugs that have minimal impact on the right heart preload and do not increase pulmonary vascular resistance. Vasodilation caused by propofol may have reduced the preload on the right heart. If a patient has a right-to-left shunt at the atrial septal level, the shunt volume may increase further. During anesthesia induction, propofol should be avoided or administered cautiously since propofol can cause significant vasodilation and the right heart preload reduction. Among the inhaled anesthetics, halothane significantly inhibits myocardial contractility, especially in infants under 6 months of age. Therefore, halothane is not recommended for anesthesia in TR patients.

36.5.3 Anesthetic Management After CPB

Although the right heart function is usually improved after valvuloplasty surgery, right heart failure can still happen in some TR patients, and positive inotropic drugs are needed to support right ventricular contractile function. Dopamine and norepinephrine are commonly used for this purpose. Using a relatively low ventilation pressure can facilitate the venous return and improve the right heart afterload. Furthermore, maintaining mild hyperventilation is beneficial for reducing pulmonary vascular resistance and avoiding an increase in right ventricular afterload.

36.6 Conclusion

In summary, the keys of anesthetic management during valvuloplasty surgery in a TR child include maintaining sufficient right heart preload, keeping the heart rate around age-related normal upper limit, and avoiding an increase in pulmonary vascular resistance. Mild hyperventilation may be beneficial for pulmonary vascular resistance reduction. In this case, the anesthesiologist successfully treated right heart failure using positive inotropic drugs and adjusting the respiratory parameters (Bo Li).

37 Anesthetic Management of Aortic Valve Commissurotomy in a Neonate with Aortic Valve Stenosis

Wei Ji

Abstract

A 28-day-old male neonate presented with cyanosis, skin rash, and lethargy. Echocardiography indicated "congenital aortic valve stenosis." After endotracheal intubation, mechanical ventilation support, and appropriate medical therapy, an emergent aortic valve commissurotomy was scheduled under general anesthesia. Aortic valve stenosis not only causes the increase of the left ventricular afterload and myocardial oxygen demand but also reduces the forward blood flow and results in inadequate perfusion of the systemic and coronary circulations. The survival of neonates with severe aortic valve stenosis hinges upon the patency of the arterial duct and the pulmonary to aorta artery shunting, which results in differential cyanosis, metabolic acidosis, and myocardial ischemia. In this case, the key to anesthetic management is to maintain the patency of the arterial duct, optimize the balance between myocardial oxygen supply and demand, and preserve myocardial function.

W. Ji (✉)
The National Children's Medical Center (Shanghai), Department of Anesthesiology of Shanghai Children's Medical Center, Shanghai Jiao Tong University School of Medicine, Shanghai, China
e-mail: jiwei@scmc.com.cn

Congenital aortic valve stenosis (AVS), also known as congenital aortic stenosis (AS), is referred to as an obstruction of the left ventricular outflow tract (LVOT) due to a congenital valve malformation. The bicuspid aortic valve malformation characterized by fusion of valve leaflets is the most common AVS, accounting for 50–60% of AVS cases. Also, alterations such as valve leaflet thickening, morphological irregularities, and mucoid degeneration can cause AVS. While the majority of AVS patients remain asymptomatic until middle to old age, urgent surgical interventions are often required in neonates or infants with severe aortic stenosis. Due to the substantial reduction of forward blood flow through the aorta valve orifice, the maintenance of effective blood volume in systemic circulation and patient survival relies on the patency of the arterial duct and the shunt from the pulmonary artery to the aorta. Such patients are predisposed to develop heart failure, hypotension, and acidosis because the deoxygenated blood from the arterial duct anterogradely perfuses into the descending aorta and results in pronounced cyanosis in the lower body (differential cyanosis) and inadequate perfusion of vital organs. The retrograde perfusion of deoxygenated blood into the coronary arteries coupled with aortic stenosis-induced afterload elevation aggravates myocardial ischemia and increases the incidence of arrhythmia and sudden death. Anesthetic management of neonates with severe AVS undergo-

J. Zheng et al. (eds.), *Selected Pediatric Cardiovascular Surgery Anesthesia Cases*, https://doi.org/10.1007/978-981-96-5614-1_37

ing emergency corrective surgery is intricate and high risk. This chapter reported the anesthetic management of aortic valve commissurotomy in a neonate with AVS.

37.1 Case Presentation

The patient is a 28-day-old male neonate weighing 3.5 kg. He was born full-term without any history of asphyxia requiring resuscitation. Upon birth, auscultation revealed a heart murmur. Echocardiography demonstrated bicuspid aortic valve malformation with severe stenosis, patent ductus arteriosus (PDA), atrial septal defect (ASD, type II), severe pulmonary arterial hypertension (PAH) accompanied by tricuspid regurgitation (TR), mild mitral regurgitation (MR), and left ventricular hypertrophy. The patient presented with symptoms of tachypnea, feeding difficulties, and excessive sweating. These symptoms deteriorated recently. He was transferred to the Cardiac Intensive Care Unit (CICU) for further treatment.

Physical examination: The patient was breathing rapidly, 45 times/min. A grade IV/VI systolic murmur was heard between the second and third ribs along the left sternal border. Pulse oxygen saturation (SpO_2) was 78% with air breathing.

Laboratory tests: HCT 31.6%, PaO_2 36.7 mmHg, $PaCO_2$ 61.0 mmHg. The functions of liver, kidney, and coagulation were within normal range.

Electrocardiogram (ECG): Sinus rhythm, T wave changes, QT interval prolongation.

Chest X-ray: Enlarged heart shadow, increased lung markings, and slightly reduced transparency in both lung fields.

Echocardiography: Bicuspid aortic valve with severe stenosis (pressure gradient 108 mmHg), ASD of type II, MR, PAH, and PDA.

Preoperative diagnosis: AVS, mitral valve insufficiency. Aortic valve commissurotomy and closure of the ductus arteriosus under general anesthesia were proposed.

37.2 Anesthetic Management

The patient was transferred from the CICU to the operating room with the support of mechanical ventilation and intravenous infusions of norepinephrine at a rate of 0.05 μg/(kg·min) and prostaglandin E_1 at a rate of 5.0 ng/(kg·min). Ventilation was maintained in pressure-controlled ventilation-volume guaranteed (PCV-VG) mode with an oxygen flow rate of 1.0 L/min and a fraction of inspired oxygen (FiO_2) of 30%. Tidal volume (VT) was set at 35 mL, inhalation to exhalation ratio (I:E) of 1:2, positive end-expiratory pressure (PEEP) of 4.0 cm H_2O, and end-tidal CO_2 pressure ($ETCO_2$) maintained between 45 and 55 mm Hg. Invasive arterial blood pressure (ABP) was recorded at 69/40 mm Hg, central venous pressure (CVP) at 11 cm H_2O, heart rate (HR) at 135 beats/min, and pulse oxygen saturation (SpO_2) at 99%. Anesthesia was induced with midazolam 0.5 mg, sufentanil 5.0 μg, and rocuronium 2.0 mg via a peripheral vein. Anesthesia was maintained by continuous infusion of propofol 4.0 mg/(kg·h), sufentanil 2.0 μg/(kg·h), and rocuronium 0.5 mg/(kg·h) with intermittent inhalation of sevoflurane. Sodium acetate Ringer's solution was infused via the femoral vein. Cerebral oxygen saturation, rectal temperature, and urine output were continuously monitored during the operation. Preoperative blood gas test results are detailed in Table 37.1. Cardiopulmonary bypass (CPB) was initiated after heparinization. The ascending aorta was clamped, and a cardioplegic solution was injected at the root to terminate cardiac activity. The PDA was ligated. The aortic valve showed bicuspid valve malformation. The fused aortic valve commissure was cut apart. Upon aortic clamp release, spontaneous heartbeat resumed immediately with sinus rhythm and HR at 120 beats/min. Under the support of intravenous infusions of epinephrine at 0.05 μg/(kg·min) and dopamine at 5.0 μg/(kg·min), ABP was maintained around 41/32 mm Hg. Then, norepinephrine at 0.02 μg/(kg·min) was added to increase myocardial contractility. After the inferior vena cava was unclamped, pres-

Table 37.1 Intraoperative blood gas test results

Time point	HCT %	pH	PaO_2 mm Hg	$PaCO_2$ mm Hg	BE mmol/L	Na^+ mmol/L	K^+ mmol/L	Ca^{2+} mmol/L	Cl^- mmol/L	Lac mmol/L
Pre-operation	39.3	7.32	68.7	65.4	5.25	133	3.6	1.23	101	1.1
During operation	29.5	7.431	185.5	42.5	2.49	134	3.8	1.32	99	1.6

sure-controlled ventilation (PCV) was resumed with VT at 6–8 mL/kg and respiratory rate (RR) at 24 times/min. Intravenous infusion of norepinephrine at 0.1 μg/(kg·min) was supplemented, and epinephrine was increased to 0.1 μg/(kg·min). ABP was gradually stabilized around 73/43 mm Hg. Postoperative transesophageal echocardiography revealed that there was no residual shunt in the PDA. The aortic valve flow velocity was 4.34 m/s. The aortic valve pressure gradient was 75 mm Hg. The mitral valve regurgitation was moderate. The ABP remained stable after CPB was weaned off. Intravenous administration of protamine was initiated after modified ultrafiltration. Intraoperative blood gas monitoring results are detailed in Table 37.1. Pulmonary artery pressure was directly measured at 42/17(28) mm Hg, and ABP was 84/50(63) mm Hg. Sonoclot Analyzer tested coagulation function and showed activated clotting time (ACT) of 136 s (normal range: 100–155 s), clot rate (CR) of 6.0 (normal range: 9–35), and platelet function (PF) of 2.6 (normal range: >1.5). Recombinant human coagulation factor VIIa at 0.3 mg was intravenously administrated to facilitate hemostasis. Autologous blood (50 mL) was reinfused, and 50 mL of urine was collected after ultrafiltration. Before leaving the operating room, HR was 125 beats/min, ABP was 80/45 mm Hg, and CVP was 10 cm H_2O. The sternal closure was delayed. The patient was subsequently transferred to the CICU under mechanical ventilation support.

37.3 Postoperative Outcome

After admission to the CICU, the child was placed on continuous mechanical ventilation in IPPV + SIMV mode. Dopamine and norepinephrine were continuously administered to maintain hemodynamic stability. Sternal closure was conducted on postoperative day 3. The endotracheal tube was removed on postoperative day 4, and the child was discharged 2 weeks after the operation.

37.4 Review of Knowledge Points

37.4.1 Arterial Duct-Dependent Congenital Heart Disease

Arterial duct-dependent congenital heart diseases refer to a group of congenital heart diseases (CHD) that pose significant threats to the survival and quality of life of affected children, necessitating reliance on the patency of the arterial duct to maintain systemic and pulmonary blood circulation, which is mainly classified into left heart obstruction-type CHD, right heart obstruction-type CHD, and complete transposition of the great arteries (TGA). In children with left heart obstruction-type CHD, the forward blood flow from the left heart is reduced, and the pulmonary artery blood is required to drain into the aorta via PDA to maintain adequate blood pressure and organ perfusion below the site of obstruction. Conversely, in children with right heart obstruction-type CHD, the pulmonary blood flow is substantially reduced, resulting in less oxygenated blood passing through the lungs and inadequate tissue oxygen supply. Therefore, diverting aortic blood into the pulmonary artery via PDA is necessary. TGA represents a unique form of CHD where systemic and pulmonary circulations do not communicate. The systemic circulation lacks oxygenated blood from the pulmonary circulation, resulting in an inadequate tissue oxygen supply. Communicating systemic and pulmonary circulation via PDA becomes essential in managing TGA.

In children with arterial duct-dependent congenital heart disease, closure or obstruction of the arterial duct can precipitate the risk of cardiac arrest or death. Before surgery, every precaution should be taken to maintain the patency of the arterial duct. This includes avoiding high concentrations of inhaled oxygen or using cyclooxygenase inhibitors such as ibuprofen and indomethacin. If necessary, prostaglandin E can be administered to sustain the patency of the arterial duct.

37.4.2 Differential Cyanosis

During fetal development, the arterial duct is a crucial conduit for blood flow between the aorta and pulmonary artery. Typically, it undergoes functional closure approximately 10–15 h after birth and anatomical closure around 3 months after birth. In certain cases of CHD, where the arterial duct fails to close, blood tends to shunt from the aorta to the pulmonary artery. Prolonged high-pressure blood flow from the aorta into the pulmonary artery will lead to pulmonary arterial hypertension. Eventually, the pulmonary arterial pressure may approach or exceed that of the aorta, resulting in pulmonary arterial blood reflux into the aorta. This phenomenon causes a significant discrepancy in oxygen saturation levels between the upper and lower body, known as differential cyanosis. Moreover, in neonates or infants with left heart obstruction-type CHD, there is a substantial reduction in aortic pressure and forward blood flow from the left ventricle. To maintain blood pressure and organ perfusion below the site of obstruction, blood from the pulmonary artery must be diverted to the aorta through the arterial duct. This diversion also results in a marked disparity in oxygen saturation levels between the upper and lower body, leading to the manifestation of differential cyanosis.

37.5 Discussion

37.5.1 Preoperative Evaluation and Preparation

Preoperative evaluation should be prioritized in children with AVS to assess the type and severity of AVS, myocardial contractility, myocardial ischemia, the patency of PDA, and the presence of arrhythmias. Differential cyanosis serves as a significant indicator of severe AVS.

During the preoperative period, it is required either to avoid inhalation of a high concentration of oxygen or to use cyclooxygenase inhibitors such as ibuprofen and indomethacin to prevent the closure of the arterial duct. For those children with prostaglandin therapy to maintain patency of the PDA, attention should be paid to preventing respiratory depression, and mechanical ventilation support is preferred. Tachycardia or bradycardia should also be avoided before surgery. Given the substantial increase in afterload in children with AVS, tachycardia can significantly elevate myocardial oxygen consumption and precipitate heart failure before surgery. Conversely, low diastolic pressure and short diastolic time can markedly reduce the subendocardial perfusion and exacerbate myocardial ischemia. Bradycardia in these children can also be fatal. To ensure adequate cardiac output, increasing the transvalvular pressure across the aorta is necessary, ultimately resulting in a notable increase in myocardial oxygen consumption.

Newborns with severe AVS may also experience cardiogenic shock before surgery, which leads to end-organ damage, myocardial ischemia, acidosis, and, ultimately, death. In this case, the child showed signs of cardiogenic shock before surgery. We used prostaglandin E 1 to maintain the opening of the arterial duct. Intravenous infusion of norepinephrine was used to raise blood pressure. Mechanical ventilation support and symptomatic treatment measures were also provided and other.

37.5.2 Anesthetic Management During Surgery

The anesthetic management of CHD children with AVS should pay special attention to maintaining sufficient left ventricular preload and myocardial contractility, sinus rhythm, and near-normal basic heart rate. A certain degree of afterload and diastolic pressure should be maintained to avoid insufficient coronary artery perfusion, and a sufficiently high pulmonary artery wedge pressure should be maintained to ensure sufficient right-to-left shunt.

Anesthesia induction involves the administration of etomidate in combination with a high dose of opioids and non-depolarizing muscle relaxants, which help reduce myocardial contractility inhibition and peripheral vasodilation. Propofol and inhaled anesthetics should be avoided during induction due to their potential to induce severe hypotension. Throughout the maintenance phase of anesthesia, continuous infusion of high doses of opioids can be employed with intermittent supplements of low concentration of sevoflurane inhalation. This approach ensures adequate depth of anesthesia and less circulatory depression.

Before surgical valve correction, tachycardia induced by stress stimuli should be avoided. The stress stimuli should be terminated first, and then the anesthesia depth should be deepened. Short-acting β_1 receptor blocker esmolol can also be used to reduce tachycardia due to rapid onset and short duration without affection of postoperative CPB weaning. It is a good choice for quickly reducing tachycardia in children with AVS. At the same time, hypotension caused by peripheral vasodilation should be avoided. Small doses of norepinephrine and an appropriate amount of fluid should be used to maintain blood pressure at pre-induction. If myocardial contractility is suspected to decrease, positive inotropic drugs such as dopamine can be chosen. In this case, anesthesia was induced with etomidate and a large dose of sufentanil titrated. Before CPB establishment, norepinephrine and prostaglandin were continuously infused to increase peripheral vascular resistance, open PDA, and maintain coronary artery perfusion. In addition, cerebral oxygen saturation monitoring can help to detect early cerebral ischemia.

Regarding ventilation management, it is advisable to utilize low-concentration oxygen (30%), low PEEP, and maintain normal $ETCO_2$ levels to prevent a reduction in pulmonary vascular resistance and subsequent decrease in right-to-left shunting. This approach helps to avoid reducing systemic diastolic pressure and ensures adequate perfusion of the coronary arteries and other vital organs. In this case, the ventilation mode and parameters in the CICU were continuously used. Blood gas analysis revealed mild hypercapnia, facilitating right-to-left shunting across the arterial duct.

37.5.3 Anesthetic Management After CPB

After surgical correction of AVS, the child is prone to have high dynamics and hypertension in the left ventricle after weaning from CPB. Using vasodilators alone to lower blood pressure can significantly reduce diastolic pressure, increase pulse pressure difference, cause reflex tachycardia, and cause subendocardial ischemia. Supplemental esmolol may be more reasonable for lowering blood pressure while avoiding tachycardia and the risk of myocardial ischemia. If there is a decrease in myocardial contractility after surgery, positive inotropic drugs such as dopamine and epinephrine can be used to improve myocardial contractility. Although vasopressin helps maintain diastolic pressure, it may affect the tissue perfusion of the intestinal organs. The significant increase in afterload can lead to decreased left ventricular function, so its use must be weighed against the benefits.

37.6 Conclusion

In summary, the anesthetic management of children with AVS should be determined based on the type of surgery and the severity of the condition. During anesthetic management, special attention should be paid to the opening of the arterial duct before surgical correction, the balance of myocardial oxygen supply and demand, and the protection of myocardial function (Wei Ji).

38 Anesthetic Management of Bentall Procedure for a Child with Bicuspid Aortic Valve and Ascending Aorta Dilation

Ming Zhu

Abstract

A 13-year-old boy presented with an aggravated respiratory infection and orthopnea and was diagnosed with bicuspid aortic valve malformation, severe aortic valve insufficiency, and ascending aortic dilation. Despite in-hospital treatment with cardiac support, diuretics, and aggressive anti-infection therapy, the therapeutic effect was unsatisfactory. He later developed severe left heart failure, and the hemodynamics could not be maintained. He underwent an emergency Bentall procedure. The key points of anesthesia for such patients include avoiding drastic blood pressure fluctuations during surgery, minimizing aortic valve regurgitation to maintain cardiovascular homeostasis, and actively maintaining myocardial contractility postoperatively to balance myocardial oxygen supply and demand.

The Bentall procedure, also known as "aortic valve-containing artificial vascular ascending aortic replacement surgery," is commonly used in adults to treat ascending aortic aneurysms or dissections combined with aortic valve disease. Still, there is a lack of corresponding surgical and anesthetic management experience in children. This chapter reports the anesthetic management of a child with bicuspid aortic valve (BAV) malformation and ascending aortic dilation who underwent the Bentall procedure.

M. Zhu (✉)
The National Children's Medical Center (Shanghai), Department of Anesthesiology of Shanghai Children's Medical Center, Shanghai Jiao Tong University School of Medicine, Shanghai, China
e-mail: zhuming@scmc.com.cn

38.1 Case Presentation

The patient was a 13-year-old boy with a height of 145 cm and weight of 32 kg. Two weeks before admission, he developed a cough and expectoration due to the respiratory infection. The cough worsened later, and he could not sleep at night due to the cough, which was accompanied by shortness of breath and dyspnea. These symptoms were partially relieved by orthopneic position. He felt fatigue and a reduction in exercise tolerance. He also felt shortness of breath and fatigue after climbing up one to two floors or walking 5–10 min on the ground.

Physical examination: Blood pressure (BP): 97/37 mm Hg, heart rate (HR): 135 beats/min, respiratory rate (RR): 40 times/minute, pulse oxygen saturation (SpO_2): 98% with nasal cannula oxygen respiratory, fine rales in both lungs at auscultation, grade III/VI diastolic murmur at the aortic valve auscultation area.

Chest X-ray: Pulmonary infiltration and pleural effusion on both sides.

J. Zheng et al. (eds.), *Selected Pediatric Cardiovascular Surgery Anesthesia Cases*,
https://doi.org/10.1007/978-981-96-5614-1_38

Electrocardiogram (ECG): Sinus tachycardia, ST segment changes.

Echocardiography: Bicuspid aortic valve malformation (BAV), severe aortic valve regurgitation, mild to moderate mitral and tricuspid regurgitation, pulmonary hypertension, left atrium and left ventricle enlargement, left ventricular ejection fractions (LVEF) 62.84%, ascending aorta dilation.

Chest CT: Ascending aorta dilation, pericardial effusion, pleural effusion on both sides, pulmonary infiltration.

Laboratory tests: CK-MB 1.8 μg/L, cTnI 0.14 μg/L, NT-pro BNP 4992 pg/mL.

Diagnosis: BAV, heart failure, pneumonia, pleural effusion.

After the boy was admitted, a series of therapeutic measures were administrated, including high-flow oxygen inhalation, pleural puncture to remove effusion, dopamine to increase cardiac contractibility, and antibiotics to control infection. However, the patient still had difficulty breathing. The urine output was decreased to 700 mL/24 h. The blood lactate level was increased to 5.4 mmol/L. Emergency endotracheal intubation and mechanical ventilation support were conducted while the dosage of dopamine was increased and epinephrine was added. Although the blood lactate level was once reduced to 1.6 mmol/L after the treatment, hemodynamic stability could not be maintained. Emergency Bentall surgery was performed.

38.2 Anesthetic Management

The patient was brought into the operating room with endotracheal intubation and PCV-VG mode mechanical ventilation support; epinephrine and dopamine were continuously infused at 0.1 μg/(kg·min) and 7.5 μg/(kg·min), respectively. The gas flow rate was set at 2 L/min, fraction of inspired oxygen (FiO_2) 50%, tidal volume (VT) 6–8 mL/kg, RR 18 times/minute, inspiratory time to expiratory time (I:E) 1:2. End-tidal carbon dioxide ($ETCO_2$) was maintained at 35–40 mm Hg. ECG, artery blood pressure (ABP), SpO_2, central venous pressure (CVP), NIRS (near-infrared spectroscopy), cerebral oxygen saturation, and rectal and tympanic temperature were monitored during surgery.

Basic vital monitoring: ABP 115/52 mm Hg, HR 120 beats/min, SpO_2 100%, CVP 15 cm H_2O. Artery blood gas analysis showed that the serum potassium was 2.82 mmol/L (Table 38.1). The patient was administered 10% KCl 3 mL in replacement fluid to correct low serum potassium. General anesthesia was maintained by intravenous infusion of propofol 4.0 mg/(kg·h), sufentanil 2.0 μg/(kg·h), rocuronium 0.6 mg/(kg·h), and sevoflurane intermittent inhalation. In addition, methylprednisolone 80 mg, ulinastatin 300,000 U, and tranexamic acid 300 mg were intravenously given before the establishment of cardiopulmonary bypass (CPB).

CPB was established after injection of heparin (3 mg/kg). The portion of the aorta from the ascending aorta root to the aortic arch was found to be significantly dilated with aneurysmal changes, and the diameter was 5 cm. Endocarditis-like changes on aortic valve leaflets appeared, visible excrescences on the right coronary valve ventricular surface, and a destroyed valve ring-valve sinus structure were also found. After the aortic valve leaflets were cut off, the autologous pericardial patch was used to repair the destroyed area via a tension reduction technique. The continuity of LVOT-ascending aortic endocardium was reconstructed, and the left and right coronary arteries were slightly dissected and implanted on the artificial conduit. Under deep hypothermic circulatory arrest, the proximal aortic arch and brachiocephalic artery were trimmed and anastomosed to the artificial conduit end-to-end. The original aortic wall was sutured to wrap the artificial conduit, and the residual cavity was treated with a window to the right atrial appendage (Fig. 38.1).

After the aorta cross-clamp was released, the heart automatically resumed sinus rhythmic beating. The transesophageal echocardiography showed good aortic valve opening and closing activities, reduced left ventricular wall contractibility, and mild to moderate tricuspid regurgitation. Dopamine 5.0 μg/(kg·min) and epinephrine 0.08 μg/(kg·min) were continuously infused to

Table 38.1 Intraoperative blood gas test result

Time point	pH	20.4	$PaCO_2$ (mm Hg)	BE (mmol/L)	HCT (%)	K^+ (mmol/L)	Ca^{2+} (mmol/L)	Cl^- (mmol/L)	Lac (mmol/L)	HCO_3^- mmol/L)
Before CPB	7.493	308	32	0.92	26.9	2.63	1.099	103	1.3	24
After modified ultrafiltration	7.425	229	31.8	−3.43	26.5	2.4	0.96	104	2.9	

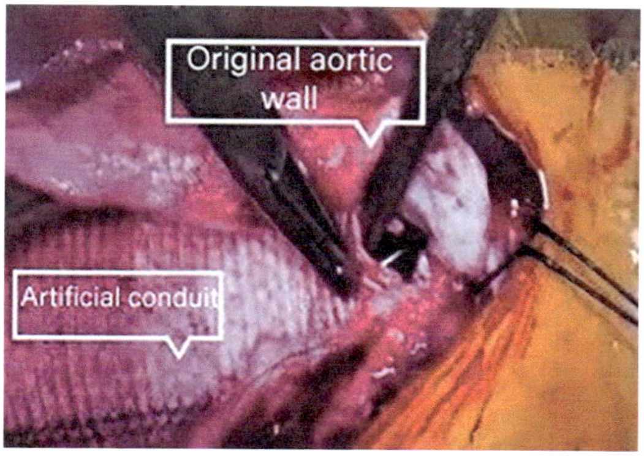

Fig. 38.1 The original aortic wall was sutured to wrap the artificial conduit

maintain the hemodynamic stability. The withdrawal from CPB was smooth. Protamine was given to neutralize heparin after modified-ultrafiltration ACT was 123 s after heparin neutralization. The artery blood gas analysis was rechecked (Table 38.1). Calcium gluconate 500 mg and 10% KCl 3 mL were intravenously given according to the artery blood gas analysis result. Packed RBCs 150 mL, FFPs 100 mL, and coagulation factor complex 300 IU were also intravenously infused.

After surgery, delayed sternal closure was performed. The patient was transported back to the cardiac intensive care unit (CICU) with endotracheal intubation. When leaving the operating room, ABP was 89/55 mm Hg, HR was 107 beats/min, and CVP was 16 cm H_2O.

38.3 Postoperative Outcome

The total CPB time was 145 min, the aortic cross-clamping time was 96, and the deep hypothermic circulatory arrest (DHCA) time was 10. The patient experienced postoperative low cardiac output and acute kidney injury (AKI) after returning to the CICU, which was improved by adjustment of cardiac function, peritoneal dialysis, and continuous renal replacement therapy, the condition improved. The endotracheal tube was removed, replaced with nasal cannula oxygen on postoperative day 4, and transferred back to the general ward on postoperative day 11. Three months later, he was successfully discharged from the hospital.

38.4 Review of Knowledge Points

38.4.1 Bicuspid Aortic Valve Malformation

Pediatric aortic valve disease mainly includes BAV, congenital valve stenosis, and valve insufficiency. Other pediatric aortic valve disease includes valve destruction caused by infective endocarditis and iatrogenic aortic valve insufficiency after congenital ventricular septal defect repair. BAV can lead to progressive loss of effective function of the aortic valve.

A previous study reported that 50–80% of children with BAV have abnormal aortic valve function, which includes 78.3% of valve stenosis, 15.6% of valve insufficiency, and 4% of both stenosis and insufficiency. In addition, the male-to-female ratio is about 3:1. The normal aortic valve consists of the left coronary cusp, right coronary cusp, and non-coronary cusp, forming a tricuspid valve structure. The main feature of BAV is the presence of two unequal-sized cusps, the larger of which is usually formed by the fusion of two normal cusps. BAV often coexists with aortic diseases, and ascending aortic dilation is the most common coexistence of aortic diseases. The pathogenesis of aortic disease caused by BAV is still controversial. In addition to the molecular mechanisms, hemodynamic and genetic mechanisms may also contribute to the pathogenesis of aortic disease in children with BAV.

38.4.2 Surgical Indications and Main Methods

BAV-related ascending aortic dilation can cause aortic dissection, even rupture. Therefore, regular follow-up and evaluation are required to optimize the timing of surgery. Surgical treatment is the main method for treating BAV and related aortic diseases. According to the newest ACC/AHA guidelines and indications for surgical treatment: If the BAV patients have an aortic sinus or ascending aorta diameter > 5.5 cm, proactive surgery treatment is recommended even without related symptoms. If the BAV patients have an aortic root or ascending aorta diameter at 5.0–5.5 cm and a family history of aortic dissection, proactive surgery treatment is also recommended. For those BAV patients who need to undergo valve surgery due to aortic stenosis or insufficiency, an ascending aorta replacement can be performed simultaneously if the aortic root or ascending aorta diameter is greater than 4.5 cm. The Bentall procedure involves the replacement of the aortic valve, aortic root, and ascending aorta with a valved artificial blood vessel and left and right coronary artery transplantation.

38.5 Discussion

38.5.1 Preoperative Assessment and Preparation

Due to aortic valve insufficiency, blood can be refluxed into the left ventricle, which increases the left ventricular volume overload, compensatory dilation, myocardial hypertrophy, and subendocardial ischemia.

Due to diastolic regurgitation, the diastolic pressure will drop, and the pulse pressure difference will become larger, reducing myocardial perfusion and increasing the risk of left heart failure.

The increased left ventricular end-diastolic pressure will lead to an increase in left atrial pressure, pulmonary congestion, and pulmonary hypertension in the end. This patient had severe aortic valve insufficiency caused by BAV and was further aggregated by respiratory tract infection, which showed the symptoms of left heart failure such as orthopnea and reduction of exercise tolerance before surgery. Both preoperative left heart failure and pulmonary artery pressure increase are high-risk factors during the perioperative period, which increases the risk of anesthesia. After admission, the patient's general condition was improved with homeostasis by cardiac and pulmonary function support, which made comprehensive preparation during the preoperative period.

38.5.2 Intraoperative Anesthetic Management

Before CPB is established, significant blood pressure fluctuation and aneurysm rupture must be avoided. It is better to maintain a relatively fast heart rate and lower afterload during anesthesia to minimize regurgitation and increase cardiac ejection, which is similar to the anesthetic management of aortic valve insufficiency. A faster heart rate can shorten the diastolic period, reduce the regurgitation fraction, and significantly increase the forward cardiac output. Mild afterload reduction can increase forward blood flow and reduce end-diastolic ventricular pressure, which helps to increase the myocardial blood supply. Therefore, we maintained HR at more than 90 beats/min and avoided using large doses of vasoconstrictors in this case. Furthermore, it is necessary to maintain the diastolic pressure not lower than 30 mmHg.

In addition, insufficient blood volume should be considered if hypotension occurs during the operation since the patient was treated with diuretics before surgery. Potassium was supplemented because the blood gas analysis showed that blood potassium was only 2.82 mol/L. In addition, DHCA was required to be used for large blood vessel surgery. Brain protection is crucial since, in the short and long term, neurological complications still occur after DHCA surgery in some patients. In this case, selective cerebral perfusion (SCP) technology was conducted to reduce or avoid brain damage caused by circulatory arrest. Furthermore, both routine rectal temperature monitoring and tympanic temperature monitoring were used. Tympanic temperature can reflect real-time changes in brain temperature, which helps avoid the recovery too quick and too high during rewarming. In addition, we also used cerebral NIRS monitoring to monitor the change in cerebral tissue oxygen saturation. It is necessary to control the shift of cerebral tissue oxygen saturation value within 20% of the baseline value to avoid brain perfusion insufficiency.

The focus of anesthetic management after heartbeat restarts includes myocardial contractibility and postoperative bleeding. Myocardial ischemia and contractility reduction frequently occur after the heartbeat restarts since the Bentall procedure involves the treatment of the coronary arteries complicated with long-time CPB and preoperative cardiac dysfunction. Therefore, it is necessary to perform intensive ECG monitoring and transesophageal echocardiography, which can help early find the myocardial ischemia and contractility reduction. Once the myocardial ischemia and contractility reduction occurs, nitroglycerin can be given to dilate the coronary arteries. In contrast, dopamine, epinephrine, and other positive inotropic drugs are given to improve myocardial contractibility.

Postoperative bleeding is the most common and dangerous complication in Bentall surgery, which often occurs at anastomotic sites. Therefore, it is better for the surgeons to keep the original aortic wall, wrap the artificial blood vessel with the original aortic wall, and perform draining from the aorta to the right atrium from the outside of the artificial blood vessel, all of which can help to reduce the possibility of post-operative surgery-related bleeding to the lowest. Considering the unfavorable effects of long-time CPB and deep hypothermia on coagulation, tranexamic acid was preventively administrated before surgery, and prothrombin complex and fresh frozen plasma were administrated after surgery to supplement coagulation factors. In addition, we rechecked the activated clotting time ACT after heparin neutralization by protamine to guide the dosage of protamine.

38.5.3 Postoperative Anesthetic Management

Like other aortic angioplasties, optimal aortic reconstruction and coronary artery treatment determine the patient's outcome. The key points of postoperative anesthetic management include postoperative bleeding management, sufficient coronary artery blood supply, and proactive cardiac function maintenance.

Generally, 1–2% of such patients have signs of preoperative myocardial infarction. Therefore, nitroglycerin, corticosteroid, and creatine phosphate can be used to ensure coronary artery blood supply, alleviate myocardial ischemia, and thus maintain necessary cardiac function after surgery. The positive inotropic drugs are mainly used to provide myocardial contractility and sufficient perfusion of important organs, which is very important for pediatric patients with preoperative left heart failure and insufficient perfusion of important organs.

Bicuspid aortic valve malformation is one of the most common risk factors for infective endocarditis. Therefore, active anti-infection after surgery is very helpful for preventing pulmonary infection and endocarditis.

38.6 Conclusion

In summary, the anesthetic management of the Bentall procedure for a child with bicuspid aortic valve and ascending aorta dilation requires adequate preoperative preparation and a comprehensive and in-depth understanding of the hemodynamic changes during the perioperative period. Brain protection during CPB, intensive cardiac and coagulation function monitoring, and management after surgery are the keys to ensuring the safety and success of the Bentall procedure in pediatric patients (Ming Zhu).

39 Anesthetic Management of Left Ventricular Outflow Tract Evacuation Surgery in a Child with Cardiac Rhabdomyosarcoma

Jiaping Zhang

Abstract

A 15-month-old male infant, who was found to have a cardiac mass during the fetal period, was re-examined after birth and showed cardiac rhabdomyoma (possible?). The mass gradually became larger with the growth and development, resulting in left ventricular outflow tract stenosis. He was scheduled for cardiac rhabdomyoma resection and left ventricular outflow tract evacuation surgery. When the left ventricular outflow tract is obstructed, the diastolic period is relatively shortened, the left ventricular myocardium becomes hypertrophy, the compliance at the end of diastole is reduced, the pressure at the end of diastole is increased, and the filling of the left ventricle is hindered. In addition, left ventricular myocardial hypertrophy can also lead to myocardial coronary vascular remodeling, resulting in a decrease in myocardial blood supply per unit volume, especially a reduction of endocardial blood supply. How to improve or maintain coronary blood supply as much as possible and reduce myocardial oxygen consumption is the focus of perioperative management.

J. Zhang (✉)
The National Children's Medical Center (Shanghai), Department of Anesthesiology of Shanghai Children's Medical Center, Shanghai Jiao Tong University School of Medicine, Shanghai, China
e-mail: zhangjiaping@scmc.com.cn

Cardiac rhabdomyoma is the second most common benign cardiac tumor after myxoma and the most common primary cardiac tumor in children. Most patients are not found until the cancer enlarges to cause cardiac cavity obstruction or valve orifice obstruction, thereby affecting normal cardiac function, which increases the risk of surgery and anesthesia. This chapter reports the anesthetic management of a case of cardiac rhabdomyoma with left ventricular outflow tract obstruction undergoing cardiac tumor resection and left ventricular outflow tract (LVOT) evacuation surgery.

39.1 Case Presentation

The patient was a 15-month-old boy with a weight of 12.5 kg. During routine prenatal check-ups, a possible cardiac mass was detected in the fetus. Further echocardiography after birth confirmed the presence of a cardiac mass, possibly a rhabdomyoma. During the follow-up, the child showed no cyanosis, growth and development delay, feeding difficulties, history of recurrent respiratory infections, or decreased activity. This examination revealed a cardiac tumor occupying the LVOT and mild aortic valve regurgitation.

Physical examination: The child was conscious without obvious abnormalities in mental response. There was no cyanosis in the lips and extremities. Auscultation revealed slightly coarse

J. Zheng et al. (eds.), *Selected Pediatric Cardiovascular Surgery Anesthesia Cases*,
https://doi.org/10.1007/978-981-96-5614-1_39

breath sounds in both lungs, but no dry or wet rales were heard. Strong heart sounds, regular heart rhythm, and grade II systolic murmur heard between the second and third ribs on the left edge of the sternum. There was no obvious enlargement of the liver and spleen. The pulse oxygen saturation (SpO_2) was 99% with air breathing.

Laboratory tests: LDH 670 U/L (elevated), neuron-specific enolase 33.8 ng/mL (elevated). Normal liver, kidney, and coagulation function.

Echocardiography: Cardiac tumor (occupying LVOT), mild aortic valve regurgitation, LVOT velocity 1.43 m/s, left ventricular ejection fraction (LVEF) 64.35%, left ventricular fractional shortening (LVFS) 33.79%.

Electrocardiogram (ECG): Normal sinus rhythm.

Preoperative diagnosis: Cardiac tumor (occupying LVOT), elective cardiac tumor resection surgery.

Thoracic CT scan (plain scan + enhancement): LVOT was occupied by a mass (rhabdomyoma), LVOT stenosis. Due to the gradually increasing trend found during follow-up, the child was admitted for further diagnosis and treatment.

Anesthesia process: No preoperative medication was given. After entering the operating room, ECG, non-invasive blood pressure (BP), and SpO_2 were monitored: BP 102/52 mm Hg, heart rate (HR) 145 beats/min, SpO_2 99%. After peripheral venous access was established, midazolam 1.2 mg, etomidate 2.0 mg, sufentanil 25 μg, and rocuronium 10 mg were intravenously administered for induction of anesthesia. After the eyelash reflex disappeared, an ID 4.0 mm cuffed endotracheal tube was intubated under direct laryngoscopy. The tube depth was 12 cm. Ventilation was controlled in PCV-VG mode with an oxygen flow rate of 1 L/min, fraction of inspired oxygen (FiO_2) of 50%, tidal volume (VT) of 120 mL, ventilation frequency of 20 times/min, and inspiratory time to expiratory time (I:E) ratio of 1:2. After intubation, right radial artery right internal jugular vein were quickly catheterized for continuous artery blood pressure (ABP) and central venous pressure monitoring. The initial CVP was 7 cm H_2O. The left femoral vein was accessed for fluid infusion, and 4.0 mL/kg of acetic acid Ringer's solution was quickly infused. During the operation, propofol 4.0 mg/(kg·h), sufentanil 2.0 μg/(kg·h), and rocuronium bromide 0.6 mg/(kg·h) were intravenously infused, and sevoflurane was intermittently inhaled to maintain the bispectral index between 40 and 60. Before the operation, tranexamic acid 10 mg/kg and Ulinastatin 120,000 U were intravenously given for antifibrinolytic and anti-inflammatory. After thoracotomy, heparin 3.0 mg/kg was intravenously given, and cardiopulmonary bypass (CPB)began after ACT >480 s.

During the operation, a tumor-like protrusion with a diameter of 1.2 cm × 1.2 cm was seen in the LVOT, which was partially adhered to the left coronary valve of the aorta. The tumor was separated and removed. The aortic valve was also explored. After the aorta cross-clamp was released, the heart automatically returned to sinus rhythm. Transesophageal ultrasound: No residual obstruction, mild aortic valve regurgitation, better than before the operation. After the vena cava cross-clamp was released, dopamine 5.0 μg/(kg·min) and epinephrine 0.03 μg/(kg·min) were intravenously infused. BP was maintained at 86/55 mm Hg, HR at 150 beats/min. After weaning off CPB, the blood pressure was stable. After ultrafiltration, protamine and thrombin were intravenously dripped to neutralize heparin and assisted hemostasis. Postoperative blood gas: pH 7.44, PaO_2 294.6 mm Hg, $PaCO_2$ 33.1 mm Hg, BE −1.55 mmol/L, HCT 32.6%, serum potassium 3.3 mmol/L, serum calcium 1.07 mmol/L, lactate 1.6 mmol/L, Hb 11.8 g/dL, HCT 32.6%. Intravenous supplement of potassium chloride 100 mg, calcium gluconate 200 mg, and autologous blood 50 mL. The intraoperative frozen section showed rhabdomyoma.

39.2 Postoperative Outcome

The operation lasted a total of 140 min, with normothermic cardiopulmonary bypass for 42 min and aortic cross-clamping for 19 min. The estimated blood loss was about 50 mL; 150 mL of acetic acid Ringer's solution and

50 mL of autologous blood were infused during the operation. The urine output was 100 mL. When leaving the room, vital signs are BP 91/50 mm Hg, HR 146 beats/min, SpO_2 100%, CVP 7 cm H_2O. After the operation, the patient was transferred to the Cardiac Intensive Care Unit (CICU) with ABP, ECG, and SpO_2 monitoring. The endotracheal tube was removed on the second day after surgery. The patient was discharged from the CICU on the fifth day after surgery and discharged from the hospital on the 8th day after surgery. Pathology report: The tumor in the LVOT was consistent with rhabdomyoma.

39.3 Review of Knowledge Points

39.3.1 Cardiac Rhabdomyoma

Rhabdomyoma accounts for 60% of cardiac tumors in newborns and infants. Some cases are diagnosed during the fetal period. Since they are formed from multiple embryonic layers, they are often considered as hamartomas rather than true neoplasms, possibly derived from embryonic cardiac myocytes. Rhabdomyomas are scattered nodular gray or yellowish-white masses ranging in size from 0.5 to 2.5 cm. They lack a true tumor capsule but are benign lesions. 90% of cases are multifocal, with a few being solitary. Rhabdomyomas often penetrate deep into the myocardial tissue or protrude into the heart chamber, causing obstruction of the heart chamber or obstruction of the valve orifice at the corresponding site, thereby affecting cardiac function. Changes in cardiac rhythm can occur when the primary mass involves the conduction bundle.

Intracavitary rhabdomyomas with significant symptoms have surgical indications. Surgery is not recommended for infants with no symptoms or only mild symptoms. The principle of surgical treatment is to relieve obstructive symptoms, protect ventricular and valve function, and prevent damage to the conduction bundle. Although rhabdomyomas have no capsule, they have clear boundaries, and surgical removal can be complete. Surgery is difficult when the tumor involves the main branches of the coronary arteries, the annulus, or the conduction system. There are reports of successful surgical removal of cardiac rhabdomyoma in neonates a few days after birth. However, not all patients have surgical indications. Fenoglio and others divided patients into three prognostic groups: The first group is stillbirths or deaths within 24 h after birth, with the main damage inside the heart, possibly dying from cardiac blood flow obstruction, accounting for the majority of those unfavorable for surgery. The second group is another extreme situation: patients with no clinical findings attributed to the heart, dying from noncardiac causes; these patients often have nodular sclerosis but rarely need treatment due to lack of intracavitary damage. The third group is tumors that are not large enough to cause death but extensive enough to cause cardiac symptoms and signs. These lesions are favorable for diagnosis, and patients are suitable for treatment. Foster and others recommend surgical removal of intracavitary obstructions causing hemodynamic damage. Still, they do not advocate for the removal of multiple intramural tumors to correct low cardiac output states because the tumors are benign, so only the intracavitary part is removed, and more thorough removal methods are not advocated, with long-term follow-up supporting the effectiveness of this approach.

The natural course varies greatly among individuals. It was previously believed that newborns or infants with cardiac rhabdomyoma would die from congestive heart failure or sudden death. Many asymptomatic patients may not be detected in early life, and there is evidence that rhabdomyomas do not undergo mitosis after birth, with a few reports of spontaneous regression of the tumor. In fact, the tumor's size and its growth location determine the course and possible outcomes. Because these tumors are often multifocal and extensive, the long-term effects are poor, and surgery is difficult to be effective.

39.4 Discussion

39.4.1 Preoperative Assessment and Preparation

The preoperative assessment and preparation focus on determining the size and location of cardiac rhabdomyoma, the obstruction of the cardiac chamber or valve orifice, and cardiac function. In this case, the cardiac rhabdomyoma was located at the LVOT with narrowed LVOT. The anesthetic management should focus on stabilizing hemodynamics and maintaining myocardial contractility during the perioperative period. Preoperative preparation includes a thorough understanding of the medical history and an accurate assessment of surgical anesthesia risk. For this patient, we focused on echocardiography, electrocardiogram, CT, MRI, and related laboratory tests and assessed the child's cardiac function status and anesthesia risk. In this case, the cardiac rhabdomyoma caused the narrowing of LVOT; the flow rate was 1.43 m/s in the left ventricular outflow tract, which could easily cause hemodynamic fluctuations during surgery, so vasoactive drugs should be prepared.

39.4.2 Intraoperative Anesthetic Management

In this case, it is better to follow the principle of pediatric cardiac anesthesia during the induction and maintenance of anesthesia. All of the selected anesthetics have the minimal impact on the cardiac function. Anesthesia was induced with intravenous midazolam, etomidate, sufentanil, and rocuronium and maintained with propofol, sufentanil, and rocuronium during surgery. Sevoflurane concentration was adjusted based on the BIS value to maintain a stable heart rate and blood pressure while ensuring the depth of anesthesia.

LVOT obstruction not only prolongs the systolic time but also correspondingly shortens the diastolic filling time and reduces left ventricular filling. Long-term LVOT obstruction can cause left ventricular hypertrophy, which, on the one hand, reduces end-diastolic compliance and increases end-diastolic pressure, further reducing left ventricular filling. On the other hand, increased systolic pressure increases myocardial oxygen consumption. In addition, ventricular hypertrophy leads to coronary vascular remodeling and coronary vessel reduction per unit volume, which reduces the myocardial blood supply per unit volume, especially the endocardial blood supply, due to the increased distance of endocardial vessels. Therefore, perioperative management should focus on optimizing coronary blood supply and reducing myocardial oxygen consumption. We have made the following adjustments:

1. Heart rate: The decrease in heart rate can prolong the diastolic time and reduce the myocardial oxygen consumption. Still, a heart rate that is too low can easily lead to a decrease in cardiac output due to the narrowed LVOT. Therefore, it is better to maintain the heart rate at the normal baseline level during surgery. In this case, the heart rate was maintained at around 120 beats per minute.
2. Heart rhythm: Due to decreased left ventricular compliance, the left ventricular end-diastolic volume mainly depends on the increase of left atrium contraction (30–40%). Therefore, maintaining normal sinus cardiac rhythm is particularly important for hemodynamic stability. Atrial fibrillation, ventricular fibrillation, and ventricular tachycardia should be avoided.
3. Preload: Higher left ventricular contractibility and sufficient volume load are required to maintain normal cardiac output due to the obstruction of LVOT. Therefore, patients with LVOT are very sensitive to fluid volume deficiency. As mentioned above, the left ventricular end-diastolic volume also depends on the contraction of the left atrium. Therefore, a slightly higher preload should be maintained

during surgery to avoid a severe decrease in blood pressure and volume preload associated with anesthesia, volume deficiency, drugs, etc. Hypotension can cause myocardial blood supply insufficiency and, in turn, exacerbates the vicious cycle of hypotension. In this case, appropriate volume replacement was given after induction to correct the fasting-related volume deficiency.

4. Afterload: The afterload in patients with LVOT is relatively increased and fixed. Therefore, coronary perfusion pressure should be maintained, and low diastolic pressure should be prevented or avoided.
5. Myocardial contractility: During the compensatory period of a patient with LVOT, the myocardial contractility is usually normal or even a little higher than normal. Small doses of positive inotropic drugs may be useful for patients with congestive heart failure, but the increase in myocardial oxygen consumption should be avoided. In this case, a large dose of fentanyl-based anesthesia method was chosen to reduce the dose of sedative drugs under BIS monitoring, alleviate the inhibitory effect of anesthetic drugs on the cardiovascular system, and make hemodynamics more stable.
6. Use of drugs: Hypotension before bypass can be treated with small doses of α receptor agonists such as norepinephrine. Although the obstruction of LVOT is relieved after CPB, positive inotropic drugs may still be needed to enhance myocardial contractility due to the impact of CPB. Dopamine 3.0–5.0 μg/(kg·min) and epinephrine 0.01–0.1 μg/(kg·min) are reasonable choices.

39.4.3 Anesthetic Management After CPB

The patient's hemodynamics were relatively stable during the induction and maintenance of anesthesia; considering the patient's young age, dopamine 5.0 μg/(kg·min) and epinephrine 0.03 μg/(kg·min) were still given intravenously to enhance myocardial contractility after CPB.

39.5 Conclusion

This case mainly focused on anesthetic management of an infant's left ventricular outflow tract obstruction. Maintaining appropriate myocardial contractility and avoiding severe hypotension and tachycardia during surgery can effectively balance myocardial oxygen supply and demand and prevent myocardial ischemia and hypoxia (Jiaping Zhang).

40 Anesthetic Management of Right Ventricular Outflow Tract Obstruction Relieving Surgery in a Child with Right Ventricular Myocardial Hemangioma

Jiaping Zhang

Abstract

A 6-year-old boy was found to have a heart murmur during a clinic visit for a fever. Echocardiography indicated a mass in the right ventricle (possible tumor) and right ventricular outflow tract obstruction (RVOTO). He was scheduled for cardiac tumor resection and right ventricular outflow tract (RVOT) relieving surgery. The postoperative pathology result indicated myocardial hemangioma. RVOTO can increase the right ventricular afterload and cause secondary myocardial hypertrophy and cardiac dysfunction. Severe RVOTO can result in hypoxemia due to reduced pulmonary blood flow. The anesthetic management of such children should focus on reducing the right ventricular afterload, maintaining sufficient preload, and preserving cardiac function.

Primary cardiac tumors in children are relatively rare, with an autopsy incidence rate of 0.01–0.50%. Over 90% of primary cardiac tumors are benign. Almost half of the tumors are rhabdomyomas, followed by fibromas, intrapericardial teratomas, myxomas, and hemangiomas. Cardiac hemangiomas are the least common primary cardiac tumors in children. The cancer's nature, size, and location determine the clinical symptoms and signs. There are currently no unified surgical indications for pediatric cardiac tumors. For children with significant blood flow obstruction, arrhythmia, and malignant cardiac tumors, surgical treatment is necessary. This chapter reports the anesthetic management of a child with right ventricular myocardial hemangioma for cardiac tumor resection and right ventricular outflow tract (RVOT) relieving surgery.

40.1 Case Presentation

The patient was a 6-year-old boy with a weight of 20 kg. He was brought to a local hospital for fever treatment 10 days ago. A heart murmur was found during a physical examination. Echocardiography indicated hypertrophic obstructive cardiomyopathy. The fever subsided after 3 days of anti-infective therapy. Upon further inquiry into the medical history, the child had chest pain after exercise, which was not clearly described, but it could be relieved after rest. There was no obvious decrease in exercise tolerance, no wheezing or shortness of breath, and normal growth and development. He was admitted to our cardiology ward for further diag-

J. Zhang (✉)
The National Children's Medical Center (Shanghai), Department of Anesthesiology of Shanghai Children's Medical Center, Shanghai Jiao Tong University School of Medicine, Shanghai, China
e-mail: zhangjiaping@scmc.com.cn

J. Zheng et al. (eds.), *Selected Pediatric Cardiovascular Surgery Anesthesia Cases*,
https://doi.org/10.1007/978-981-96-5614-1_40

nosis and treatment, with the primary diagnosis of hypertrophic cardiomyopathy.

Physical examination: The child was conscious and had a normal mental response. Coarse breath sounds in both lungs without rales. The heart rhythm was regular, the heart sounds were strong, and a grade III blowing systolic murmur could be heard at the 2–3 intercostal spaces on the left edge of the sternum. The pulse oxygen saturation (SpO_2) was 99% with room air.

Laboratory tests: NT-pro BNP 141 pg/mL. Normal Liver, kidney, and coagulation function.

Echocardiography: Moderate echo mass (possible tumor) in the right ventricular cavity. Ventricular septum thickening. RVOT obstruction (pressure difference 31 mm Hg). Normal left heart systolic function. No pericardial effusion.

Electrocardiogram (ECG): Sinus bradycardia, incomplete right bundle branch block, right ventricular hypertrophy, high and pointed T waves in some leads.

Cardiac magnetic resonance: A mass extending from the right ventricular anterior wall to the ventricular septum, rich blood supply, sarcoma (possible).

Preoperative diagnosis: Cardiac tumor, RVOT obstruction. The patient was transferred to the cardiothoracic surgery ward for elective cardiac tumor resection and RVOT relieving surgery.

40.2 Anesthetic Management

The patient did not take any preoperative medications. After entering the operating room, ECG, noninvasive blood pressure (BP), and SpO_2 were routinely monitored: BP 117/72 mm Hg, heart rate (HR) 115 beats/min, SpO_2 99%. After the peripheral venous access was established, 2.0 mg of midazolam, 6.0 mg of etomidate, 40 μg of sufentanil, and 12 mg of rocuronium were intravenously administered for the induction of anesthesia. After the eyelash reflex disappeared, an ID 5.0 mm cuffed tracheal tube was intubated under direct laryngoscopy with a depth of 15 cm. Pressure-controlled ventilation-volume guaranteed mode was used for mechanical ventilation with the following parameters: oxygen flow rate 1 L/min, fraction of inspired oxygen (FiO_2) 50%, tidal volume (VT) 160 mL, respiration rate (RR) 20 times/min, and inspiratory to expiratory (I:E) time ratio 1:2. Preoperative blood gas analysis time: pH 7.44, PaO_2 77.9 mm Hg, $PaCO_2$ 31.6 mm Hg, BE −1.5 mmol/L, Hb 12.5 g/dL, HCT 38.5%, serum potassium 4.6 mmol/L, serum calcium 1.27 mmol/L, lactate 1.3 mmol/L. The FiO_2 and ventilator parameters were adjusted based on the blood gas analysis results.

After endotracheal intubation, the left radial artery and the right internal jugular vein were quickly catheterized for artery blood pressure (ABP) and central venous pressure (CVP) monitoring, respectively. The CVP value was 11 cm H_2O. The left femoral vein was accessed for rapid fluid replacement. During the operation, propofol 4.0 mg/(kg·h), sufentanil 2.0 μg/(kg·h), and rocuronium 0.6 mg/(kg·h) were intravenously infused by an intravenous pump, and sevoflurane was intermittently inhaled to maintain Bispectral Index (BIS) at 40–60. Before the skin incision, 10 mg/kg of tranexamic acid and 200,000 U of Ulinastatin were intravenously administered. After the sternum was opened, 3.0 mg/kg of heparin was intravenously given. Cardiopulmonary bypass (CPB) began after ACT >480 s.

During the operation, a right ventricular mass below the anterior leaflet of the tricuspid valve was seen, which was tightly connected to the surrounding myocardium. The right ventricular outflow tract was partially obstructed due to the mass. The mass at RVOT was partially resected to improve RVOT's blood flow. After the aortic cross-clamping was released, the heart automatically resumed heart beating and sinus rhythm. Transesophageal echocardiography indicated no residual obstruction. Mechanical ventilation was resumed after the vena cava cross-clamping was released. Dopamine 5.0 μg/(kg·min) was intravenously infused to maintain ABP around 80/50 mm Hg and heart rate around 120 beats/min. CPB was smoothly weaned off. Protamine was intravenously given to neutralize heparin based on the dosage ratio of 1:1. Approximately 1 U of thrombin was used to assist hemostasis. Postoperative blood gas analysis results: pH 7.51, PaO_2 304 mm Hg, $PaCO_2$ 28 mm Hg, BE 0.4 mmol/L, Hb 11.5 g/dL, HCT 35.3%, serum potassium 4.3 mmol/L, serum calcium 1.08 mmol/L, lactate 1.1 mmol/L. Two hundred milligram of calcium gluconate was intravenously infused.

40.3 Postoperative Outcome

The operation lasted 120 min in total, with normothermic CBP for 34 min and aortic cross-clamping for 15 min. The estimated blood loss was about 50 mL. The urine output was 100 mL. Ringer's acetate solution 250 mL autologous salvaged blood 50 mL, and frozen plasma 100 mL was intravenously infused. Upon leaving the operating room, ABP was 96/57 mm Hg, HR was 128 beats/min, SpO_2 was 100%, and CVP was 11 cm H_2O. The patient was transported to the Cardiac Intensive Care Unit (CICU) with endotracheal intubation after the operation. The endotracheal tube was removed on the postoperative day 2. The patient was discharged from the CICU on postoperative day 3 and transferred back to the Department of Cardiology on postoperative day 7 for fever treatment. The patient was discharged from the hospital on the postoperative day 25. Pathological results: proliferative vascular components were seen between the striated muscles with irregular and unevenly thickened vessel walls. The endothelial cells showed no obvious atypia, which was consistent with intramuscular hemangioma. Hemangioma components were seen at the edge of the biopsy tissue.

40.4 Review of Knowledge Points

40.4.1 Cardiac Hemangioma

Cardiac hemangiomas are extremely rare and are usually characterized by benign vascular tumors or malformations composed of matured vessels. They are divided into three types based on their histological characteristics: nonspecific type hemangiomas, capillary hemangiomas, and cavernous hemangiomas. The capillary hemangiomas are composed of small, thin-walled vessels, which often originate or cluster around larger nourishing vessels. Cavernous hemangiomas are frequently located in the myocardial walls, with large, dilated vascular lumens, uneven wall thickness, and widespread blood pools. Nonspecific type hemangiomas usually lack the typical structure of capillary and cavernous hemangiomas, which are typically composed of a mixture of malformed arteriovenous structures. Therefore, nonspecific type hemangiomas are also called arteriovenous malformations.

Cardiac hemangiomas can occur in any heart chamber. They appear as multiple anechoic areas within the myocardium on two-dimensional echocardiography. Similar to pericardial teratomas, these tumors often coexist with serous pericardial effusion. Although most of these benign tumors are found incidentally, some can cause arrhythmias or obstructive symptoms. Any size of asymptomatic hemangiomas can be followed up with a series of echocardiograms, but small, well-defined, symptomatic hemangiomas still need to be surgically removed. Furthermore, for those symptomatic hemangiomas with diffuse involvement of the myocardium, a heart transplant may even be required.

40.5 Discussion

40.5.1 Preoperative Assessment and Preparation

The size and location of cardiac hemangiomas determine the severity of the disease. Common complications include arrhythmia, ventricular outflow tract obstruction, valvular diseases, cardiac dysfunction, cardiogenic shock, and heart failure caused by tumor rupture. Cardiac hemangiomas can also cause restrictive cardiac dysfunction due to the pericardial effusion.

In this case, the preoperative cardiac ultrasound indicated a mass in the right ventricular cavity with RVOT obstruction. ECG and NT-pro BNP indicated right ventricular dysfunction. All of these suggested that the patient needs to be surgically treated.

40.5.2 Intraoperative Management of Anesthesia

RVOT obstruction increases the afterload of the right ventricle and causes secondary hypertrophy, further exacerbating RVOT obstruction. On the other hand, with the worsening of RVOT obstruction, pulmonary blood flow decreases, and the balance of ventilation–perfusion ratio is impaired. In the end, hypoxemia occurs.

The goal of anesthetic management is to reduce the right ventricular afterload and increase the right ventricular forward blood flow by lowering PVR, including increasing FiO_2, moderate hyperventilation, and lower mean airway pressure. Hypoxia, acidosis, and sympathetic excitement will significantly increase pulmonary vascular resistance. During the operation, an appropriate depth of anesthesia should be maintained to avoid sympathetic excitement. It is better to maintain a higher PaO_2 and $PaCO_2$ at 30–35 mm Hg through ventilation management.

Furthermore, sufficient blood volume is necessary to maintain the left ventricular preload and avoid aggravating the RVOT obstruction.

For those patients with right ventricular hypertrophy, blood pressure should be maintained within the normal range to avoid myocardial ischemia caused by hypotension.

40.5.3 Anesthetic Management of Post-cardiopulmonary Bypass

Reducing pulmonary vascular resistance after surgery is also necessary since the right ventricular afterload must still be reduced. In addition, positive inotropic drugs may be needed to support the right ventricular function. Dobutamine 5–10 μg/(kg·min) or dopamine 5–10 μg/(kg·min) does not increase PVR while providing strong positive inotropic support. Milrinone can also be considered since it can increase cardiac contractility, improve myocardial diastolic function, and reduce PVR.

In addition, surgery itself may cause arrhythmia or conduction block. A permanent pacemaker may occasionally be needed.

40.6 Conclusion

The anesthetic management of children with right ventricular hemangiomas and RVOT obstruction should focus on the reduction of right ventricular afterload and the maintenance of sufficient preload. The cardiac function should be actively supported after the surgically removes the tumor, and the RVOT obstruction is relieved (Jiaping Zhang).

Anesthetic Management of Cardiac Tumor Resection in a Child with Left Atrial Myxoma

41

Jianwei Zhang

Abstract

A 6-year-old boy presented with lethargy and reduced physical endurance. He was diagnosed with left atrial myxoma (LAM) and mitral regurgitation and scheduled for cardiac tumor resection under general anesthesia. LAM often causes mitral obstruction, regurgitation, left heart failure, and secondary pulmonary hypertension. The key to anesthetic management of this surgery should focus on the cardiac function and timely detection and treatment of arrhythmias.

Cardiac myxoma is a type of primary cardiac tumor. Around 82–90% of primary cardiac tumors in children are benign. Among them, rhabdomyomas are the most common cardiac tumors, which account for 50.7%, and myxomas account for 21.5%. Over 75% of myxomas originate in the left atrium, located at the edge of the mitral valve annulus or the oval fossa of the atrial septum, 20% of myxomas originate in the right atrium, and 5% of myxomas originate in the ventricles. The clinical manifestations of myxomas vary widely due to the fact that they may grow and protrude into the heart chamber and their fragile tissue characteristics. They can often lead to acute hemodynamic changes and peripheral vascular embolism, which pose great challenges to perioperative management and usually require special attention. This chapter reports the anesthetic management of cardiac tumor resection surgery in a child with left atrial myxoma and mitral regurgitation.

J. Zhang (✉)
The National Children's Medical Center (Shanghai), Department of Anesthesiology of Shanghai Children's Medical Center, Shanghai Jiao Tong University School of Medicine, Shanghai, China
e-mail: zhangjianwei@scmc.com.cn

41.1 Case Presentation

A 6-year and 8-month-old boy was 21.0 kg in weight. He was naturally born at full term without a history of asphyxia at birth. Echocardiography showed left atrial myxoma and mitral regurgitation. He was admitted to the ward with "left atrial myxoma (LAM) and mitral regurgitation (MR)."

Physical examination: The boy's general condition was normal, with clear consciousness and a good mental state. The bilateral lung sounds were symmetrical without rales. Heart sounds were powerful and rhythmic, and II/VI murmurs could be heard in the precordial area. P2 was not hyperactive. The abdomen was soft, and the extremities were warm.

Laboratory tests: Routine blood test: C-reactive protein (CRP) 3 mg/L, white blood cell (WBC) 8.87×10^9/L, neutrophils 55.8%, red

J. Zheng et al. (eds.), *Selected Pediatric Cardiovascular Surgery Anesthesia Cases*,
https://doi.org/10.1007/978-981-96-5614-1_41

blood cell count (RBC) 5.22 × 10^{12}/L, hemoglobin (Hb) 131 g/L, platelet count 137 × 10^9/L.

Liver and kidney function: Serum total bilirubin (TBIL) 18.7 μmol/L, direct bilirubin (DBIL) 8.6 μmol/L, alanine transaminase (ALT) 80 IU/L, blood urea nitrogen (BUN) 9.3 mmol/L.

Coagulation function: Activated partial thromboplastin time (APTT) 26.6 s, prothrombin time (PT) 20.5 s, antithrombin (AT) 74.0%.

N terminal pro B type natriuretic peptide (NT-ProBNP) 6254 pg/mL, procalcitonin 3.67 ng/mL.

Echocardiography: ① There was a mass in the left atrium with a size of 5 cm (length) × 2.2 cm and attached to the left atrial side of the atrial septum at the base. The mass swung with large ranges during the cardiac cycle and could protrude into the left ventricle during diastole. ② Mitral valve forward flow speed 1.75 m/s, moderate regurgitation, 2 streams of regurgitation with the wider one 0.44 cm. ③ Mild to moderate tricuspid valve regurgitation (TR) with the wider one 0.32 cm, negative aortic valve regurgitation.

Preoperative diagnosis: LAM, MR, tricuspid regurgitation (TR). Elective cardiac tumor resection surgery was scheduled.

41.2 Anesthetic Management

The patient did not take any preoperative medications. After entering the operating room, the vital signs were routinely monitored before anesthesia with noninvasive blood pressure (BP) 115/80 mm Hg, heart rate (HR) 115 beats/min, and pulse oxygen saturation (SpO_2) 97%. Anesthesia was induced with intravenous bolus doses of 1.0 mg midazolam, 6.0 mg etomidate, 40 μg sufentanil, and 15 mg rocuronium. An ID 5.5 mm cuffed endotracheal tube was intubated under a visual laryngoscope with a tube depth of 16 cm. Pressure-controlled ventilation-volume guaranteed (PCV-VG) mode was used with respiratory parameters setting as oxygen flow rate 1 L/min, fraction of inspired oxygen (FiO_2) 50%, tidal volume (VT)150 mL, respiratory rate (RR) 20 breaths/min, and inspiratory to expiratory time (I:E) ratio 1:2. During the operation, the end-tidal carbon dioxide partial pressure ($ETCO_2$) was maintained at 35–40 mm Hg by adjustment of RR and VT. During induction, there was no significant change in the child's vital signs. After anesthesia induction, the right radial artery and left internal jugular vein were catheterized under ultrasound guidance to continuously monitor invasive blood pressure (ABP) and central venous pressure (CVP).During the operation, general anesthesia was maintained by continuous intravenous infusion of 5.0 mg/(kg·h) propofol, 2.5 μg/(kg·h) sufentanil, and 0.6 mg/(kg·h)rocuronium combined with 1% sevoflurane inhalation. The operation was performed under cardiopulmonary bypass (CPB) support. A 6 cm × 6 cm mucinous tissue was seen through the atrial septal incision, which was removed. Then the atrial septal defect was closed. The heart automatically resumed beating and sinus rhythm after aortic cross-clamp release. Dopamine and epinephrine were infused at 5.0 μg/(kg·min) and 0.05 μg/(kg·min), respectively. ABP was maintained at 90–100/50–55 mm Hg, HR at 100 beats/min, SpO_2 at 99%, and CVP at 6 cm H_2O. The child's vital signs were kept stable, and then he was successfully weaned off CPB.

41.3 Postoperative Outcome

The operation lasted for 155 min in total, with an estimated blood loss of about 50 mL and a urine output of 60 mL. A total of 200 mL of sodium acetate Ringer's solution and 50 mL of red blood cells were transfused. Postoperative blood gas analysis results showed: pH 7.4, PaO_2 78 mm Hg, $PaCO_2$ 45 mm Hg, BE 1.4 mmol/L, HCT 37.2%, K^+ 3.8 mmol/L, Ca^{2+} 0.9 mmol/L, Lac 1.7 mmol/L. After the operation, the child was transferred to the Cardiac Intensive Care Unit (CICU) under the monitoring of ABP, ECG, and SpO_2 with endotracheal intubation. The postoperative pathology indicated a left atrial mucinous tumor. The endotracheal tube was successfully removed on postoperative day 6, and the patient was discharged from the CICU on postoperative day 3 and from the hospital on postoperative day 7.

41.4 Review of Knowledge Points

Atrial myxoma is a type of primary cardiac tumor. The exact cause is still unclear. About 10% of myxomas are autosomal dominant inherited diseases, namely Carney's syndrome (a syndrome composed of myxoma, skin pigmentation, and multiple endocrine tumors). At the same time, the remaining cases seem to be sporadic. It originates from mesenchymal cells under the endocardium with multidirectional differentiation potential.

Histological manifestation: Characteristic star-shaped and spindle-shaped cells exist on the acidic mucopolysaccharide matrix with oval nuclei and thin-walled capillaries around them. As the tumor grows, it protrudes into the heart like a polypoid mass, often with a tumor pedicle attached to the atrial septum or atrial wall, and the tumor moves with the cardiac cycle.

Clinical manifestation: The clinical manifestations of atrial myxoma vary greatly, from asymptomatic to life-threatening, depending on the size, location, and activity of the tumor. The main manifestations are hemodynamic changes, peripheral vascular embolism, and systemic symptoms. Left atrial myxoma often causes mitral valve obstruction, regurgitation, left heart failure, and secondary pulmonary hypertension. Therefore, once cardiac myxoma is diagnosed, surgery should be performed as soon as possible to avoid embolism and sudden death.

41.5 Discussion

41.5.1 Preoperative Assessment and Preparation

The aim of anesthetic management for children with atrial myxoma is to maintain perioperative hemodynamic stability (e.g., prevent the tumor body from blocking the atrioventricular valve) and prevent thrombus shedding throughout the entire perioperative period.

Before surgery, the patient's condition should be thoroughly understood. If there are infections, poor heart function, etc., preoperative anti-infection, diuresis, improvement of heart function, etc. should be performed. Surgery should be performed when the child's symptoms and overall condition are improved. Knowing the special position that causes blood flow obstruction symptoms and the habitual position of self-relief is important. Do not change positions suddenly during surgery preparation, transferring, and moving the child, and always pay attention to changes in circulatory function. After entering the operating room, try to adopt their habitual position and continuously monitor the child's hemodynamic changes. If the tumor body blocks the mitral valve, immediately adopt the head-low right-side position to relieve the obstruction.

Preoperative preparation includes vasoactive drugs, defibrillation, and resuscitation equipment, etc. In addition, attention should be paid to the dosage of preoperative medication due to excessive preoperative medicines that may lead to severe hypoxemia if long-term pulmonary congestion and limited respiratory function exist. For this child, we focused on the preoperative symptoms and echocardiogram of the child and assessed the cardiac function status and anesthesia risks. The child had no preoperative valve obstruction and habitual body position, no thromboembolism symptoms, no infection, etc., and cardiac function level I. The diagnosis of the child's myxoma was clear, and the general condition was acceptable, so the surgery was carried out.

41.5.2 Anesthetic Management During Surgery

The induction of anesthesia in children with myxoma should be stable. The changes in position should be avoided as much as possible during the induction of anesthesia. Surgeons and CBP perfusionists should always be on standby in case of severe blood flow obstruction for emergency establishment of CBP. The anesthetics for induction with significant myocardial suppression should be avoided. Since most of the left atrium in this child was occupied by the tumor, the heart rate was very important to maintain the hemodynamic stability. A large dose of sufentanil may cause bradycardia, thus the dose should be appropriately reduced during induction. Suppose there is a dramatic drop in BP, a slowdown in HR, or a sharp rise in CVP during the operation which is not clearly related to anesthesia. In that case, it should be highly suspected that the mitral valve is obstructed, and action should be taken to lower the head and establish CBP as soon as possible. After the aortic cross-clamp is released, we should alert for arrhythmias and changes in the nervous system (such as pupil changes). During the operation, the fluid volume and speed should be controlled based on transesophageal echocardiography and CVP to avoid pulmonary edema and excessive blood volume caused by overhydration. In addition, respiratory management should be strengthened, and diuresis should be used when necessary to prevent edema. Also, hypoalbuminemia, anemia, arrhythmia, and electrolyte and acid–base balance disorders should be actively corrected. Transesophageal echocardiography and changes in the ST segment of the ECG can help early detection of coronary artery embolism. Electroencephalogram (EEG) monitoring can detect cerebral embolism early.

The method of anesthetic management in the present case refers to the methods for pediatric cardiac surgery anesthesia. The selected drugs have little impact on the cardiac function. The induction of anesthesia was performed by intravenous injection of midazolam, etomidate, sufentanil, and rocuronium. General anesthesia was maintained by continuous infusion of propofol, sufentanil, rocuronium, and 0.6 MAC sevoflurane inhalation during the operation. The speed of propofol infusion was adjusted based on the changes in heart rate and blood pressure to maintain a stable heart rate and blood pressure while satisfying the depth of anesthesia. After induction, the radial artery and internal jugular vein catheterization were quickly established, routine ECG monitoring was conducted during the operation, and the changes in ABP and CVP were closely monitored. The operation went smoothly without significant hemodynamic changes, arrhythmias, or manifestations of myocardial ischemia. After the aortic cross-clamp was released, pupil changes, cerebral oxygen saturation, and ECG monitoring were checked carefully. No pupil abnormalities were found, and there were no signs and symptoms of cerebral and coronary ischemia. After the operation, the surgical effect, cardiac function status, and volume status were evaluated by transesophageal echocardiography.

In terms of extracorporeal circulation, cardiac myxoma in children is fragile and prone to embolism during venous catheterization or CBP. Therefore, in addition to installing an arterial micro-emboli filter during CBP, the blood reservoir with a micro-emboli filter should also be installed to filter the blood drawn back by the left and right heart suction devices before entering the oxygenator. Because these children may have reduced levels and activity of plasma antithrombin III, they may develop heparin resistance. The ACT value may quickly drop due to the faster heparin metabolism during CBP, especially at the start of rewarming. Therefore, ACT should be closely monitored during surgery, and heparin should be added at times when the ACT value does not meet the standard. Fresh frozen plasma or antithrombin III should be given if necessary.

In terms of surgery, special attention should be paid to avoid the shedding of tumor fragments during the operation. The operation should be as gentle as possible, and strong touches and rough operations on the heart should be avoided. Before the left atrium is opened to remove the tumor, the mitral valve orifice should be blocked with saline gauze. When the tumor is removed, the fragments should be cleaned up in time. Any remaining tumor fragments should be checked after myxoma removal. Try to remove the tumor completely and rinse thoroughly with a large amount of physiological saline. If it is possible, the filters at both the arterial and venous ends (not placed in this case) should be placed. After the operation, the saline injection test and transesophageal echocardiography is used to evaluate the valve regurgitation. For those suspected of mitral valve insufficiency, the sizes of the mitral valve leaflets and orifice should be carefully checked during the operation and corrected simultaneously.

41.6 Conclusion

In summary, the clinical manifestations of children with atrial myxoma are diverse and varied. A thorough and detailed preoperative assessment should be performed before surgery. If it is diagnosed, preoperative preparations should be fully made, and surgery should be performed as soon as possible. During the operation, it is better to use drugs that have less impact on circulation and maintain hemodynamic stability under careful monitoring (Jianwei Zhang).

42 Anesthetic Management of Modified Morrow Surgery in a Child with Hypertrophic Obstructive Cardiomyopathy

Yingying Ji

Abstract

A 16-year-old girl with hypertrophic obstructive cardiomyopathy (HOCM) was admitted to our hospital for elective left ventricular outflow tract (LVOT) surgical myectomy. LVOT obstruction will be worsened by increased myocardial contractility, decreased ventricular volume, and lower blood pressure. Therefore, the key points of anesthetic management include inhibiting the myocardial contractility and increasing the preload and afterload to avoid LVOT obstruction.

Hypertrophic cardiomyopathy (HCM) is mainly characterized by asymmetric ventricular wall hypertrophy, often involving the interventricular septum, which usually results in a smaller ventricular cavity, reduced left ventricular blood filling, and decreased diastolic compliance. HOCM can be diagnosed when the interventricular septum is markedly hypertrophic, obstructs the LVOT, and causes a pressure gradient across the LVOT beyond 30 mm Hg. HOCM is a common cause of sudden death in young people and can lead to heart failure at any age. The patients with HOCM are at high perioperative risk, and the focus of anesthetic management is to avoid the exacerbation of LVOT obstruction.

42.1 Case Presentation

A 16-year-old girl with 69 kg in weight was born by cesarean section at full term without asphyxia. She was diagnosed with HCM 6 years ago due to shortness of breath and exercise intolerance. She has been followed up for a long period of time and has been taking propranolol to keep the disease under control. She felt that her shortness of breath after exercise had worsened, and her exercise tolerance had further decreased in the last 6 months. She was admitted to our hospital because the echocardiogram showed significant hypertrophy of ventricular septal and LVOT (pressure gradient >100 mm Hg).

Physical examination: The girl is lucid and in good spirits. Her heart rate (HR) is 80 beats/min, and her noninvasive blood pressure (BP) is 120/75 mm Hg. There is no cyanosis, but slightly coarse breath sounds are heard in bilateral lungs. A grade IV systolic murmur is heard between the second and fourth ribs at the left sternal border. There is no obvious enlargement of the liver and spleen. The extremities are warm without edema.

Laboratory tests: Routine blood tests, coagulation function, and liver and kidney function are unremarkable. NT-proBNP: 4336 pg/mL.

Y. Ji (✉)
The National Children's Medical Center (Shanghai), Department of Anesthesiology of Shanghai Children's Medical Center, Shanghai Jiao Tong University School of Medicine, Shanghai, China
e-mail: jiyingying@scmc.com.cn

J. Zheng et al. (eds.), *Selected Pediatric Cardiovascular Surgery Anesthesia Cases*,
https://doi.org/10.1007/978-981-96-5614-1_42

Electrocardiogram (ECG): Sinus rhythm, first-degree atrioventricular block, left atrial enlargement, biphasic T wave in avf lead.

Echocardiography: Significant thickening of both ventricular septal and ventricular walls, left ventricular outflow tract obstruction (pressure gradient >100 mm Hg), muscular ventricular septal defect (VSD), mild to moderate mitral regurgitation, normal left ventricular systolic function, impaired ventricular diastolic function, pericardial effusion.

Chest X-ray: Heart shadow enlargement, increased lung markings.

Cardiac MRI: Hypertrophic obstructive cardiomyopathy, multiple abnormal delayed twinning of the left ventricular myocardium, LVOT narrowed.

Preoperative diagnosis: HOCM, VSD. Modified Morrow surgery was scheduled.

42.2 Anesthetic Management

The girl did not take any preoperative medications. After she was transported to the operating room, routine monitoring included blood pressure, ECG, and pulse oxygen saturation (SpO_2). The peripheral vein and the left radial artery were catheterized before the induction of anesthesia. Basic vital signs: invasive arterial blood pressure (ABP) 132/70 mm Hg, HR 80 beats/min, and SpO_2 100%. Anesthesia was induced with intravenous bolus doses of 2.0 mg midazolam, 6.0 mg etomidate, 70 μg sufentanil, and 50 mg rocuronium. After losing the eyelash reflex, An ID 7.0 mm cuffed endotracheal tube was intubated under a visual laryngoscope, and the tube was fixed 22 cm away from the incisors. The girl was ventilated with pressure-controlled ventilation-volume guaranteed (PCV-VG) mode and ventilator parameters: gas flow rate 2 L/min, a fraction of inspired oxygen (FiO_2) 50%, tidal volume (VT) 380 mL, respiratory rate (RR) of 12 times/min, inspiratory to expiratory (I:E) time ratio of 1:2, positive end-expiratory pressure (PEEP) 4 cm H_2O. The end-tidal carbon dioxide ($ETCO_2$) was maintained at 35–40 mm Hg by adjusting VT and RR. The blood gas analysis results are shown in Table 42.1.

After the induction of anesthesia, the right great saphenous vein and the right internal jugular vein were catheterized. The central venous pressure (CVP), bispectral index (BIS), body temperature, and urine output were continuously monitored during the operation. General anesthesia was maintained by continuous intravenous infusion of 5.0 mg/(kg·h) propofol, 1.5 μg/(kg·h) sufentanil, 0.6 mg/(kg·h) rocuronium, and combined with sevoflurane inhalation. The sevoflurane concentration was adjusted to maintain the girl's HR at about 70 beats/min, ABP about 100/60 mm Hg, and BIS 40–60. Sodium acetate Ringer's solution 300 mL was infused to maintain CVP <12 cm H_2O.

After the establishment of CPB and aortic cross-clamp, it was found that the ventricular septum became significantly thick. The surgeon decided to perform the modified Morrow procedure. A parallel incision was made along the thickened ventricular septum below the right coronary valve towards the apex, removing the hypertrophic muscle bundle. After the aortic cross-clamp release, the heart automatically resumed beating and sinus rhythm. Transesophageal echocardiography (TEE) showed: The blood flow velocity in the left ventricular outflow tract was 2.5 m/s. The pressure gradient was 25.6 mm Hg, and the regurgitation of the second and third tricuspid valves was mild. HR was maintained at 83 beats/min and ABP at 103/55 mm Hg with dopamine infusion at 5.0 μg/(kg·min), norepinephrine at 0.05 μg/(kg·min). After ultrafiltration, protamine was intravenously given to neutralize heparin; intraoperative blood gas analysis results are shown in Table 42.1. According to the blood gas analysis results, 500 mg of calcium gluconate was given. Three hundred milliliter autologous salvaged blood, and 100 mL plasma was transfused. The sternum was closed after sufficient hemostasis.

Table 42.1 Intraoperative blood gas test results

Time point	Hb (g/dL)	HCT (%)	pH	PaO_2 (mm Hg)	$PaCO_2$ (mm Hg)	BE (mmol/L)	Na^+ (mmol/L)	K^+ (mmol/L)	Cl^- (mmol/L)	Ca^{2+} (mmol/L)	Lac (mmol/L)
After induction	12.5	39.4	7.4	156	33	2.6	136	3.7	107	1.1	1.2
After stopping extracorporeal	9.4	28.9	7.4	348	33	0.1	141	3.9	106	1.0	0.6

42.3 Postoperative Outcome

The operation lasted for 285 min in total, with a CPB time of 95 min and an aortic cross-clamp time of 67 min. The patient was intubated and transferred to the pediatric Cardiac Intensive Care Unit (CICU) with continuous infusion of vasoactive drugs and continuous monitoring of ABP and ECG. On the third postoperative day, low cardiac output and hypoxemia occurred. Extracorporeal membrane oxygenation (ECMO) was utilized to support the stability of hemodynamics. The severe arrhythmia was still persistent the next day, and it was difficult to maintain the hemodynamic stability. Due to multiple organ failures and abnormal dynamic EEG performance, her parents abandoned the treatment. At last, the patient died after ECMO was withdrawn.

42.4 Review of Knowledge Points

42.4.1 Pathophysiology of HCM

The ventricular septal hypertrophy leads to LVOT stenosis. Systolic anterior motion (SAM) of the anterior mitral caused by the venture effect can exacerbate stenosis or even obstruction. The degree of LVOT obstruction varies with cardiac beats in patients with HOCM. Myocardial hypertrophy reduces ventricular diastolic compliance and increases left ventricular end-diastolic pressure, which prevents left ventricular filling. Increased myocardial contractility and hypovolemia can exacerbate LVOT obstruction, so the key to anesthetic management is maintaining sinus rhythm and preload. In addition to LVOT obstruction and mitral regurgitation, the pathophysiology of HOCM may also include diastolic dysfunction, myocardial ischemia, and arrhythmias, all of which can have adverse implications during anesthesia and surgery.

42.4.2 Clinical Manifestations of HCM

The typical clinical signs of patients with HCM are associated with the LVOT obstruction. Cardiac auscultation reveals a systolic murmur between the apex of the heart and the left parasternal border. The murmur becomes stronger with the aggravation of LVOT obstruction, which commonly includes gesture changes from squatting, sitting, and supine gestures to standing gestures during the Valsalva maneuver and compensatory increase of myocardial contraction following the premature ventricular contractions or after the use of nitroglycerin.

42.4.3 Anatomy and Classification of HCM

HCM is a condition characterized by hypertrophy of the left ventricle. The most commonly hypertrophic site is an anterior septal basal segment and left ventricular anterior wall. It is possibly ascribed to genetic disorders. The peak pressure gradient over 30 mm Hg at rest was considered an LVOT obstruction.

42.4.4 Treatment of HCM

β-Receptor blockers and calcium channel blockers are the primary therapeutic medicines for patients with HCM. β-Blockers can reduce myocardial contractility, relieve ventricular outflow tract obstruction, and decrease myocardial oxygen consumption and heart rate. If the patients cannot tolerate β-blockers, calcium channel blockers can be recommended. Propafenone and amiodarone can be used to treat rapid arrhythmias.

Surgical treatment is recommended for those children with symptoms that are unresponsive to pharmacologic therapy and obstruction with gradients ≥50 mm Hg at rest or with physiologic provocation (exercise). Classical surgical therapies include the Morrow surgery, modified Morrow surgery, and interventional septal ablation. Numerous national and international cohort studies have confirmed that long-term survival time after the surgical treatment, including the classic Morrow surgery and the more commonly received modified Morrow surgery, is similar to that of the general population. Interventional septal ablation surgery is more appropriate for older children with uncomplicated left ventricular pathology, hypertrophy mainly confined to the basal septum, appropriate anatomy of the septal perforating arteries, and those who cannot tolerate or refuse surgery. Newer surgeries include percutaneous myocardial septal radiofrequency ablation and percutaneous puncture endocardial septal radiofrequency catheter ablation. Although these surgeries have the advantages of less trauma, faster recovery, and fewer complications, they are difficult to perform, and their long-term effects require further follow-up.

42.5 Discussion

42.5.1 Preoperative Assessment and Preparation

Patients with HOCM are commonly presented with exertional dyspnea, chest pain, palpitations, and syncope. Sudden cardiac death, heart failure, and thromboembolism are the three main causes of death in children. Sudden cardiac death is often associated with fatal arrhythmias. Every anesthesiologist should assess the cardiac function and anesthetic risks based on the patient's clinical symptoms, degree of obstruction, and history of arrhythmias. NYHA III, in this case, remains an important indicator for assessing the patient's cardiac function and treatment outcome. In addition to the present medical history, it is also necessary to know the patient's past medical history, including arrhythmia, syncope, and sudden death history in her family members. Preoperative echocardiography and MRI examination can help to find diastolic dysfunction and myocardial fibrosis, which is very important for an anesthesiologist to make an appropriate management plan to minimize the exacerbation or adverse outcomes.

It is recommended that the β-blockers should be continuously used to control heart rate and blood pressure before surgery. Prolonged fasting should be avoided as much as possible, and adequate fluids should be taken to avoid hypotension. At the same time, the preload reduction may reduce the left ventricular volume and increase the risk of ventricular outflow tract obstruction. Preoperative medication may be used if the child is anxious.

42.5.2 Intraoperative Anesthetic Management

In this case, arterial catheterization and ABP monitoring were established before the induction of anesthesia. Under continuous ABP monitoring, general anesthesia was induced by slowly titrating the use of sufentanil, etomidate, and rocuronium to reach a satisfactory depth of anesthesia for endotracheal intubation and avoid large heart rate fluctuations and blood pressure. Pretreatment with intravenous injection of metoprolol or esmolol can reduce the stress response caused by intubation. Vasopressors such as phenylephrine can be used to treat hypotension, improve myocardial perfusion, and relieve ventricular outflow tract obstruction. Anesthesia was maintained by continuous infusion of sufentanil, propofol, rocuronium, and sevoflurane inhalation. BIS was monitored to ensure the appropriate depth of anesthesia. Intraoperative anesthetic management aims to maintain sinus rhythm, adequate preload and afterload, as well as suppress sympathetic stimulation. Inadequate anesthesia, hypovolemia, tachycardia, and large hemodynamic fluctuations can exacerbate LVOT obstruction and should be avoided.

After the aortic cross-clamp release and the heartbeat resumes, it should be very careful to use agents with β-adrenergic activity, such as dopamine, dobutamine, or isoproterenol, due to their heart-racing effects. Acute episodes of atrial fibrillation should be immediately reversed with direct current cardioversion rather than pharmacologic rate control because the ventricular filling is mainly dependent on atrial contraction. TEE has been recommended for use in patients with HOCM before or after cardiac surgical procedures, which is useful in evaluating the degree of LVOT obstruction and mitral regurgitation. In addition, the monitoring of the intravascular status by measurement of inferior vena cava size and collapse conditions caused by inspiration combined with the assessment of myocardial contractibility can help to assess the ventricular preload and afterload, which are the two critical factors to prevent the exacerbation of LVOT obstruction. In this case, TEE was used to evaluate the surgical effect, cardiac function, and volume status to guide the use of vasoactive drugs and volume supplementation before successfully weaning off CBP.

The preoperative volume status in this patient was not evaluated by ultrasound, and the fluid replacement was also not guided by ultrasound. If the conditions permit, invasive monitoring such as pulmonary artery catheter and Pulse index Continuous Cardiac Output (PiCCO) should be used to assess the child's cardiac function and volume status.

42.6 Shortcomings and Limitations

The preoperative volume status in this patient was not evaluated by ultrasound, and the fluid replacement was also not guided by ultrasound. If the conditions permit, invasive monitoring such as pulmonary artery catheter and PICCO should be used to assess the child's cardiac function and volume status.

42.7 Conclusion

Due to the specific pathophysiology of HOCM, diastolic dysfunction, myocardial ischemia, arrhythmia, etc., complications are easy to occur during the perioperative period. The key to anesthetic management in patients with HOCM is to choose the anesthetic drugs that have the least effect on heart rate and blood pressure to use appropriate vasopressors, maintain intravascular volume and sinus rhythm, monitor continuously, and assess the tissue perfusion to avoid exacerbation of LVOT obstruction and minimize the perioperative adverse outcomes (Yingying Ji).

43 Anesthetic Management of Coronary Artery Transplantation in an Infant with Anomalous Left Coronary Artery from the Pulmonary Artery

Yunan Song

Abstract

A 9-month-old boy was diagnosed by echocardiography with anomalous origin of the left coronary artery from the pulmonary artery. The left ventricular ejection fraction was 22%. After coronary artery transplantation, low cardiac output developed, and a left ventricular artificial assist (LVAD) was urgently installed. Perioperative cardioprotection is particularly important for children with low cardiac function. With the recent development of extracorporeal circulation technology, LVAD has been increasingly used in children with severe postoperative low cardiac output and significantly reduces the early postoperative mortality in such children.

The anomalous left coronary artery from the pulmonary artery (ALCAPA) refers to a congenital malformation in which the left coronary artery abnormally originates from the pulmonary artery. In contrast, the right coronary artery normally arises from the aorta. It is the most common and clinically significant anomalous coronary artery origin type. The incidence is about 1/300,000, accounting for 0.25–0.5% of the total incidence of congenital heart disease. ALCAPA is classified into infantile and adult types. The clinical symptoms depend on the formation of collateral vessels between the left and right coronary arteries. This report described the anesthetic management of a case of infantile ALCAPA with preoperative low cardiac function undergoing coronary artery transplantation.

43.1 Case Presentation

The patient was a 9-month-old male with a height of 72 cm and a weight of 7.3 kg. He was diagnosed with a left coronary artery originating from the pulmonary artery after examination at a local hospital due to fever and cough. The child was delivered by cesarean section at 38 weeks +2 days of gestation with a birth weight of 2.85 kg and an unknown postnatal Apgar score. The child had a history of upper respiratory tract infection and pneumonia. He was on mixed feeding without feeding difficulties. He had shortness of breath after feeding, excessive sweating at ordinary times, and delayed weight gain.

Physical examination: Conscious, body temperature 37.1 °C, heart rate (HR) 158 beats/min, blood pressure (BP) 90/52 mm Hg, respiratory rate (RR) 25 times/min. No lips and extremities cyanosis.

Y. Song (✉)
The National Children's Medical Center (Shanghai), Department of Anesthesiology of Shanghai Children's Medical Center, Shanghai Jiao Tong University School of Medicine, Shanghai, China
e-mail: songyunan@scmc.com.cn

J. Zheng et al. (eds.), *Selected Pediatric Cardiovascular Surgery Anesthesia Cases*,
https://doi.org/10.1007/978-981-96-5614-1_43

Specialized examination: Enlarged heart with dull heart sounds, arrhythmia, class III murmur in the precordial region, coarse breath sounds in both lungs without rales, soft abdomen without pressure pain, enlarged liver with one finger below the costal margin, no edema in the limbs.

Past history: Repeated upper respiratory tract infections and pneumonia.

Laboratory tests: Normal blood routine test, normal liver and kidney function, NT-proBNP 1965 pg/mL, Troponin I 0.02 μg/mL.

Electrocardiogram (ECG): Sinus tachycardia, ST-T changes, deep Q wave on aVL lead, QRS complex widening.

Chest X-ray: Enlarged heart shadow, thickened lung texture.

Echocardiography: Left ventricular ejection fraction (LVEF) 22%, left atrium enlargement, the spherical dilation of the left ventricle, diffuse reduction of left ventricular contractility, the left coronary artery was open to the inner wall of the pulmonary artery, the internal diameters of the left and right coronary arteries were 0.19 centimeters, no significant widening of the pulmonary artery, normal cardiac valves activity. The papillary muscles were in normal position, with the tendon cords thickening. Mild mitral regurgitation (MR) and no atrial or ventricular shunting.

Chest CT: Left coronary artery opening in the medial wall of the pulmonary artery and distal left bronchial stenosis.

Preoperative diagnosis ALCAPA, MR, heart failure. Left coronary artery reconstruction and pulmonary artery patch expansion angioplasty were planned.

43.2 Anesthetic Management

The patient's basic HR was 160 beats/min, BP was 85/48 mm Hg, and pulse oxygen saturation (SpO_2 95%). Midazolam 0.1 mg/kg, sufentanil 2.0 μg/kg, etomidate 0.2 mg/kg, and rocuronium 0.6 mg/kg were administered intravenously for the induction of anesthesia and endotracheal intubation. Pressure-controlled ventilation (PCV) mode was used for mechanical ventilation with tidal volume (VT) of 8–10 mL/kg, RR 24 times/min. End-tidal carbon dioxide ($ETCO_2$) was maintained at 40–45 mm Hg. The radial artery was catheterized to monitor invasive arterial pressure (ABP); the initial ABP was 80/42 mm Hg. A double-lumen central venous catheter was inserted into the right internal jugular vein for central venous pressure (CVP) monitoring and vasoactive drugs infusion; the initial CVP was 8–10 cm H_2O. A femoral vein was catheterized for fluid replacement. General anesthesia was maintained by continuous infusion of sufentanil 2.5 μg/(kg·h), rocuronium 0.6 mg/(kg·h), and propofol 4.0 mg/(kg·h).

After the aorta was dissected for aortic cannulation, the ABP suddenly dropped to 55/28 mm Hg, with a tendency to fall further and significant ST-segment depression; the depression amplitude was beyond 2 mV. Intravenous infusion of dopamine 7.5 μg/(kg·min) was started immediately. ABP was increased to 62–70/38–45 mm Hg with significant improvement of ST segment depression. After heparinization, the aorta and vena cava were cannulated, and 15–20 mL of crystalloid was given through the aortic cannula to maintain CVP at 10 cm H_2O. Cardiopulmonary bypass (CPB) was started after ACT >380 s. Under mild hypothermic CBP support, left coronary artery transplantation was performed. The left coronary artery opening was located on the posterior wall of the pulmonary artery. The left coronary artery opening was cut off like a button and implanted into the aortic root. The pulmonary valve sinus was repaired by a pericardial patch and sutured to the distal pulmonary artery. MR was not treated. The aortic cannula for CBP was 12 gauge, and the superior vena cava and inferior vena cava cannulas were all 18 gauge. A single 380 mL infusion of HTK cardioplegia solution was sequentially infused for 78 min of aortic cross-clamp time, 42 min of parallel time, and 123 min of total CBP time.

After the aorta cross-clamp was released, the ventricular fibrillation occurred. Epical defibrillation was initially conducted with 0.5 J/kg. Epinephrine 0.02 μg/(kg·min) and dopamine 5.0 μg/(kg·min) were started for continuous infusion to increase myocardial contractility and blood pressure. The sinus rhythm resumed 2 min after defibrillation with ABP 40/32 mm Hg. After the vena cava cross-clamp was released, mechanical ventilation was resumed with PCV mode, VT 6–8 mL/kg, RR 24 times/min. During the parallel period, the CBP flow was maintained at 100–120 mL/min, HR 170–175 beats/min. The left atrial pressure was measured at 12 mm Hg by placing the left atrial catheter. Dopamine was adjusted to 7.5 μg/(kg·min), the dose of epinephrine was gradually adjusted to 0.1 μg/(kg·min), and norepinephrine 0.1 μg/(kg·min) was continuously infused. The CBP flow was gradually reduced. The blood pressure was gradually increased and maintained around 70/38 mm Hg, CVP 12 cm H_2O, and left atrial pressure 11 mm Hg. After weaning off CBP, modified ultrafiltration was conducted. Protamine was intravenously given at a ratio of 1.2:1 to neutralize heparin after modified ultrafiltration. Artery blood gas analysis result: pH 7.35, Lac 2.1 mmol/L, Ca^{2+} 0.95 mmol/L. Continuous infusion of $CaCl_2$ 10 mg/(kg·h) through a left atrial pressure catheter was performed to avoid the unintended occurrence of tissue necrosis caused by the infiltration of high concentrations of calcium into the subcutaneous tissue. The cold precipitate, prothrombin complex, etc. were given to enhance coagulation function through femoral venous access. During the operation, 100 mL of autologous blood was collected and 30 mL of red blood cell suspension was given during hemostasis to maintain HCT 35%. After ultrafiltration, 50 mL of urine was collected. A right ventricular pacing lead was placed and connected to a temporary pacemaker for standby. The sternum was closed with delay after the operation. When leaving the operating room, HR was 152 beats/min, ABP was 78/39 mm Hg, CVP was 10 cm H_2O, and left atrial pressure was 11–12 mm Hg. The patient was transferred to the Cardiac Intensive Care Unit (CICU) under ABP monitoring and manual bag ventilation.

43.3 Postoperative Outcome

After admission to the CICU, mechanical ventilation was continued with IPPV+SIMV mode and PEEP 10 cm H_2O. He was treated with creatine phosphate for myocardial nutrition, low molecular heparin for anticoagulation, and antibiotics for anti-infection. Seventeen hours after surgery, recurrent ventricular tachycardia and fibrillation occurred with ABP 35/30 mm Hg, left atrial pressure higher than 25 mm Hg, NT-proBNP 4853 pg/mL, and C Troponin I 7.74 μg/mL. Epical defibrillation and cardiac compressions were immediately conducted after bedside chest opening. The doses of norepinephrine and epinephrine were increased to 0.15 μg/(kg·min)and 0.3 μg/(kg·min), respectively, but the resuscitation was not effective. A left ventricular assist device (LVAD) was immediately installed with a flow rate of 80 mL/kg. The epinephrine was reduced to 0.1 μg/(kg·min). Iloprost was inhaled to reduce pulmonary vascular resistance, right ventricular afterload, and left ventricular preload. The ECG showed sustained rapid junctional tachycardia. Amiodarone 10 μg/(kg·min) was initially infused. During LVAD assistance, ventricular fibrillation recurred, and epical defibrillation at 1 J/kg was conducted. Four days later, the cardiac function was improved, the LVAD was removed, and the sternum was closed. Peritoneal dialysis was used to facilitate homeostasis. The dosage of cardiovascular drugs was adjusted according to the real situation. The child's cardiac function was gradually stabilized. On the postoperative day 22, he was transferred back to the general ward.

43.4 Review of Knowledge Points

43.4.1 Pathophysiology of ALCAPA

Rich collateral circulation formations exist between the normal right coronary artery (RCA) and the anomalous originated left coronary artery (LCA) in patients with ALCAPA. The RCA supplies blood to the LCA through the collateral vessels. Normally, the pulmonary artery resistance is significantly lower than the coronary arteries. So, part of the blood flow from the LCA enters the pulmonary artery, resulting in blood thief. Due to the physiological pulmonary artery hypertension in the neonatal period, most children are asymptomatic within 2 months after birth. As the pulmonary artery resistance decreases with age, the left coronary artery flow gradually reduces, which results in varying degrees of myocardial ischemic injury and heart failure. If not treated surgically in time, about 90% of children will die within 1 year.

43.4.2 Types of ALCAPA

ALCAPA can be categorized into infantile and adult types. The infantile type of ALCAPA has few or no coronary collaterals, so symptoms appear a few days to weeks after birth. Patients develop severe myocardial ischemia, left ventricular dilatation, and dysfunction. Ischemia of the papillary muscles of the left ventricle leads to mitral valve insufficiency. If the infantile type of ALCAPA is left untreated, the patient may die quickly. In adult-type ALCAPA, which accounts for 10–15% of cases, the collateral vessels of the right coronary artery provide adequate blood flow to the anomalously originated left coronary artery. When the patient's right coronary artery system dominantly develops, and the opening of the left coronary artery originating from the pulmonary artery is small simultaneously, the patient may survive to adulthood. The rate of sudden death in this small group of patients is estimated to be 80–90% at their average age of 35 years.

43.4.3 Surgical Treatment for ALCAPA

The surgical treatment of ALCAPA is based on different anatomical features, including direct coronary artery grafting to the aortic root, extending the coronary arteries using autologous tissues to reduce the anastomotic tension or create pulmonary artery tunnels to complete coronary artery transplantation using the Takeuchi technique. Whether mitral regurgitation should be managed remains controversial. Some people believe that mitral regurgitation in most patients does not require surgical treatment except for structural mitral valve abnormalities. Other people believe that the reduction of mitral regurgitation can effectively promote the early recovery of heart function after ALCAPA surgery. In contrast, untreated mitral regurgitation increases the rate of reoperation in patients. So valvuloplasty is recommended for those patients with moderate to severe mitral regurgitation.

43.5 Discussion

43.5.1 Preoperative Assessment and Preparation

With regard to the timing of surgery in patients with ALCAPA, the widely accepted international consensus is that the diagnosis of ALCAPA is a clear indication for surgery regardless of the development of coronary collateral circulation or the presence of clinical symptoms. The patient's cardiac function should be thoroughly evaluated. Patients with severe congestive heart failure often have delayed growth and have difficulty in achieving age-related height and weight. Laboratory tests such as NT-pro BNP can help determine the degree of heart failure and predict postoperative cardiac risks. Cardiac ultrasound, CT, and MRI are performed to assess cardiac systolic and diastolic function, valve regurgitation, and the presence of other congenital heart defects that require management. In patients with poor cardiac function (LVEF <30%), preoperative medication should be administered, and cardiac function should be aggressively adjusted. Mechanical assist devices should be prepared intraoperatively. Early postoperative ventricular assist may promote early recovery of cardiac function.

43.5.2 Intraoperative Anesthetic Management

1. Anesthesia induction and maintenance. In this case, the patient had a preoperative spherical enlargement of the left ventricle with an LVEF of 22%. Laboratory and imaging examinations indicated severe cardiac dysfunction. The anesthetic drugs should be chosen to

avoid depressing myocardial contractility, heart rate, and blood pressure. Patients often cannot tolerate high concentrations of inhaled anesthetics as they can cause a sharp drop in blood pressure, so inhaled anesthesia induction is not recommended. Sufentanil has a more stable cardiovascular effect and is more suitable as an option for anesthesia induction. Blood pressure and electrocardiogram should be closely monitored, and drugs should be administered in a titrated manner. Fluid supplementation is recommended not to exceed 4 mL/kg of physiological requirement. Hyperventilation should be avoided before CBP, and $ETCO_2$ should be maintained at about 40 mm Hg to stabilize pulmonary vascular resistance. Avoid inadequate coronary perfusion due to sudden drops in pulmonary artery pressure. All patients should be prepared for defibrillation in advance.

2. Myocardial protection during CBP. Comprehensive measures need to be taken to protect the myocardium during CBP. The left atrial drain should be placed before bypass to reduce left ventricular pressure and avoid myocardial ischemia effectively. Hypothermia is an effective method to reduce the metabolic rate of cardiomyocytes. Combined ultrafiltration during and after CBP can greatly reduce myocardial edema. After CBP initiation, the blood from the superior and inferior vena cava flows back to the oxygenator, which results in a significant reduction of blood flow to the right ventricle-pulmonary artery trunk and a significant drop in pulmonary artery perfusion pressure. So, the blood flow of the left coronary artery supplied by the pulmonary artery also decreases accordingly. At the same time, the energy consumption of the beating heart at this time will aggravate myocardial damage. Therefore, cross-clamping the aorta and pulmonary arteries immediately after CBP initiation is recommended to stop the heartbeat before subsequent operations. Shortening the time of parallel circulation after CBP initiation may be more beneficial in shortening the ischemic time of left ventricular myocardial cells. In addition, it is of utmost importance that the surgeon should be familiar with the pathologic anatomy of an abnormally located left coronary artery. The key to the reimplantation of the left coronary artery is to prevent stenosis and myocardial ischemia caused by the coronary artery deformation. Postoperative electrocardiogram monitoring can reflect the blood supply effect of the left coronary artery.
3. Hemodynamic management after the release of aortic cross-clamp. The principle of hemodynamic management after ALCAPA surgery in children is to maintain appropriate preload, improve coronary blood supply, and appropriately enhance myocardial contractility. After the aortic cross-clamp is released, ventricular fibrillation and arrhythmias are likely to occur due to myocardial ischemia and reperfusion injury, as well as myocardial stunning and hibernation. These situations should be proactively managed, and the sinus rhythm should be restored immediately. Continuous amiodarone infusion or low-dose esmolol can control the heart rate for persistent ventricular fibrillation and supraventricular tachycardia. However, when β-blockers are administered to children, attention should be paid to their impact on blood pressure and HR since low HR can significantly reduce cardiac output in pediatric patients. Excessive volume loading should be avoided in children with dilated ventricles and weakened myocardial contractility. At the same time, epinephrine could be used to enhance myocardial contractility. Norepinephrine has a peripheral vasoconstrictor effect and can significantly increase diastolic blood pressure but has less effect on increasing heart rate than epinephrine. Children with low blood pressure after surgery can be given continuous intravenous infusion. Comprehensive hemodynamic monitoring during surgery, including left atrial pressure, cardiac output, peripheral vascular resistance, and myocardial contractility, is recommended to optimize the medication regimens. Blood gas analysis and urine output should be actively tested to maintain acid–base balance and homeostasis.

43.5.3 Postoperative Anesthetic Management

1. Low cardiac output syndrome (LCOS). The peak incidence of low cardiac output syndrome occurs within 24 h after ALCAPA. Dramatic changes in hemodynamics in the early postoperative period cause absolute or relative oxygen insufficiency, poor perfusion of vital organs, the internal environment disturbances, which further result in oliguria, blood lactate level elevation, acidosis, central venous oxygen saturation decrease, pulmonary congestion, and cardiac index <2–2.2 L/(min·m^2). Continuous urine output <0.5 mL/(kg·h) for 4 h is considered as oliguria. The appearance of pathological Q waves on the ECG suggests myocardial infarction. Left atrial pressure > 15 mm Hg, blood lactate value >5 mmoL/L, and ejection fraction <45% all indicate left ventricular dysfunction. Using indirect hemodynamic parameters to assess LCOS is often not accurate enough. Bedside echocardiography and continuous cardiac output monitoring can help detect low cardiac output early after surgery. Although the normal coronary blood supply has been reconstructed after surgery, some children have difficulty in weaning off CBP assistance. High doses of epinephrine and other positive inotropic drugs are required for postoperative maintenance. Positive inotropic drug score: epinephrine μg/(kg·min) × 100 + dopamine μg/(kg·min) × 1 + milrinone μg/(kg·min) × 10 > 20 suggests severe condition. The risk of sudden ventricular fibrillation or even sudden death in the early postoperative period is quite high.
2. Application of left ventricular assist device (LVAD). After ALCAPA surgery, children with a positive inotropic drug score > 20 and persistent tachycardia or pathologic Q waves, as well as oliguria, progressively higher blood lactate values, left ventricular systolic dysfunction suggested by bedside ultrasound, and ejection fractions of <30% are all indications for installation of an LVAD. LVAD assistance can reduce LV work and assist LV pumping function so that the LV can be rested in the early postoperative period and get through the acute postoperative LV dysfunction stage. Therefore, aggressive implementation of LVAD may be the first choice for perioperative myocardial protection in ALCAPA, if available, and may be the most effective way to save a child's life. Right ventricular function is an important factor affecting the success of LVAD application. Suppose the child has severe pulmonary hypertension with high pulmonary vascular bed resistance. In that case, the right ventricle will have a reduced volume of blood entering the pulmonary circulation, and the right ventricle will not be able to provide sufficient cardiac output for the LVAD. So, the circulatory blood flow will be limited. In this case, drugs such as inhaled Iloprost should be used to reduce right ventricular afterload. The use of small doses of dopamine and epinephrine can help improve right ventricular function. If the right ventricular function cannot ensure left ventricular cardiac output, ECMO assistance must be conducted. Optimal assisted circulatory flow should be controlled at 100–120 mL/(kg·min) since excessive flow can increase the risk of right heart failure. The systolic function of the left ventricle should be continuously monitored and generally maintained. The infant's blood pressure should be at 60 mm Hg, left atrial pressure should be <10 mm Hg, and then the dose of vasoactive drugs is gradually decreased. When the auxiliary flow rate is reduced to 30–50 mL/(kg·min), the systolic pressure is stable at 65 mm Hg, and the left atrial pressure < 10 mm Hg, an attempt can be made to withdraw the LVAD. Before withdrawal of LVAD aid, the dose of positive inotropic drugs should be increased appropriately, the tube should be clamped, and the LVAD should be withdrawn after observation of the clinical indicators for 1–2 h.

43.6 Conclusion

Surgical manipulation and LVAD can cause cardiomyocyte degenerative edema and ischemia-reperfusion injury, which may further reduce left ventricular systolic function. Severe arrhythmias and heart failure may occur after surgery. Comprehensive assessment of cardiac function and timely installation of an LVAD is an effective strategy to reduce mortality during acute left ventricular failure (Yunan Song).

Anesthetic Management of Coronary Artery Fistula Repair Surgery in an Infant with Right Coronary Artery–Right Ventricular Fistula

44

Yunan Song

Abstract

A 9-month-old boy underwent surgery for a right coronary artery–right ventricular fistula. Due to the left-to-right shunt, the volume of the pulmonary circulation was overloaded with a dysfunctional right ventricle. He was susceptible to myocardial perfusion insufficiency due to coronary artery "blood theft" and decreased diastolic pressure. Therefore, the key to perioperative management in such patients should focus on blood volume management, right ventricular function protection, and myocardial oxygen supply and oxygen consumption balance.

Coronary artery fistula (CAF) is the congenital abnormal communication between the left and right coronary arteries with the heart or large vessels. It is a congenital heart malformation formed by abnormal cardiovascular development in the embryonic period. It is relatively rare and accounts for 0.26–0.4% of congenital heart diseases. CAF can originate from various coronary arteries, but the right CAF is more common, accounting for 50–60% of CAF cases. CAF often opens to the right cardiac system, such as the right atrium (19–26%), right ventricle (14–40%), pulmonary artery (15–20%), and coronary sinus (7%), but also seen in the left ventricle (2–19%) and left atrium (5–6%). CAF with high fractional flow may lead to myocardial ischemia, congestive heart failure, and pulmonary hypertension. In this situation, emergency surgery is required. This chapter reports the anesthetic management of CAF repair surgery in an infant with right coronary artery–right ventricular fistula.

44.1 Case Presentation

A 9-month-and-29-day-old boy, 75 cm in height and 9.5 kg in weight, was born at full term. After birth, a heart murmur was detected during a physical examination. No cyanosis, growth retardation, or feeding difficulties have occurred since birth. There was a history of multiple respiratory infections and decreased mobility. The child was regularly followed up at the local hospital. He was admitted to our hospital for surgical treatment of the right coronary artery–right ventricle fistula detected by an echocardiogram.

Physical examination: Body temperature 36.8 °C, pulse 148 bpm, respiratory rate (RR) 32 bpm, blood pressure (BP) 92/37 mm Hg. The patient was conscious, had normal development, and had average nutrition. Specialized physical

Y. Song (✉)
The National Children's Medical Center (Shanghai), Department of Anesthesiology of Shanghai Children's Medical Center, Shanghai Jiao Tong University School of Medicine, Shanghai, China
e-mail: songyunan@scmc.com.cn

J. Zheng et al. (eds.), *Selected Pediatric Cardiovascular Surgery Anesthesia Cases*,
https://doi.org/10.1007/978-981-96-5614-1_44

examination: No cyanosis, steady breathing, coarse breath sounds without rales in both lungs and slightly weak breath sounds on the right side. Strong heart sounds, regular heart rhythm, grade II systolic murmur between the second and third ribs on the left edge of the sternum, accentuated P2. The liver was not palpable below the ribs. Extremities were warm without edema.

Chest CT: Bronchial obstruction was seen in the right upper lobe with patchy, dense, fuzzy shadows, and the two lower lobes were fuzzy in texture and uneven in transparency. The viscera and atria were correctly positioned with normal pulmonary venous return. The presence or absence of a septal shunt was not clearly demonstrated, and the left atrium was slightly enlarged. The left and right ventricles were not enlarged, and there was no significant narrowing of the left and right ventricular outflow tracts. Coronary artery origin was normal. A right coronary artery–right ventricle fistula was formed with an opening of approximately 2.8 mm (Figs. 44.1 and 44.2).

Echocardiography: A branch originating from the right coronary artery about 0.93 cm from the opening ran tortuously along the atrioventricular groove from the front to the back and below the right atrium and drained into the right ventricle below the anterior leaflet of the tricuspid valve.

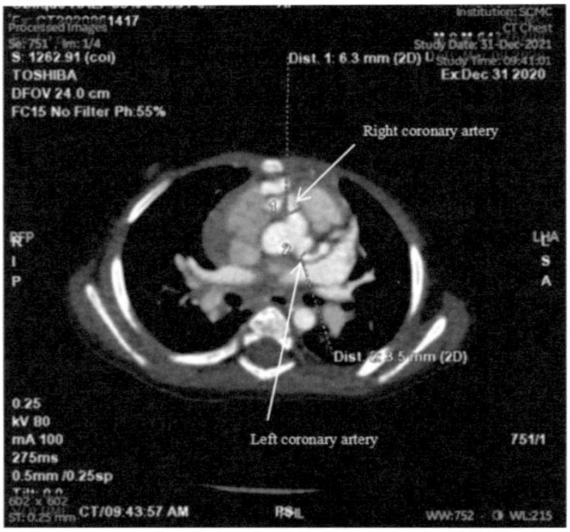

Fig. 44.1 Preoperative cardiac CT. The proximal ends of the left and right coronary arteries are approximately 3.5 mm × 2.9 mm and 6.3 mm × 6.0 mm, respectively

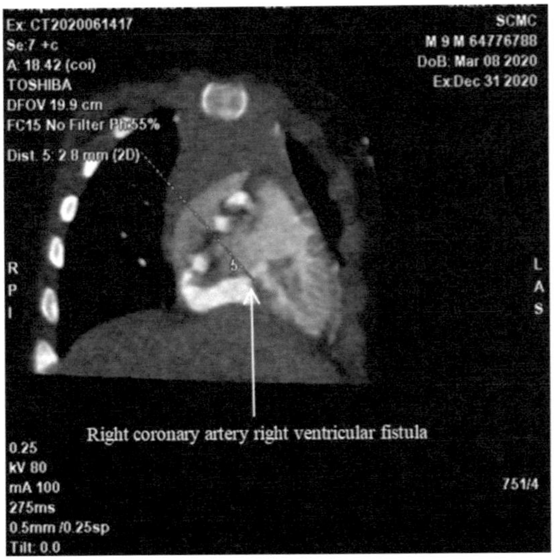

Fig. 44.2 Preoperative cardiac CT. Right coronary artery–right ventricular fistula, the fistula opening is about 2.8 mm

The widest inner diameter of the fistula was about 0.89 cm, the width of the blood flow bundle at the fistula opening was about 0.30 cm, and the continuous blood flow speed was 4.04 m/s. The tips of the tricuspid valve leaflets were slightly thick with mild regurgitation and multiple regurgitation bundles; the wider bundle was 0.25 cm, and the regurgitation speed was 2.5 m/s. The atrial septum and ventricular septum were intact.

44.2 Anesthetic Management

The child drank 0.5 mg/kg of midazolam syrup 30 min before entering the operating room. After falling asleep, the child was brought into the operating room. The basic heart rate (HR) was 125 bpm, BP was 86/40 mm Hg, and pulse oxygen saturation (SpO_2) was 98%. After the induction of anesthesia with intravenous administration of 0.1 mg/kg midazolam, 2.0 μg/kg sufentanil, 0.2 mg/kg etomidate, and 0.6 mg/kg rocuronium, endotracheal intubation was conducted. A 4 mm inner diameter cuffed endotracheal tube was intubated to a depth of 11 cm. Mechanical ventilation was conducted in the pressure-controlled ventilation-volume guaranteed (PCV-VG) mode with ventilator parameters setting as tidal volume (VT) 6–8 mL/kg, RR 20–24 times/min, peak airway pressure (PIP) around 20 cm H_2O. The end-tidal carbon dioxide ($ETCO_2$) was maintained at 35–45 mm Hg. Anesthesia was maintained with sufentanil 2.5 μg/(kg·h), rocuronium 0.6 mg/(kg·h), and propofol 4.0 mg/(kg·h). The radial artery was catheterized for invasive arterial pressure monitoring, and a double-lumen central venous was catheterized in the right internal jugular vein for central venous pressure (CVP) monitoring. The basic CVP was 8–10 cm H_2O. The femoral vein was catheterized for fluid replacement. During the operation, dopamine 3.0–5.0 μg/(kg·min) and norepinephrine 0.02 μg/(kg·min) were intermittently infused based on blood pressure. The invasive arterial pressure was maintained at 80–85/45–50 mm Hg, heart rate at 130 ± 10 bpm, CVP 13 cm H_2O, SpO_2 98%. The CAF was ligated without cardiopulmonary bypass (CBP) through a median sternotomy incision. During the operation, the right coronary artery was found to be significantly enlarged. The proximal opening of the fistula was found in the middle segment of the right coronary artery along the atrioventricular groove. The fistula was ligated with a 10-gauge wire near the opening of the right coronary artery. Intraoperative blood gas analysis (FiO_2 40%): pH 7.3, PaO_2 196.8 mm Hg, $PaCO_2$ 41.4 mm Hg, HCT 30.8%, BE −1.4 mmol/L, Lac 1.0 mmol/L. Postoperative transesophageal echocardiography showed no residual shunting. The chest was closed in layers. The patient was transferred back to the Cardiac Intensive Care Unit (CICU) with endotracheal intubation.

44.3 Postoperative Outcome

The operation lasted 90 min. The estimated blood loss was 20 mL. The urine output was 100 mL. About 150 mLof Ringer's acetate and 50 mL of erythrocyte suspension were infused during the operation. The blood gas analysis under FiO_2 40% condition in CICU: $PaCO_2$ 35.4 mm Hg, PaO_2 180.4 mm Hg, HCT 32.3%, Lac 0.9 mmol/L, Hb 10.8 g/dL. Mechanical ventilation was conducted in SIMV mode. The patient was weaned from the ventilator on the postoperative day 2. The internal environment was maintained stable. The electrolyte disorders were corrected in time.

44.4 Review of Knowledge Points

44.4.1 Pathophysiology

The hemodynamic impact of CAF depends primarily on the location and diameter of the fistula, the resistance of the anomalous coronary artery, and the pressure gradient between the involved cardiac chambers and vessels. Large CAF may cause coronary artery dilatation or even aneurysms, which further leads to ischemia in the distal coronary artery supply area.

A left-to-right shunt is present in more than 90% of cases. If a left-to-right shunt occurs, it increases the volume load of the right heart, pulmonary vascular bed, left atrium, and left ventricle, leading to left ventricular hypertrophy, dilation, and heart failure. If the shunt enters the left heart system, it will increase the volume load of the left atrium or ventricle. In cases where the fistula enters the left ventricle, shunting generally only occurs during diastole. In contrast, those entering the left atrium exhibit continuous shunting, developing pathophysiologic changes similar to aortic valve closure insufficiency. A prominent feature is a significant decrease in diastolic blood pressure.

44.4.2 Surgical Methods

Both surgical and catheter techniques can be used to close the fistula. However, percutaneous catheter closure is only successfully performed in carefully selected cases with short disease duration, no tortuosity, single fistula, and no complications. Surgery under CBP is a routine method for cardiac surgeons. But CBP can also cause many side effects, such as longer recovery time, postoperative cognitive dysfunction, etc. In recent years, minimally invasive surgical treatment for CAF in children has been reported, but it is only suitable for children with a single CAF, easily exposed locations, and those without other abnormalities such as aneurysms.

44.5 Discussion

44.5.1 Preoperative Assessment and Preparation

Although no significant coronary artery dilatation or aneurysm occurred, there existed a pathophysiologic basis for coronary blood theft and coronary perfusion insufficiency. Decreased diastolic pressure may adversely affect myocardial perfusion. The persistent left-to-right shunt increased the heart's volume load and pulmonary blood flow, which caused frequent pulmonary infections and left atrial enlargement. The preoperative fluid infusion should be appropriately controlled to avoid further increase in volume load. A thorough preoperative echocardiography should be performed to determine the location of the fistula, the size of the shunt tract, diastolic and systolic function of the right ventricle. Pulmonary artery pressures should be carefully assessed. Significant ST-T changes on the ECG should be noted as an indication of myocardial ischemia. In children with preoperative pulmonary infections, a protective lung ventilation strategy during anesthetic management should be considered to protect the respiratory function.

44.5.2 Intraoperative Anesthetic Management

The surgical approach for CAF can be conducted with or without CBP, depending on the size of the fistula, the degree of shunting, and the presence of intracardiac malformations. Surgery without CBP has less impact on the overall cardiac function of the patient. The perfusion of the coronary arteries depends on the coronary perfusion pressure and the duration of diastole. To improve the balance of myocardial oxygen supply and consumption, the following aspects should be noted during intraoperative anesthetic management: ① Maintain an age-appropriate heart rate and adequate ventricular diastolic time to prevent tachycardia from increasing myocardial oxygen consumption; ② maintain normal or slightly high diastolic pressure, which is beneficial for improving coronary blood supply; and ③ Apply appropriate vasoactive drugs to improve myocardial contractility.

44.5.3 Postoperative Anesthetic Management

For those patients with large shunt and heart failure before surgery, it is necessary to improve myocardial contractility and provide sufficient preload after surgery. For those patients with large shunts, pulmonary congestion, and pulmonary artery pressure increase before surgery, it is necessary to decrease the pulmonary artery pressure and right ventricular afterload and maintain appropriate systemic circulation resistance to minimize cardiac work and oxygen consumption. Much attention should be paid to the changes in postoperative electrocardiograms to detect early signs of poor coronary artery perfusion, myocardial ischemia, or even myocardial infarction.

44.6 Conclusion

The pathophysiology of CAF varies dynamically, which is related to the resistance at both ends of the fistula and the shunt site. Careful preoperative assessment is crucial for anesthetic management. In addition, CAF can be operated in a variety of ways. Transesophageal echocardiography can provide important details such as the location of the fistula and coronary artery dilatation, and assessment of the degree of myocardial ischemia. Paying close attention to the progress of surgical procedures and pathophysiologic changes can facilitate the detection of complications in time (Yunan Song).

Anesthetic Management of the Corrective Surgery in Child with Double Aortic Arch

45

Yanhui Huang

Abstract

A 10-month-old female infant was diagnosed with a double aortic arch by cardiac ultrasound and CT scan. She was scheduled to undergo corrective surgery under general anesthesia. She had obvious wheeze after birth, with pulse oxygen saturation (SpO_2) of 92%. Children with double arch often have tracheal stenosis and tracheomalacia due to vascular ring compression, so preoperative airway assessment, selection of appropriate tracheal tube, induction methods of anesthesia, and enhanced airway management during the perioperative period are important. In addition, invasive arterial blood pressure monitoring both in the upper and lower limbs should be established according to surgical needs.

Congenital double aortic arch (DAA) is the most common vascular malformation in congenital vascular rings. Because the left and right aortic arches simultaneously encircle and compress the trachea and esophagus to form a complete ring, children will experience wheezing, shortness of breath, difficulty swallowing, etc. It is necessary to ligate the smaller arch in the left or right aortic arches to resolve the compression of the vascular ring on the trachea and esophagus and alleviate the clinical symptoms. The tracheal stenosis caused by the vascular ring compression brings challenges to the perioperative anesthesia. This chapter reports the anesthetic management of one infant with a double aortic arch undergoing radical surgery for the vascular ring.

45.1 Case Presentation

The patient was a 10-month-and-28-day-old female with a weight of 7.4 kg. The patient has been wheezing since birth. An echocardiography at a local hospital indicated a congenital right aortic arch and aberrant left subclavian artery. She was regularly followed up due to her young age at the time. She was admitted to our hospital for surgery this time.

Physical examination: Mild rapid breathing, pulse oxygen saturation (SpO_2) 92%, coarse breath sounds in both lungs, regular heart rhythm.

Laboratory tests: Normal blood routine test, normal coagulation, liver and kidney function.

Chest X-ray: No abnormalities in the thoracic skeleton and chest wall soft tissues, no displacement of the mediastinum and trachea, mild heart shadow enlargement, and multiple lung markings.

Y. Huang (✉)
The National Children's Medical Center (Shanghai), Department of Anesthesiology of Shanghai Children's Medical Center, Shanghai Jiao Tong University School of Medicine, Shanghai, China
e-mail: huangyanhui@scmc.com.cn

J. Zheng et al. (eds.), *Selected Pediatric Cardiovascular Surgery Anesthesia Cases*,
https://doi.org/10.1007/978-981-96-5614-1_45

Electrocardiogram (ECG): Sinus rhythm, slightly elevated T wave.

Cardiac ultrasound: Double aortic arch, the inner diameter of the transverse part of the right arch was 0.89 cm, the inner diameter of the isthmus was 0.81 cm, the blood flow speed of the right descending aorta was 1.4 m/s, the left arch seems to be occluded at the distal end of the left subclavian artery after it gave off the left common carotid artery and the left subclavian artery, the inner diameter of the transverse part of the left arch was 0.43 cm and the inner diameter of the isthmus was 0.34 cm.

Chest CT (plain scan + enhancement): The spiral scanning and three-dimensional reconstruction showed that the mediastinum was basically centered, the trachea became narrowed at the level of the aortic arch, the size of the narrowed site was about 3.5 mm × 3.0 mm, the proximal end was about 5.3 mm × 4.8 mm, the bronchi were unobstructed, the lung window had shown normal lung texture. Double arch, right descending aorta, the diameter of the right arch was about 8.6 mm, the left arch and the arch descending part became narrowed; the arch part was about 3.8 mm, the isthmus part was about 2.0 mm, the descending aorta had a Kommerell diverticulum (Fig. 45.1).

Preoperative diagnosis: Double aortic arch, aberrant subclavian artery. The vascular ring correction and aortic arch plasty surgery were scheduled.

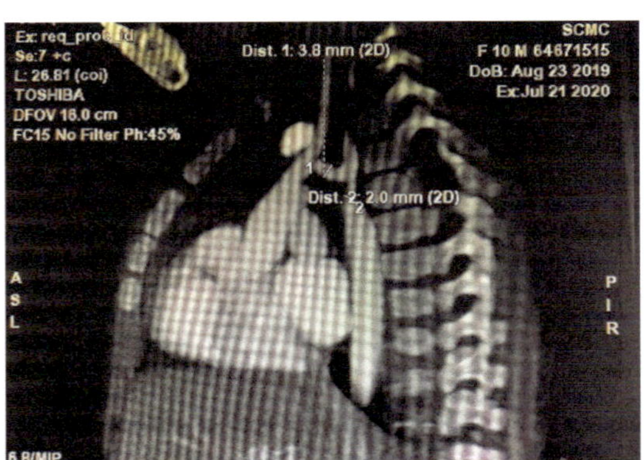

Fig. 45.1 Preoperative heart CT of the patient

45.2 Anesthetic Management

The patient did not take any preoperative medication. After entering the operating room, ECG, noninvasive blood pressure (BP), and SpO_2 monitoring were conducted with a basic heart rate (HR) of 133 beats/min, BP 89/47 mm Hg, and SpO_2 92%. Midazolam 1.0 mg, etomidate 2.0 mg, and sufentanil 10 μg were injected intravenously after the peripheral vein was accessed. Once the mask-assisted ventilation could provide a normal oxygen supply, rocuronium 4.0 mg was given for skeletal muscle relaxation, and then an ID 4.0 mm cuffed endotracheal tube was intubated under the assistance of a visual laryngoscope. A fiber bronchoscope with an outer diameter of 2.2 mm confirmed that the head end of the tracheal tube had passed through the tracheal stenosis segment and above the tracheal carina. At this time, the tube insertion depth was 12.5 cm. The tracheal tube was then properly fixed. Pressure-controlled ventilation (PCV) mode was used with respiratory parameters set as peak inspiratory pressure (PIP) less than 20 cm H_2O, 2 L/min oxygen flow rate, 50% fraction of inspired oxygen (FiO_2), 25 breaths/min respiratory rate (RR), and 1:2 (inspiratory to expiratory time) I:E ratio. Tidal volume (VT) could reach 70 mL when PIP was 18 cm H_2O, SpO_2 could reach 98%, and end-tidal carbon dioxide partial pressure ($ETCO_2$) fluctuated around 37 mm Hg. After induction of anesthesia, the left radial artery, right femoral artery, and right internal jugular vein were quickly catheterized to monitor invasive artery blood pressure (ABP) and central vein pressure (CVP) and the rapid fluid infusion. The patient was then placed in the right lateral decubitus position. After routine disinfection and draping, the left paravertebral nerve block at the T4 level was performed with 0.2% ropivacaine 4.0 mL under ultrasound guidance. General anesthesia was maintained with intravenous infusion of 4.0 mg/(kg·h) propofol, 1.0 μg/(kg·h) sufentanil, and 0.6 mg/(kg·h) rocuronium, which was combined with sevoflurane inhalation.

The airway pressure and respiratory rate were adjusted to maintain $ETCO_2$ within the range of 35–45 mm Hg during the left posterolateral thoracic thoracotomy. The patient's blood pressure dropped below 80 mm Hg after thoracotomy, and a small dose of dopamine 3.0 μg/(kg·min) was administered via intravenous pump infusion to maintain hemodynamic stability.

Before sternal closure, lung recruitment maneuvers were conducted. The ventilator parameters were adjusted, and the arterial blood gases were checked. The results showed: pH 7.32, PaO_2 98.6 mm Hg, $PaCO_2$ 40.3 mm Hg,BE −5.03 mmol/L, HCT 30.7%, Hb 10.3 g/dL, K^+ 3.42, Ca^{2+} 1.198, Cl^- 109.6, Lac 0.9 mmol/L. Metabolic acidosis was corrected with 5% sodium bicarbonate 10 mL. The patient was transferred to the cardiac intensive care unit (CICU) with endotracheal intubation when surgery was finished.

45.3 Postoperative Outcome

The endotracheal intubation was successfully removed, and the patient was transferred back to the general ward with nasal oxygen inhalation on postoperative day 1. The patient was discharged from the hospital on postoperative day 6.

45.4 Review of Knowledge Points

45.4.1 Embryological Basis of DAA

DAA is the most common type of vascular ring disease, which occurs when the left and right fourth pairs of arterial arches coexist during embryonic development. Both pairs of aortic arches originate from the ascending aorta, bypass the trachea and esophagus on both sides, then merge into the descending aorta at the back and form a true ring that encircles the trachea and esophagus, as shown in Fig. 45.2.

45.4.2 Pathological Anatomy and Clinical Manifestations of DAA

The anatomical structure of DAA mainly consists of the left and right aortic arches, each giving rise to their respective subclavian arteries and common carotid arteries. Generally speaking, about 75% of double aortic arches are right arch dominant, about 20% are left arch dominant, and about 5% are balanced. Usually, blood circulates in both the left and right aortic arches of DAA, but there are cases where one side of the aortic arch is closed, with 40% being the right aortic arch open and the left

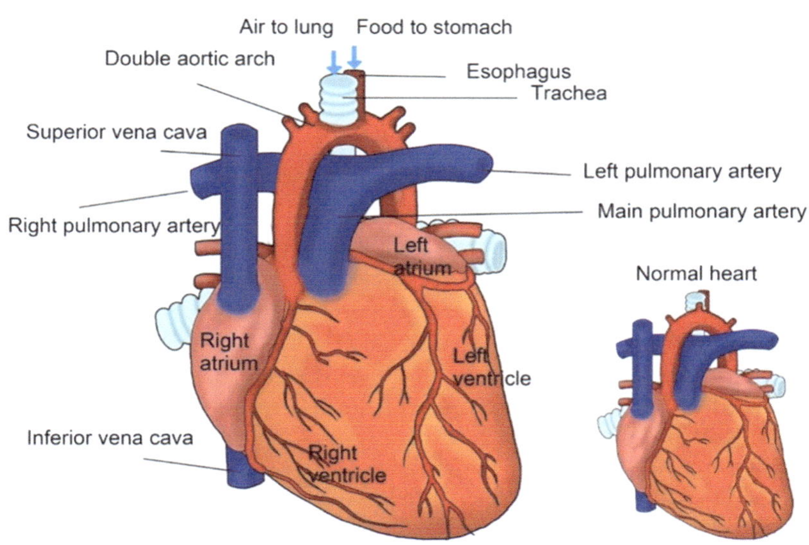

Fig. 45.2 Double aortic arch and normal heart

aortic arch closed. Conversely, about 20% of cases have the left aortic arch open and the right aortic arch closed. Clinical symptoms of DAA can manifest within the first month after birth. Early tracheal compression is common, such as severe coughing, recurrent lung infections, wheezing, and shortness of breath. If the trachea is severely compressed and causes respiratory distress, tracheal intubation and mechanical ventilation are required to maintain oxygenation. Difficulty swallowing liquid food due to esophageal compression is less common in patients, but difficulty swallowing solid food becomes relatively obvious as the patient's age increases.

45.4.3 Diagnosis and Treatment of DAA

The traditional methods for preliminary assessment of DAA are chest radiographs, barium meals, and echocardiograms. However, the exact anatomy of aortic arch malformations and their relationship with adjacent structures can only be accurately located through cross-sectional imaging techniques, such as multi-detector computed tomography (MDCT) or magnetic resonance imaging (MRI). As MRI examinations require more time and usually need to be completed under sedation or anesthesia, and MRI does not provide tracheal anatomical image as clear as CT imaging, most DAA patients choose to have a CT scan before surgery. Enhanced scanning with MDCT can display abnormalities of the aortic arch and tracheal lesions. Furthermore, it can also provide clear 3D visualization of vascular anatomy from multiple angles and provide helpful information for determining a detailed surgical plan. For DAA patients, MDCT has now become an excellent method for the preoperative and postoperative diagnostic evaluation of DAA. Bronchoscopy is a necessary diagnostic tool for direct, dynamic assessment of the trachea and bronchi, it can not only show the degree of extrinsic compression, but it can also determine the level and degree of tracheal stenosis and determine whether there is a complete tracheal ring or tracheomalacia. Furthermore, it can also be used to assess the surgical effect postoperatively. Most DAA patients have clinical symptoms, and they should be scheduled to receive surgery as soon as possible once the diagnosis is confirmed. The left posterolateral thoracotomy is commonly used, and the secondary aortic arch is dissected between the subclavian artery and the descending aorta. The occlusion test at the expected severed location of the secondary arch should first be conducted to ensure there is no change in the blood pressure and oxygen saturation of the upper and lower limb arteries, and then the secondary arch is severed.

45.5 Discussion

45.5.1 Preoperative Assessment and Preparation

Airway assessment is the key part of the preoperative assessment for children with DAA. In this case, the preoperative airway CT (plain scan + enhancement) showed that the tracheal stenosis existed at the level of the aortic arch with a diameter of about 3.5 mm × 3 mm at the narrowest location. Usually, extrinsic compression-induced tracheal stenosis usually does not affect the pass of the tracheal tube through the narrow part, so we still chose an ID 4.0 mm cuffed tracheal tube according to the infant's age and prepared an ID 3.5 mm cuffed tracheal tube at the same time. The infant's baseline SpO_2 was 92%, which may be related to recurrent respiratory infections. In order to prevent the infant's hypoxia from worsening, no preoperative sedative drugs were given.

45.5.2 Induction of Anesthesia

For children with tracheal compression caused by DAA, awake intubation is the safest intubation method theoretically, but it is actually not feasible in uncooperative pediatric patients. Inhalational induction with sevoflurane is a safer and more feasible method of anesthesia induction for the patient with DAA by maintaining sufficient depth of anesthesia and spontaneous breathing. Muscle relaxants are usually given after endotracheal intubation, and sufficient oxygenation is maintained by mechanical positive pressure ventilation. However, rapid induction with intravenous anesthetics and muscle relaxants can also be performed for tracheal intubation, assuming mask-assisted ventilation can guarantee normal oxygenation. Our team adopted the second induction method with rapid induction of anesthesia and early airway security.

45.5.3 Airway Management

The depth of intubation is particularly important in such patients. The depth of the tracheal tube should ensure that the tracheal tube passes the tracheal stenosis to prevent difficulty in the positive pressure ventilation and single lung ventilation must also be avoided caused by too deep intubation. The position of the tracheal tube can be confirmed with the help of bronchoscopy. The tracheal tube can be inserted into one bronchus first, and then the tracheal tube can be slowly withdrawn until the lung breath sounds are heard on both sides if there is no bronchoscopy. When the lung breath sounds change from one side to symmetrical on both sides, it indicates that the tracheal tube is close to the tracheal carina, which can be considered an ideal intubation position, and then the tube can be fixed. Children with double aortic arch generally undergo surgery in the lateral position. During the process of changing position, there is a possibility that the position of the tracheal tube may become too deep, causing single-lung ventilation. Once single lung ventilation occurs, as long as ventilation is normal and can ensure the oxygen supply of the child, it can be left untreated, and the position of the tracheal tube should be re-determined when the operation is finished.

45.5.4 Artery and Vein Pathways

Due to the risk of sudden massive bleeding during DAA surgery, our team established the internal jugular and femoral vein pathways so that vasoactive drugs could be infused through the internal jugular vein and fluids could be quickly infused through the femoral vein. During the operation, the infant's blood pressure dropped once without major bleeding, which was considered to be the impact of surgical manipulation. After reminding the surgeon to operate carefully and intravenous pump dopamine, the blood pressure rose to the normal range. The surgical plan for this infant was to ligate the left arch. In order to assist in determining the accurate position of the left arch ligation, our team established blood pressure monitoring of the left radial artery and right femoral artery to reflect the effect of the occlusion test and ensure that the blood supply to the upper and lower limbs of the infant was normal after the left arch ligation.

45.5.5 Perioperative Analgesia

The infant underwent left thoracotomy surgery in the right lateral position. In order to improve intraoperative analgesia and reduce stress response and the dosage of perioperative opioids, general anesthesia combined with epidural anesthesia is a common anesthesia method. However, considering that paravertebral block can achieve similar analgesic effects with epidural anesthesia and less damage, our team used the long-acting local anesthetic ropivacaine for paravertebral block to enhance perioperative analgesia.

45.6 Conclusion

In summary, airway compression is the most prominent issue in children with DAA. So, preoperative airway assessment is particularly important. In addition to improving perioperative airway management, it is also important to assist the surgeon in conducting the occlusion tests to ensure the success of the surgery (Yanhui Huang).

46 Anesthetic Management of Surgical Correction of Pulmonary Artery Sling with Ventricular Septal Defect in an Infant

Bin Xue

Abstract

A two-month-old female infant was diagnosed with pulmonary artery sling and tracheal stenosis due to postnatal wheezing. She was admitted to our hospital and scheduled to undergo left pulmonary artery reconstruction, tracheoplasty, and ventricular septal defect (VSD) repair. Pulmonary artery sling refers to the abnormal route of the left pulmonary artery, which comes from the back of the right pulmonary artery and forms a vascular ring as it crosses the right main bronchus in a semicircular manner and passes in front of the esophagus and behind the trachea to reach the left lung hilum. Approximately 50% of children with pulmonary artery sling have other cardiovascular and tracheal malformations, such as congenital tracheal stenosis. The abnormal routed left pulmonary usually can cause tracheal compression and result in airway obstruction, respiratory distress, and even life-threatening situations in severe cases. Preoperative selection of appropriate endotracheal tubes based on whether the child has tracheal stenosis and the degree of compression, rational intraoperative anesthetic management, and correct postoperative airway management are the key to successful anesthetic management and surgery.

Pulmonary artery sling (PAS) is a very rare congenital vascular ring malformation with an incidence rate of about 0.95/10,000. Children with PAS often have other cardiac malformations, such as ventricular septal defect (VSD), atrial septal defect (ASD), patent ductus arteriosus (PDA), persistent left superior vena cava, etc. At the same time, children with PAS often have congenital tracheal malformations, such as tracheal stenosis. The abnormally routed left pulmonary artery (LPA) often compresses the surrounding trachea, which may cause tracheal stenosis and respiratory symptoms such as coughing, wheezing, stridor, and dyspnea. The severity of children with PAS and airway problems depends on the severity of tracheal stenosis and intracardiac malformations. It does not increase the risk of tracheal surgery while correcting other intracardiac malformations at the same time. Furthermore, it may also be beneficial to the child's recovery. This chapter reports the anesthetic management of a case of an infant with PAS and VSD undergoing left pulmonary artery reconstruction, tracheoplasty, and ventricular septal defect repair surgery.

B. Xue (✉)
The National Children's Medical Center (Shanghai), Department of Anesthesiology of Shanghai Children's Medical Center, Shanghai Jiao Tong University School of Medicine, Shanghai, China
e-mail: xuebin@scmc.com.cn

J. Zheng et al. (eds.), *Selected Pediatric Cardiovascular Surgery Anesthesia Cases*,
https://doi.org/10.1007/978-981-96-5614-1_46

46.1 Case Presentation

The patient was a 2-month-old girl with 3.9 kg in weight. She was naturally born at full term without a history of asphyxia. Wheezing occurred after birth. Cardiac ultrasound and CT indicated pulmonary artery sling with tracheal stenosis 1 month ago. The patient was brought to our outpatient clinic 6 days ago and was admitted to our hospital with pulmonary artery sling and tracheal stenosis.

Physical examination: The child was conscious without cyanosis. Wheezing with slightly coarse breathing sounds in both lungs. Three concave signs were not found. Pulse oxygen saturation (SpO_2) was 98% with air breathing.

Laboratory tests: Hemoglobin 93 g/L, hematocrit 32%, normal liver, kidney, and coagulation function.

Electrocardiogram (ECG): Right ventricular hypertrophy (possible).

Echocardiography: LPA abnormally originates from the right pulmonary artery (RPA), ASD (II) 3.8 mm, VSD 5.4 mm (perimembranous fusion type) with some tricuspid valve tissue attached. The shunting was diffuse. Left-sided aortic arch, the enlarged coronary sinus, persistent left superior vena cava, the flow speed of pulmonary artery branches was increased (the flow speed of LPA was 2.86 m/s, the flow speed at the beginning of RPA was 3.47 m/s, and the distal flow speed was 2.21 m/s).

Chest CT: Tracheal bifurcation at T5 level, lower trachea narrowing with the narrowest diameter about 0.5 mm × 0.5 mm, the left superior vena cava flows back into the coronary sinus, patent foramen ovale (PFO), enlarged left atrium, perimembranous VSD about 3.6 mm, enlarged left ventricle. The left pulmonary artery originates from the beginning of the right upper pulmonary artery branch, bypasses the back of the trachea, and runs above the left bronchus.

Preoperative diagnosis: Pulmonary artery sling, tracheal stenosis, VSD, PFO. The patient was scheduled to undergo left pulmonary artery reconstruction + tracheoplasty + VSD repair under general anesthesia.

46.2 Anesthetic Management

The patient did not take any preoperative medications. After entering the operating room, ECG, noninvasive blood pressure (BP), and SpO_2 were monitored. Baseline vital signs: BP 68/42 mm Hg, heart rate (HR) 130 beats/min, SpO_2 99%. After the peripheral vein was accessed, 0.5 mg of midazolam, 1.0 mg of etomidate, 8.0 μg of sufentanil, and 2.4 mg of rocuronium were intravenously administered for the induction of anesthesia. After the eyelash reflex disappeared, an ID 3.5 mm cuffed endotracheal tube was intubated with video laryngoscopy assistance; the intubation depth was 10 cm. Pressure control (PCV) mode was adopted with 2 L/min oxygen flow rate, 50% fraction of inspired oxygen (FiO_2), 15 cm H_2O peak inspiratory pressure (PIP), 36 mL VT, 24 times/min respiratory rate (RR), 1:2 inspiratory to expiratory (I:E) time ratio. After intubation, tidal volume (VT) was found to be very low, while the end-tidal carbon dioxide partial pressure ($ETCO_2$) increased continuously, even reaching a maximum of 70 mm Hg. We adjusted PIP to 24 cm H_2O and increased RR quickly. $ETCO_2$ was slightly reduced and maintained at about 60 mm Hg.

After intubation, invasive arterial pressure (ABP), central venous pressure (CVP), bispectral index (BIS), and cerebral tissue oxygen saturation (rSO_2) monitoring were quickly established. Vital signs after intubation: ABP 65/43 mm Hg, HR 142 beats/min, SpO_2 98%, CVP 13 cm H_2O, rSO_2 70%. During the operation, propofol 4.0 mg/(kg·h), sufentanil 2.0 μg/(kg·h), and rocuronium 0.5 mg/(kg·h) were intravenously infused for the maintenance of general anesthesia. At the same time, 0.5–1.0 MAC sevoflurane was intermittently inhaled to maintain the BIS value at 40–60. The results of intraoperative artery blood gas analysis results were shown in Table 46.1.

Before the operation, tranexamic acid 10 mg/kg and ulinastatin 100,000 U was intravenously administrated for antifibrinolysis and anti-inflammation. Heparin 3 mg/kg was intravenously administrated after thoracotomy. Cardiopulmonary bypass (CPB) was initiated

Table 46.1 Intraoperative blood gas test results

Time point	pH	Hb (g/dL)	HCT (%)	PaO_2 (mm Hg)	$PaCO_2$ (mm Hg)	BE (mmol/L)	Na^+ (mmol/L)	K^+ (mmol/L)	Cl^- (mmol/L)	Ca^{2+} (mmol/L)	Lac (mmol/L)
Post-intubation	7.2	8.6	25.5	210.2	73.8	−0.94	136	3.6	106	1.33	<1
Post-ultrafiltration	7.33	11.2	33.7	518.6	48.4	−1.3	143.4	4.1	100.7	1.21	1.0

after activated clotting time (ACT) >480 s. After aortic cannulation, the patient experienced hypotension, arrhythmia, and significant ST segment depression, which was considered to be caused by the excessive depth of aortic cannulation. ABP and HR quickly returned to normal after the adjustment of aortic cannulation. The pericardial patch was used to suture and close VSD under the support of CPB. After the aortic cross-clamp was released, the heart automatically resumed beating and sinus rhythm. Dopamine 5.0 μg/(kg·min) was intravenously infused with ABP maintained at 42/35 mm Hg and HR at 112 beats/min. Epinephrine 0.02 μg/(kg·min) was added to maintain ABP at 55/41 mm Hg and HR at 120 beats/min. After the vena cava cross-clamp was released, mechanical ventilation was resumed in PCV mode with 2 L/min oxygen flow rate, 50% FiO_2, 18 cm H_2O PIP, 38 mL VT, 24 times/min RR, and an I:E ratio of 1:2. The pulmonary artery was first dissected under CBP parallel circulation. The left pulmonary artery was separated from the right pulmonary artery, and the left pulmonary artery was finally anastomosed with the main pulmonary artery. The trachea was longitudinally incised at the proximal and distal ends for slide anastomosis. The anastomosis was wrapped by the pericardial patch without leakage. Fiberoptic bronchoscopy showed that the anastomosis was unobstructed. Transesophageal echocardiography revealed a cardiac ejection fraction of 68%, pulmonary artery flow velocity of 0.7 m/s, and no residual shunt around the VSD patch. CPB flow was adjusted and gradually withdrawn. BP and HR were stable after CPB. After modified ultrafiltration, protamine 15 mg (1.2:1) was intravenously dripped to neutralize heparin. Hemocoagulase 0.5 U was used to assist hemostasis. The artery blood gas analysis was rechecked (Table 46.1), among which pH was 7.33 and Ca^{2+} was 1.21 mmol/L. RR was increased to 26 times/min and calcium gluconate 100 mg was slowly infused to supplement calcium ions. The dosage of vasoactive drugs and inhaled anesthetics was adjusted according to ABP. About 30 mL of autologous salvaged blood was transfused to maintain ABP around 82/50 mm Hg and HR 120–130 beats/min. After adequate hemostasis, the sternum was closed.

46.3 Postoperative Outcome

The operation lasted for 255 min in total, with a mild hypothermia bypass time of 154 minutes and an aortic cross-clamping time of 24 min. The estimated blood loss was about 30 mL. The urine output was 90 mL. During the operation, 50 mL of Ringer's acetate solution and 30 mL of autologous salvaged blood were transfused. The intraoperative lactate level remained within the normal range. At the end of the surgery, ABP was 85/54 mm Hg; HR was 123 beats/min, SpO_2 was 100%, CVP was 8 cm H_2O, rectal temperature was 36.5 °C, and rSO_2 was 65%. Under the monitoring of ABP, ECG, and SpO_2, the patient was transferred to the pediatric Cardiac Intensive Care Unit (CICU) with endotracheal intubation. The endotracheal tube was removed on the postoperative day 6. The patient was discharged from the CICU on postoperative day 8 and discharged from the hospital on postoperative day 19.

46.4 Review of Knowledge Points

46.4.1 Pulmonary Artery Sling

PAS is a rare congenital cardiovascular malformation characterized by the abnormal origin of LPA from RPA running between the trachea and esophagus. The abnormal LPA can compress the trachea and lead to tracheal stenosis. PAS often presents with various respiratory symptoms as the initial symptoms, including cough, shortness of breath, difficulty breathing, wheezing, recurrent respiratory infections, etc. The course of the disease is usually lengthy and recurrent. Furthermore, the effect of drug treatment is relatively poor. The severity of clinical symptoms mainly depends on the degree of tracheal and bronchial stenosis. About 90% of children with PAS show respiratory symptoms before they are 1 year old. About 30% of children with PAS have congenital heart defects, among which VSD,

ASD, and PDA are more common. In addition, it can also be accompanied by Tetralogy of Fallot, double outlet right ventricle, etc. Some are accompanied by other types of vascular rings, such as aberrant left subclavian artery and right-sided aortic arch with aberrant left subclavian artery.

In 1988, Wells and others classified PAS into type I (normal tracheal bifurcation position and angle) and type II (lower tracheal bifurcation position and increased angle) based on the position and angle of the tracheal bifurcation. Depending on whether the bronchus supplies the right upper lobe, it could be classified into subtypes A and B. The right upper lobe supplied by the normal right main bronchus is type A, as provided by the tracheal bronchus is type I B, and delivered by the underdeveloped right main bronchus is type II B, which is often accompanied by underdevelopment of the right lung.

46.4.2 Classification and Diagnostic Criteria of Tracheal Stenosis

Based on clinical symptoms and radiological diagnosis, the degree of tracheal stenosis in PAS is divided into three types: mild (occasional or no symptoms), moderate (persistent respiratory symptoms, but no respiratory distress), and severe (severe respiratory symptoms, respiratory distress, and even need for ventilator assistance).

The Hoffer grading method is used to evaluate the length of tracheal stenosis: Grade I is localized stenosis with the length of tracheal stenosis less than 50% of the total length of the main trachea. Grade II is long-segment stenosis, with the length of tracheal stenosis accounting for 50–80% of the total length of the main trachea. Grade III is diffuse stenosis with the length of tracheal stenosis greater than 80% of the total length of the main trachea. The COTTON grading method is often used to evaluate the degree of tracheal stenosis: stenosis less than 70% is grade I, stenosis 70–90% is grade II, stenosis greater than 90% is grade III, and complete obstruction is grade IV.

46.4.3 Slide Tracheoplasty

It is the safest surgical method for long-segment tracheal stenosis, which includes first cutting at the midpoint of tracheal stenosis, then opening the anterior wall of the upper tracheal end and the posterior wall of the lower tracheal end, and trimming the upper and lower tracheal ends into a tongue shape and slide them together at last. This method uses autologous tracheal tissue and a tracheal ring to ensure the integrity of the tracheal wall. The diameter of the trachea after anastomosis is twice the original size. The postoperative anastomosis is stable, and it maintains normal tracheal mucosa, which may greatly reduce the possible growth of tracheal granulation tissue.

46.5 Discussion

46.5.1 Preoperative Assessment and Preparation

Most tracheal stenosis in children with PAS is localized tracheal stenosis, which is usually caused by LPA compression. Long-segment tracheal uniform stenosis may be caused by intrauterine developmental abnormalities related to tracheal softening or membranous cartilage deficiency, which may form a ring-sling complex malformation. During the preoperative diagnostic process, imaging examinations, especially cardiac and large vessel CTA, multi-slice spiral CT, and cardiovascular magnetic resonance imaging (MRI), can clearly display the anatomical structure of the trachea and bronchial tree. Carefully reviewing the imaging data before surgery and evaluating the location and degree of airway stenosis is helpful for selecting a tracheal tube and determining the appropriate intubation depth. For children with bronchial stenosis or bronchial bridge, the selection of tracheal tube can be calculated according to the normal age. For those children with mild tracheal stenosis and airway stenosis near the carina, the tracheal tube selection is similar to the normal age children. The tracheal tube is first selected according to the normal age calculation because the airway stenosis is near the glottis. When insertion is obstructed, we could use the smaller size. Try to choose a larger tracheal tube to ensure ventilation. For severe tracheal stenosis, it is necessary to measure the transverse diameter of the stenotic segment according to the imaging data to choose the appropriate tracheal tube. The cuffed tracheal tube is the preferred choice unless the stenosis is severe. It is conducive to ventilation with the larger inner diameter of the tracheal tube. The patient, in this case, had no respiratory distress, cyanosis, or hypoxia before surgery. Therefore, this patient was classified as mild tracheal stenosis. In addition, the stenotic segment was located at the lower part of the trachea. Therefore, we chose an ID 3.5 mm cuffed endotracheal tube, and ID 2.0–3.5 mm endotracheal tubes were all prepared in advance.

46.5.2 Intraoperative Anesthetic Management

Since children with PAS may have a difficult airway, an emergency airway plan should be made before anesthesia. For patients with severe tracheal stenosis, muscle relaxants should be avoided as much as possible. Tracheal intubation can be performed under spontaneous breathing after intravenous induction combined with topical anesthesia. This case was mild tracheal stenosis, and the stenotic segment was located at the lower part of the trachea, so the patient was induced with routine anesthetics and methods by intravenous bolus injection of midazolam, etomidate, sufentanil, and rocuronium.

Compared with volume-controlled ventilation (VCV) mode, PCV mode is more conducive to the uniform distribution of gas in the lungs and can avoid lung injury caused by high airway pressure in VCV mode. Positive end-expiratory pressure ventilation (PEEP) cannot be recommended due to the increased airway pressure and alveolar pressure, negatively impacting pulmonary circulation resistance. This case had good airway compliance before intubation, but airway resistance was significantly increased, and VT was significantly reduced after endotracheal intubation. Then, $ETCO_2$ was subsequently increased, which may be due to ① bronchospasm induced by tracheal carina stimulation from the tip of the endotracheal tube, which is mediated by acetylcholine release from postganglionic cholinergic nerve fibers, and ② the increased airway resistance is caused by airway area reduction. The former cause can be relieved by sevoflurane inhalation, which can play a role in relaxing the tracheal smooth muscle. We must immediately adjust the respiratory parameters for the latter case by increasing PIP and RR. If this situation is not handled in time, it may cause hypoxia and even suffocation death due to insufficient ventilation in the child.

During the operation, general anesthesia was maintained by intravenous infusion of sufentanil, propofol, and muscle relaxants. At the same time, sevoflurane was intermittently inhaled to maintain sufficient anesthesia depth to suppress the pulmonary vasoconstriction caused by surgical stimulation. If necessary, nitroglycerin can be intravenously dripped to reduce pulmonary artery pressure based on real situations, which can benefit surgical operations. Anticholinergic drugs can also be used to reduce airway secretions during the operation.

Airway secretions should be promptly sucked out to reduce the risk of airway spasms after tracheoplasty. The depth of the endotracheal tube should be adjusted according to the surgeon's needs. Violent operations that could damage the anastomosis should be avoided.

46.6 Conclusion

In summary, careful preoperative assessment of the location and degree of tracheal stenosis, selection of an appropriate endotracheal tube, detailed preparation of an emergency airway plan for difficult airways, selection of reasonable ventilation management strategies, optimal anesthetics combination for sufficient anesthesia depth without minimal hemodynamic suppression during the operation, and proper airway management after the operation are important factors for the successful anesthetic management in children with PAS undergoing pulmonary artery sling surgery (Bin Xue).

47 Anesthetic Management of Vascular Ring Correction Surgery in a Child with Kommerell's Diverticulum

Jingjing Lv

Abstract

A 2-year-old girl was diagnosed with the right aortic arch and subclavian artery pseudoaneurysm (Kommerell's diverticulum) during the fetal period. She had been followed up since birth and was scheduled for vascular ring correction surgery. In such cases, Kommerell's diverticulum may cause compression of the trachea and esophagus. Furthermore, cerebral hypoxia may happen due to the cross-clamping of the left common carotid artery and subclavian artery to help resection of the diverticulum and anastomosing of the subclavian artery to the carotid artery. Therefore, anesthetic management should focus on assessing and managing airway stenosis and cerebral oxygen monitoring during the perioperative period.

Kommerell's diverticulum is one extremely rare type of vascular ring formed by the remnant fourth dorsal aortic arch, which is characterized by the dilated proximal aberrant right or left subclavian artery associated with either right or left aortic arches. Kommerell's diverticulum can cause compression of the trachea and esophagus and thus cause dyspnea, dysphagia, etc., compression symptoms, which require early surgery to relieve the compression. This chapter reports the perioperative management of anesthesia in a 2-year-old child with Kommerell's diverticulum for vascular ring correction surgery.

47.1 Case Presentation

A 2-years and 5-month-old girl was 87 cm in height and 14 kg in weight. She was born full-term without a history of asphyxia. Fetal ultrasonography showed the right aortic arch and subclavian artery pseudoaneurysm. She had been followed up since birth. For further treatment, she was admitted to our hospital with an echocardiographic diagnosis of right-sided aortic arch, possible aberrant left subclavian artery, and normal left heart systolic function.

Physical examination: The girl was conscious and normally responsive. Symmetrical respiratory sounds in bilateral lungs without rales and shortness of breath. Normal skin appearance without edema and cyanosis. The heart sounds were strong and regular without obvious heart murmurs. The abdomen was soft, and the limbs were warm.

Laboratory tests: Normal routine blood test and normal liver, kidney, and coagulation functions.

J. Lv (✉)
The National Children's Medical Center (Shanghai), Department of Anesthesiology of Shanghai Children's Medical Center, Shanghai Jiao Tong University School of Medicine, Shanghai, China

J. Zheng et al. (eds.), *Selected Pediatric Cardiovascular Surgery Anesthesia Cases*,
https://doi.org/10.1007/978-981-96-5614-1_47

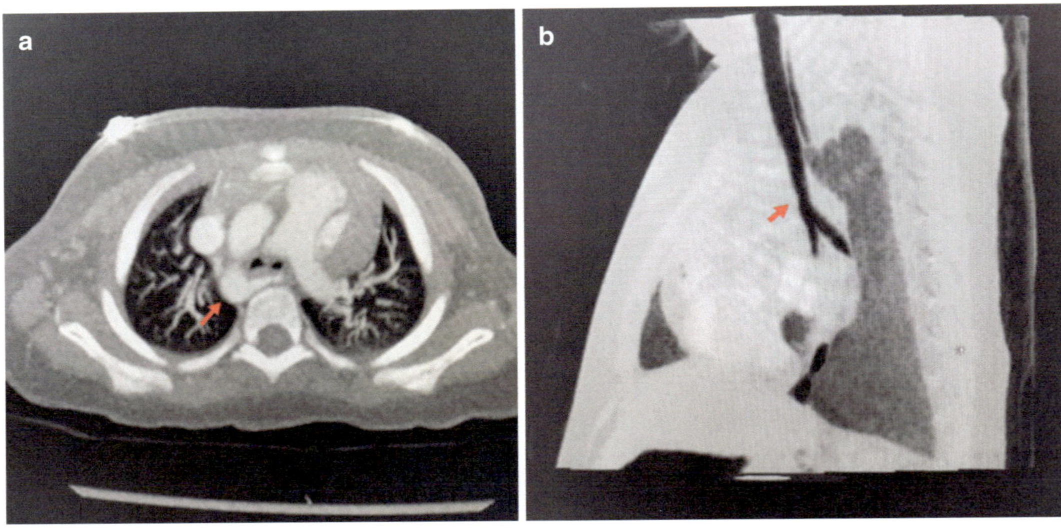

Fig. 47.1 The patient's chest CT. (**a**) The red arrow shows the Kommerell's diverticulum; (**b**) the red arrow shows the slightly narrowed area of the trachea

Chest CT: Vascular ring including the right-sided aortic arch, aberrant left subclavian artery, left patent ductus arteriosus (PDA) ligament, descending aortic Kommerell's diverticulum, mild stenosis of the trachea above the carina (Fig. 47.1a, b).

Preoperative diagnosis: Right-sided aortic arch, aberrant left subclavian artery, Kommerell's diverticulum. Elective vascular ring correction surgery was scheduled.

47.2 Anesthetic Management

The child did not take any preoperative medications. After entering the operating room (OR), routine monitoring was performed. Noninvasive blood pressure (BP) was 90/50 mm Hg, heart rate (HR) was 122 beats/min, and pulse oxygen saturation (SpO_2) was 99%. The anesthesia was induced by intravenous bolus injection of 1.5 mg midazolam, 5.5 mg etomidate, 28 μg sufentanil, and 9.0 mg rocuronium. After the eyelash reflex disappeared, an ID 4.5 mm cuffed endotracheal tube was intubated under direct laryngoscopy with a tube depth of 13 cm.

Pressure-controlled ventilation-volume guaranteed (PCV-VG) mode was used with the respiratory parameters setting as: oxygen flow rate 1 L/min, fraction of inspired oxygen (FiO_2) 40%, tidal volume (VT) 120 mL, respiratory rate (RR) 20 breaths/min, positive end-expiratory pressure (PEEP) 3 cm H_2O, and inspiratory to expiratory time ratio (I:E) 1:2. The end-tidal carbon dioxide partial pressure ($ETCO_2$) was around 42 mm Hg. Arterial blood gas analysis results showed: PH 7.338, $PaCO_2$ 44 mm Hg, PaO_2 140.9 mm Hg, HCT 33%, Na^+ 140 mmol/L, K^+ 3.56 mmol/L, Cl^- 108 mmol/L, Ca^{2+} 1.3 mmol/L.

After endotracheal intubation, the left radial artery and left femoral artery were first catheterized for simultaneous invasive blood pressure (ABP) monitoring in the upper and lower extremities under ultrasound guidance. The right jugular vein was then catheterized under ultrasound guidance for continuous monitoring of central venous pressure (CVP) and vasoactive drug infusion. The left great saphenous vein was also catheterized for rapid fluid replacement. The regional cerebral oxygen saturation (rSO_2) monitoring was conducted on the left forehead. General anesthesia was maintained by intravenous infusion of 4.0 mg/(kg·h)propofol, 2.0 μg/(kg·h) sufentanil, and 0.5 mg/(kg·h) rocuronium and intermittent inhalation of 1% sevoflurane.

During the operation, surgical exploration showed that the aortic arch was right-sided, the aberrant left subclavian artery originated from the descending aorta, the initial part of the aberrant left subclavian artery was enlarged to form a Kommerell's diverticulum, and the PDA ligament was 3 mm in diameter, all of them formed a large vascular ring together. The PDA ligament was ligated and severed. The root of the diverticulum was ligated with the diverticulum resected. The left subclavian artery was severed and connected with the left common carotid artery via end-to-side anastomosis. The anastomosis orifice was 8 mm. During the period of carotid artery cross-clamping, rSO_2 dropped from 64% to 50%. FiO_2 was quickly increased; $ETCO_2$ was maintained at a slightly high level while BP was maintained stable. Then, rSO_2 was soon improved. The vital signs were stable during the operation.

47.3 Postoperative Outcome

The operation lasted approximately 85 min in total, with the left carotid artery cross-clamping for 25 min. The estimated blood loss was about 20 mL. The urine output was 50 mL. About 300 mL of Ringer's acetate solution was infused during the operation. There was no blood products were transfused. After the operation, the patient was transferred to the cardiac surgery intensive care unit (CICU) with continuous monitoring of ABP, ECG, and SpO_2. The endotracheal tube was successfully removed, and she was transferred out of CICU on postoperative day 2. She was discharged from the hospital 1 week later.

47.4 Review of Knowledge Points

47.4.1 Definition and Classification

Kommerell's diverticulum is a type of aortic diverticulum, accounting for most aortic diverticulum. Salomonowitz et al. divided the aortic diverticulum into three types: ① Right aortic arch combined with aberrant left subclavian artery (most common); ② left aortic arch combined with aberrant right subclavian artery; and ③ aortic diverticulum at the junction of the aortic duct, duct diverticulum (but this category is not considered to be Kommerell's diverticulum). According to the initial nomenclature, when the aortic diverticulum is combined with the aberrant subclavian artery, it is called Kommerell's diverticulum.

47.4.2 Surgical Treatment

The occurrence of severe esophageal or tracheal compression symptoms in a child is a clear surgical indication for this type of disease. Once it is diagnosed, surgery should be performed as soon as possible. However, children with this condition often have no symptoms and are accidentally discovered through chest CT scans. Because this type of disease is relatively rare, there is currently no consensus on the surgical indications for asymptomatic Kommerell's diverticulum in children. Our center currently advocates for surgery as soon as possible after diagnosis, regardless of the presence of symptoms. Reports have pointed out that there is a 19–53% chance of rupture and dissection in the diverticulum with poor prognosis regardless of the presence of symptoms. Thus, many cardiothoracic surgeons choose surgical correction rather than conservative treatment. In adult patients, the surgical procedures often include graft replacement of the descending aorta with in situ subclavian artery reconstruction or graft replacement of the descending aorta with aortic arch subclavian artery bypass or total arch replacement. In children, the common surgical procedure is diverticulum resection with subclavian artery-carotid artery anastomosis through the left thoracotomy.

47.5 Discussion

47.5.1 Preoperative Assessment and Preparation

Kommerell's diverticulum often coexists with a vascular ring, which can cause compression of the airway and esophagus, leading to symptoms such as wheezing, cyanosis, shortness of breath, feeding difficulties, and developmental delays. The respiratory symptoms caused by airway compression are more likely to occur in children than adults due to the less rigid trachea. Due to the presence of vascular ring compression and tracheal stenosis in these children, the key to anesthetic management should focus on thorough preoperative airway assessment and preparation as well as intraoperative ventilation management to keep the airway open. In this case, the trachea was slightly narrowed above the carina with an anterior–posterior diameter of about 4.0 mm. The bronchi were unobstructed. Therefore, there were no preoperative airway obstruction symptoms in this patient. The narrowed part of the trachea did not affect the tracheal intubation and ventilation since the normal ID 4.5 mm cuffed tracheal tube was easily intubated with a depth of 13 cm, and the airway resistance was within the normal range after the induction of anesthesia. The arterial blood PaO_2 and $PaCO_2$ were normal range during the operation.

47.5.2 Intraoperative Anesthetic Management

The surgical procedure for such pediatric patients often involves diverticulum resection and left subclavian artery-left common carotid artery anastomosis without CPB in a lateral position. During the operation, the left radial artery catheterization for ABP monitoring was conducted to assess the patency of vascular anastomosis by comparing the ABP differences before and after surgical correction. The upper extremity ABP before and after surgical correction was basically the same, around 75/53 mm Hg. Monitoring right upper or lower extremities, ABP can accurately and reliably reflect the patient's blood pressure during the partial cross-clamping of the left common carotid artery and left subclavian artery, which was maintained at about 95/56 mm Hg. After the artery cross-clamping was released, the arterial blood gas analysis should be reviewed in time the internal environment should be adjusted, and the blood pressure drop caused by the release of acidic substances should be avoided. Studies have shown that the Willis circle is incomplete in 50–85% of cases. Since long-term low rSO_2 values can lead to cognitive dysfunction, prolonged length of hospital stay, and perioperative cerebrovascular accidents, it is very important to monitor the changes in left and right brain blood flow and rSO_2 when brain blood flow decreases.

The blood flow to the left common carotid artery must be temporarily blocked during the anastomosis. Therefore, insufficient blood supply to the left brain can occur without insufficient blood flow support from the Willis Circle or other sources. The neurological complications after the cardiac and carotid surgeries can be avoided by monitoring rSO_2 due to the early detection of cerebral oxygen supply-demand imbalance. It was previously reported that the left forehead rSO_2 dropped from 60% to 40% after the left common carotid artery cross-clamping. The forehead rSO_2 dropped from 64% to 50% in the present case after the left common carotid artery cross-clamping. After the increase of FiO_2, the maintenance of slightly high-level $ETCO_2$, and short-time use of dopamine 5.0 μg/(kg·min) before the left common carotid artery cross-clamping, rSO_2 was improved soon. During the vascular anastomosis, BP was maintained at about 90/50 mm Hg without vasoactive drugs, $ETCO_2$ was maintained at around 40–50 mm Hg, and FiO_2 was increased to 100%. The patient's rSO_2 was maintained at about 58%. The patient recovered well after the operation without any significant neurological complications. The long-term neurological complications were also not found during the postoperative follow-up. Therefore, it is necessary to monitor rSO_2 changes in such patients undergoing vascular ring correction surgery.

47.6 Conclusion

In summary, it is essential to conduct a detailed preoperative airway assessment due to the potential compression of the airway and esophagus to ensure the safety of anesthesia. If there exists tracheal stenosis, the location and severity of tracheal stenosis should be assessed in detail, such as whether it is necessary first to correct the tracheal stenosis before the vascular ring correction, whether it affects tracheal intubation, mechanical ventilation, etc. In addition, intraoperative monitoring and management should be strengthened. Cerebral rSO_2 monitoring can help to prevent postoperative cerebral injuries and other complications caused by cerebral ischemia and hypoxia (Jingjing Lv).

48 Anesthetic Management of Tricuspid Valvuloplasty Surgery in a Child After Ventricular Septal Defect Repair

Jingjing Lv

Abstract

A 10-year-old boy who underwent ventricular septal defect repair 8 years ago was diagnosed with severe tricuspid regurgitation and was scheduled for tricuspid valvuloplasty surgery. The right heart was significantly enlarged due to long-term tricuspid regurgitation. Preoperative arrhythmia and right heart failure occurred. The risk of cardiac rupture and arrhythmia before the establishment of cardiopulmonary bypass during the secondary thoracotomy is significantly increased due to severe adhesion. The perioperative anesthetic management should focus on maintaining the hemodynamic stability, preventing the factors that worsen right heart function, and improving the right heart function.

Tricuspid regurgitation (TR) refers to the reflux of blood from the right ventricle into the right atrium through the incompletely closed tricuspid valve, which is usually secondary to the right ventricular dilation and right ventricular hypertension caused by severe pulmonary hypertension or right ventricular outflow tract obstruction. It can also be secondary to ventricular septal defect (VSD) occlusion or post-thoracotomy, which is a relatively rare postoperative complication of such surgeries. However, long-term reflux can cause severe heart failure and endanger life. This chapter reports the anesthetic management of tricuspid valvuloplasty surgery in a child with severe TR and heart failure after VSD repair.

48.1 Case Presentation

A 10-year-old and 6-month-old boy was 138 cm in height and 27.5 kg in weight. He was naturally born at full term without a history of asphyxia at birth. He underwent VSD repair surgery at a local hospital 8 years ago. He came to our hospital due to abnormal postoperative follow-up results. Echocardiography indicated severe TR. He was admitted to the ward with "incomplete closure of the tricuspid valve after ventricular septal defect repair surgery".

Physical examination: The patient was conscious and responsive without obvious abnormalities. No cyanosis. The bilateral lung sounds were symmetrical and coarse. Irregular heart rhythm and II/VI systolic murmurs at the precordial area. Hyperactive P2 sound. No obvious discomfort at rest but shortness of breath after activities. The heart function grade III and ASA classification IV.

J. Lv (✉)
The National Children's Medical Center (Shanghai), Department of Anesthesiology of Shanghai Children's Medical Center, Shanghai Jiao Tong University School of Medicine, Shanghai, China
e-mail: lvjingjing@scmc.com.cn

J. Zheng et al. (eds.), *Selected Pediatric Cardiovascular Surgery Anesthesia Cases*,
https://doi.org/10.1007/978-981-96-5614-1_48

Routine blood test: White blood cell counts 4.12×10^9/L, neutrophil percentage 32.5%, red blood cell counts 3.68×10^{12}/L, hemoglobin 113.0 g/L, platelet count 170×10^9/L.

Coagulation function: APTT 35.7 s, PT 14.6 s.

Liver and kidney function were basically normal.

Echocardiography: Post-VSD surgery with no obvious residual shunt, severe TR, huge right atrium, and normal left ventricular systolic function.

Cardiac magnetic resonance imaging indicated post-VSD surgery, severe TR, huge right atrium and right ventricle, and narrowed anteroposterior diameter of the right bronchus. Left ventricular ejection fraction (LVEF) 52.5%, stroke volume (SV) 27.2 mL, left ventricular end-diastolic volume (LVEDV) 51.84 mL, right ventricular ejection fraction (RVEF) 45.5%, stroke volume (SV) 177.9 mL, and right ventricular end-diastolic volume (RVEDV) 390.8 mL.

Electrocardiography (ECG): Ectopic rhythm, atrial fibrillation, complete right bundle branch block, possible right ventricular hypertrophy.

Preoperative diagnosis: Incomplete closure of the tricuspid valve after VSD surgery. Elective tricuspid valvuloplasty surgery was scheduled.

48.2 Anesthetic Management

After entering the operating room, the vital signs were routinely monitored with non-invasive blood pressure (BP) 112/65 mm Hg, heart rate (HR) 86 beats/min with atrial flutter rhythm, and pulse oxygen saturation (SpO_2) 100%. Continuous invasive arterial pressure (ABP) monitoring was conducted before the induction of anesthesia. Then, 2.0 mg midazolam, 6.0 mg etomidate, 10 mg ketamine, 25 μg sufentanil, and 15 mg rocuronium were administered intravenously titrated for the induction of anesthesia. After the eyelash reflex disappeared, an ID 6.5 mm cuffed endotracheal tube was intubated under direct laryngoscopy with a tube depth of 18 cm. Pressure-controlled ventilation-volume guaranteed (PCV-VG) mode was used with respiratory parameters setting as: oxygen flow rate 1 L/min, fraction of inspired oxygen (FiO_2) 50%, tidal volume (VT) 250 mL, respiratory rate (RR) 16 breaths/min, positive end-expiratory pressure (PEEP) 3 cm H_2O, and inspiratory to expiratory time ratio (I:E) 1:2. During the operation, the end-tidal carbon dioxide partial pressure ($ETCO_2$) was maintained at 35–45 mm Hg by RR adjustment. During the operation, general anesthesia was maintained by continuous intravenous infusion of 4.0 mg/(kg·h) propofol, 2.0 μg/(kg·h) sufentanil, and 0.5 mg/(kg·h) rocuronium and intermittent sevoflurane inhalation to maintain BIS at 40–60. The internal jugular and femoral veins were catheterized under ultrasound guidance to continuously monitor central venous pressure (CVP) and infusion of vasoactive drugs and fluids. Baseline CVP was 19 cm H_2O. The operation was performed under cardiopulmonary bypass (CPB) support. During the operation, the right atrium, right ventricle, and tricuspid annulus were found to be enlarged. The tricuspid valve could not be fully closed. The anterior chordae tendineae were missing. Attempts were unsuccessful in reducing the annulus, chordae tendineae, and papillary muscles and creating double holes. Eventually, the tricuspid leaflets were sutured together with a pad to form a clover shape. The water injection test showed a significant improvement in TR. The patent oval foramen was preserved. The heart automatically resumed beating and sinus rhythm after aortic cross-clamp release. Dobutamine and norepinephrine were intravenously infused to maintain ABP at 100–110/50–55 mm Hg. Transesophageal echocardiography was used to evaluate the surgical outcome. CPB was successfully weaned off after a gradual reduction of CPB flow. Protamine was used to neutralize heparin at a ratio of 1:1. Arterial blood gas analysis result was rechecked, electrolytes were adjusted, and acid–base balance was maintained. One hundred milliliter of autologous blood was infused in total. After adequate hemostasis, the chest was closed layer by layer. The CPB time was 165 min. The aortic cross-clamping time was 111 min. The estimated blood loss was about 50 mL. Theurine output was 500 mL. A total of 250 mL of sodium acetate

Ringer's solution and 100 mL of hydroxyethyl starch were transfused.

48.3 Postoperative Outcome

The child was transferred to the cardiac surgery intensive care unit (CICU) with continuous monitoring of ABP, ECG, and SpO_2. The endotracheal tube was successfully removed on the postoperative day 3. The patient was discharged from the CICU on postoperative day 7 and from the hospital on postoperative day 14.

48.4 Review of Knowledge Points

48.4.1 Etiology and Pathophysiology of TR

Primary (or organic) TR is caused by congenital or acquired abnormalities of the valve itself, accounting for 15–20%; Secondary (or functional) TR is due to deformation of the tricuspid valve caused by pressure and/or volume load in the right heart chamber. Secondary TR is much more common than primary TR, accounting for 80–85%. The most common causes of functional tricuspid regurgitation are right heart enlargement, left heart dysfunction, and mitral valve diseases, followed by dilated cardiomyopathy, pulmonary hypertension, and atrial fibrillation. Atrial fibrillation is currently considered one of the independent risk factors for functional tricuspid regurgitation. During atrial fibrillation, as the electrophysiology and mechanical activity of the atrium are disordered and the atrium loses its regular autonomous contraction and relaxation, blood cannot be filled and discharged normally, resulting in blood stasis, atrial enlargement, leading to annular enlargement, and then valve regurgitation. In this case, the child had secondary tricuspid regurgitation after ventricular septal defect repair surgery. Long-term reflux leads to excessive volume load in the right ventricle, right atrium, and ventricle enlargement, right heart failure, and atrial fibrillation; the right atrium and right ventricle enlargement further aggravate tricuspid regurgitation.

48.4.2 Treatment of TR

It is generally thought that functional TR can be improved by diuretic-based drug treatment. However, recent evidences show that long-term chronic TR causes excessive volume load in the right ventricle, which can lead to irreversible right ventricular myocardial injury, and satisfactory tricuspid valve repair or replacement can reduce the mortality. Therefore, the importance of TR treatment has been increased. More and more tricuspid valve surgeries are conducted. In recent years, transcatheter valve intervention has rapidly developed. Under the drive of transcatheter aortic valve replacement (TAVR), transcatheter repair and replacement of the tricuspid valve have also developed. However, due to the special structure of the tricuspid valve, the development and innovation of devices play a key role in technology development.

48.5 Discussion

48.5.1 Preoperative Preparation and Evaluation

Preoperative preparation requires multidisciplinary cooperation to fully assess the child's cardiopulmonary function status and whether there is acute right heart failure, arrhythmia, etc., including anesthesiology, cardiology, respiratory medicine, and intensive care unit. Special attention should be focused on peripheral tissue edema, jugular vein dilation, hepatosplenomegaly, ascites symptoms. The patient's cardiac function can be evaluated by ECG, chest X-ray, echocardiogram, magnetic resonance, etc. The preoperative cardiac function can be adjusted by internal medicine treatment. With sufficient preoperative evaluation and preparation, the risk of perioperative complications can be minimized.

In this case, the patient showed a significant decrease in activity tolerance before surgery, shortness of breath after activity, arrhythmia, and atrial fibrillation. Echocardiography and cardiac MRI indicated a large right atrium and right ventricle, with right heart dysfunction. Before the operation, the child was advised to reduce activity and was treated with amiodarone. The child did not show obvious symptoms of right heart failure, such as lower limb edema and hepatosplenomegaly. Therefore, the diuretic and inotropic drugs were not used before the operation. The anesthesiologist conducted a thorough preoperative assessment, formulated a complete anesthesia plan based on the child's own hemodynamic characteristics, and prepared for various cardiovascular events. Preoperative communication and education relieved the child's anxiety and reduced myocardial oxygen consumption. After entering the room, continuous arterial blood pressure monitoring was established in a conscious state, making titrated medication possible and ensuring hemodynamic stability during induction. Considering that this child underwent secondary thoracotomy with preoperative atrial fibrillation, the risk of serious arrhythmias during the adhesion dissection was significantly increased. Therefore, a defibrillator and external defibrillation electrodes were prepared before the operation for timely defibrillation or electrical cardioversion.

48.5.2 Intraoperative and Postoperative Anesthetic Management

The goal of intraoperative anesthetic management is to maintain the right heart function. All factors that may increase pulmonary vascular resistance and potentially worsen right heart function should be avoided. The fast-onset anesthetics with minimal circulatory impact can be used for the induction of anesthesia. Adequate sedation and analgesia were required to reduce the pulmonary vascular resistance. During the maintenance of anesthesia, attention should be paid to the adjustment of anesthesia depth to avoid insufficient anesthesia, which may lead to sympathetic excitement and pulmonary vascular resistance increase. Excessive deep anesthesia should also be avoided in case of excessive circulatory suppression. Insufficient ventilation can increase the risk of hypoxemia, hypercapnia, and atelectasis, leading to increased pulmonary vascular resistance. However, high airway pressure and positive end-expiratory pressure during surgery can also increase pulmonary vascular resistance and worsen right heart function. Therefore, for such patients, the goal of intraoperative ventilation management should focus on minimizing the ventilation pressure and positive end-expiratory pressure level while ensuring hypoxemia and hypercapnia do not occur. The process of anesthesia induction was smooth without significant hemodynamic changes in this case. To reduce the pulmonary vascular resistance and increase the forward blood flow of the right ventricle, PaO_2 and $ETCO_2$ were maintained at 100–120 mm Hg and 35–40 mm Hg, respectively, by adjusting ventilator parameters based on respiratory function monitoring and blood gas analysis. After the aorta cross-clamp was released, dobutamine and norepinephrine were intravenously infused to enhance cardiac contractibility and increase blood pressure, further improving brain and coronary artery perfusion. If the postoperative hemodynamics is unstable, cardiac assist devices can be considered for use. In this case, the hemodynamics were maintained stable by the proactive use of vasoactive drugs after surgery, and the patient was safely transferred to the intensive care unit for further monitoring and treatment.

The vasoactive drugs and mechanical ventilation support continued to be used after the operation. Pulmonary infection and atelectasis should be avoided, which can increase pulmonary vascular resistance and right heart load. Amiodarone, inotropes, and diuretics continued to be used for symptomatic treatment. The child recovered very well after the operation.

48.6 Conclusion

In summary, proactive preoperative preparation and management, rational use of positive inotropic drugs and vasoactive drugs, appropriate respiratory support, avoiding factors that exacerbate right heart failure, and maintaining hemodynamic stability are keys to the perioperative management of children with right heart failure (Jingjing Lv).

49 Anesthetic Management of Right Ventricle-Pulmonary Artery Conduit Replacement in a Child After Radical Surgery for Tetralogy of Fallot

Yingying Ji

Abstract

A 9-year-old boy underwent tetralogy of Fallot (TOF) correction and arterial duct closure surgery at 6 months old. He was admitted to our hospital due to worsening cyanosis of the lips, shortness of breath, and eyelid and facial edema after the respiratory tract infection. He was treated with inotropes, diuretics, and mechanical ventilation. He underwent right ventricle-pulmonary artery conduit replacement after the cardiac function was improved. In this case, the anesthetic management should focus on adjusting preoperative cardiac function, infection control, intraoperative monitoring, rational use of inotropes and fluid replacement, and avoiding aggravation of right heart dysfunction.

Tetralogy of Fallot (TOF) is the most common type of cyanotic congenital heart disease. The long-term survival rate of children with TOF has been greatly increasing with the continuous improvement of surgical procures. However, the residual obstruction of the right ventricular outflow tract (RVOT) after surgery is still the most common reason for reoperation cardiac surgery in children with TOF. Reoperation cardiac surgery increases the risk of heavy bleeding and arrhythmia. The anesthesiologist in charge should make a detailed contingency plan. For those patients with chronic right heart failure caused by RVOT obstruction, the key point of anesthetic management is to reduce the right ventricular afterload and maintain the right ventricular function.

49.1 Case Presentation

The patient was a 9-year-old and 6-month-old boy with 21.6 kg in weight. He was born at 32 weeks of gestation via hasten parturition. He experienced a history of asphyxia resuscitation after birth, and a heart murmur was heard. Echocardiography further clarified the diagnosis of TOF. He underwent TOF correction surgery for patent ductus arteriosus (PDA) closure in 2012. He was followed up regularly until 2017. Prior to this surgery, cyanosis of the lips, eyelids, and face edema, shortness of breath with paroxysmal cough, and yellow sputum occurred, which indicated the acute exacerbation of chronic heart failure caused by the respiratory tract infection. Carbon dioxide retention remained significantly high after high-flow oxygen therapy. So, it was

Y. Ji (✉)
The National Children's Medical Center (Shanghai), Department of Anesthesiology of Shanghai Children's Medical Center, Shanghai Jiao Tong University School of Medicine, Shanghai, China
e-mail: jiyingying@scmc.com.cn

J. Zheng et al. (eds.), *Selected Pediatric Cardiovascular Surgery Anesthesia Cases*,
https://doi.org/10.1007/978-981-96-5614-1_49

determined to conduct the endotracheal intubation and bedside mechanical ventilation support. The mechanical ventilation parameters were set as a fraction of inspired oxygen (FiO_2) 60%, positive end-expiratory pressure (PEEP) 6 cm H_2O, respiratory rate (RR) 23 times/min, and peak inspiratory pressure (PIP) 19 cm H_2O. Cefotaxime was given for anti-infection treatment. After dopamine was intravenously infused to maintain blood pressure and furosemide for diuresis to reduce the heart preload, the vital signs became stable, and the cyanosis was improved. After 9 days of mechanical ventilation supportive treatment, he was successfully withdrawn from the ventilator, and elective right ventricle-pulmonary artery conduit replacement surgery was scheduled.

Physical examination: The patient was conscious, had shortness of breath, had no respiratory retractions, pulse oxygen saturation (SpO_2) 94–98% under face mask oxygen supplement, heart rate (HR) 128 beats/min, and grade III–IV systolic murmur. Facial and limb edema, hepatomegaly with three fingers below the ribs, peripheral cyanosis, capillary refill test 3 s, scoliosis, normal limb muscle tone.

Laboratory tests: Routine blood tests, coagulation, and liver and kidney function were all within normal ranges.

Echocardiography: Post-TOF surgery, no obvious residual shunt, main pulmonary artery flow speed increase with proximal flow speed 1.0 m/s, distal flow speed 2.25 m/s, left pulmonary artery stenosis, mild to moderate tricuspid regurgitation, reduced right ventricular systolic activity, normal left ventricular systolic function.

Cardiac CT: Post-TOF surgery, relative stenosis at the origin of the left pulmonary artery, distal dilatation, right pulmonary artery dilatation.

Chest X-ray: Left mediastinal deviation, large cardiac shadow, blurred lung markings.

Preoperative diagnosis: Acute exacerbation of chronic heart failure, dyspnea, bronchitis, post-TOF surgery, postoperative scoliosis. Elective RVOT reconstruction surgery was scheduled.

49.2 Anesthetic Management

The patient did not take any preoperative medications. He was transferred to the operating room from the pediatric Cardiac Intensive Care Unit (CICU) with catheterization of the right internal jugular vein and left femoral vein. Norepinephrine 0.05 μg/(kg·min) was continuously infused to maintain hemodynamic stability. Non-invasive blood pressure (BP), electrocardiogram (ECG), and SpO_2 were routinely monitored upon entering the operating room. The basic vital signs are BP 107/52 mm Hg, HR 105 beats/min, and SpO_2 98%. Anesthesia was induced by intravenous bolus injection of midazolam 2.0 mg, etomidate 4.0 mg, sufentanil 20 μg, and rocuronium 20 mg. After losing the eyelash reflex, an ID 6.0 mm cuffed endotracheal tube was intubated under a visual laryngoscope and fixed 18 cm away from the incisors. The pressure-controlled ventilation (PCV) mode was adopted with an oxygen flow rate of 2 L/min, FiO_2 50%, PIP13 cm H_2O, RR 13 times/min, inspiratory-to-expiratory time ratio (I:E) 1:2, PEEP 4 cm H_2O. Auscultation revealed asymmetric lung sounds with slightly light left lung sounds (due to the pressure from the scoliosis).

After the endotracheal intubation, the left radial artery was catheterized for continuous artery blood pressure (ABP) monitoring. The central venous pressure (CVP) was monitored from the right jugular vein. Body temperature and Bispectral Index (BIS) were also monitored. Blood gas analysis and coagulation test were checked after anesthetic induction and before separation from cardiopulmonary bypass. Vital signs after anesthetic induction: ABP 100/65 mm Hg, HR 75 beats/min, CVP 10 cm H_2O, BIS 43. General anesthesia was maintained by continuous intravenous infusion of 4.0 mg/(kg·h) propofol, 2 μg/(kg·h) sufentanil, and 0.5 mg/(kg·h) rocuronium. Intermittent inhalation of sevoflurane maintains BIS at 40–60. The ventilator parameters were adjusted based on the blood gas analysis results to maintain the partial pressure

Table 49.1 Intraoperative blood gas test results

Time point	Hb (g/dL)	HCT (%)	pH	PaO_2 (mm Hg)	$PaCO_2$ (mm Hg)	BE (mmol/L)	Na^+ (mmol/L)	K^+ (mmol/L)	Cl^- (mmol/L)	Ca^{2+} (mmol/L)	Lac (mmol/L)
Pre-extracorporeal	14.4	45.9	7.5	210.5	29.6	7.0	137.2	3.6	100.5	1.1	1.2
Post-extracorporeal stop	10.3	31.3	7.5	319.0	28.8	4.1	138.3	3.4	105.3	1.0	1.2

of end-tidal carbon dioxide ($ETCO_2$) at 35–40 mm Hg.

CPB was established after systemic heparinization and cannulations of the femoral artery and vein. The artificial blood vessel made by a 20 mm GTX conduit with three artificially sutured vessel leaflets of the pericardial patch was used to connect the bifurcation of the left and right pulmonary arteries and the original RVOT incision. At the end of the surgery, the pulmonary artery was catheterized under direct vision to measure the pulmonary artery pressure. The pulmonary artery pressure was 30/18 mm Hg, while ABP was 100/60 mm Hg. Mild hyperventilation was maintained to reduce the pulmonary vascular resistance. Dopamine (5.0 μg/(kg·min)) was intravenously infused to enhance myocardial contractility and maintain hemodynamic stability. Transesophageal echocardiography (TEE) was used to assess the surgical effect and cardiac function. TEE showed no residual shunt and no residual obstruction. RVOT flow speed was 0.8 m/s, and pulmonary artery flow speed was 1.4 m/s. Mild tricuspid and aortic valve regurgitation. After modified ultrafiltration, protamine was intravenously given to neutralize heparin with 1:1 ratio. Intraoperative blood gas analysis results are shown in Table 49.1. The coagulation function test showed ACT 98 s and CR 23. According to the blood gas analysis results, 300 mg of calcium gluconate was given. Two milliliter plasma and 100 mL red cell suspension were transfused. At the end of the surgery, HR was 68 beats/min, and ABP was 102/55 mm Hg. The sternum was closed after satisfied hemostasis.

49.3 Postoperative Outcome

The operation lasted for 235 min, with a CPB time of 100 min. The patient was transferred to the CICU with endotracheal intubation, continuous infusion of vasoactive drugs, and continuous monitoring of ABP, ECG, and SpO_2. Postoperative norepinephrine, dopamine, and milrinone were used to maintain hemodynamic stability. The endotracheal tube was removed on the postoperative day 7. The patient was discharged from the CICU on postoperative day 14 and from the hospital on postoperative day 27.

49.4 Review of Knowledge Points

49.4.1 Surgical Treatment of TOF

Once a child is diagnosed with TOF, cardiac surgery should be considered. According to the development of the pulmonary artery, patients with TOF who meet the criteria for single-stage surgery should undergo single-stage radical surgery. Otherwise, palliative surgery should be conducted. Currently, the most commonly used palliative surgical methods include modified Blalock–Taussig shunt, central shunt, and RVOT patch augmentation. RVOT residual obstruction is the most common reason for reoperation after the radical surgery of TOF. The best repair strategy for children with TOF remains controversial. The size of the pulmonary valve annulus, the timing of surgery, and whether transvalvular repair is necessary are still determined by using the reference nomogram of the pulmonary valve annulus diameter. Techniques for pulmonary valve replacement include allogeneic valve replacement, valved conduit replacement, in situ implantation of a biological valve, and RVOT reconstruction with GTX.

49.4.2 Impact of Long-Term Complications After TOF Surgery on Anesthetic Management

Right heart volume overload can occur after TOF surgery in the presence of pulmonary valve insufficiency, tricuspid regurgitation, or residual shunting. Suppose there is also a stenosis of the pulmonary artery or a residual obstruction of the right ventricular outflow tract causing an excessive pressure right heart overload. In that case, there will be a superimposed effect. Over time, the long-term presence of volume and pressure overload in the right heart will cause the right ventricular myocardium to thicken, compliance to deteriorate, and eventually, right heart failure. Therefore, these children need to undergo cardiac magnetic resonance, echocardiography, and even exercise testing to assess the status of right heart function before surgery.

49.5 Discussion

49.5.1 Preoperative Assessment and Preparation

The patient had a long history of shortness of breath and cyanosis after TOF surgery. Based on the preoperative clinical symptoms, signs, laboratory tests, and imaging results, he was diagnosed with chronic cardiac dysfunction. Therefore, anesthetic management aims to maintain hemodynamic stability, improve cardiac and respiratory function, and maintain organ perfusion. In this case, adequate preoperative preparation, including anti-infection, inotropes, and diuresis, was conducted to improve cardiovascular function. RVOT reconstruction was scheduled after the infection was well controlled and cardiovascular function was stabilized. In addition, we also focused on the effects of spinal scoliosis on anesthetic management. The child's neck bent backward and was relatively fixed with limited mobility. Although the growth valve had been placed, the scoliosis was still significant, which could make intubation difficult. The child had a good mouth opening. After rapid intravenous induction and satisfied mask ventilation, we decided to conduct oral intubation under visual laryngoscopy. The ventilator parameters were appropriately adjusted to maintain the partial pressure of carbon dioxide in the blood at 35–45 mm Hg and avoid pulmonary resistance increase and right heart failure worsening.

49.5.2 Intraoperative Anesthetic Management

The anesthetic strategy used in this child was similar to other pediatric cardiac anesthesia. The anesthetics with less impact on cardiac function were chosen for the induction and maintenance of anesthesia. In this case, anesthesia was induced with intravenous bolus injection of midazolam, etomidate, sufentanil, and rocuronium. Anesthesia was maintained with intravenous infusion of propofol, sufentanil, and rocuronium and intermittent inhalation of sevoflurane to maintain BIS at 40–60 and avoid tachycardia caused by light anesthesia.

Patients with right heart failure are very sensitive to the increase of preload and pulmonary resistance, which can cause acute exacerbation of right heart failure. Restrictive fluid input, appropriate inotropes to increase myocardial contractility, and reduced pulmonary vascular resistance can improve cardiac output and tissue perfusion. In addition to the basic monitoring of ECG, SpO_2, $ETCO_2$, temperature, urine output, ABP, CVP, and BIS were also monitored. The ventilator parameters were adjusted to avoid CO_2 accumulation and mean airway pressure increase, further increasing the right ventricle afterload. In addition, the pulmonary artery was catheterized under vision for direct pulmonary artery pressure monitoring. Transesophageal echocardiography was used to assess the surgical effect and cardiac function status to guide the use of vasoactive drugs and volume replacement. The entire surgical procedure was uneventful, without massive bleeding or arrhythmia. After the RVOT augmentation by a patch, dopamine was given to increase HR and BP. Dopamine can provide inotropic support while the pulmonary arterial resistance is not increased. Suppose the patient's pulmonary arterial pressure is high. In that case, milrinone can be combined with a loading dose of 50 μg/kg and maintenance dose of 0.5–1.0 μg/(kg.min), which may reduce the pulmonary artery pressure, enhance the myocardial contractility, and improve the myocardial diastolic function. If the blood pressure is still low, epinephrine or norepinephrine can be considered to maintain blood pressure and perfusion.

49.6 Shortcomings and Limitations

If conditions allow, the mini-invasive monitoring (Most Care®, LIDCO hemodynamic monitors) of pulmonary artery pressure, stroke volume, cardiac output, peripheral vascular resistance, and myocardial contractility can be used to facilitate hemodynamic management during surgery and improve the postoperative outcomes.

49.7 Conclusion

In conclusion, the anesthetic management for children with RVOT obstruction after TOF surgery and preoperative symptoms of right heart failure should focus on the maintenance of hemodynamic stability by using anesthetics with less impact on cardiovascular function. Furthermore, proactive regulation of the preoperative cardiac and pulmonary functions, closely monitoring hemodynamic changes, rational use of inotropes and fluid replacement, and avoiding the aggravation of right heart dysfunction during surgery should be implemented to ensure tissue sufficient perfusion, protect the function of the major organs, and reduce the perioperative mortality (Yingying Ji).

Anesthetic Management of Malignant Arrhythmia during Re-thoracotomy

50

Yingying Tao

Abstract

A 7-year-old boy with complex congenital heart disease characterized by double outlet right ventricle (DORV), ventricular septal defect (VSD), atrial septal defect (ASD), coarctation of the aorta (CoA), and patent ductus arteriosus (PDA) underwent arterial switch surgery (ASO) + VSD repair + ASD repair + PDA ligation + CoA correction surgery 6 years ago. During a recent follow-up, echocardiography demonstrated supravalvular aortic anastomosis stenosis. The patient was scheduled for surgical treatment. Malignant arrhythmia occurred during the thoracotomy, which was successfully managed and quickly returned to normal. For patients undergoing re-thoracotomy, the key to anesthetic management should focus on the prevention and preparation for various potential accidents and quick response to these emergent accidents.

The treatment of complex congenital heart disease (CHD) poses a huge challenge for cardiovascular surgeons and their team members. With the increase in surgical complexity, lowering the ages of patients, and higher diversity of surgeries, more and more complex congenital heart diseases require staged surgical treatment and(or) reoperation for postoperative complications. The number of re-thoracotomies is increasing year by year. The most common and troublesome events for anesthesiologists during re-thoracotomy include malignant arrhythmias requiring defibrillation or synchronized cardioversion, unexpected major bleeding, or anticipated difficulties in thoracotomy requiring femoral artery–venous bypass support to finish the operation. This case reports the key issues of anesthetic management for sudden malignant arrhythmia in a child undergoing re-thoracotomy.

50.1 Case Presentation

A 7-year-old boy with 24.5 kg in weight, G1P1, naturally delivered at full term without asphyxia. He was diagnosed with double outlet right ventricle (DORV, SDD type), subpulmonary ventricular septal defect (VSD), coarctation of the aorta (CoA), hypoplastic descending aortic arch, patent ductus arteriosus (PDA), and pulmonary artery dilation by fetal echocardiography at a local hospital. He was referred to our hospital for further treatment and underwent ASO + VSD repair + ASD repair + PDA ligation + CoA correction surgery in 2014. The patient was regu-

Y. Tao (✉)
The National Children's Medical Center (Shanghai), Department of Anesthesiology of Shanghai Children's Medical Center, Shanghai Jiao Tong University School of Medicine, Shanghai, China
e-mail: taoyingying@scmc.com.cn

J. Zheng et al. (eds.), *Selected Pediatric Cardiovascular Surgery Anesthesia Cases*,
https://doi.org/10.1007/978-981-96-5614-1_50

larly followed up after the surgery. He was in good general condition with normal growth, development, and good activity tolerance. There was no dyspnea or cyanosis. During a regular follow-up in July 2020, the patient's echocardiography demonstrated residual obstruction of the aortic anastomosis (pressure difference was 73 mm Hg). The flow velocity of the pulmonary anastomosis was increased. Enhanced cardiac CT examination demonstrated stenosis of both the supra valvular aortic anastomosis and the origin of the right pulmonary artery, a slightly small size of the proximal part of the left lower pulmonary vein, etc. The patient was admitted to our hospital and scheduled for elective surgery after completing preoperative examinations to relieve the residual obstruction.

Physical examination: Normal growth and development, clear consciousness, no obvious cyanosis of the lips when breathing calmly, pulse oxygen saturation (SpO_2) at room air, a noticeable surgical scar on the chest, clear lung sounds, no obvious rales, strong heart sounds, heart murmurs, the abdomen is soft, no obvious enlargement of the liver and spleen, warm extremities, no edema.

Laboratory tests: Normal routine blood test and normal liver, kidney, and coagulation function.

Electrocardiogram: Sinus arrhythmia, incomplete right bundle branch block, right ventricular hypertrophy.

Echocardiography: Post-ASO surgery for DORV/VSD/ASD/CoA/PDA; no obvious residual shunt, residual obstruction of the aortic anastomosis (pressure difference 7 3 mm Hg), increased flow speed of the pulmonary artery anastomosis, increased flow speed of the descending aorta.

Enhanced cardiac CT scan: Narrowing at the anastomosis above the aortic valve, dilation of the aortic sinus, small descending part of the aortic arch, narrowing at the origin of the right pulmonary artery, small proximal part of the left lower pulmonary vein, etc.

To relieve the patient's narrowing of the aortic valve and right pulmonary artery, an elective operation was scheduled.

50.2 Anesthetic Management

The patient took midazolam syrup 0.5 mg/kg for sedation 30 minutes before surgery in the waiting area of the operating room (OR). After entering the OR, the basic vital signs were monitored with blood pressure (BP) 100/65 mm Hg, heart rate (HR) 96 beats/min, and SpO_2 99%. Anesthesia was induced with intravenous bolus doses of 2.5 mg midazolam, 7.0 mg etomidate, 50 μg sufentanil, and 20 mg rocuronium. After the patient's eyelash reflex disappeared, an ID 5.5 mm cuffed endotracheal tube was intubated under a visual laryngoscopy with a depth of 16 cm. Pressure control ventilation (PCV) mode was used with the following respiratory parameters set as 2 L/min oxygen flow rate, 50% fraction of inspiration O_2 (FiO_2), 15 cm H_2O inspiratory pressure, 24 times/min respiratory rate (RR), and 1:2 inspiratory time to expiratory time (I:E) ratio, intraoperative tidal volume (VT) between 150 and 200 mL, and end-tidal carbon dioxide ($ETCO_2$) between 35 and 40 mm Hg. After intubation, invasive arterial blood pressure (ABP, right dorsal pedal artery, and right radial artery) and central venous pressure (CVP, right internal jugular vein) monitoring were quickly established, and the left femoral vein was accessed for rapid fluid replacement afterward. Intraoperatively general anesthesia was maintained by continuous intravenous infusion of 4.0 mg/(kg·h) propofol, 2.0 μg/(kg·h) sufentanil, and 0.5 mg/(kg·h) rocuronium with 1–2% sevoflurane intermittent inhalation. After intubation, the blood pressure was 100/60 mm Hg, HR was 100 beats/min, CVP was 10 cm H_2O, and SpO_2 was 97%. The ABP in the upper and lower extremities was 111/66 mm Hg and 103/63 mm Hg, respectively. There was no significant difference in ABP between the upper and lower extremities.

Surgical disinfection and draping areas included the right inguinal area for emergent right femoral artery and vein cannulation. A median sternum incision was conducted, and a pendulum saw was used to cut the sternum. Severe adhesions between the pericardium and the sternal tissues were found, and hard to dissect the adhesive tissues. While the adhesive tissues were being carefully separated by the surgeons, an obvious ventricular fibrillation suddenly occurred. The ABP in the upper extremity also reduced dramatically. The lowest ABP was 70/38 mm Hg. The surgery was immediately stopped, and 30 J defibrillation (nonsynchronous) was applied to the patient. The patient's heart rhythm soon returned to sinus rhythm; the ABP recovered to 86/40 mm Hg. The patient's arterial blood gas analysis showed: pH 7.44, PaO_2 210 mm Hg, $PaCO_2$ 38 mm Hg, BE 1.07, K^+ 3.5 mmol/L, Ca^{2+} 1.04 mmol/L, Lac 1.1 mmol/L, HCT 33.0%. Shortly after the defibrillation, the surgeons continued the dissection of adhesive tissues and established cardiopulmonary bypass (CPB), found the narrowing regions at the anastomosis of the aortic and right pulmonary artery were found and enlarged with bovine pericardial patches. The left pulmonary artery was explored and found to be 10 mm in diameter. After the aortic cross-clamp was released, the heart automatically resumed beating in sinus rhythm. Dopamine 5.0 μg/(kg·min) and norepinephrine 0.05 μg/(kg·min) were administered to maintain the child's invasive arterial pressure at 85–95/45–55 mm Hg and heart rate at 85–92 beats/min. Transesophageal echocardiography showed no residual shunting or obstruction after opening the aorta. After the separation from CPB, the boy's blood pressure gradually resumed with systolic pressure greater than 100 mm Hg. The dose of norepinephrine was adjusted to 0.025 μg/(kg·min). Arterial blood gas analysis showed pH 7.37, PaO_2 228 mm Hg, $PaCO_2$ 42 mm Hg, BE −1.0 mmol/L, K^+ 5.1 mmol/L, Ca^{2+} 1.1 mmol/L, Lac 1.2 mmol/L, HCT 35.9%. After the surgery, the patient was transferred to the cardiac intensive care unit (CICU) with endotracheal intubation for further observation and treatment.

50.3 Postoperative Outcome

The surgery lasted a total of 210 min, with aortic cross-clamp for 60 min and CPB for 90 min. The estimated blood loss urine output was about 200 mL and 300 mL, respectively. Ringer's acetate solution 200 mL, hydroxyethyl starch 100 mL, and red blood cells 150 mL were intravenously infused. At the end of the surgery, the ABP was 86/40 mm Hg. HR was 122 beats/min, SpO_2 was 90%, CVP was 9 cm H_2O, and rectal temperature was 36.5 °C. The patient was transferred to the CICU with endotracheal intubation under ABP, ECG, and SpO_2 monitoring. On the second day after surgery, the endotracheal tube was removed. The SpO_2 was maintained at 95–98% with nasal cannula oxygen respiration. On the fifth day after surgery, the patient was transferred to the general surgery ward without inotropic and vasoactive drug support. The boy was discharged from the hospital on the eighth day after surgery.

50.4 Review of Knowledge Points

50.4.1 Characteristics of Re-thoracotomy

Re-thoracotomy in congenital heart surgery can be divided into planned and unplanned. Planned re-thoracotomy are mainly for the staged treatment of infants and complex congenital heart diseases, while unplanned re-thoracotomies are mainly for residual or new heart malformations that need surgical treatment, including short-term postoperative complications such as bleeding, long-term complications such as residual shunting, regurgitation, or secondary lesions.

Heart and vascular structures are most prone to be injured during re-thoracotomy before the establishment of CPB, which may require defibrillation, vasoactive drug treatment, emergency fluid replacement, or nonselective establishment of the femoral vein-to-artery cannulation for CPB support to maintain hemodynamic stability. All of these are defined as major injuries (MI). It has been reported that the risk of MI in children undergoing re-thoracotomy is significantly increased to 6–10%.

In addition to the type of primary cardiac malformations, the surgical procedure and pathophysiological changes of the first surgery, the number of surgeries, and the timing of re-thoracotomy all determine the risk level of re-thoracotomy in the child with CHD. For those children who have undergone three or more times of cardiac surgeries, the perioperative mortality rate will definitely increase due to the severe mediastinal adhesion and compromised cardiac function. Remarkably, the difficulty of median sternotomy will be significantly increased if re-thoracotomy is performed within 6–12 months after the first surgery because the vascular and tissue adhesions are most severe at this time and can affect the long-term outcome. Generally speaking, the longer the interval between the re-thoracotomy and the previous surgery, the less severe the tissue and vascular adhesion, and the lower the risk of bleeding and other related complications during surgery. In addition, the patient's ventricular function should be carefully evaluated before re-sternotomy, especially for those with regurgitant valve diseases, which cause persistent ventricular enlargement and functional impairment; the prognosis is usually poor.

50.4.2 Taussig-Bing Anomaly (TBA)

TBA was first reported by Taussig-Bing in 1949 as a particular type of DORV, which has recently been increasingly understood and recognized. The widely accepted definition of TBA now is a nonrestrictive ventricular septal defect below the pulmonary valve, the pulmonary artery originates from both ventricles, the ascending aorta is in parallel with the pulmonary trunk without a spiral relationship, there is a single or bilateral conus below the great arteries with or without a fibrous connection from the pulmonary artery to the mitral valve. If the patients with TBA are not treated in a timely manner, they will finally suffer from pulmonary congestion, early onset pulmonary hypertension, and obstructive pulmonary vascular disease. Therefore, it currently tends to perform anatomical correction in the neonatal period. In 1981, Freedom and others first reported using arterial switch operation (ASO) to treat TBA, which has gradually become the mainstream surgical treatment. Patients with TBA often have other malformations, such as aortic arch anomalies, including coarctation, hypoplasia, and interruption of the arch, as well as common coronary artery malformations, all of which increase the difficulty of surgery and the possibility of postoperative complications. In China, the 2020 expert consensus recommends that the best time for surgery for patients with TBA is at 2–3 months of age.

For those surgically treated TBA patients, the 10-year re-intervention rate is 25–53%. The main reasons for re-intervention are right ventricular outflow tract and pulmonary artery re-obstruction, new sub-aortic stenosis or anastomotic stenosis, arch anastomotic re-obstruction, new aortic valve regurgitation, residual ventricular septal defect closure, pacemaker implantation, and coronary artery re-implantation.

The incidence of aortic anastomotic re-obstruction after ASO in children with TBA is 5.4–44%. Some patients will develop periaortic valve fibrous ridges that grow with age during follow-up. The mechanism of periaortic valve fibrous ridges formation after ASO is still unclear, surgical removal of these fibrous ridges is necessary. Arch anastomotic stenosis is also common. The possible causes may include patch tissue calcification and narrowing, lack of growth potential of the artificial patch, and residual stenotic segment tissue limiting the growth of the anastomosis. In addition, studies have shown that about 15% of surviving TBA patients need to be re-intervened at the level of the right ventricular outflow tract and pulmonary artery 10 years after the ASO. Therefore, it is now believed that abnormal anatomical structures that may cause right ventricular outflow tract stenosis should also be completely removed during ASO, such as hypertrophic conus tissue and patch enlargement of the right ventricular outflow tract.

50.5 Discussion

In this case, the patient received a high-risk re-thoracotomy process due to complex preoperative conditions and difficult surgical procedures, all of which pose great challenges to anesthetic management. For anesthesiologists, detailed preoperative assessment and anesthesia preparation are the keys to ensuring smooth and safe management of surgery.

50.5.1 Preoperative Assessment and Preparation

Before surgery, comprehensive imaging examinations, including echocardiography, computed tomography (CT), and magnetic resonance imaging (MRI), should be performed in order to determine the possibility of a high risk of cardiac or major vascular injury during the re-thoracotomy process. Extremely enlarged right atrium or right ventricle, thickened aorta adjacent to the sternum, external pipeline, and coronary artery running behind the sternum may underlie the high risk of cardiac or major vascular injury during the re-thoracotomy process. It will be of great help for the surgeons to make a precise preoperative plan based on the 3D reconstruction of the heart and mediastinal structures during a CT scan. In pediatric CHD cases, especially those with cyanotic congenital heart disease tend to develop abundant collateral vessels because of the strong developmental potential of the vasculatures. Large systemic-pulmonary collaterals increase the risk of re-thoracotomy. Secondly, it is also very important to evaluate the preoperative function of the liver and kidney and the electrolyte levels and give corresponding preoperative treatment in time, which can help to reduce the possibility of intraoperative arrhythmia. It is better to make a preparation for immediate peripheral vessel cannulation (commonly femoral artery and vein cannulation) before thoracotomy to facilitate the establishment of emergency CPB. Therefore, it is recommended to assess peripheral vessels through ultrasound or CT imaging before surgery, especially for those patients who have undergone multiple surgeries or have a history of femoral artery and vein catheterization. These patients may encounter great challenges when emergency artery and vein cannulation is needed.

50.5.2 Anesthetic Management During Operation

General anesthesia with endotracheal intubation is required for those patients undergoing re-thoracotomy. The key to anesthetic management should focus on the prevention and preparation for various potential MI accidents and quick response to these emergent accidents during thoracotomy.

1. Placement of external defibrillation electrode pads before anesthesia
   It is recommended that the external defibrillation electrode pads should be placed on the lateral chest wall and ready to be immediately used for those patients undergoing re-thoracotomy, which is beneficial for anesthesiologists to timely and effectively treat the sudden occurrence of malignant arrhythmias such as ventricular fibrillation, especially when thoracic surgeons cannot easily dissect the adhesive tissue. They cannot perform rapid open-chest defibrillation or when it is difficult to place temporary defibrillation paddles due to surgical disinfection drapes. External defibrillation can be quickly conducted through the pre-set defibrillation electrode pads. In addition, routine use of electrocautery for hemostasis during surgery can help the surgeons to get a clear surgical field; special attention should be paid to the effects of electrocautery on the heart rate and rhythm. It is better to use the electrocautery quickly and decisively to avoid arrhythmia or ventricular fibrillation.
2. Peripheral vascular cannulation
   In addition to the disinfection and draping in the surgical incision, the possible sites for peripheral vascular cannulation, such as the femoral artery and vein for emergency CPB support, should also be disinfected and draped. Some studies showed that routine cannulation of the femoral vessels for CPB could make the re-thoracotomy safer and simpler for congenital heart diseases. The small femoral arteries and veins in children make cannulation much more difficult. Even though

the cannulation procedure is successfully performed, it is still difficult to achieve full flow during CPB sometimes, and these patients are more likely to have lower limb vascular complications. It is only recommended the cannulation of the femoral artery and vein is conducted in advance in infants with high-risk and low weight who are predicted to have MI. Therefore, the peripheral CPB can be quickly established when MI suddenly happens. After the sternum is opened and the heart and major vessels are clearly dissected, peripheral vascular cannulation should be converted to central intubation as soon as possible to avoid related complications.

3. Preparation of blood products
   Coagulation dysfunction is very common during re-thoracotomy in children with complex congenital heart diseases and more common in cyanotic children with abundant collateral circulation, which is caused by extensive sternal adhesion dissection and long CPB time. Before the surgery, sufficient blood products should be prepared, including platelets, prothrombin complex, factor VII, cold precipitate, plasma, red blood cells, etc. The blood products should be transfused based on the progress of the operation and changes in the patient's condition.

50.6 Shortcomings and Limitations

NIRS brain, kidney, and intestine monitoring was not performed in this case. For children undergoing re-thoracotomy, accurate and real-time monitoring of the perfusion of the brain and vital organs would be helpful for us to assess the effects of MI on the patients and direct the subsequent management.

50.7 Conclusion

In conclusion, re-thoracotomy for congenital heart disease is a complex and arduous task, requiring an accurate grasp of surgical indications, solid surgical techniques, and perfect perioperative anesthetic management. Reducing risks and mortality in re-thoracotomy depends on the cooperation of multiple disciplines, including cardiac surgery, radiology, anesthesia, and critical care medicine (Yingying Tao).

51 Anesthetic Management of Delayed Sternal Closure After Neonatal ASO Surgery

Siyi Zhou

Abstract

A 3-day-old newborn underwent an emergency arterial switch operation (ASO) for transposition of the great arteries on the first day of birth. Delayed sternal closure was performed due to postoperative low cardiac output and unstable hemodynamics. On the third day after surgery, the infant's vital signs were stable. It was scheduled to perform sternal closure. Infants requiring delayed sternal closure are often newborns or preterm infants shortly after complex cardiovascular correction surgery, which makes anesthetic management extremely challenging.

With the development of pediatric congenital heart disease surgery, all of the complex congenital heart diseases, including the transposition of the great arteries, can be surgically corrected. However, the mismatch between the heart and the mediastinum caused by cardiopulmonary bypass-related myocardial edema and the reduction of cardiac output related to myocardial contractility can result in various postoperative complications. Delayed sternal closure (DSC) is a relatively safe and effective method to prevent the sternum from compressing the enlarged heart and hemodynamic instability due to myocardial edema. After the hemodynamics has been significantly improved, a second stage of sternal closure can dramatically enhance the early survival rate of young and low-weight patients after cardiac surgery. This chapter reports the anesthetic management of a neonate who underwent delayed sternal closure after ASO surgery.

S. Zhou (✉)
The National Children's Medical Center (Shanghai), Department of Anesthesiology of Shanghai Children's Medical Center, Shanghai Jiao Tong University School of Medicine, Shanghai, China
e-mail: zhousiyi@scmc.com.cn

51.1 Case Presentation

A 3-day-old male infant with 50 cm in height and 3.6 kg in weight was born via in vitro fertilization and cesarean section at full term. There was no history of asphyxia at birth. An echocardiogram during the fetal period indicated transposition of the great arteries. An emergency arterial switch operation (ASO) was performed on the day of birth, which lasted 3 h. Maintaining the infant's blood pressure when the sternum was closed was very difficult. Then, delayed sternal closure was conducted after a comprehensive assessment. The infant was transferred to the Cardiac Intensive Care Unit (CICU) with an endotracheal tube for further treatments by cardiac support, diuresis, anti-infection, and maintenance of fluid and electrolyte balance. On the third day after the operation, the infant's edema in chest tissue subsided gradually, hemodynamics was slightly sta-

J. Zheng et al. (eds.), *Selected Pediatric Cardiovascular Surgery Anesthesia Cases*,
https://doi.org/10.1007/978-981-96-5614-1_51

bilized. Re-closure of the sternum was conducted under general anesthesia to avoid infection.

Physical examination: The infant was intubated with mechanical ventilation, sedation, and analgesia. The ventilator parameters were set as follows: fraction of inspired oxygen (FiO_2) of 40%, tidal volume (VT) of 30 mL, respiratory rate (RR) of 28 breaths/min, and positive end-expiratory pressure (PEEP) of 6 cm H_2O. Epinephrine 0.1 μg/(kg·min) and norepinephrine 0.15 μg/(kg·min) were intravenously infused. The lung sounds are clear without rales at auscultation. The cardiac rhythm is regular. The abdomen was soft by palpation without touching the liver under the ribs. The extremities of the baby were warm without edema. Pulse oxygen saturation (SpO_2) was 98%. The heart rate(HR) is 150 beats/min, and invasive arterial blood pressure (ABP) is 75/43 mm Hg.

Laboratory tests: C-reactive protein 11.6 mg/L, white blood cell count $41.2^9 \times 10^9$/L, platelet count 131×10^9/L, hemoglobin 142 g/L, neutrophils 85×10^9/L, PT 12.4 s, APTT 41.2 s, TT 19.5 s. NT-proBNP 8970 pg/mL.

Chest X-ray (bedside): Endotracheal tube in place, increased lung markings, slightly enlarged cardiac silhouette.

Echocardiography (bedside): Post-ASO, no significant residual obstruction, no significant obstruction at the anastomosis.

Preoperative diagnosis: Delayed chest closure after ASO, elective surgery of sternal closure.

51.2 Anesthetic Management

The infant was mechanically ventilated and maintained with epinephrine 0.1 μg/(kg·min) and norepinephrine 0.15 μg/(kg·min)during transporting to the operating room. After entering the operating room, pressure-controlled ventilation-volume guaranteed (PCV-VG) mode ventilation from the CICU was continuously used with ventilation parameters set as follows: oxygen flow rate 1 L/min, FiO_2 50%, VT30 mL, RR 28 breaths/min, PEEP 5 cm H_2O, I:E ratio 1:2. The vasoactive drugs was continuously infused. Vital signs were continuously monitored: ABP 70/40 mm Hg, sinus rhythm, heart rate (HR) 154 beats/min, SpO_2 99% (FiO_2 50%). Anesthesia was induced by administering etomidate 0.6 mg, sufentanil 5.0 μg, and rocuronium bromide 2.0 mg. Anesthesia was maintained by intravenous infusion of propofol 3.0 mg/(kg·h), rocuronium bromide 0.6 mg/(kg·h), sufentanil 2.0 μg/(kg·h), intermittent inhalation of sevoflurane to maintain BIS at 40–60. Blood gas analysis was performed after anesthesia (Table 51.1), and calcium gluconate 200 mg was slowly infused.

The original incision along the midline of the sternum was used as the entry point after skin disinfection. No obvious abnormal secretions were observed in the thoracic cavity. The hemostatic device was carefully removed, and the adhesions around the heart were fully dissected. The thoracic cavity was then rinsed with warm saline. No obvious bleeding points were found. The sternum was closed layer by layer. The patient's vital signs were stable without obvious circulatory fluctuations, and the airway pressure was slightly higher than before the sternum was closed. After the operation, the patient was transferred to the CICU under mechanical ventilation and vasoactive drug support.

Table 51.1 Intraoperative blood gas analysis results

Hb	HCT	pH	PaO_2	$PaCO_2$	BE	Na^+	K^+	Cl^-	Ca^{++}	Lac
11.6	36.9	7.52	255.7	32.3	4.3	140	3.6	118	0.65	1.3

51.3 Postoperative Outcome

The operation lasted a total of 60 min. About 30 mL of compound electrolyte solution was infused with an estimated blood loss of about 5 mL and a urine output of 10 mL. Epinephrine 0.1 μg/(kg·min) and norepinephrine 0.15 μg/(kg·min) were continuously infused throughout the procedure. Postoperative ABP was 79/48 mm Hg, HR was 158 beats/min, SpO_2 was 99%, CVP was 10 cm H_2O, and rectal temperature was 36.4 °C. Diaphragmatic plication surgery was performed on the fourth day after sternum closure because it was difficult to wean off mechanical ventilation. On the sixth day after surgery, the endotracheal tube was removed. On the 9th day after surgery, the patient was discharged from the ICU, and on the 16th day after surgery, the patient was discharged from the hospital.

51.4 Review of Knowledge Points

51.4.1 Delayed Sternal Closure

Delayed sternal closure is one of the most effective methods to improve the early postoperative survival rate of children with complex congenital heart disease, especially those of young age and low weight, which was first used in cardiac surgery in 1975 by Riahi. It is mainly a temporary measure for postoperative hemodynamic instability, severe arrhythmia, uncontrollable bleeding at the incision and/or anastomosis site due to myocardial edema, cardiac chamber enlargement, etc. After the patient's myocardial edema subsides and hemodynamics stabilize, a second-stage sternum suture is performed, providing time and conditions for treating postoperative coagulation abnormalities.

Currently, there is no unified method to close the sternum. Some trimmed hard plastic pipes into a "工" shape and inserted into the middle of the sternum. Some trimmed the core of a 5–10 cm syringe into an "II" shape and placed it in the middle of the sternum, and some used a sternum spreader, which can adjust the spreading distance at any time to make it easy to clear blood clots. The spread distance should not cause hemodynamic instability. Surgical active bleeding should be stopped. To prevent pericardium, mediastinum, sternum, and skin infections, diluted iodophor solution or antibiotic solution can be added to the pericardium, and the fluid in the pericardium should be replaced regularly. The incision is sealed with a transparent disinfectant surgical patch, which is convenient for observing cardiac activity, bleeding, and drainage in the CICU.

51.5 Discussion

51.5.1 Preoperative Assessment and Preparation

The incidence of DSC after ASO in newborns is relatively high. These patients all require mechanical ventilation and have poor cardiopulmonary reserve. A careful preoperative assessment should be conducted, including ventilator parameters setting, SpO_2 monitoring, blood gas analysis, chest radiographs, etc., to detect and manage abnormalities early. The patient should be kept calm and avoid excessive stimulation to ensure that the tracheal intubation was appropriately fixed. The suction needed to be gentle and aseptic. At the same time, appropriate-sized masks and bags should be prepared for emergencies such as tube slippage. In addition, patients after DSC surgery strongly depend on vasopressors, and the circulatory system needs to be closely monitored during transfer to maintain hemodynamic stability. Anesthesiologists must be familiar with the patient's available venous access to ensure all intravenous infusion catheters and infusion pumps are working properly.

51.5.2 Anesthetic Management

It was better to keep the ventilation mode and parameter settings in the CICU just after the patient entered the operating room. Then, the parameter settings were adjusted according to the patient's current situation. H_2O PEEP

(5 cm) was used to maintain alveolar opening and prevent lung collapse during anesthesia. Anesthetics with less suppression of hemodynamics, such as etomidate, sufentanil, and sevoflurane, were chosen for induction and maintenance. Induction of anesthesia was conducted under continuous invasive arterial monitoring, closely observing changes in hemodynamic parameters and slowly titrating the medications to avoid hemodynamic fluctuations. For children with unstable circulatory status, a small dose of ketamine can be used for induction. After the child's vital signs were stable, a blood gas analysis was checked to understand the child's fluid, electrolyte, and other inner environment levels timely. Symptomatic treatment should be given promptly. The mechanism of temperature regulation in newborns is immature and easily affected by environmental temperature. Therefore, special attention should be paid to the temperature of the thoracic lavage fluid and the environmental temperature during surgery. We used a warm air blanket to keep the child warm throughout the surgery. In addition, blood glucose levels in newborns should be regularly checked and should not be less than 2.6 mmol/L.

During sternal closure, special attention should be paid to the indications of cardiac compression, such as tachycardia or bradycardia, blood pressure drop >10–12 mm Hg, central venous pressure increase, cardiac output decrease, etc. Once these indications occur, immediate communication with the surgeon should be made, and vasoactive drugs should be adjusted in time. If necessary, the thoracic cavity should be opened, and the sternal closure surgery should be postponed. The child's lung compliance was lower after sternal closure and the airway pressure might be increased as a result, so the ventilator parameters should be adjusted in time. In addition, special attention should be paid to fluid replacement and urine output in young and low-weight children to avoid insufficient or excessive fluid replacement.

51.6 Shortcomings and Limitations

Literature reports that children with DSC after complex congenital heart surgery are more likely to develop renal dysfunction. In this case, we could not monitor the child's renal perfusion in real time, which needs improvement.

51.7 Conclusion

In conclusion, children with DSC usually have a poor cardiopulmonary reserve. The anesthetic management is very challenging, which should be based on the special physiological characteristics of complex congenital heart correction surgery. Close intraoperative monitoring, rational use of vasoactive drugs, and timely adjustment of ventilator parameters can be helpful to those children who undergo delayed thoracic closure after congenital heart surgery (Siyi Zhou).

Anesthetic Management of Emergency Pericardiotomy in a Child After Open-Heart Surgery

52

Lihong Jin

Abstract

A 3-month-old female infant was found to have a large amount of pericardial effusion by cardiac ultrasound due to restlessness, rapid breathing, and increased heart rate on the 18th day after atrial septal defect and ventricular septal defect repair surgery. She was scheduled for an emergency pericardiotomy. A large amount of pericardial effusion can compress the heart, which restricts the ventricular diastolic filling, reduces the venous return, and decreases the cardiac output and blood pressure. In severe cases, it can lead to pericardial tamponade and acute circulatory failure. Cardiac compression symptoms can be effectively alleviated by effusion draining. The goal of anesthetic management for children with large amounts of pericardial effusion is to maintain sufficient cardiac output by avoiding the occurrence of bradycardia, hypotension, hypovolemia, and myocardial suppression. Due to the sharp increase of blood return to the heart after pericardial decompression, the risk of congestive heart failure is significantly increased. Therefore, the anesthesiologist should be particularly vigilant for the possible occurrence of congestive heart failure.

L. Jin (✉)
The National Children's Medical Center (Shanghai), Department of Anesthesiology of Shanghai Children's Medical Center, Shanghai Jiao Tong University School of Medicine, Shanghai, China
e-mail: jinlihong@scmc.com.cn

Pericardial effusion is one of the common complications after pediatric cardiac surgery, with an incidence rate of 10–20%, of which 1% of patients with large amounts of pericardial effusion require pericardiotomy. The pressure in the pericardial cavity with a large amount of effusion can be significantly increased, which will compress the heart and even cause the pericardial tamponade, posing a higher anesthesia risk. This chapter reports the anesthetic management of emergency pericardiotomy in a child with a large amount of pericardial effusion after pediatric cardiac surgery.

52.1 Case Presentation

The patient was a 3-month-old female with a weight of 3.6 kg. She was found to have a large amount of pericardial effusion by cardiac ultrasound on the 18th day after atrial septal defect (ASD) and ventricular septal defect (VSD) repair surgery because of restlessness, rapid breathing, and increased heart rate (HR).

Physical examination: The patient was conscious and restless, HR 170 beats/min, blood pressure 72/59 mm Hg, respiratory rate (RR) 40 breaths/min, pulse oxygen saturation (SpO_2) 95%

J. Zheng et al. (eds.), *Selected Pediatric Cardiovascular Surgery Anesthesia Cases*,
https://doi.org/10.1007/978-981-96-5614-1_52

with oxygen flow rate 2 L/min by nasal cannula. Coarse breath sounds in both lungs, distant heart sounds. The abdomen is soft; the liver is not palpable under the ribs, and normal limb movement without edema.

Laboratory tests: Routine blood tests, coagulation tests, and liver and kidney function tests showed no significant abnormalities.

Cardiac ultrasound: Post VSD/ASD/pulmonary stenosis (PS) surgery, no significant residual shunting, slightly enlarged right atrium, slightly thickened right ventricular wall, left ventricular hypertrophy, acceptable left ventricular wall contraction activity, left ventricular ejection fraction 83%. Large amount of pericardial effusion, the depth of diaphragmatic surface 0.66 cm, near the apex of the diaphragm 2 cm, apical part 0.62 cm, right posterior atrioventricular groove 0.52 cm, right ventricular sidewall 1.0 cm, left posterior atrioventricular groove 0.90 cm, left ventricular sidewall 2.21 cm, left ventricular posterior wall 1.13 cm, multiple fibrous cord-like echoes can be seen.

Preoperative diagnosis: Post VSD/ASD/PS surgery, a large amount of pericardial effusion. Emergency pericardiocentesis was scheduled.

52.2 Anesthetic Management

The patient did not take any preoperative medication. She was transferred to the operating room with peripheral venous access from the ward. After the establishment of vital signs monitoring, Ketamine 5 mg was intravenously administered, and the right femoral artery was catheterized for invasive arterial pressure (ABP) monitoring after the patient fell asleep. The ABP was 72/62 mm Hg, HR was 174 beats/min, and SpO_2 was 99% with mask oxygen inhalation. General anesthesia was induced by intravenous administration of sufentanil 5.0 μg and rocuronium 2.5 mg. An ID 3.5 mm cuffed endotracheal tube was intubated under direct laryngoscopy with a tube depth of about 11 cm. Pressure-controlled ventilation (PCV) mode was used with respiratory parameters set as: oxygen flow rate 2 L/min, fraction of inspired oxygen (FiO_2) 50%, peak inspiratory pressure (PIP) 20 cm H_2O, RR 26 breaths/min, inspiratory to expiratory time (I:E) ratio 1:2. The end of tidal carbon dioxygen ($ETCO_2$) was maintained around 42 mm Hg by the adjustment of PIP and RR. The right internal jugular vein was catheterized under ultrasound guidance for rapid fluid replacement, vasoactive agent infusion, and central venous pressure (CVP) monitoring. General anesthesia was maintained by intravenous infusion of propofol 2.0 mg/(kg·h), sufentanil 2.5 μg/(kg·h), rocuronium 0.6 mg/(kg·h), and 1–2% sevoflurane intermittent inhalation.

After the induction of anesthesia, the blood pressure dropped to 65/55 mm Hg; HR rose to 185 beats/min, and CVP 20 cm H_2O. Dopamine 5.0 μg/(kg·min) was immediately initiated. The result of arterial blood gas analysis: pH 7.51, PaO_2 119 mm Hg, $PaCO_2$ 50.9 mm Hg, BE 16.6, HCT 34.4%, K^+ 3.4 mmol/L, Ca^{2+} 1.13 mmol/L, Lac 0.8 mmol/L. The RR was adjusted to 30 breaths/min to remove the accumulated CO_2.

After rapid disinfection and draping, a subxiphoid pericardiocentesis was performed, and 150 milliliters of blood fluid were slowly drawn out. The ABP quickly recovered to 75/42 mm Hg with HR reduction to 160 beats/min and CVP reduction to 12 cm H_2O. The dopamine infusion was stopped.

52.3 Postoperative Outcome

The surgery lasted a total of 30 minutes, with an estimated blood loss of about 10 mL and a urine output of 5 mL. Forty milliliter of acetate ringer's solution was infused. Before leaving the operating room, ABP was 84/56 mm Hg, HR 153 beats/min, SpO_2 100%, CVP 11 cm H_2O, and rectal temperature 37.2 °C. The child was transferred to the Cardiac Intensive Care Unit with endotracheal intubation under ABP, ECG, and SpO_2 monitoring.

52.4 Review of Knowledge Points

52.4.1 Pathophysiology of Pericardial Effusion

A small amount of pericardial effusion usually does not affect the hemodynamics, but as the effusion increases, the pressure in the pericardial cavity also increases and causes hemodynamic changes. The severity of pericardial effusion is usually related to the speed of effusion increase, the amount of effusion, the nature of the effusion, the age of the child, and the primary disease. When the pericardial effusion increases slowly, even a large amount of it only causes a slight increase in pericardial cavity pressure, and the child can tolerate it well. But when the pericardial effusion continues to grow and exceeds a certain range, it will compress the heart. Usually, a small amount (<100 mL) of pericardial effusion does not cause a significant increase in pericardial cavity pressure. Still, if a small amount of fluid grows rapidly, it can also cause cardiac tamponade due to the rapid increase in pericardial cavity pressure in a short time.

When the pericardium is filled, the ventricular diastolic filling is obstructed, and venous return is also obstructed, leading to a decrease in cardiac output, a drop in blood pressure, and ultimately leading to acute circulatory failure or even cardiac arrest.

52.4.2 Diagnosis of Cardiac Tamponade

52.4.2.1 Clinical Diagnosis

1. For children with low blood pressure, jugular vein distension, pulsus paradoxus, tachycardia, dyspnea, or severe respiratory distress, the possibility of children with pericardial tamponade should be considered.
2. Other symptoms include low QRS complex voltage, electrical alternate, and cardiac silhouette enlargement on chest X-ray imaging.

52.4.2.2 Imaging Diagnosis

For children suspected of pericardial tamponade, echocardiography is the preferred diagnostic method and should be performed immediately. Cardiac CT and MRI are not routinely used for the diagnosis of pericardial tamponade. Still, they can be used to rule out the possibility of mediastinal or pulmonary comorbidities in children with a large amount of pericardial effusion.

Once the echocardiography indicates the occurrence of pericardial effusion, the following should be carefully examined: full inferior vena cava with reduced diameter change rate during respiration; cardiac compression (collapse of the right atrium and right ventricle are the most common clues for diagnosing pericardial tamponade); changes in mitral and tricuspid Doppler blood flow velocity curves with respiratory movement; paradoxical movement of the interventricular septum; cardiac swing sign. Regardless of the amount of pericardial effusion, the possibility of pericardial tamponade should be considered when the above echocardiographic manifestations occur.

52.5 Discussion

52.5.1 Preoperative Assessment and Preparation

The risk of anesthetic management mainly depends on the effects of pericardial effusion on the heart and circulation. The focus of preoperative assessment is to clarify whether the child has cardiac compression symptoms and whether there is pericardial tamponade. Typical symptoms of pericardial tamponade include hypotension, jugular venous distension, pulsus paradoxus, tachycardia, dyspnea, severe respiratory distress, etc. Bedside echocardiography can be used to evaluate the amount of pericardial effusion, judge whether the heart is compressed, and identify pericardial tamponade earlier.

In this case, the child showed restless, rapid breathing, HR increase, and normal blood pressure with decreased pulse pressure before surgery. Furthermore, the echocardiography indicated a large amount of pericardial effusion. All of which showed a large amount of pericardial effusion instead of pericardial tamponade and the heart function was in a compensatory state. Considering the recent history of congenital heart surgery, an evaluation of the surgical effect should also be included. The child's echocardiography indicated normal heart function without residual shunt at the anastomosis.

Considering the child's age, overall condition, and surgical procedure, it may be safer for the child to undergo pericardiotomy and drainage under general anesthesia. Anesthesia and mechanical ventilation may disrupt the inherent compensation mechanism of the heart and lead to circulatory failure, so anesthesia should be performed under strict hemodynamic monitoring. In addition, the resuscitation drugs and the emergency equipment, including defibrillators, should be prepared in advance.

52.5.2 Intraoperative Anesthetic Management

The goal of hemodynamic management in children with a large amount of pericardial effusion is to maintain a slightly fast HR and sufficient preload to ensure adequate cardiac output and avoid hypotension.

The large amount of pericardial effusion can impair the diastolic function of the child's heart and affect the venous return. Therefore, the cardiac output mainly depends on the compensatory increase of heart rate, which is very fragile. The induction of anesthesia is very challenging. Improper anesthesia induction can cause severe arrhythmia, even cardiac arrest. General anesthesia must be conducted with optimal anesthetics with minimal effects on the hemodynamics and a small dosage of anesthetics with slow titration under strict hemodynamic monitoring.

In this case, invasive arterial pressure monitoring was first established under basic ketamine anesthesia. Then the induction of anesthesia was conducted by intravenous administration of sufentanil and rocuronium. Ketamine combined with sufentanil can effectively suppress the hemodynamic fluctuations caused by laryngoscopy and tracheal intubation while avoiding bradycardia, hypotension, and significant myocardial suppression. A low concentration of sevoflurane inhalation during surgery will not cause significant heart rate drop and hypotension and can provide good hemodynamic stability for anesthesia maintenance.

The ventricular filling and cardiac output can only be maintained by an effective pressure gradient between the systemic vein and the right atrium considering the cardiac compression and venous return obstruction caused by the large amount of pericardial effusion. Therefore, it is necessary to maintain satisfactory preload and myocardial contractility with an appropriate volume of fluid supplementation and small doses of positive inotropic drugs during the operation. Mechanical ventilation can increase the intrapleural pressure and reduce venous return. Therefore, it is better to use mechanical ventilation with a lower average airway pressure as much as possible to ensure sufficient oxygenation and ventilation. Relatively fast ventilation frequency and smaller tidal volume can be used to minimize the average airway pressure.

In addition, surgical operations can induce arrhythmia. Therefore, it is very important to maintain close communication and cooperation with the surgeon during the operation. If severe arrhythmia occurs, the operation should be suspended, and symptomatic treatment should be given in time. When draining a large amount of pericardial effusion, attention should be paid to the drainage speed to avoid violent fluctuations in hemodynamics.

Once the cardiac compression is relieved, the return blood volume increases sharply. The hemodynamic status usually undergoes huge changes. Children with preoperative cardiac dysfunction may develop congestive heart failure, which requires extra vigilance. Appropriate cardiac support can be conducted if it is necessary.

52.6 Conclusion

Children with a large amount of pericardial effusion are at risk of cardiac tamponade during surgery. The effects of pericardial effusion on the heart and circulation should be fully evaluated before anesthesia. Before the cardiac compression is relieved, higher sympathetic tension should be maintained. Furthermore, the induction of anesthesia should be extremely cautious to avoid the occurrence of bradycardia, hypotension, low blood volume, and even cardiac arrest. The cardiac function should be closely monitored with reasonable use of cardiovascular active drugs after the operation (Lihong Jin).

53 Anesthetic Management of Bypass Surgery with Artificial Blood Vessel in a Child with Multiple Large Arteritis

Hongbin Gu

Abstract

A 12-year-old boy presented with a 4-year history of unexplained hypertension accompanied by chest tightness and other complaints. After careful examination by vascular ultrasound, cardiac ultrasound, and cardiac MRI, he was diagnosed with aortitis and descending aortic stenosis. He was scheduled to undergo bypass surgery with general anesthesia. During the operation, the abdominal aorta was found to be significantly narrowed at the diaphragm, and the vessel wall was stiff. The artificial blood vessel was anastomosed to the abdominal aorta and the ascending aorta along their right-sided walls, respectively. In such cases, the key point of anesthetic management is to maintain blood pressure at an appropriate preoperative level, adequate perfusion pressure without drastic changes in cardiac preload and afterload, and avoid further supersession of the function of cardiac and cerebral vessels by drugs. Other severe potential accidents should also be avoided and treated immediately. To better support bypass surgery in children with multiple large arteritis, the anesthesiologist team members should fully understand the abnormal anatomic structure, the disease's stage and pathophysiology, and the functions of vital organs.

Multiple large arteritis, also known as Takayasu's arteritis (TA), is a chronic autoimmune disease mainly affecting the largest blood vessels, including the aorta, pulmonary artery, and branches. TA is one type of large vessel vasculitis, which is common in Asia and South America young females and can cause multiple arterial stenosis. Once TA progresses to the occlusive stage, ischemia and damage will occur in these tissues and organs supplied by the affected arteries, which results in diminished or completely lost function.

TA can be classified into four categories based on the location of the lesion: type I: large vessel vasculitis involves the aortic arch and its major branches. Type II: large vessel vasculitis is restricted to the descending and abdominal aortas; type III: large vessel vasculitis combines the characteristics of types I and II, and type IV: large vessel vasculitis includes the pulmonary artery.

More than half of children with TA do not react well to medication therapy and must receive surgical treatment to restore the blood flow supply. Open surgical correction of stenotic arteries is preferred because of its high long-term patency rate. However, there is a significantly increased incidence of perioperative cardiovascular and

H. Gu (✉)
The National Children's Medical Center (Shanghai), Department of Anesthesiology of Shanghai Children's Medical Center, Shanghai Jiao Tong University School of Medicine, Shanghai, China
e-mail: guhongbin@scmc.com.cn

J. Zheng et al. (eds.), *Selected Pediatric Cardiovascular Surgery Anesthesia Cases*,
https://doi.org/10.1007/978-981-96-5614-1_53

cerebrovascular complications, which include (1) aortic regurgitation, arterial aneurysm rupture, and related hemodynamic changes and (2) severe ischemia in the limbs, heart, brain, etc. In addition to the imaging examination for objective evaluation of organic abnormalities, blood pressure measurement is also necessary. Surgical corrective procedures include end-to-end anastomosis following the removal of the stenotic segment, patch aortic grafting, and artificial blood vessel bypass surgery. This chapter reports a case of type II TA for ascending and abdominal aortic bypass surgery under general anesthesia.

53.1 Case Presentation

The 12-year-old child had an elevated blood pressure about 4 years. Noninvasive blood pressure (BP) in the upper right lower extremities ranged between 140 and 150/80 and 90 mm Hg. The patient had a faster heart rate (HR) and chest discomfort. Ultrasonography of lower extremity arteries: abnormal blood flow spectrum, low blood flow speed, proximal vascular stenosis (possible). Renal ultrasonography: obscure imaging at the openings of bilateral renal main arteries, little dot-like blood flow, which might indicate congenital developmental renal artery stenosis (possible). Echocardiography: aortic stenosis, mild mitral and tricuspid regurgitation, and normal left ventricular systolic function. The patient's general condition was improved after treatment with metoprolol. He was admitted to our hospital for large vessel vasculitis and descending aortic stenosis. Bypass surgery with artificial blood vessels was scheduled.

Physical examination: Good general condition, HR 100 beats/min, respiratory rate 20 times/min, the right upper extremity BP 147/83 mm Hg, the left upper extremity BP 155/86 mm Hg, and right lower extremity 98/55 mm Hg, and left lower extremity 119/73 mm Hg.

Abdominal ultrasonography: Normal imaging in liver, gallbladder, pancreas, spleen, kidneys, and adrenal glands.

Laboratory tests: Routine blood tests, liver and kidney function, coagulation function, and blood gas were almost normal.

Electrocardiogram (ECG): Sinus rhythm and S-T segment alterations.

Cardiac MRI: Long-segment descending aortic stenosis, large vessel vasculitis, collateral vessel formation, left ventricular hypertrophy with higher myocardial mass index, moderate mitral regurgitation, normal size of left and right ventricles, mild dilated ascending aorta, normal development in the descending portion of aortic arch, no apparent stenosis in the ascending aorta or patent ductus arteriosus, long segment stenosis in the distal portion of thoracic aortic stenosis(53.6 mm) and with a narrowest diameter of 5.0 mm, unsmooth thoracic aortic intima, thickened and calcified intima wall of thoracic aorta, dilated intercostal and intrathoracic arteries, normal development of the pulmonary trunk and the left and right pulmonary arteries.

Echocardiography: Mild mitral and tricuspid regurgitation, thoracic aortic stenosis, left ventricular hypertrophy, slightly enlarged left ventricle, normal left ventricular systolic function, concordant atrioventricular connections, intact ventricular septum, and normal left ventricular outflow tract.

Abdominal computed tomography angiography (CTA): Narrowed and stiff abdominal aorta, especially in the distal portion below the liver, unsmooth thoracic aortic intima with irregular thickness, obscure branches of the celiac trunk, barely visible superior mesenteric artery, long-segment descending aortic stenosis with the narrowest section about 5.2 mm × 7.8 mm, multiple filling defects in descending aortic lumen, stenosis and calcification in origin and middle segment of the right iliac artery, normal filling of bilateral renal artery lumens, insufficient blood filling at the thoracic aorta, partial filling defect. The inner diameter of the abdominal aorta behind the liver was about 9.5 mm. The narrowest diameter of the abdominal aorta below the liver was 5.8 mm. The maximum velocity (V max) was 74 cm/s, and the minimum velocity (V min) was 10 cm/s. The

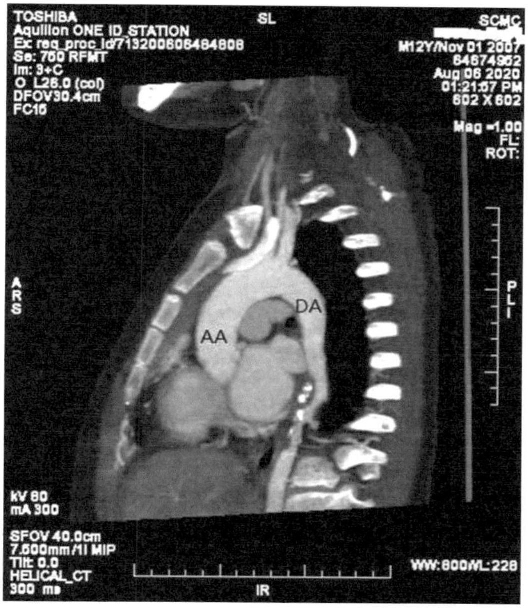

Fig. 53.1 Abdominal CTA. *AA* ascending aorta, *DA* descending aorta

resistance index (RI) is 0.87. These results were similar to the alterations of large vessel vasculitis (Fig. 53.1).

Preoperative diagnosis: TA.

53.2 Anesthetic Management

Intranasal dexmedetomidine 1.0 μg/kg was administrated 30 min before the induction of anesthesia.

Routine monitoring was performed after the patient was transported to the operating room. The noninvasive blood pressure (NBP) was 145/95 mm Hg in the left upper extremity, HR 80 beats/min, and a pulse oxygen saturation (SpO_2) of 98%. Anesthesia was induced with 0.2 mg/kg of etomidate, propofol, 3.0 mg/kg, rocuronium, 0.6 mg/kg, and sufentanil, 2.5 μg/kg. After the eyelash reflex disappeared, an ID 7.0 mm cuffed endotracheal tube was intubated under a fibrotic bronchoscope at a depth of 18 cm. Subsequently, SIMV-PCV-VG ventilation mode was chosen with RR at 20 times /min, tidal volume (VT) at 8 mL/kg, peak inspiratory pressure (PIP) approximately at 15 mm Hg, synchronous trigger sensitivity at −4 cm H_2O, oxygen flow rate at 2 L/min, fraction of inspired oxygen (FiO_2) at 50%, inspiratory time to expiratory time (I:E) ratio at 1:2, positive end-expiratory pressure (PEEP) at 4 cm H_2O, and intraoperative end-tidal carbon dioxide ($ETCO_2$) at 45–50 mm Hg.

After intubation, invasive arterial catheterization was conducted in both the upper and lower extremities for continuous artery blood pressure (ABP) monitoring Most Care® device. At the same time, the right internal jugular vein was catheterized for central venous pressure (CVP) monitoring was monitored using a 5 F–8 cm double-lumen deep venous catheter. Additionally, Bispectral Index (BIS) monitoring and INVOS regional tissue oxygen saturation (rSO_2) monitoring (renal area) were conducted. The right femoral vein was accessed for rapid fluid replacement. Tranexamic acid 10 mg/kg was infused before skin incision. During the operation, anesthesia was maintained with a combination of propofol 3.0–4.0 mg/(kg·h), dexmedetomidine 1.0 μg/(kg·h), sufentanil 2.0 μg/(kg·h), and rocuronium 0.6 mg/(kg·h), along with sevoflurane intermittent inhalation. The BIS values were maintained at 45–50. Nicardipine 0.5–1 μg/(kg·min) was administered to regulate blood pressure. The initial left upper extremity ABP was 150/95 mm Hg, while the left lower extremity ABP was 95/65 mm Hg. The cardiac index (CI) was 3.5 L/min·m^2, left ventricular pressure rising rate (dp/dt) was 1.2 mm Hg/ms, stroke volume variation (SVV) was 10.5%, HR was 85 beats/min, CVP was 8 cm H_2O, and renal area rSO_2 was 90%. During the operation, if the cardiac index (CI) drops to 2.00, dp/dt falls below 0.8 mm Hg/ms, and the left upper extremity ABP drops to 120/60 mm Hg, nicardipine should be discontinued. Instead, norepinephrine at 0.05 μg/(kg·min) and dopamine at 5.0 μg/(kg·min) should be intravenously administered. Additionally, fluid replacement should be accelerated if stroke volume variation (SVV) is equal to or greater than 13%. Blood gases were monitored every 30 min to 1 h throughout the operation (Table 53.1). A packed red blood cell of 150 mL was transfused during the operation. Electrolytes were supplemented based on blood

Table 53.1 Intraoperative blood gas test results

Time point	pH	PaO_2 (mm Hg)	$PaCO_2$ (mm Hg)	BE (mmol/L)	HCT (%)	K^+ (mmol/L)	Ca^{2+} (mmol/L)	Lac (mmol/L)	Cl^- (mmol/L)	Hgb (g/dL)	HCO_3^- mmol/L
Admission	7.46	288.3	38	−3.1	37.5	3.2	1.10	1.5	107	12.5	19.5
During surgery	7.43	240	37.4	−4.9	38.1	3.7	1.12	1.8	110	13.1	17.8
Discharge	7.40	331	31.3	−4.4	32.5	3.1	1.14	1.3	112	11.8	19.3

gas test results, including 300 mg of calcium gluconate and 0.5 g of potassium chloride. Body temperature was monitored, and active warming measures, such as warm air blankets and fluid warming, were provided.

The thoracoabdominal incision was adopted to expose both the thoracic and abdominal compartments. It was found that a segment of significantly narrowed abdominal aorta passed through the diaphragm with a stiff vessel wall. After the distal portion of the abdominal aorta was separated free, a 30 cm long, 12-thread Gore-Tex vessel was chosen to make end-to-side anastomoses with the abdominal aorta and the ascending aorta through the left diaphragm along their right-sided walls. The preoperative upper extremity ABP was 150/80 mm Hg, and the lower extremity ABP was 80/68 mm Hg. After the bypass surgery, the upper extremity ABP was 100/60 mm Hg, and the lower extremity ABP was 90/63 mm Hg.

After the operation, the patient was transferred to the Cardiac Intensive Care Unit (CICU) with endotracheal intubation and invasive blood pressure monitoring. Upon returning to the CICU, dopamine and norepinephrine were continuously administered for hemodynamic stability, which was adjusted based on cardiac output, ABP, HR, and SpO_2. The hemodynamics remained stable after the operation without symptoms of dizziness, blackouts, and blood-steal phenomena.

Intraoperative transesophageal echocardiography showed: slight hypertrophy of the interventricular septum and left ventricular wall, reduced left ventricular contractibility, left ventricular and septal muscle contraction is mildly isotropic, mild aortic valve regurgitation with regurgitation jet width of 0.22 cm, normal opening of atrioventricular valve, slightly thickened mitral valve tip and displaced closing point, mild to moderate mitral valve regurgitation with multiple regurgitation jets. The jet width was 0.32 cm. Mild to moderate tricuspid valve regurgitation with a regurgitation jet of 0.35 cm and a regurgitation velocity of 2.92 m/s.

Postoperative angiography results indicated: Normal development of the pulmonary artery and normal return of the pulmonary veins, unobstructed external pipeline at the anastomosis between the ascending aorta and abdominal aorta, stenotic changes in the distal thoracic aorta with the narrowest diameter of approximately 2.88 mm. The diameter above narrowest portion was approximately 8.31 mm.

The endotracheal tube was removed on postoperative day 1 and discharged from the CICU on postoperative day 3. One week later, he was discharged from the hospital.

53.3 Review of Knowledge Points

TA is characterized by high blood pressure in the upper extremities and low blood pressure in the lower extremities. The pressure gradient between the upper and lower extremities mainly depends on the location and degree of stenosis, as well as the collateral formation. The hypertension in TA patients is mainly caused by renal artery stenosis, followed by aortic stenosis. Suppose the narrowed portion is severe, close to the heart, and without sufficient collateral formation. In that case, the afterload of the left ventricle can be significantly increased, which will result in left ventricular hypertrophy and heart failure. Heart failure is the primary cause of death after TA surgery. Preoperative immunosuppressive treatment can effectively induce a non-active period, significantly reduce the mortality rate, and further prevent surgical stimulation-induced vasculitis, which can lead to recurrent or aggravated vascular re-narrowing.

53.4 Discussion

53.4.1 Preoperative Assessment and Preparation

When assessing children with TA, it is important to assess the function of vital organs, the hypertension level, and the related complications. TA is a rare condition in clinical practice, which often results in tissue ischemia or multiple organ failure due to widespread vascular involvement. Before surgery, it is important to ensure multidisciplinary consultations to correctly guide perioperative medication and regularly assess the patient's condition by surgeons and rheumatology immunologists. This will help achieve a standardized, refined, and comprehensive diagnostic and treatment process.

Assessing and optimizing the patient's overall condition before surgery is essential. This includes evaluation and optimization of the upper and lower extremities blood pressure, overall vascular condition, liver and kidney function, coagulation function, medical treatment process, TA typing, in active or inactive period, and related complications. It is important to evaluate the renal function if renal vessels are involved completely. For those patients with corticosteroid treatment, it is also important to evaluate the function of the adrenal cortex and determine whether supplemental corticosteroids are needed during the perioperative period. The patient's overall condition stability and disease activity should also be evaluated.

The choice of anesthesia protocols should be based on the child's general condition and the type of surgery. Regional anesthesia and analgesia should be used cautiously. The sympathetic nerves are blocked by spinal anesthesia, which can cause "blood stealing" and hypotension and result in ischemia in vital organs such as the brain, intestines, and kidneys. General anesthesia is less likely to cause severe hypotension compared to spinal anesthesia. Therefore, spinal anesthesia can only be used in children with significant differences between upper and lower extremities blood pressure after a thorough assessment of neurological function. The top concern of anesthesia in TA patients is maintaining hemodynamic stability and avoiding significant blood pressure fluctuations. A sudden increase in blood pressure could result in cerebral hemorrhage, cerebral infarction, myocardial dysfunction, and postoperative brain dysfunction. If the child's organ perfusion has already been compromised, the administration of high doses of vasoconstrictors should also be avoided. Intraoperative brain oxygen saturation and transcranial Doppler ultrasound can be used to monitor cerebral blood flow perfusion.

53.4.2 Intraoperative Anesthetic Management

The aim of intraoperative anesthetic management is to maintain sufficient tissue perfusion pressure, prevent significant changes in cardiac preload and afterload, and avoid further suppression of the cardiac and cerebral vessels by drugs. For children with pre-existing heart failure before surgery, it is important to reduce the cardiac preload and afterload during the perioperative period. Drugs and fluid therapy should be adjusted based on changes in invasive arterial pressure, central venous pressure, cardiac index, and stroke volume variation.

The lower extremity arteries are less affected than other arteries in patients with TA. Therefore, it is recommended to simultaneously monitor both the upper and lower extremities' invasive artery blood pressure if significant differences in blood pressure exist between the upper and lower extremities. The femoral artery pressure in the supine position should be used as the standard. If the pulse cannot be felt, noninvasive methods such as Doppler ultrasound blood flow signals and pulse oximetry can be used as alternatives. In this case, continuous monitoring of invasive radial and femoral artery blood pressure, intermittent monitoring of ascending aortic blood pressure, continuous monitoring of depth of anesthesia by BIS, and continuous monitoring of hemodynamics by Most Care®.

Intraoperative aortic pressure measurement is excellent for patients with TA to assess core blood pressure and hemodynamic status. Compared to peripheral arterial pressure measurement, direct aortic pressure measurement can provide a more accurate reflection of cardiac afterload and aid in determining the extent and severity of aortic lesions, which can facilitate the selection of surgical approaches. Due to the risks of multiple organ ischemia and heart failure, it is essential to consider the function of multiple organs when the balance point of blood pressure is established and regulated. During surgery, anesthesiologists must carefully manage blood pressure to prevent cerebrovascular accidents and heart failure. To achieve this, the child's blood pressure should be closely monitored during the hospitalization. During surgery, it is better to set the balance point of invasive systolic pressure at 140–160 mm Hg in the upper extremity.

In children with poorly controlled blood pressure, the cerebral blood flow autoregulation curve may be shifted to the right, and intracranial vascular resistance may be increased, which can cause more risk of cerebral ischemia once blood pressure decreases. Therefore, it is crucial to pay more attention to cerebral perfusion. Electroencephalograms, transcranial Doppler ultrasound, and near-infrared local brain oxygen tissue monitoring can be used to assess intraoperative cerebral perfusion status. During tracheal intubation, it is important to avoid overextension of the neck in children with severe carotid artery stenosis to prevent obstruction of the cerebral blood supply. Intraoperative neurological monitoring may also be considered. Our team utilizes a fibrotic bronchoscope for tracheal intubation to avoid cerebral ischemia when the neck is extended. Insufficient ventilation during surgery can cause cerebral vasoconstriction and cerebral ischemia. It is required to control $ETCO_2$ levels at 35–45 mm Hg to avoid excessive cerebral vasoconstriction.

In this case, the child underwent end-to-side anastomosis without extracorporeal circulation to complete the artificial blood vessel bypass surgery. Compared to standard artificial blood vessel replacement surgery, this procedure dramatically reduced the risks of severe hemodynamic fluctuations and extracorporeal circulation-related adverse effects. Separating the entire arterial vessel is unnecessary due to the low requirement of the surgical field, thus avoiding damage to important organs and nerves.

53.4.3 Postoperative Anesthetic Management

While the artificial blood vessel is anastomosed to the descending aorta's narrow distal end, the impact of anastomoses on the left ventricle's afterload is minimal, which reduces the risk of left heart failure. However, the child's stenosis is located after the first branch of the aorta, which is high and distant. Therefore, clamping and anastomosing of the artificial blood vessel and ascending aorta at this location may increase the afterload and severely impact the fragile heart, leading to the collapse of the child's circulation. To avoid this risk, we prepared emergency procedures and facilities after the operation, ready for the occurrence of acute heart failure at any time.

53.5 Shortcomings and Limitations

Although no adverse events occurred during the perioperative period, there were still shortcomings in the anesthetic management. Firstly, cerebral ultrasound monitoring of the middle cerebral artery was not conducted, which may help to reduce the risk of insufficient blood supply to the brain. Additionally, the brain oxygen supply was not monitored. Secondly, regional block anesthesia, such as paravertebral block, was not provided during the operation, and postoperative analgesia was solely dependent on opioids. This does not align with the original intention of providing comfortable medical treatment.

53.6 Conclusion

In the case of anesthetic management discussed above, the anesthetic management of children with multiple large arteritis should be based on the pathological characteristics of the disease itself. To ensure the safe progress of the surgery, intraoperative invasive arterial monitoring, blood gas analysis, and other real-time monitoring methods should be used. During the process of artificial blood vessel bypass surgery, it is essential to maintain the invasive blood pressure of the upper and lower extremities at the preoperative baseline level. If there is a drop in blood pressure, surgical shunting should be promptly performed, and fluid replacement and vasoactive drugs should be used to restore blood pressure quickly. Additionally, preparation for extracorporeal circulation should be made to manage possible circulatory collapse (Hongbin Gu).

Anesthetic Management of Pericardiectomy in a Child with Chronic Constrictive Pericarditis

54

Hongbin Gu

Abstract

A 7-year-old boy presented with abdominal distension for 1 year, accompanied by chest tightness after activity, inability to lie down at night, morning eyelid edema, etc. Cardiac ultrasound and digital subtraction angiography (DSA) examinations suggested increased pressure in the inferior vena cava, right atrium, right ventricle, etc. Based on clinical manifestations, constrictive pericarditis was suspected, and pericardiectomy was planned under general anesthesia. In cases such as this, anesthesia should focus on a thorough preoperative assessment and the implementation of appropriate management strategies before and after pericardial stripping surgery. During the operation, selecting suitable invasive monitoring and effective vascular access is important, as well as administering appropriate vasoactive drugs and fluid therapy based on the monitoring indicators to maintain circulatory function stability after pericardial stripping and prevent circulatory collapse. For children undergoing surgery for constrictive pericarditis, the entire medical team needs to focus on the cause of the disease, clearly communicate the surgical steps, and establish good medical connections.

H. Gu (✉)
The National Children's Medical Center (Shanghai), Department of Anesthesiology of Shanghai Children's Medical Center, Shanghai Jiao Tong University School of Medicine, Shanghai, China
e-mail: guhongbin@scmc.com.cn

Chronic constrictive pericarditis is a rare disease caused by connective tissue diseases, pericardial injury syndrome, tumors, microbial infections, or idiopathic constrictive pericarditis. The incidence rate of chronic constrictive pericarditis in the population is currently unknown. However, it is estimated that approximately 1.8% of children will develop this condition following an acute pericarditis attack.

Constrictive pericarditis is a cardiac filling disorder that results from pericardial lesions and a lack of elasticity. Chronic changes in the pericardium can lead to thickening, adhesion, calcification, and compression of the heart and large blood volume. This can limit the expansion of the heart chamber and cause a series of systemic blood circulation disorders. Symptoms and signs of heart failure, including difficulty breathing when exerting, increased venous pressure, and edema, eventually become apparent in the child. A pericardiectomy is the most effective treatment for chronic constrictive pericarditis.

Chronic constrictive pericarditis is a rare condition in children. This chapter presents a case of anesthetic management for pericardiectomy in chronic constrictive pericarditis.

J. Zheng et al. (eds.), *Selected Pediatric Cardiovascular Surgery Anesthesia Cases*,
https://doi.org/10.1007/978-981-96-5614-1_54

54.1 Case Presentation

The 7-year-old male patient, weighing 31 kg, was admitted to the hospital due to abdominal distension of unknown origin, persisting for 1 year. He also reported chest tightness after physical activity, inability to lie flat at night, eyelid edema in the morning, and mild edema in both lower limbs. The abdominal puncture ascites smear revealed no tumor cells or microbial infection. The patient was tentatively diagnosed with abdominal effusion to be investigated and admitted for treatment. The patient's usual medication includes ambrisentan 2.5 mg orally once daily, Furosemide 20 mg once daily, and Spironolactone 20 mg once daily. Following admission, all necessary examinations were conducted, and the patient received cardiac strengthening treatment, fluid restriction, and diuresis to maintain a negative balance of intake and output. The medical team also planned to perform pericardiectomy under general anesthesia.

During the physical examination, the patient exhibited eyelid edema, mild edema in both lower limbs, and an abdominal circumference of 70 cm. The patient's vital signs were recorded as follows: temperature of 36.5 °C, pulse rate of 95 beats per minute, and respiratory rate of 24 breaths per minute. The patient was alert and responsive, with a heart rate of 95 beats per minute, regular rhythm, and strong heart sounds. No murmurs were detected. The abdomen was soft with no palpable masses or tenderness, including no rebound tenderness. The liver was 5 cm below the ribs and 6 cm below the xiphoid process, while the spleen was not palpable below the ribs. Normal bowel sounds were present. The neurological examination yielded negative results.

Laboratory examination: ALT 33 U/L, AST 52 U/L, ALP 231 U/L, CK-MB 26 U/L, TP 84.7 g/L, ALB 56.2 g/L, TBIL 20.8 μmol/L, Na^+ 132.1 mmol/L, K^+ 4.92 mmol/L, TC 3.8 mmol/L; blood, urine, and stool routine normal. Thyroid function monitoring is normal. NT-proBNP >30,000 pg/mL. Blood gas analysis: pH 7.35, $PaCO_2$ 42 mm Hg, PaO_2 101 mm Hg, Lac 4.7 mmol/L, red blood cell-specific volume 33.7%, SBE −1.7, Hb 10.9 g/dL.

Electrocardiogram: Sinus rhythm, T wave changes.

CT shows that the inferior vena cava near the right atrium was widened, the diaphragm, the lower esophageal wall, and part of the intestinal wall were unevenly thickened. The liver was enlarged, and the parenchyma showed diffuse density abnormalities. The inferior vena cava near the heart and the main trunk of the hepatic vein were also thickened. There was a small amount of effusion under the liver capsule. Pleural effusion was present in both thoracic cavities, with more on the right side. The interlobular septa of both lungs were thickened, and there was localized emphysema in the lower lobe of the right lung.

The abdominal ultrasound revealed a hypoechoic area with a maximum anterior–posterior diameter of about 58 mm around the liver, spleen, and within the pelvic cavity, indicating pelvic effusion.

The cardiac ultrasound was mentioned. The patient's condition was characterized by right atrial dilation, severe tricuspid regurgitation, and slight left deviation of the interventricular septum.

The DSA examination revealed a pressure of 26 mm Hg in the middle segment of the inferior vena cava, smooth walls of the right and middle hepatic veins with no apparent narrowing or stenosis, a pulmonary artery pressure of 40 mm Hg, a right atrial pressure of 33 mm Hg, and a right ventricular pressure of 34 mm Hg. The left ventricular ejection fraction is 64%. The pulmonary artery is thickened, and no shunting was found.

Liver biopsy: The liver parenchyma showed diffuse density abnormalities, hepatocyte swelling, and deformation.

54.2 Anesthetic Management

Prior to the operation, the child received intranasal dexmedetomidine 1.0 μg/kg. Once calmed, the child was placed supine and taken to the operating room. Upon arrival, routine monitoring revealed noninvasive blood pressure (NBP) of 102/65 mm Hg, heart rate (HR) of 95 beats/min, and pulse oxygen saturation (SpO_2) of 98%. Anesthesia was induced and maintained using etomidate 0.2 mg/kg, propofol 3.0 mg/kg, rocuronium 0.6 mg/kg, and sufentanil 2.5 μg/kg. Following the disappearance of the eyelash reflex, we performed direct laryngoscopy and inserted an ID 5.5 mm cuffed endotracheal tube to a depth of 15.5 cm. We then provided ventilation support in SIMV-PCV-VG mode with a respiratory rate of 20 breaths/min, tidal volume (VT)maintained at 8 mL/kg, pressure control at approximately 15 mm Hg, synchronous trigger sensitivity at −4 cm H_2O, oxygen flow rate at 2 L/min, fraction of inspired oxygen (FiO_2) at 50%, inspiratory time to expiratory time (I:E) ratio at 1:2, positive end-expiratory pressure (PEEP) at 4 cm H_2O, and intraoperative end-tidal carbon dioxide ($ETCO_2$) at 35–45 mm Hg.

Following intubation, we established invasive arterial pressure using a 22 G left radial artery and Most Care® hemodynamic monitoring. We also monitored central venous pressure using a 5 F–8 cm double-lumen deep vein catheter in the right internal jugular vein and used Bispectral Index (BIS) monitoring. The left femoral vein was also for pressure measurement using a 20 G–5.1 cm catheter for rapid fluid replacement. Tranexamic acid 10 mg/kg was infused intravenously before the skin incision. During surgery, propofol was administered intravenously at 3.0–4.0 mg/(kg·h), along with sufentanil 2.0 μg/(kg·h) and rocuronium 0.6 mg/(kg·h). Sevoflurane inhalation was also used to maintain anesthesia, while the BIS value was kept between 45 and 50. The patient's initial arterial blood pressure was 110/62 mm Hg, with a cardiac index of 2.9 L/(min·m^2), a left ventricular pressure rise rate of 0.79, a stroke volume variation of 11.2%, a heart rate of 115 beats/min, a central venous pressure of 18 cm H_2O, and a left femoral vein pressure of 28 cm H_2O. During surgery, the cardiac index dropped to 2 L/(min·m^2), the left ventricular pressure rise rate dropped to 0.3, and the arterial blood pressure dropped to 85/40 mm Hg. Norepinephrine 0.05 μg/(kg·min) and dobutamine 5.0 μg/(kg·min)were administered innately, and fluid replacement was accelerated when SVV $\geq$ 13%. Furosemide 1 mg/kg was administered, and norepinephrine was increased to 0.1 μg/(kg·min) and dobutamine to 7.5 μg/(kg·min) after complete release of the pericardium and vena cava entrance. Blood gas levels were monitored every 30 min to 1 h throughout the surgery (Table 54.1). No red blood cell suspension was transfused during the procedure. Electrolytes, specifically calcium gluconate 300 mg, were supplemented based on blood gas results. Body temperature was closely monitored, and active warming measures, such as warm air blankets and fluid warming, were administered.

Table 54.1 Intraoperative blood gas test results

Time point	pH	PaO_2 (mm Hg)	$PaCO_2$ (mm Hg)	BE (mmol/L)	HCT (%)	Na^+ (mmol/L)	K^+ (mmol/L)	Ca^{2+} (mmol/L)	Lac (mmol/L)	Cl^- (mmol/L)L	Hgb g/dL
Admission	7.41	359	46	−3.92	36.2	147	3.91	1.04	1.0	104	11
Discharge	7.49	338	45	−2.2	34.2	137	4.07	1.14	1.1	106	10.8

54.3 Postoperative Outcome

A median sternotomy was performed to access the chest, revealing significant thickening of the pericardium, which was heavily adhered to the heart. Careful dissection was performed around the right atrium, right ventricle, and apex of the heart and gradually around the superior and inferior vena cava, resulting in a pericardiectomy. The operation lasted a total of 105 mins, with an estimated blood loss of approximately 30 mL and a urine output of 150 mL. A total of 650 mL of Ringer's acetate was infused, and the lactate level remained within the normal range. At the end of the operation, the blood pressure was 102/65 mm Hg, heart rate was 113 beats/min, SpO_2 was 99%, rectal temperature was 36.3 °C, the pressures of the superior and inferior vena cava dropped to 17 cm H_2O and 26 cm H_2O respectively, and transesophageal echocardiography showed that the atrial septum was in the middle. There was no obstruction in the atrial and pulmonary veins.

Following the operation, the patient was transferred to the Cardiac Intensive Care Unit (CICU) with an endotracheal tube. The patient was monitored using invasive blood pressure (ABP), electrocardiogram (EKG), and SpO_2. Upon returning to the CICU, the patient continued to receive maintenance doses of dopamine and norepinephrine. The dose of vasoactive drugs was adjusted based on cardiac output, BP, HR, and SpO_2. The patient was discharged from the CICU on the third day after the endotracheal tube was removed and from the hospital 1 week later.

The pathological results showed a pericardial cyst with wall-like growth, mild fibrous tissue hyperplasia, focal degeneration, mild interstitial vascular hyperplasia, dilation, and congestion, accompanied by inflammatory cell infiltration.

54.4 Review of Knowledge Points

Chronic constrictive pericarditis is characterized by the loss of reserve capacity in the pericardium, which restricts ventricular expansion. The diseased pericardium causes a separation of intrathoracic and intracardiac pressures during the respiratory cycle, resulting in a lack of synchronization between the two pressures. This leads to enhanced interaction between the left and right ventricles. It is important to note that this description is objective and avoids any biased or figurative language.

Echocardiography reveals respiratory-related changes in the position of the interventricular septum and blood flow Doppler flow velocity. The myocardium exhibits distinctive diastolic characteristics and systolic strain. Invasive hemodynamic examination is the gold standard for evaluation, requiring careful recording of the right and left ventricle pressures and using catheters that can measure pressure with high fidelity at the tip.

Constrictive pericarditis typically presents as diastolic heart failure. Diagnosis requires a detailed history and physical examination, precise cardiac imaging, and invasive hemodynamic evaluation due to the pathologic inelastic pericardium restricting cardiac filling and leading to unique hemodynamic abnormalities. While some children with constrictive pericarditis can be relieved by anti-inflammatory therapy, others require pericardiectomy.

Children with chronic constrictive pericarditis may present with severe preoperative conditions and poor cardiac function. They are at risk of severe hypotension, massive bleeding, congestive heart failure, malignant arrhythmia, and even cardiac arrest during surgery. Additionally, they may experience low cardiac output after surgery. Maintaining objectivity and avoiding biased language when discussing their condition and treatment is essential. Therefore, the Anesthetic management of these children requires special attention. When formulating an anesthesia plan for a child, it is essential to carefully consider preoperative assessment and examination, anesthesia induction, maintenance, and perioperative management. This is especially important for children who require pericardial drainage surgery.

Additionally, precise subject-specific vocabulary should be used when it conveys the meaning more precisely than a similar nontechnical term. No new content should be added to the text.

Anesthetic management should use drugs and techniques that minimize the impact on heart rate, systemic vascular resistance, venous return, and myocardial contractility.

54.5 Discussion

54.5.1 Preoperative Assessment and Preparation

Ensure a comprehensive and complete assessment of the child's overall condition, clarifying the possible causes of pericarditis. Determine the presence of pericardial friction or dull heart sound, tachycardia, hypotension, paradoxical pulse-distended jugular veins, and other manifestations of hemodynamic damage. Assess for thrombosis, low blood oxygen saturation, difficulty breathing, dizziness, and chest pain. Laboratory tests should include hematology tests, coagulation function tests, electrolyte tests, liver function tests, kidney function tests, chest X-ray, CT scan or MRI examination, and echocardiography. In addition to routine monitoring, invasive arterial blood pressure monitoring is essential preoperatively. Establishing a central venous channel is unnecessary and should not delay urgent pericardial surgery.

Constrictive pericarditis is a chronic disease that can cause damage to multiple systems and organs, often leading to anemia, hypoalbuminemia, pleural and abdominal effusion, heart failure, and electrolyte disorders. The preoperative general condition is typically poor. It is important to note that any subjective evaluations have been excluded from this description. To prepare for surgery, it is essential to focus on preoperative cardiac strengthening, diuretic control of heart failure, water and electrolyte disorders correction, and transfusion of an appropriate amount of concentrated red blood cells to correct anemia above 90 g/L. If necessary, albumin supplementation can also be considered.

Additionally, maintaining a certain depth of sedation preoperatively can help to reduce myocardial oxygen consumption. Preoperative optimization of blood volume is crucial. If preoperative hemodynamic damage, such as hypotension, is caused by increased intracardiac pressure, anesthetic treatment should follow the principles of cardiac tamponade treatment.

Predictors of low survival rate include preoperative poor liver and kidney function, high pulmonary artery pressure, abnormal left ventricular systolic function, lower body edema, hyponatremia, and older age. The perioperative mortality rate for this disease ranges from 6% to 12%. In cases where children have extensive myocardial atrophy/fibrosis, the perioperative mortality rate can increase to 40%. The main complications include acute cardiac dysfunction and ventricular wall rupture. Performing surgery as soon as possible can lead to a long-term survival rate after pericardial stripping surgery that is consistent with the survival rate of the general population. Furthermore, due to the subtle differences in surgical methods, the anesthesiologist should conduct multidisciplinary case discussions to confirm the anesthesia and surgical plans with the entire team.

54.5.2 Intraoperative Anesthetic Management

Before anesthesia induction, prepare adequate resuscitation fluids, including blood, and various types of vasoactive drugs such as norepinephrine and epinephrine, as well as defibrillators. During anesthesia induction, aim to minimize the suppression of circulation. These patients exhibit a prolonged systemic circulation time, slower onset of drug action, and require slow induction in small doses under strict blood pressure and electrocardiogram monitoring to avoid induction-induced hypotension and sudden heart rate drop. It is vital to avoid blindly increasing the dose of the drug to deepen anesthesia and cause circulatory suppression. When there are no contraindications, such as significant respiratory difficulty, obesity, facial deformity, or noncooperation of the child, sevoflurane inhalation induction can be used. It is essential to avoid coughing during the induction process and maintain spontaneous ventilation. If hemodynamics deteriorates during the induction process, surgery should be performed quickly after intubation.

This patient's anesthesia induction and maintenance involved medication methods specific to pediatric cardiac surgery. Selected drugs with minimal impact on cardiac function were used. General anesthesia was induced with endotracheal intubation and maintained with opioids (such as sufentanil), rocuronium, and propofol. Low-flow sevoflurane inhalation was also used to achieve minimal circulatory impact and maintain stable anesthesia. The hemodynamic goals for patients in such cases should be to maintain preload, contractility, and heart rate (preferably in sinus rhythm). Avoiding high positive-pressure ventilation and minimizing inspiratory pressure to prevent significant hemodynamic deterioration is essential. The use of nitrous oxide should also be avoided. During surgery, it is recommended that continuous intravenous infusion of vasoconstrictors be administered to maintain hemodynamic stability. However, it is essential to consider the adverse consequences of excessive vasoconstriction, which may decrease overall cardiac output.

Anesthetic management should follow the same protocol as heart valve disease treatment during surgery. Pericardial stripping surgery is a lengthy procedure that often results in significant blood loss and fluid loss, which may necessitate intravenous infusion of blood products. Additionally, direct mechanical stimulation of the heart can lead to arrhythmia. Therefore, for this patient, essential monitoring such as electrocardiogram, pulse oxygen saturation, end-tidal carbon dioxide, body temperature, and urine output were supplemented with invasive blood pressure and central venous pressure monitoring. Most Care® monitor was used to monitor stroke volume, peripheral vascular resistance, cardiac circulation efficiency, maximum pressure gradient, stroke volume variability, and pulse pressure variability during surgery. During intraoperative analysis, invasive blood pressure, central venous pressure, and stroke volume variation (SVV) trends are comprehensively examined. If the cardiac index significantly drops and is accompanied by a decrease in blood pressure, small doses of norepinephrine and dobutamine are combined to increase myocardial contractility and improve cardiac output.

Intraoperative fluid control is also essential. Infusion speed should be controlled during the operation based on ABP, SVV, cardiac index (CI), central venous pressure (CVP), etc. Following the principle of equal volume infusion or blood transfusion is essential before complete pericardial stripping. After stripping, the infusion should be limited to prevent an increase in heart blood volume, which can cause heart enlargement, pulmonary edema, and heart failure.

Ventilation management should also be considered. During mechanical ventilation, it is recommended to adopt permissive hypercapnia with an $ETCO_2$ range of 45–55 mm Hg to maintain adequate ventilation. Furthermore, lung-protective ventilation strategies reduce average airway pressure and prevent increased intrapleural pressure. These include low FiO_2 ($\leq 60\%$), low TV (6–8 mL/kg), optimal PEEP (higher than the lower inflection point of the P–V curve by 2 cm H_2O), and manual re-expansion. It is important to avoid further decreasing cardiac output.

Post-pericardiectomy treatment requires careful management to prevent acute congestive heart failure. Due to the increase in venous return, the already atrophied myocardium cannot adapt. During the operation, controlling fluid intake based on CVP, ABP, HR, urine output, and SVV is essential. Additionally, cardiac diuretics can be administered, and the patient can be positioned head-high-foot-low to prevent an increase in venous return and subsequent heart failure or pulmonary edema. When the narrowed pericardium is removed, there is a risk of persistent low cardiac output due to the already atrophied myocardium and sudden increase in venous return. Creatine phosphate can be administered to protect cardiac function.

54.5.3 Postoperative Anesthetic Management

Children with constrictive pericarditis may have poor lung compliance due to factors such as pleural effusion, intra-abdominal hematoma, or slow circulation. Additionally, postoperative arrhythmias, such as supraventricular tachycardia, low cardiac output, and pericardial effusion, are common. It is essential to consider these factors when treating children with constrictive pericarditis. Therefore, after the operation, patients should be transferred to the CICU for 1–2 days of mechanical ventilation treatment. Diuretic, cardiotonic, and vasodilator therapy should be administered, and electrolyte and acid–base balance should be checked regularly. Maintaining a balance of fluid intake and excretion is crucial, as well as aggressively protecting vital organ function while closely monitoring changes in cardiac rhythm. In addition to long-acting opioids, consider the use of local anesthetic infiltration or regional nerve blocks, such as intercostal and/or paravertebral blocks, for postoperative analgesia.

54.6 Shortcomings and Limitations

Although this case was successful, it is essential to note that the clinical manifestations of constrictive pericarditis and restrictive cardiomyopathy are very similar. They share common pathophysiological characteristics, including bilateral ventricular diastolic dysfunction, increased bilateral atrial pressure, and decreased cardiac output at rest. However, it is crucial to differentiate between the two diseases as their treatments are completely different. While pericardiectomy may cure constrictive pericarditis, treatment options for restrictive cardiomyopathy are limited, often requiring heart transplantation. Accurately distinguishing between constrictive pericarditis and restrictive cardiomyopathy has significant clinical implications for guiding further treatment. The clinician did not provide a precise differential diagnosis examination for the two conditions in this case.

54.7 Conclusion

Chronic constrictive pericarditis anesthetic management should prioritize preoperative assessment and communication with a multidisciplinary team. Anesthetics with minimal impact on circulatory function should be selected. The use of invasive monitoring should be rational, and positive inotropic drugs and volume supplementation should be correctly administered to achieve optimal perioperative outcomes (Hongbin Gu).

Anesthetic Management of Coronary Artery Bypass Grafting Under Cardiopulmonary Bypass in a Child with Kawasaki Disease

55

Huiyan Hou

Abstract

A 16-year-old girl with a history of Kawasaki disease experienced chest tightness and pain without obvious cause recently, and the symptoms became worse after physical exertion. Preoperative examinations showed coronary artery stenosis with a giant coronary artery thrombus. She underwent giant thrombus removal from the left coronary artery and anastomosis of the left internal mammary artery with the obtuse marginal branch under cardiopulmonary bypass. The anesthetic management should balance myocardial oxygen supply and demand and maintain myocardial contractibility during the perioperative period.

Kawasaki disease (KD) is a common autoimmune systemic vasculitis disease in childhood. KD often occurs in children under 5 years old. The medium and small blood vessels, especially the coronary arteries, are often involved, which can be the main cause of acquired heart disease in children. The coronary artery lesions caused by KD can result in coronary aneurysmal dilation, thrombosis, lumen stenosis, and even complete occlusion, which causes the reduction of coronary blood flow and the imbalance of myocardial oxygen supply and demand. When the myocardial oxygen consumption is increased, the patient may experience precordial pain and even myocardial infarction. This chapter reports the anesthetic management of one case of KD undergoing coronary artery bypass surgery under cardiopulmonary bypass.

55.1 Case Presentation

The patient was a 16-year-old girl with 63 kg in weight and 155 cm in height. Three months ago, she experienced chest tightness and pain without any obvious cause, which became worse after physical exertion. The echocardiography at a local hospital indicated a mass in the left atrium, possibly due to KD. One month ago, cardiac magnetic resonance imaging (MRI) showed dilation of the left coronary artery trunk and the left circumflex branch with local aneurysm formation and visible thrombus, left ventricular myocardial ischemia, which was considered to be caused by KD. Angiography demonstrated a giant aneurysmal dilation at the origin of the left circumflex branch with thrombus and calcification, mild stenosis following the aneurysmal dilation, and unclear display of the left coronary artery trunk. The patient was generally healthy without cyanosis and a history

H. Hou (✉)
The National Children's Medical Center (Shanghai), Department of Anesthesiology of Shanghai Children's Medical Center, Shanghai Jiao Tong University School of Medicine, Shanghai, China
e-mail: houhuiyan@scmc.com.cn

J. Zheng et al. (eds.), *Selected Pediatric Cardiovascular Surgery Anesthesia Cases*,
https://doi.org/10.1007/978-981-96-5614-1_55

of recurrent respiratory infections. She experienced normal appetite and significant physical endurance reduction recently. She was admitted to our hospital with the diagnosis of coronary artery aneurysm/coronary thrombus for further treatment.

Physical examination: The patient was conscious and had normal breathing without cyanosis, clear lung sounds in both lungs without dry or wet rales, regular heart rhythm, and strong heart sound without an obvious murmur. The liver and spleen were not palpable under the ribs. The extremities were warm without edema.

Laboratory tests: Platelet distribution width 15.9%. Liver and kidney function: Globulin 33.4 g/L, c Troponin I 0.03 μg/L. NT-proBNP 182 pg/mL.

Electrocardiogram (ECG): Sinus rhythm with atrial premature beats.

Chest X-ray: No abnormalities were seen in the soft tissues of the thoracic skeleton and chest wall. The mediastinum and trachea were centered without displacement. The mediastinum was not widened, and an oval, slightly high-density heart shadow was seen. Both diaphragms were intact, both costophrenic angles were sharp, and the lung markings were increased.

24-h dynamic ECG: Total number of heartbeats: 103,819 times, supraventricular beats: 779 times, slowest heart rate: 50 beats/minute, fastest heart rate: 144 beats/minute, average heart rate: 74 beats/minute, longest RR interval 1.24 s. Diagnosis: Sinus rhythm, junctional premature beats, sinus arrhythmia, T wave changes with rapid heartbeat, ST segment changes.

Echocardiography: The positions and connections of the heart are normal without obvious atrial and ventricular enlargement and acceptable left ventricular wall contraction activity. No widening of the aorta and pulmonary artery. Acceptable opening activity of pulmonary valve and atrioventricular valve. Intact atrial septum and ventricular septum. Left aortic arch. A medium uneven echo mass shadow of 2.51 cm × 3.51 cm was found on the posterior lateral wall of the left atrium, which protruded into the left atrium. There was no effect on the pulmonary vein blood flow. Left atrial occupancy, normal left ventricular contractibility.

Cardiac CT: Spiral CT scanning and three-dimensional reconstruction showed that the mediastinum was basically located within the central thoracic cavity. There were no obvious abnormal signal shadows in both lungs. Situs solitus of the atrium and visceral organs. Normal return of both pulmonary vein and vena cava. Unclear atrial septum shunting and slightly enlarged right atrium. Concordant atrioventricular connection and ventricular-aortic connection. The ventricular septum seemed to be intact. The left and right ventricles were slightly enlarged. No stenosis was seen in the left and right ventricular outflow tracts. Left aortic arch without obvious patent ductus arteriosus and aortic stenosis. The root of the left coronary artery was dilated with a diameter of 15.4 mm. The whole left circumflex branch was dilated with a root diameter of 7.1 mm, but no dilation in the left anterior descending branch was seen. Aneurysmal enlargement with 31.4 mm × 48.2 mm at the entrance of the left atrioventricular groove was seen with calcification of the vascular wall during the CT plain scan. Thrombus formation was seen inside. The diameter of the left circumflex branch at the atrioventricular groove was 12.6 mm. Normal pulmonary artery trunk and the left and right pulmonary artery branches develop. The diameter of the descending aorta at the diaphragm level was 14.7 mm.

Cardiac MRI: A cardiac MRI sequence scan showed the mediastinum was basically located within the central thoracic cavity. There were no obvious abnormal signal shadows in both lungs. Situs solitus of the atrium and visceral organs. Normal return of both pulmonary vein and vena cava. Unclear atrial septum shunting and slightly enlarged right atrium. Concordant atrioventricular connection and ventricular-aortic connection. The ventricular septum seemed to be intact. The left and right ventricles were slightly enlarged. No stenosis was seen in the outflow tract of the left and right ventricles. Left aortic arch without obvious patent ductus arteriosus and aortic stenosis. The root of the left coronary artery was dilated with a diameter of 17.6 mm. The left circumflex branch was dilated with a root diameter of 8.5 mm, but no dilation in the left anterior descending branch was seen. Aneurysmal enlargement with 31.5 mm × 44.6 mm at the entrance of the left atrioventricular groove with inside thrombus formation. The diameter of the left circumflex branch at the atrioventricular groove was 12.6 mm. Normal pulmonary artery trunk and the left and right pulmonary artery branches develop. There was no obvious abnormal local myocardial movement.

Coronary angiography: Ascending aortic angiography showed that the right coronary artery's origin, morphology, and running pathway were normal. The origin of the left coronary artery was not clearly shown. There are no obvious abnormalities in the morphology and the running pathway of the left anterior descending branch. Aneurysmal enlargement of 50.4 mm × 28.7 mm was seen at the origin of the left circumflex branch with inside thrombosis and calcification formation. The left circumflex branch became slightly narrow after aneurysmal enlargement. The contrast was seen at the distal end. The main trunk of the left coronary artery was not clear; the clinical history of KD should be combined.

Preoperative diagnosis: Left coronary artery dilation, left coronary artery aneurysm, coronary thrombosis. Elective coronary artery bypass grafting (CABG) under extracorporeal circulation was scheduled.

55.2 Anesthetic Management

The patient did not take any preoperative medications. Upon entering the operating room, basic vital signs were closely monitored with cuff blood pressure (BP) at 122/68 mm Hg, heart rate (HR) at 102 beats/min, and pulse oxygen saturation (SpO_2) at 99%. Anesthesia was induced by intravenous bolus injection of midazolam 3.0 mg, propofol 110 mg, sufentanil 50 μg, and rocuronium 35 mg. Once the eyelash reflex disappeared, an ID 7.0 mm cuffed endotracheal tube was intubated under direct laryngoscopy. The tube depth was fixed at 21 cm after verification of the appropriate position by bilateral auscultation of the lungs. The patient was ventilated with pressure-controlled ventilation (PCV) mode with ventilation parameters set as oxygen flow rate 2 L/min, inspired oxygen fraction (FiO_2) 50%, tidal volume (VT) 400 mL, respiratory rate (RR) 15 times/min, inspiratory to expiratory (I:E) time ratio 1:2. The end-tidal carbon dioxide ($ETCO_2$) was maintained around 35–45 mm Hg during surgery.

After intubation, the right radial artery was quickly catheterized to monitor invasive arterial blood pressure (ABP) continuously. The right jugular vein was catheterized with a 5 F double-lumen central venous catheter for central venous pressure (CVP) monitoring and infusion of vasoactive drugs. Anesthesia was maintained by continuous infusion of sufentanil 2.0 μg/(kg·h), propofol 4.0 mg/(kg·h), and rocuronium 0.5 mg/(kg·h). Sevoflurane concentration was adjusted to maintain a stable heart rate and blood pressure. Sodium acetate Ringer's solution of 400 mL was intravenously infused. Vasoactive drugs such as dopamine, nitroglycerin, and epinephrine were prepared preoperatively. Preoperative blood gas analysis results are shown in Table 55.1.

The left internal mammary artery was first dissected for later use. Purse-string sutures were placed in the right atrial appendage and ascending aorta, heparin was administered through the right atrial appendage. Cannulas were inserted into the ascending aorta and right atrial appendage to establish cardiopulmonary bypass (CBP). Under CBP parallel circulation, the inferior vena

Table 55.1 Intraoperative blood gas test results

Time point	Hb (g/dL)	HCT (%)	pH	PaO_2 (mm Hg)	$PaCO_2$ (mm Hg)	BE (mmol/L)	Na^+ (mmol/L)	K^+ (mmol/L)	Cl^- (mmol/L)	Ca^{2+} (mmol/L)	Lac (mmol/L)
Entry	14.6	43.1	7.42	354.7	36.2	0.9	138	3.7	105	1.13	1.4
Exit	10.1	30.6	7.41	281.2	34.7	2.2	139	4.2	106	1.1	1.7

cava and superior and inferior vena cava were cannulated. The cardioplegic solution was infused anterogradely from the aortic root and retrogradely from the coronary sinus to cause cardiac arrest after the ascending aorta was cross-clamped. During surgery, aneurysmal dilation was observed at the origin of the left coronary artery with a diameter of 1.5 cm and length of 3 cm. The left anterior descending artery was patent, but the circumflex artery was occluded by a large thrombus measuring 6 cm × 3 cm. The opening of the obtuse marginal branch was nearly occluded.

The thrombus was completely removed by incising the circumflex branch. The vessel wall and the distal end of the occluded circumflex branch were sutured. The left internal mammary artery (inner diameter 2 mm) was anastomosed with the distal end of the obtuse marginal branch (inner diameter 1.5 mm). The dilated origin of the left coronary artery was resected, and the aorta and pulmonary artery were connected. The aortic clamp was released after the heart was de-aired. The cardiac incision was continuously sutured. The heart spontaneously resumed beating and sinus rhythm. Vasoactive drugs such as milrinone 0.5 μg/(kg·min), nitroglycerin 0.5 μg/(kg·min), dopamine 5.0 μg/(kg·min), and norepinephrine 0.02 μg/(kg·min) were intravenously infused to maintain hemodynamics stability. The superior and inferior vena cava cannulation and ascending aorta were removed after separation from CBP. Albumin was intravenously infused. Arterial blood gas after CBP separation is shown in Table 55.1. The vasoactive drugs continued to be used after the patient was transferred to the pediatric Cardiac Intensive Care Unit (CICU) under ABP, ECG, and SpO_2 monitoring with the endotracheal tube in place.

55.3 Postoperative Outcome

The patient recovered well after surgery. The tracheal tube was removed on postoperative day 2. Then the child's vital signs stabilized, and the child was transferred to a general ward.

55.4 Review of Knowledge Points

55.4.1 Pathophysiology

KD is an acute febrile rash disease with unknown cause so far. The severe pathological change of KD is characterized by systemic vasculitis, mainly involving large and medium vessels. The coronary arteries are also often involved and cause coronary artery aneurysm, thrombosis formation, lumen narrowing, and even complete occlusion, all of which can cause the reduction of coronary artery blood flow and the imbalance between myocardial oxygen supply and demand, which further results in ischemic heart disease, myocardial infarction, and even sudden death. Coronary artery lesions are one of the major complications of KD, manifested as coronary artery dilation, coronary aneurysms, and coronary artery stenosis.

55.4.2 Balance of Myocardial Oxygen Supply and Demand

Myocardial oxygen supply is mainly determined by arterial blood oxygen content and coronary artery blood flow. The arterial blood oxygen content mainly depends on hemoglobin concentration, blood oxygen saturation, and oxygen partial pressure. Meanwhile, the ratio of coronary perfusion pressure to coronary vascular resistance determines coronary artery blood flow. Metabolic products of myocardial metabolism, autonomic nerve tension, endocrine hormone levels, and coronary anatomy can all affect coronary vascular resistance, while hemodynamic factors mainly determine coronary perfusion pressure. HR, myocardial contractility, and ventricular wall tension determine myocardial oxygen consumption, among which HR is the most important impact factor. Ventricular wall tension is affected by factors such as ventricular internal pressure (afterload), ventricular cavity size (preload), and wall thickness. Therefore, it is necessary to maintain an appropriate coronary perfusion pressure while avoiding the increase in myocardial oxygen consumption.

55.5 Discussion

55.5.1 Preoperative Evaluation and Preparation

The preoperative evaluation of children with coronary artery diseases mainly includes two aspects: the balance of myocardial oxygen supply and demand and the cardiac pumping function. Due to the symptoms of unstable angina and New York Heart Association (NYHA) classification of heart failure II in this case, oral midazolam syrup 0.5 mg/kg was taken for preoperative sedation (the maximum dose should not exceed 15 mg) to avoid the emotional fluctuations and reduce stress response.

Due to the long-term use of anticoagulant drugs in children with KD, it is necessary to stop aspirin therapy 1 week before surgery and low molecular weight heparin therapy 12 h before surgery to avoid the occurrence of intraoperative coagulation dysfunction.

Preparation of intraoperative monitoring: ECG monitor is a must for patients with KD since it cannot only monitor the heart rate and rhythm but can also help to detect the early signs of myocardial ischemia, especially by V5 lead, which can detect various perioperative arrhythmias and myocardial ischemia as high as 75%. Respiratory and oxygenation indicators included SpO_2, VT, RR, $ETCO_2$, and peak inspiratory pressure (PIP). Temperature monitoring includes nasopharyngeal temperature, bladder or rectal temperature. Other monitoring includes ABP, CVP, coagulation function, urine output, and transesophageal echocardiography.

55.5.2 Intraoperative Anesthetic Management

The principle of anesthetic induction for children with coronary artery diseases is to choose a reasonable combination of drugs and doses based on the patient's specific situations, avoid significant hemodynamic fluctuations, maintain the balance of myocardial oxygen supply and demand, and provide sufficient perfusion of important organs.

It is necessary to maintain hemodynamic stability during the maintenance of anesthesia. The BP and HR should not fluctuate significantly with the changes in surgical stimulation. For those patients with good cardiac function before surgery, considering the sufficient urine output, homeostasis, no metabolic disorder, and venous oxygen saturation (SvO_2) >70%, it is not necessary to handle if the heart rate is around 60 beats/min before CBP, but attention should be paid to control the fluid volume to avoid excessive blood volume. For those patients with poor cardiac function who need higher sympathetic tension to maintain cardiac output, medications with significant inhibition on the myocardium should be avoided. In addition, positive inotropic drugs should be used if it is necessary.

The key points of anesthetic management of CABG under CBP are as follows:

1. Myocardial protection and perfusion of vital organs: Cold blood cardioplegia is usually perfused via cannulation at the aortic root for most children undergoing CABG. For those with severe coronary artery disease, antegrade and retrograde perfusion can be conducted via cannulation at the aortic root and coronary sinus to enhance myocardial protection. The protection of other vital organs during CBP is mainly determined by hypothermia and relatively high perfusion pressure (50–80 mm Hg). It is better to maintain SvO_2 above 75%.
2. Management of hypotension and hypertension during CBP: Due to various factors, the perfusion pressure is often low (30–40 mm Hg) after the initiation of CBP, which can be generally maintained at an acceptable level by increasing CBP flow. If the blood pressure remains low, it can be managed by α receptor agonists through CBP, such as phenylephrine 0.5–1.0 μg/kg, often yield satisfactory results. However, it should be noted that the response to phenylephrine varies among pediatric patients. Hypertension during CBP can usually be managed by the deepening of anesthesia and/or using vasodilators.
3. Post-CBP management: Post-CBP management mainly includes the use of positive ino-

tropic drugs, vasodilators, β receptor blockers, or calcium channel blockers, which are one of the important aspects of anesthetic management in the patient undergoing CABG.

① Patients with coronary artery disease are often accompanied by varying degrees of heart failure due to myocardial ischemia, myocardial infarction, or ventricular aneurysms, which necessitates the use of positive inotropic drugs to enhance myocardial contractility during anesthetic management. However, any positive inotropic drug will increase myocardial oxygen consumption. Therefore, for older patients undergoing CABG, the indications for positive inotropic drug use are: pulmonary artery wedge pressure (PCWP) >16 mm Hg (mean arterial pressure (MAP) <70 mm Hg, or systolic pressure (SBP) <90 mm Hg), cardiac index (CI) <2.2 L/(min·m^2), SvO_2 < 65%. The choice of positive inotropic drugs includes dobutamine, dopamine, epinephrine, milrinone, etc.

② Nitroglycerin dilates coronary arteries, reduces myocardial oxygen consumption, and reduces pulmonary artery pressure and PCWP, which is recommended to be used during the anesthesia of patients with coronary artery diseases, especially in cases of hypertension, high PCWP, acute left or right ventricular dysfunction, etc. It is worth noting that early tolerance to nitroglycerin can be easily developed.

③ β-Receptor blockers such as esmolol and metoprolol are beneficial for patients with coronary artery diseases, which can be selected based on the patient's specific conditions. Due to the negative inotropic and chronotropic effects of β-receptor blockers, they should be titrated based on close hemodynamic monitoring. Once the heart rate significantly decreases, β-receptor blockers should be stopped immediately. For those patients who highly depend on sympathetic tension and rapid heart rate to maintain cardiac output, β-receptor blockers should be avoided as they can easily induce heart failure.

④ Calcium channel blocker diltiazem can dilate the coronary arteries, prevent coronary artery spasms, increase coronary blood flow, and improve myocardial ischemia. It has no significant inhibitory effect on myocardial contractility and can be used for total arterialized CABG (i.e., all graft vessels used during coronary bypass surgery are arterial vessels). The dosage is 1–3 μg/(kg·min). The dihydropyridine class of calcium channel blockers, nicardipine, is also commonly used in patients with total arterialization.

55.6 Shortcomings and Limitations

In this case, cerebral function was not monitored during the surgery. If conditions permit, oxygen saturation monitoring of vital organs should be conducted to provide more effective help for postoperative functional recovery.

55.7 Conclusion

This patient was in good general condition with preoperative NYHA class II, indicating good tolerance to anesthesia and surgery. Therefore, the invasive arterial blood pressure monitoring from the radial artery was established after the induction of anesthesia. Papaverine was intravenously injected to prevent vascular spasm before the dissection of the internal mammary artery and the establishment of CBP, which can occasionally cause hypotension, for which attention should be paid. Anesthetic management during surgery can refer to the management strategies of adult coronary heart disease undergoing CABG. There are a few cases of pediatric CABG, but this patient's surgery went smoothly. The key point of anesthetic management is to use drugs to maintain coronary perfusion pressure without increasing myocardial oxygen consumption and to be fully prepared for the treatment of intraoperative complications, which includes the readily available positive inotropic drugs and standby CBP support team in case of need (Huiyan Hou).

Anesthetic Management of Potts Shunt Surgery in a Child with Idiopathic Pulmonary Hypertension

56

Lihong Jin

Abstract

A 3-year-old boy was admitted to the local hospital due to a lack of appetite and fatigue for over a month. Pulmonary arterial hypertension (PAH) was found a half month ago. He was diagnosed with idiopathic pulmonary arterial hypertension (IPAH) after other causes were ruled out. Oral sildenafil and bosentan were used to control IPAH. He was transferred to our hospital. Cardiac catheterization indicated severe PAH (pulmonary artery pressure/systemic circulation pressure = 0.81) and right heart failure. During hospitalization, the child repeatedly suffered from pulmonary hypertension crises. He was treated with intravenous milrinone and treprostinil, but pulmonary artery pressure (PAP) did not significantly decrease. After multidisciplinary consultation, he was scheduled for a Potts shunt surgery, in which the left pulmonary artery was anastomosed to the descending aorta. Perioperative management of PAH was key to the success of Potts shunt surgery.

The etiology of IPAH remains unknown. IPAH is characterized by an unexplained persistent increase in PAP and progressive right heart failure. Patients with IPAH suffer from the risk of sudden death. Furthermore, the prognosis is poor; the mortality rate is high. The median survival time of children with IPAH is only 10 months before the targeted drugs for PAH treatment can be used in the clinic. Tremendous progress has been made in the development of targeted drugs for PAH treatment over the last decade, but the prognosis of IPAH is still very poor. Apart from lung transplantation, atrial septostomy is one of the surgical treatments for IPAH. However, it may cause systemic hypoxia, which is not conducive to the patient's growth and development. Therefore, Potts shunt surgery connecting the pulmonary artery and descending aorta has become a new choice for the treatment of IPAH. This chapter reports the anesthetic management of Potts shunt surgery in a child with IPAH.

56.1 Case Presentation

The patient was a 3-year-old and 7-month-old boy with 90 cm in height and 14.3 kg in weight. He was diagnosed with IPAH for over half a month due to poor appetite and fatigue for over a month. After admission, he received oral sildenafil and bosentan dual-targeted drug treat-

L. Jin (✉)
The National Children's Medical Center (Shanghai), Department of Anesthesiology of Shanghai Children's Medical Center, Shanghai Jiao Tong University School of Medicine, Shanghai, China
e-mail: jinlihong@scmc.com.cn

J. Zheng et al. (eds.), *Selected Pediatric Cardiovascular Surgery Anesthesia Cases*,
https://doi.org/10.1007/978-981-96-5614-1_56

ment. A cardiac catheterization examination was conducted under general anesthesia. The heart rate (HR) suddenly dropped to 50 beats/min during the sputum suction process, and the peripheral arterial pulsation could not be touched, indicating that a pulmonary arterial hypertension crisis (PHC) might occur. After cardiopulmonary resuscitation, vital signs were stabilized. Then, the patient was transferred to the Cardiac Intensive Care Unit (CICU) for further treatment. After admission to the CICU, dexmedetomidine was used for sedation. Treprostinil (Remodulin) 30 ng/(kg·min) and milrinone 0.5 μg/(kg·min) were continuously infused to reduce PAH. Swan–Ganz catheter was inserted via the right internal jugular vein to monitor PAP, but PAP was not significantly reduced by dual-targeted drug treatment. Therefore, the patient decided to receive Potts shunt surgery after consultation with multidisciplinary experts.

Physical examination: The child was under sedation treatment with consciousness and a Ramsay score of 5. He breathed spontaneously with a facemask oxygen supply of 2.0 L/min, respiratory rate (RR) 32 breaths/min, pulse oxygen saturation (SpO_2) 100%, heart rate (HR) 80 beats/min, PAP fluctuated between 130/81(98) mm Hg and 76/33(50) mm Hg, PAP and systemic circulation pressure ratio fluctuates between 0.69 and 1.34. Coarse breath sounds without rales in both lungs. Heart sounds were strong; the heart rhythm was regular, with III/VI grade murmur in the second intercostal space on the left edge of the sternum. The abdomen was soft, the liver and spleen were not palpable under the ribs, and there was no shifting dullness and no edema in all four limbs.

Laboratory tests: Hemoglobin 92 g/L, hematocrit 28.9%, total protein 56.7 g/L. There are no obvious abnormalities in liver and kidney function. Antithrombin was 81%, NT-proBNP was 8100 pg/mL.

Cardiac ultrasound: The right atrium and ventricle were enlarged significantly, and the interatrial and interventricular septum leaned to the left. Widened pulmonary artery, mild pulmonary artery valve regurgitation with regurgitation speed 4.15 m/s, pressure difference 68.7 mm Hg. Mild mitral valve regurgitation with regurgitation beam width 0.2 cm. The tip of the tricuspid valve was slightly thickened and curled, with mild to moderate tricuspid valve regurgitation with a regurgitation speed of 4.54 m/s and a pressure difference of 82.6 mm Hg.

Cardiac MRI: Significant right atrium and ventricle enlargement, reduced right ventricular systolic function, right ventricular ejection fraction 34.4%, right ventricular end-diastolic volume 107.88 mL/m^2.

Cardiac catheterization: Descending aortic pressure was 108/59 mm Hg, PAP was 88/42 mm Hg (PAP and systemic circulation pressure ratio = 0.81), descending aortic oxygen saturation was 99.6% (under oxygen), pulmonary circulation blood flow/systemic circulation blood flow (Qp/Qs) = 1, pulmonary vascular resistance index was 14.40 WU/m^2, negative pulmonary vasodilation test.

Preoperative diagnosis: PAH, heart failure, PHC.

56.2 Anesthetic Management

The patient did not take any preoperative medication. The left femoral artery and vein were already catheterized in the CICU. Swan–Ganz catheter was also placed in the CICU via internal jugular vein. Treprostinil 30 ng/(kg·min) was continuously infused into the operating room. After entering the operating room, an electrocardiogram (ECG), pulse oxygen saturation (SpO_2), invasive arterial pressure (ABP), and PAP monitoring were immediately established; routine monitoring revealed ABP of 103/46 mm Hg, HR of 104 beats/min, and SpO_2 of 90%. General anesthesia was induced by intravenous bolus injection of etomidate 3.0 mg, sufentanil 20 μg, and rocuronium 10 mg in a titrated manner through the femoral vein. After the eyelash reflex disappeared, an ID 4.5 mm cuffed endotracheal tube was intubated under direct laryngoscopy with an endotracheal tube depth of 14 cm. Pressure-controlled ventilation (PCV) mode was used with oxygen flow rate 2 L/min, fraction of inspired oxygen (FiO_2) 100%, peak of inspiratory pressure (PIP) 20 cm H_2O, RR 20 breaths/min, inspiratory to expiratory (I:E) time ratio 1:2, The partial pressure of carbon dioxide in artery blood ($PaCO_2$) was maintained at 30–35 mm Hg by adjustment of ventilator parameters based on blood gas analysis results.

After intubation, the right radial artery and left internal jugular vein were quickly catheterized for upper ABP monitoring and central venous pressure (CVP) monitoring. Upper and lower limb ABP, upper and lower limb SpO_2, CVP, and regional renal tissue oxygen saturation (rSO_2) monitoring were also included during surgery. General anesthesia was maintained by continuous infusion of propofol 2.0 mg/(kg·h), sufentanil 2.5 μg/(kg·h), and rocuronium 0.5 mg/(kg·h). In addition, 1–2% sevoflurane was intermittently inhaled. ABP suddenly dropped to 70/35 mm Hg after the induction of anesthesia. Norepinephrine 0.02 μg/(kg·min) infusion was initiated immediately. ABP recovered to 103/46 mm Hg, PAP 98/44 mm Hg, HR 81 beats/min, CVP 10 cm H_2O, upper and lower limb SpO_2 100%, renal area rSO_2 88%.

Extracorporeal circulation was established via the right internal jugular vein and artery cannulation. Potts shunt surgery was conducted under parallel circulation in the right lateral decubitus position. An 8# Gortex tube connected the left pulmonary artery and descending aorta. After the Potts shunt was established, dopamine 5.0 μg/(kg·min) and norepinephrine 0.05 μg/(kg·min) were intravenously infused. The dosage of treprostinil was reduced to 10 ng/(kg·min) to maintain stable blood pressure. Extracorporeal circulation was successfully weaned off. Transesophageal echocardiography indicated bidirectional shunting in the Potts conduit. The arterial blood gas analysis was performed on the upper and lower limbs (Table 56.1). Protamine neutralized heparin (1:1). The sternum and neck incisions were closed after satisfactory hemostasis.

Table 56.1 Comparison of preoperative and postoperative parameters

	Preoperative	Postoperative
Upper limb blood pressure (mm Hg)	103/46	133/62
Lower limb blood pressure (mm Hg)	104/45	128/60
PAP (mm Hg)	100/44	Removed during surgery
Upper limb oxygen saturation (%)	100	100
Lower limb oxygen saturation (%)	100	100
Upper limb oxygen partial pressure (mm Hg)	122	203
Lower limb oxygen pressure (mm Hg)	136	142
Renal oxygen (%)	88	88

56.3 Postoperative Outcome

The operation lasted 330 min in total, with an estimated blood loss of about 150 mL and urine output of 50 mL. About 150 mL of acetate Ringer's solution and 50 mL of autologous salvaged blood were infused. Postoperative vital signs: ABP 99/61 mm Hg, HR 83 beats/min, SpO_2 100%, CVP 8 cm H_2O, rectal temperature 37.2 °C. Under ABP, ECG, and SpO_2 monitoring, the patient was transferred to the CICU with controlled ventilation by a simple resuscitation bag. Treprostinil was discontinued 2 h after surgery. The ventilator was removed 19 h after surgery. The patient was discharged from the CICU on postoperative day 8 and discharged from the hospital on postoperative day 18. Postoperative SpO_2 in the upper and lower limbs was maintained at 82–100% and 69–100%, respectively, with an oxygen saturation difference of 2–14%.

56.4 Review of Knowledge Points

56.4.1 Potts Shunt Surgery

Willis J. Potts first reported the Potts shunt procedure in 1946, in which he conducted the first descending aorta-pulmonary artery anastomosis using sidewall occlusion technology without extracorporeal circulation support. The traditional Potts shunt procedure established a left-to-right shunt for children with pulmonary artery stenosis. It reduced pulmonary blood flow to ensure pulmonary artery blood supply and systemic oxygenation. In 2004, Blanc performed a reverse Potts shunt procedure for two children with PAH after transposition of the great arteries correction surgery, which was the first attempt to treat PAH with the Potts shunt.

Potts shunt procedure connects the left pulmonary artery and the descending aorta through an external conduit to establish an unrestricted shunt between the systemic and pulmonary circulation and reduce right ventricular afterload from the above systemic pressure to the systemic pressure level. Currently, the indications of the Potts shunt procedure for the treatment of PAH are limited to non-stable refractory PAH in children. However, it is considered a promising palliative surgery for right ventricular decompression, reducing the dependence on targeted drugs and extending the waiting time for lung transplantation.

After the Potts shunt procedure, left-to-right shunting may occur when PAP is lower than aortic pressure, which may increase left ventricular volume load, exacerbate left atrioventricular valve regurgitation, and aggravate pulmonary vascular diseases. In 2019, Rosenzweig and others first reported the unidirectional valved Potts shunt in clinical practice, which optimized right-to-left shunting and avoided potential complications of bidirectional shunting.

The cardiac function was extremely poor in children with end-stage PAH, and it is hard to suffer from surgical trauma. A new type of Potts shunt based on cardiac catheterization technology is under clinical translation, including radiofrequency perforation technology, needle puncture technology, and stent placement via an arterial catheter.

The current mortality rate of Potts shunt procedure is still as high as 15–20%. The largest pediatric cohort study on IPAH undergoing Potts shunt procedure included 24 children; 3 children died, one died during surgery, and two died from postoperative hypertensive crisis after termination of vasodilation treatment. A total of 21 survivors all received PAH treatment. Their cardiac function was improved with the New York Heart Association (NYHA) Classification of class I–II. During an average of 2 years (3 months-14 years) of follow-up, the functional status of all survivors was significantly improved.

56.5 Discussion

56.5.1 Preoperative Assessment and Treatment

Compared with the general population, children with PAH have an increased risk of cardiac arrest and sudden death during the perioperative period. The perioperative mortality rate is positively correlated with the degree of PAH. There were multiple risk factors associated with high mortality in this case, which included rapid progression of symptoms that cannot be recovered, the WHO classification of pulmonary hypertension: category III or IV, elevated brain natriuretic peptide levels, severe right ventricular enlargement or dysfunction, and pulmonary artery average pressure exceeding 3/4 of systemic blood pressure. So, the anesthetic risk of this patient was extremely high. Although this case was conducted under extracorporeal circulation support, the sudden increase in PAP and lung oxygenation was also affected by the lung lobe compression of surgical operations; the risk was still very high before and after extracorporeal circulation, especially during anesthetic induction.

Potts shunt procedure creates a passage between the systemic and pulmonary circulation. The direction of the shunt was determined by the difference of resistance on both sides. To prevent “backflow” of blood from the aorta to the pulmonary artery after Potts shunt surgery, some scholars believe that the preoperative ratio of PAP to systemic circulation pressure should equal or greater than 70%. Therefore, conducting a comprehensive preoperative assessment of PAP is very important. In this case, cardiac catheter examination indicated the ratio of PAP and systemic circulation pressure was 0.81. The highest

PAP reached 1.34 times the systemic circulation pressure, so this patient was suitable for the Potts shunt procedure.

For children with severe IPAH, it can cause a significant increase in PAP if the drugs that control pulmonary hypertension are suddenly stopped and lead to a pulmonary hypertension crisis. This patient received preoperative oral bosentan and Sildenafil targeted drug treatment and continued to be used to surgical day. Intravenous infusion of milrinone at 0.5 μg/(kg·min) and treprostinil at 30 ng/(kg·min) continued to establish extracorporeal circulation.

Children with PAH should be fully sedated before surgery to avoid PAP increase caused by sympathetic excitement and pulmonary hypertension crisis.

56.5.2 Intraoperative Anesthetic Management

1. Perioperative management of PAH is the key to the success of the Potts shunt procedure.

During the perioperative period, all of the factors that can increase PAP and trigger PHC should be avoided, which include hypoxia, acidosis, sympathetic excitement, and hypothermia.

The depth of anesthesia should be well controlled in this kind of patient. Adequate sedation and analgesia can prevent the hemodynamic changes and PAP increase caused by sympathetic excitement, while myocardial suppression, vasodilation, and hypotension should be avoided. Combining etomidate and anesthetic analgesics, such as fentanyl or sufentanil, and careful titration of medications can provide good hemodynamic stability with the least direct impact on HR, myocardial contractility, peripheral vascular resistance, or venous capacity. High dosages of anesthetic analgesics can effectively alleviate the increased pulmonary vascular resistance (PVR) caused by surgical stimulation.

Controlled ventilation can reduce the PVR and right ventricular afterload during operation. Specific measures include a high concentration of oxygen inhalation, hyperventilation to maintain $PaCO_2$ 30–35 mm Hg, and low mean airway pressure ventilation.

Pulmonary vasodilators, such as nitric oxide and iloprost, can be used in patients with severe PAH to control PAP. In this case, treprostinil continued to be used during the perioperative period.

2. Provide cardiac function support to maintain hemodynamic stability.

Severe PAH patients often suffer from subendocardial myocardial ischemia due to the imbalance of myocardial oxygen supply and demand. Low blood pressure can lead to coronary perfusion pressure reduction, which increases the risk of acute heart failure in the ischemic right ventricle. Left ventricular afterload decrease may cause the leftward shift of the interventricular septum, further restricting the function of the left ventricle and coronary perfusion. During surgery, it is necessary to maintain optimal sinus rhythm, avoid tachycardia, maximize ventricular filling to maintain cardiac output, and maintain normal to high blood pressure to ensure coronary perfusion pressure. Patients with severe PAH can usually tolerate mild hypertension well. In this case, a small dose of dopamine combined with norepinephrine was used to increase myocardial contractility, raise blood pressure, and improve myocardial perfusion pressure after the operation.

Potts shunt is usually bidirectional, which is difficult to avoid left-to-right shunt. Stable shunting may occur at the postoperative days 3–4. In this case, transesophageal echocardiography suggested bidirectional shunting in the Potts channel after the Potts shunt procedure, mainly from left to right shunting. The dose of treprostinil was reduced to avoid the increase in left-to-right shunting. The patient's hemodynamics became stabilized after the above treatments. Extracorporeal circulation support was successfully withdrawn.

3. Monitoring during anesthesia

Potts shunt is between the pulmonary artery (usually the left pulmonary artery) and the descending aorta. The systemic and pulmonary circulation resistance ratio determines the direction and amount of shunting. When PAP is higher than the aortic artery pressure, the pulmonary blood will flow to the aorta through Potts conduit and generate right to left shunting, serving as a rapid pressure relief function. Since the shunt is established at the level of the descending aorta, the blood perfusion above the shunt opening (the upper body, including brain and coronary artery perfusion) is oxygenated blood. In contrast, the blood perfusion below the shunt opening (abdominal organ and lower limb) is mixed oxygenated blood. When PAP is lower than the aortic pressure, left-to-right shunting will occur, and then the blood oxygen contents of the upper and lower limbs will be the same. Based on the physiology of Potts shunt, the status of Potts shunt can be roughly assessed by comparison of upper and lower limb SpO_2. Literature reports that the optimal difference between upper and lower limb SpO_2 is 10–15% for patients with Potts shunt.

In this case, ABP and SpO_2 were simultaneously monitored in the upper and lower limbs to assess Potts's shunt status. Postoperative blood gas analysis from upper and lower limb artery blood showed that lower limb arterial partial pressure of oxygen (PaO_2) was significantly lower than upper limb, suggesting that the deoxygenated pulmonary artery blood flowed to the descending aorta through the Potts conduit. However, SpO_2 in the upper and lower limbs was 100%; no difference in SpO_2 was observed, which may relate to pure oxygen inhalation during surgery.

Renal or intestinal rSO_2 monitoring can assess the balance of oxygen supply and demand in important abdominal organs after the Potts shunt procedure. In addition, literature reports that the difference in cerebral and renal rSO_2 after the Potts procedure can also reflect the status of the Potts shunt. In this case, renal rSO_2 was within the normal range during the perioperative period, indicating no renal ischemia or hypoxia occurred. The preoperative and postoperative renal rSO_2 was similar, which may relate to bidirectional Potts shunt, but mainly from left to right shunting.

Intraoperative transesophageal echocardiography can quickly assess the status of Potts shunt, measure PAP, and evaluate heart function.

56.6 Shortcomings and Limitations

This is the first case of using Potts shunt to treat severe PAP in children in our hospital. Therefore, our team lacks experience in surgical techniques or anesthetic management, such as evaluating Potts shunt status and rationally applying pulmonary vasodilators and vasoactive drugs.

The placement of pulmonary artery catheters in children with severe PAP is still under debate. Placement of pulmonary artery can monitor PAP in real time, timely detect and deal with PHC, but it can increase the risk of pulmonary hypertension during the placement process. In this case, a pulmonary artery catheter was placed through the right internal jugular vein before surgery, but it was removed during surgery since extracorporeal circulation was established via the right internal jugular vein and artery, which caused inconvenience to postoperative PAP monitoring. PAP can be well controlled during Potts shunt procedure under extracorporeal circulation and make the procedure safer. However, extracorporeal circulation often requires blood preloading, and nonphysiological circulation can cause lung injury. Therefore, we hope the Potts shunt procedure can be conducted without extracorporeal circulation support with the accumulation of surgical and anesthetic management experience.

56.7 Conclusion

The purpose of the Potts shunt procedure is to reduce right ventricular afterload from above systemic circulation pressure to systemic circulation pressure level without affecting the oxygen supply of the central nervous system and relieve the life-threatening right heart failure. The key to anesthetic management for the Potts shunt procedure is the management of PAP based on the pathophysiology of PAP and the principle of the Potts shunt procedure (Lihong Jin).

57 Anesthetic Management of Heart Transplantation in a Child with Fulminant Myocarditis

Liping Sun

Abstract

A 10-year-old girl was admitted to the hospital due to fulminant myocarditis. Two days after admission, her condition deteriorated, with recurrent ventricular fibrillation and cardiac arrest. Emergent extracorporeal membrane oxygenation (ECMO) was initiated for supportive treatment. There was no spontaneous return of pulse beat during ECMO support, and a heart transplant was planned. On the seventh day of ECMO support, the patient received a matched donor heart and underwent emergency heart transplant surgery. The operation succeeded, and the patient was kept intubated to the cardiothoracic surgery intensive care unit.

Fulminant myocarditis is relatively rare, with a rapid onset, fast progression, and high mortality rate. It often requires extracorporeal membrane oxygenation (ECMO) support or even heart transplantation. This chapter reports anesthetic management of a child with fulminant myocarditis undergoing heart transplantation. Postoperative management of hemodynamics and prevention of acute right heart failure in denervated transplanted hearts are the keys to anesthetic management in heart transplantation.

57.1 Case Presentation

A 10-year and 9-month-old girl with 37.7 kg in weight and 148 cm in height. She was born full-term and had well past health. The patient presented with symptoms of chest tightness, shortness of breath, and vomiting together with fever; an electrocardiogram revealed an ST elevation in the chest leads V4 to V6 with significantly elevated NT-proBNP and troponin I levels. Based on these findings, she was admitted to the hospital with a diagnosis of fulminant myocarditis. On the second day of admission, her condition deteriorated and manifested with progressively increased myocardial enzyme spectrum indicators, recurrent ventricular fibrillation, and cardiac arrest. She was then intubated and mechanically ventilated; veno-arterial ECMO (VA-ECMO) was also initiated to support her condition. However, the patient developed signs of acute kidney injury as evidenced by oliguria, rising blood lactate, and potassium levels within 12 h of ECMO; she was then put on continuous renal replacement therapy (CRRT) to support the renal function. However, despite all organ-supporting measures being used, there was no spontaneous heartbeat return.

L. Sun (✉)
The National Children's Medical Center (Shanghai), Department of Anesthesiology of Shanghai Children's Medical Center, Shanghai Jiao Tong University School of Medicine, Shanghai, China
e-mail: sunliping@scmc.com.cn

J. Zheng et al. (eds.), *Selected Pediatric Cardiovascular Surgery Anesthesia Cases*,
https://doi.org/10.1007/978-981-96-5614-1_57

Laboratory test: Several abnormal and meaningful negative indicators were observed; C-reactive protein was 7 mg/L, white blood cell count elevated at 18.86 × 10^9/L, platelet count decreased to 112 × 10^9/L, hemoglobin slightly low at 101 g/L, neutrophil count elevated at 14.98 × 10^9/L, and procalcitonin was 0.73 ng/mL. Additionally, cTNI quantitative was >50 μg/L, uric acid was 33.9 μmol/L, CREA was 69 μmol/L, TP was 86.8 g/l, TBIL was 34.6 μmol/L, AST was significantly elevated at 1713 U/L, GGT was 36 U/L, ALB was 44.6 g/L, ALT was also elevated at 666 U/L. Electrolyte levels revealed Na^+ of 148.6 mmol/L, K^+ of 4.36 mmol/L, P^{3+} of 0.86 mmol/L, and Mg^{2+} of 0.55 mmol/L. Finally, NT-proBNP was 695 pg/mL. These results indicate significant abnormalities in various biochemical markers, potentially indicating a pathological condition.

Electrocardiogram (ECG): ST elevation in lateral chest leads.

Chest CT: Possible myocardial bridge in the left anterior descending branch.

Cardiac MRI: There was enlargement of both the left and right ventricles. While the left ventricle demonstrated acceptable contractile function, the right ventricle showed impaired contraction and diastolic function.

Preoperative diagnosis: Fulminant myocarditis, heart failure, cardiogenic shock, and acute renal failure following ECMO support. After 7 days of ECMO support, a matched donor heart was found, and the child was scheduled for an emergency heart transplant.

57.2 Anesthetic Management

The child was transferred to the operating theatre with VA-ECMO support, with arterial blood pressure (ABP) at 73/68 mm Hg and no intrinsic heart rhythm. She was ventilated with the same mode and settings as in Pediatric Intensive Care Unit (PICU): PCV-VG mode, total gas flow rate of 1 L/min, inspired oxygen fraction of 35%, tidal volume (VT) of 125 mL, respiratory rate (RR) of 15 times/min, peak airway pressure of 17 mm Hg, inspiratory to expiratory ratio (I:E) of 1:2, and positive end-expiratory pressure (PEEP) of 10 cm H_2O. PICU inserted the arterial line and central venous line. A 5 Fr pulmonary artery catheter (Swan Ganz Catheter) was inserted into the right internal jugular vein inside the operating suite. For anesthetic induction, intravenous injection of etomidate 4.0 mg and sufentanil 40 μg was given. Maintenance of anesthesia was achieved through continuous infusion of sufentanil 2.0 μg/(kg·h), propofol 4.0 mg/(kg·h), and rocuronium 0.5 mg/(kg·h). Following induction, the child received methylprednisolone 500 mg and basiliximab 20 mg, along with esomeprazole 40 mg and ulinastatin 100,000 U.

The team and the patient with a mini sternotomy were ready 30 min before the arrival of the donor's heart. Intraoperatively, the diseased heart exhibited no contraction or beating. Following systemic heparinization, cannulation of the ascending aorta and superior and inferior vena cava was performed, ECMO was stopped, and cardiopulmonary bypass (CPB) was initiated. The ascending aorta was clamped, and the diseased heart was removed. The donor's heart was trimmed and implanted into the recipient's pericardial cavity. Subsequently, the left atrium, right atrium, aorta, and pulmonary artery were anastomosed in sequence using the bicaval technique, successfully completing the orthotopic heart transplant. Postoperatively, the heart was de-aired, and methylprednisolone was administered again before the aortic cross-clamp was released. Once the aortic clamp was released, the ECG revealed ventricular fibrillation, which was reverted to sinus rhythm after three defibrillation attempts with 20 J. The ST segment showed transient elevation before it returned to normal.

Dopamine (5.0 μg/kg·min), dobutamine (5.0 μg/kg·min), and epinephrine (0.02 μg/kg·min) were infused intravenously to maintain hemodynamics stability. Postoperative transesophageal echocardiography revealed no abnormalities in cardiac structure with normal cardiac contraction function. The CPB flow rate was then gradually reduced and finally stopped. After CPB, the heart rate (HR) was stabilized at 94 beats/min, with ABP of 73/68 mm Hg, central venous pressure (CVP) of 14 cm H_2O, and mean

Table 57.1 Intraoperative blood gas test results

Time point	Hb (g/dL)	HCT (%)	pH	PaO_2 (mm Hg)	$PaCO_2$ (mm Hg)	BE (mmol/L)	Na^+ (mmol/L)	K^+ (mmol/L)	Cl^- (mmol/L)	Ca^{2+} (mmol/L)	Lac (mmol/L)
Admission	8.1	29	7.38	434	28	−7.0	136	2.8	102	1.2	1.8
Stop extracorporeal circulation	10.1	26	7.46	450	32	−1.6	135	3.5	103	1.1	3.7
Exit room	10.9	23	7.47	405	31	−0.5	134	3.5	103	1.13	2.7

pulmonary artery pressure of 18 mm Hg. Modified ultrafiltration (MUF) was performed, followed by an intravenous protamine infusion at a 1.2:1 ratio to reverse the heparin effect. Additionally, 1 U of platelets and 50 mL of cell saver blood were transfused. Blood gas analysis was repeated (Table 57.1). After ensuring hemostasis, a temporary pacing lead was implanted, mediastinal and right chest drainage tubes were inserted, and the chest wall was closed in layers. The patient was then transferred to the Cardiac Intensive Care Unit (CICU) for close monitoring with mechanical ventilation assistance.

57.3 Postoperative Outcome

The surgical time was 395 min, including 300 minof bypass time, 177 min of aortic cross-clamping time, an estimated blood loss of approximately 20 milliliters, and a urine output of 100 milliliters. During the operation, the patient received 1 U of platelets and 50 milliliters of cell salvage blood transfusion. At the end of the surgery, the patient's ABP was 108/68 mm Hg, HR was 82 beats/minute, oxygen saturation (SpO_2) was 100%, CVP was 8 cm H_2O, and rectal temperature was 36.0 degrees Celsius. The patient was extubated on the postoperative 2nd day, discharged from ICU on the 14th day postoperatively, and discharged from the hospital on the 45th day. Pathological examination of the diseased heart specimen revealed diffuse edema, rupture, degeneration, and necrosis of myocardial fibers, along with hyperplasia of adipose tissue in the apex, left ventricle, and epicardium of the right heart, along with inflammatory cell infiltration.

57.4 Review of Knowledge Points

57.4.1 Fulminant Myocarditis

Fulminant myocarditis, though relatively uncommon, is an acute cardiac condition that can lead to hemodynamic instability, arrhythmias, and rapid progression to heart failure. Despite medical therapy, patients often experience persistent lactic acidosis and organ hypoperfusion, often necessitating mechanical cardiac support or heart transplantation, with a significant mortality rate. Literature showed that approximately 20% of children with fulminant myocarditis in the United States undergo ECMO treatment. However, about 40% of these children fail to wean off ECMO successfully and may require heart transplantation. ECMO does not offer a curative solution for acute fulminant myocarditis; it rather supports cardiopulmonary functions, providing time for heart function recovery or serving as a bridging measure for transplantation. Timely ECMO support can elevate the survival rate of children with acute fulminant myocarditis to about 80%, compared to only about 50% for those who do not receive ECMO support. Therefore, it is imperative to offer ECMO support to these children promptly. For children who do not show improvement in cardiac function with ECMO support, consideration should be given to the use of a left ventricular assist device (LVAD) or emergency heart transplantation.

57.4.2 Surgical Methods

There exist three surgical techniques for heart transplantation: the biatrial, bicaval, and total transplantation techniques. Each of these procedures necessitates a median sternotomy, hypothermic cardiopulmonary bypass, bicaval cannulation, and aortic cross-clamping. The crux of the operation lies in ensuring precise anastomosis alignment, preventing leakage at the anastomotic sites, and minimizing the operation duration. Notably, the surgical techniques employed during heart transplantation for children with congenital heart disease pose greater challenges. These children often require extensive reconstruction of the aorta, pulmonary artery, and vena cava to establish an unobstructed anatomical connection with the donor's heart.

57.5 Discussion

Pediatric heart transplantation primarily aims to treat end-stage cardiomyopathy, complex congenital heart disease manifesting severe heart failure/hypoxia refractory to standard measures, and irreversible heart disease unresponsive to palliative or standard curative management. Recent advancements in surgical techniques, organ harvesting and preservation strategies, immunosuppressive medications, and intricate monitoring strategies have gradually increased posttransplantation survival rates. Notably, our country's in-hospital survival rate for pediatric heart transplantation was 94.6% between 2015 and 2016, highlighting the positive impact of these advancements.

57.5.1 Preoperative Evaluation and Preparation

Anesthesiologists must possess a thorough knowledge of the pathophysiology of the child's underlying disease and the physiological nuances of the transplanted heart, conducting a thorough preoperative evaluation for pediatric heart transplantation patients. Right heart failure often leads to volume overload, hepatic congestion, portal hypertension, and impaired coagulation function in children. Prolonged low cardiac output can result in the pre-renal type of acute kidney injury. Chronic left heart leads to elevation of left ventricular end-diastolic pressure, causing pulmonary congestion and pulmonary hypertension. Children undergoing heart transplantation may already be receiving various treatments for heart failure, including pharmacological interventions and circulatory support, including ECMO.

During the preoperative visit, it is crucial to have a comprehensive understanding of the child's condition, cardiac function, laboratory tests, and other cardiac examination results. Patients on assisted ventilation, mechanical ventricular assistance, or continuous intravenous infusion of inotropes should continue receiving these treatments. Before induction, all necessary drugs and equipment should be prepared, including vasopressors, inotropes, vasodilators, antiarrhythmic agents, immunosuppressants, diuretics, hemostatic agents, anticoagulants, and specifically, milrinone, treprostinil, and inhaled nitric oxide for those with pulmonary hypertension. We should also ensure adequate blood products. Defibrillators and pacemakers should also be readily available to use.

57.5.2 Anesthetic Induction

Before anesthetic induction, obtaining a large bore intravenous vascular access is crucial. The hemodynamic goal is to maintain myocardial contractility and avoid significant fluctuation in preload and afterload. Anesthetic induction agents should be administered in small, titrated doses, with options including midazolam, ketamine, etomidate, fentanyl, or sufentanil. For patients with preoperative hemodynamic instability or those reliant on endogenous sympathetic tone, smaller dosages of ketamine may be employed for induction. Whenever possible, anesthesia induction should be performed under continuous invasive arterial pressure monitoring, followed by the insertion of central venous and pulmonary artery catheters. We should ensure strict asepsis during all invasive procedures.

57.5.3 Anesthetic Management

Intraoperative monitoring encompasses ventilation parameters monitoring, including tidal volume, ventilation frequency, airway pressure, end-tidal carbon dioxide ($ETCO_2$), SpO_2, and blood gas analysis. Cardiovascular monitoring involves ECG, ABP, CVP, etc. For patients with underlying pulmonary hypertension, the placement of a pulmonary artery catheter may be necessary. TEE has become the gold standard for monitoring pediatric cardiac surgery, enabling real-time ventricular contractility assessment, guiding vasoactive drug administration, and volume replacement. Additionally, cerebral oximetry monitoring is vital in preventing secondary brain injury due to hypoxia, ischemia, embolism, and other electrophysiological disturbances. Intraoperative coagulation function monitoring also guides the use of blood products. Other monitoring practices include urine output monitoring and body temperature monitoring. Urine output monitoring before, during, and after extracorporeal circulation is crucial for assessing kidney function, maintaining input–output balance, and effective blood volume. Hypothermia is key to providing cerebral and myocardial protection during extracorporeal circulation. Precise monitoring of continuous changes in body temperature at various sites ensures accurate implementation of cooling and rewarming.

Maintaining posttransplantation cardiovascular function should be tailored to the physiological characteristics of the transplanted heart, including:

1. The transplanted heart is denervated, resulting in a diminished response to reduced blood volume and pressure. Additionally, there is increased sensitivity to catecholamines. The transplanted heart does not exhibit a baroreceptor reflex. Instead, the cardiac output is preload-dependent based on the Frank–Starling mechanism. The cardiac output remains relatively normal when HR ranges from 90 to 120 beats/min.
2. Direct-acting drugs, such as epinephrine and isoprenaline, exert their intended effects normally. However, medications that indirectly act on the sympathetic and parasympathetic nervous systems, like ephedrine and atropine, are rendered ineffective.
3. The transplanted heart is susceptible to atrial, nodal, and ventricular arrhythmias. The electrocardiogram can show two distinct P waves and independent heart rhythms. Accurate identification of these arrhythmias can be challenging, necessitating meticulous analysis to prevent misdiagnosis. Consequently, the routine placement of a pacing lead in the transplanted heart is recommended.
4. The transplanted heart exhibits increased sensitivity to potassium ions (K^+). Thus, it is crucial to maintain serum potassium levels at a slightly lower concentration, specifically ≤3.5 mmol, to ensure optimal heart function.

Acute right heart failure is the most prevalent early complication following heart transplantation. The treatment approach encompasses several key points: excluding mechanical obstructions caused by surgical factors (e.g., pulmonary artery anastomosis narrowing); maintaining appropriate systemic vascular resistance and coronary perfusion pressure; preserving positive inotropy, which can be achieved using dobutamine, milrinone, epinephrine, and other agents; maintaining a higher concentration of inhaled oxygen with mild hypocapnia ($PaCO_2$ 32–35 mm Hg) and avoiding excessive PEEP; administering inhaled NO or intravenous treprostinil to children with pulmonary hypertension; avoiding light plane of anesthesia; and considering early utilization of right heart assist devices, such as ECMO, for refractory cases of right heart failure.

In this case, the child was diagnosed with fulminant myocarditis, experiencing rapid disease deterioration. Despite ECMO support treatment, the heart failed to recover, necessitating heart transplantation. Under continuous invasive arterial pressure monitoring and ECMO assistance, the child's anesthesia induction was conducted using drugs with minimal myocardial suppression and reduction in systemic vascular resistance, specifically etomidate and sufentanil. Administration of the anesthetic agents in a cautious, titrated approach maintained the hemodynamic stability perioperatively.

Following the heart transplant, our team conducted a comprehensive evaluation of the donor heart's contractile function, right ventricular afterload, sinus node and atrioventricular function, and volume status relying on a minimally invasive system, such as Most Care® monitoring and TEE examination. We selected appropriate vasoactive drugs and performed goal-directed fluid management according to the physiological characteristics of the transplanted heart. This approach helped us maintain heart rate, blood pressure, and preload within the ideal range.

Additionally, we adjusted the ventilation setting to control pulmonary vascular resistance, preserving right ventricular function and preventing acute right heart failure. Throughout the procedure, we actively monitored blood gas and electrolyte levels, maintaining normal physiology and keeping serum potassium levels low at normal levels.

Through our meticulous anesthetic management and surgical techniques, we successfully guided the child through the most critical surgical phase.

57.6 Shortcomings and Limitations

In this case, the child did not undergo continuous monitoring of brain and kidney perfusion using NIRS, as this would have provided valuable insights into their condition. The absence of such continuous assessments limits our understanding of the child's brain and kidney perfusion status.

57.7 Conclusion

Heart transplantation serves as an effective treatment option for pediatric end-stage cardiomyopathy, albeit posing greater challenges compared to its adult counterpart. Anesthetic management during heart transplantation necessitates comprehensive monitoring and evaluation, meticulous communication with surgeons, maintaining circulatory stability to the utmost extent possible, and preventing any potential complications (Liping Sun).

Anesthetic Management of Organ Donation (Donor) from a Postoperative Congenital Heart Disease Child

58

Ruidong Zhang

Abstract

A 9-month-old female infant was diagnosed with congenital heart disease via fetal echocardiography. After the second stage of open-heart surgery, she developed refractory ventricular fibrillation. After proactive drug treatment and extracorporeal membrane oxygenation (ECMO) support, thrombocytopenia and multiple organ failure still occurred. Considering the poor prognosis of the child, her family members ultimately decided to give up treatment and donate the child's organs. During the organ retrieval process, anesthesiologists participated in the evaluation, transportation, and clinical management of the child's organ function. The anesthesiologists also need to follow the standard procedures and technical norms to ensure the quality of the retrieved organs. They also need to be aware of the human organ retrieval and allocation system and take responsibility for promoting the healthy and sustainable development of human organ donation and transplantation.

R. Zhang (✉)
The National Children's Medical Center (Shanghai), Department of Anesthesiology of Shanghai Children's Medical Center, Shanghai Jiao Tong University School of Medicine, Shanghai, China
e-mail: zhangruidong@scmc.com.cn

Organ donation is usually classified into organ donation after brain death and organ donation after cardiac death. Studies have shown that the preoperative assessment and the selection of anesthetics for the donor can significantly impact the number of transplantable organs and the function of the organs after transplantation. This chapter reports the perioperative anesthetic management of a 9-month-old child with congenital heart disease as a donor undergoing organ donation surgery.

58.1 Case Presentation

A 9-month-old female patient with 5.6 kg in weight and 65 cm in height was diagnosed with fetal heart disease during her mother's pregnancy. Echocardiography indicated transitional atrioventricular septal defect, functional single atrium, moderate regurgitation of the common atrioventricular valve, small left ventricular outflow tract and aortic valve annulus, underdeveloped left ventricle and left atrium, aortic stenosis, underdeveloped descending aorta, persistent left superior vena cava, and pulmonary hypertension. The thoracic CT scan indicated atrioventricular septal defect, functional single atrium, aortic stenosis, proximal stenosis of the left superior vena cava, aberrant right subclavian artery, and localized pulmonary emphysema in both lungs. The patient underwent atrioventricular septal defect repair

J. Zheng et al. (eds.), *Selected Pediatric Cardiovascular Surgery Anesthesia Cases*,
https://doi.org/10.1007/978-981-96-5614-1_58

(single patch method), aortic stenosis correction (end-to-side anastomosis), and arterial duct ligation 2 months after birth. Around 7 months after discharge, she was readmitted for treatment due to residual ventricular shunting, mitral stenosis, moderate regurgitation of the mitral and tricuspid valves, and descending aorta combined with severe pulmonary hypertension. After undergoing mitral stenosis enlargement and atrial septal reconstruction, the patient developed refractory ventricular fibrillation and was treated with extracorporeal membrane oxygenation (ECMO), maintained with various vasoactive drugs, but she continued to deteriorate. She developed thrombocytopenia and multiple organ failure. Considering the poor prognosis, the team of family members decided to give up all medical treatment and proposed organ donation.

58.2 Anesthetic Management

The patient was transferred to the operating room with ECMO support. Anesthesia was induced with intravenous bolus doses of 0.1 mg/kg midazolam, 1.0 μg/kg sufentanil, and 0.6 mg/kg rocuronium, and anesthesia was maintained with an intravenous infusion of sufentanil 2.0 μg/(kg·h). After the surgical team was ready, the patient's ECMO support was stopped, and the ventilator was turned off. The patient had no spontaneous breathing, and her heart rate gradually slowed. Ten minutes later, the ECG showed a straight line. After the patient showed no pupillary light reflex and the arterial pulse disappeared, clinical death was declared, and organ donation surgery was conducted.

58.3 Review of Knowledge Points

58.3.1 Laws and Regulations Related to Human Organ Transplantation

In 2007, China promulgated its first organ transplant law, the "Regulations on Human Organ Transplantation," marking the entry of China's organ donation and transplantation work into a new era of the legal system. The only legal source of organs in China is voluntary donation by citizens. The number of organ donations in China has reached the second highest globally, but the gap between supply and demand is still severe. In 2018, to further implement the "Regulations on Human Organ Transplantation," further improve the policy of human organ allocation and sharing, and ensure the scientific and fair allocation of human organs, the National Health Commission formulated the core policies for heart and lung allocation and sharing, and issued the "Basic Principles and Core Policies for Human Organ Allocation and Sharing in China." In 2019, the National Health Commission issued the "Regulations on the Acquisition and Allocation of Donated Human Organs." The clinical data and legality documents of potential donors, donors, and their donated organs are uploaded to the China Human Organ Allocation and Sharing Computer System (website: www.cot.org.cn). The organ allocation system is used to allocate donated organs automatically. The China Human Organ Allocation and Sharing Computer System consists of three subsystems: the "Potential Human Organ Donor Identification System," the "Human Organ Donor Registration and Organ Matching System," and the "Human Organ Transplant Waitlist Appointment System." They are used to discover, identify and refer potential organ donors, register information of human organ donors, and register information of human organ transplant waitlist. The first system aims to ensure the traceability of organs, strengthen supervision, and improve donation efficiency; when new supplier information appears, the latter two systems will automatically match suitable organ recipients according to the national allocation policy, generating an orderly "matching list."

58.3.2 Anesthesia for Brain-Dead Donors

The clinical manifestations of brain-dead children include hemodynamic disorders and insufficient perfusion of tissues and organs throughout the body. In the early stages of brain death, hypertension may occur due to the release of catecholamine, but severe hypertension is not common. This may be followed by persistent hypotension, the causes of which include central sympathetic dysfunction, decreased cardiac output, severe peripheral vasodilation, and volume deficiency caused by diabetes insipidus. When hypotension occurs, fluid resuscitation should be conducted first, usually choosing normal saline or balanced salt solution. Hydroxyethyl starch is associated with renal dysfunction after transplantation, so it is not recommended for routine use. Vasoactive drugs are required if hypotension cannot be corrected by fluid resuscitation. Dopamine is usually the first choice of vasoactive drugs, but its use is limited in cases of tachycardia. Vasopressin can alleviate vasodilation, reduce the use of catecholamine, and treat diabetes insipidus, which has been commonly used recently and is becoming the first-line medication for treating hemodynamic instability in donors. Norepinephrine is also commonly used, but high dosage may cause myocardial damage and reduce the survival rate of organs after transplantation. In addition, the strategies of fluid management and vasoactive drug use have different emphases in different organ donors, which need to be carefully balanced and evaluated. For example, large amounts of fluid replacement benefit transplanted livers and kidneys. Still, they can have harmful effects on transplanted lungs because the permeability of pulmonary capillaries in brain-dead children is abnormally increased. Excessive fluid enters into the pulmonary interstitium and alveoli, which further damages the lung's ventilation function, and exacerbates pulmonary edema in the transplanted lung. Therefore, it is better to avoid excessive fluid replacement and use high-dose vasoactive drugs to reduce adverse events after lung transplantation. Colloid fluid is recommended for lung donation since it can alleviate pulmonary edema and improve gas exchange. The secretion function of the hypothalamic–pituitary–adrenal axis in brain-dead children is usually also disturbed, manifesting as deficiencies in cortisol, thyroid hormone, thyroid-stimulating hormone, antidiuretic hormone, and insulin, which can easily cause the occurrence of diabetes insipidus and other internal environment disorders. Diabetes insipidus can result in electrolyte disorders (such as hypernatremia, hypocalcemia, and hypomagnesemia), which can then induce arrhythmias. Hypernatremia is associated with adverse events after liver transplantation (>155 mmol/L) and heart transplantation (>170 mmol/L). Persistent hypernatremia can be corrected by infusing hypotonic fluid while treating diabetes insipidus with vasopressin; the blood sodium level should be maintained below 155 mmol/L. Brain-dead children often have hyperglycemia due to decreased insulin secretion and insulin resistance. The use of corticosteroids will further exacerbate hyperglycemia. Poor blood sugar control is an important factor affecting renal function after transplantation. When the blood sugar level is too high, it is recommended to use insulin to control blood sugar at 6.6–8.3 mmol/L. There is currently no consensus on the best respiratory management strategy for brain-dead organ donors. The ventilator is usually pre-set with a tidal volume of 6–8 mL/kg, PEEP 5 cm H_2O, the ventilator parameters and fraction of inspired oxygen (FiO_2) should be adjusted according to the results of blood gas analysis to maintain PaO_2 > 100 mm Hg, $PaCO_2$ 35–45 mm Hg and SpO_2 > 95%. The lung has always been considered a fragile organ. The respiratory management of potential lung donors is very important. It should avoid the occurrence of pulmonary edema and lung injury in donors as much as possible, as these conditions can reduce the number of lung donors that meet the standards. There are various reasons for pulmonary edema after brain death, which include the increase of venous blood volume and lung blood volume caused by the increased systemic vascular resistance, excessive infusion of crystalloid during fluid resuscitation, lung endothelial cell injury, and capillary rupture caused by early catecholamine release. All of them can cause and exacerbate pulmonary edema. Protective respiratory management strategies for lung donation include small tidal volume VT 6–8 mL/kg, FiO_2 < 40%, PEEP 8–10 cm H_2O, and lung recruitment maneuvers to prevent pulmonary oxygen toxicity and maintain the alveoli in an expanded state. Once the chest is opened, the ventilator parameters should be adjusted to prevent over-expansion of the alveoli. Continuous manual ventilation is required when the lung is obtained.

As the hypothalamic function of brain-dead children decreases, their temperature regulation function gradually loses. Reduced metabolic rate, decreased muscle activity, and peripheral vasodilation can all lead to persistent hypothermia. Studies have shown that maintaining a mild hypothermia of 34–35 °C in donors compared to maintaining normal body temperature (36.5–37.5 °C) can improve organ function and survival rate after kidney transplantation. When the body temperature is too high, physical cooling treatment is needed to try to keep the donor's body temperature at 34–35 °C.

Brain-dead donors still have spinal reflexes below the level of the brainstem. Therefore, spinal reflex-mediated body movement is still possible during surgery, so muscle relaxants must be used. Brain-dead children may still have pain responses under the stimulation of surgical operations, causing high blood pressure and a large release of catecholamine. To prevent potential damage to the donated organs, opioid drugs need to be used. Inhalational anesthetics (such as sevoflurane, isoflurane, and desflurane) prevent ischemia-reperfusion injury. Ischemia-reperfusion injury will further affect the function of the organ after transplantation, so inhalation anesthetics are usually used during organ transplantation surgery.

58.4 Discussion

58.4.1 Preoperative Transfer and Preparation

Before anesthesia, the donor's medical history, laboratory test results, and medications need to be fully evaluated. The donor's gas exchange situation can be understood through blood gas analysis, imaging examinations, and bronchoscopy. The donor's liver and kidney function can be understood through laboratory tests and urine output. If the donor has already used mechanical ventilation and vasoactive drugs, the anesthesiologist must continuously monitor the donor's heart rate, blood pressure, and SpO_2 during transportation. Therefore, the main task of the anesthesiologist before organ donation surgery is to accept the donor transfer from the intensive care unit to the operating room and maintain their hemodynamic stability and other physiological parameters up to standard.

58.4.2 Anesthesia for Donors After Cardiac Death

Opioids and benzodiazepines are given as appropriate before the child is disconnected from the ventilator. Cardiac arrest is carried out under the supervision of the organ procurement team, and organ procurement can be carried out only after the child has no spontaneous return of heartbeat and is declared dead after 5 min of observation. After death is declared, interventions to restore cerebral blood flow are strictly avoided. The order of organ procurement is lungs, liver, pancreas, and kidneys. When procuring the lungs, lung re-expansion should be carried out after aortic clamping, restart the ventilator, and set the tidal volume to 6–8 mL/kg, PEEP 8–10 cm H_2O. Fluid balance should be avoided when procuring kidneys.

The goal of anesthetic management in organ donation surgery is to maintain the oxygen supply and perfusion of the organs. To donate as many organs as possible and preserve organ function to the maximum extent, the United States Organ Procurement Organization jointly formulated the organ maintenance goals of donors (Table 58.1). Depending on the number and type of donated organs, an appropriate anesthetic management plan is formulated in communication with the surgical team before surgery.

Table 58.1 The organ maintenance goals of donors formulated by the United States Organ Procurement Organization

Clinical indicators	Target values
Mean arterial pressure	>60 mm Hg
Central venous pressure	5–13 cm H_2O
Left ventricular ejection fraction	>45%
Vasopressor drugs	Try to use only one type and low-dose drugs, such as dopamine ≤10 μg/(kg·min)
Oxygenation index (measurement when PEEP = 5 cm H_2O)	>300 mm Hg
Arterial blood gas analysis	pH 7.3–7.45
Blood sodium	<155 mmol/L
Blood glucose	<8.3 mmol/L
Urine output (accumulated over 4 h)	>1 mL/(kg·h)

58.5 Conclusion

Organ donation is a special medical act centered on medicine involving society, humanities, ethics, and law. Anesthesiologists evaluate the child's organ function, transportation, and clinical management during organ acquisition. When talking to family members before surgery, we should not only consider the child's condition, but we also need to fully understand and care for the feelings of the child's family members. Organ acquisition can only begin after the heart of the brain-dead donor stops beating. Only with professional level and legal and compliant work processes paying attention to humanistic care can truly protect the interests of the donor and the family and further promote the development of transplantation (Ruidong Zhang).

Anesthetic Management of Left Atrial Appendectomy in a Child with Atrial Tachycardia

59

Yingying Ji

Abstract

A 7-year-old boy with atrial tachycardia was scheduled to undergo a video-assisted thoracoscopic left atrial appendectomy. After anesthesia induction and before the start of the operation, the child had repeated atrial tachycardia with hypotension. Synchronized electrical cardioversion was not effective. The heartbeat was converted to sinus rhythm after intravenous administration of amiodarone and propafenone. During the video-assisted thoracoscopic surgery, a bronchial blocker was used to block the left lung.

Atrial tachycardia in children can occur at any age, and the clinical symptoms may not be typical. Radiofrequency ablation should be considered in children if atrial tachycardia is persistent, a poor response to medical therapy, and is accompanied by possible cardiac dysfunction. If the atrial ectopic focus recurs after radiofrequency ablation and is located in the atrial appendage, a video-assisted thoracoscopic atrial appendectomy may be performed.

Y. Ji (✉)
The National Children's Medical Center (Shanghai), Department of Anesthesiology of Shanghai Children's Medical Center, Shanghai Jiao Tong University School of Medicine, Shanghai, China
e-mail: jiyingying@scmc.com.cn

59.1 Case Presentation

A 7-year-old and 11-month-old boy with 27.5 kg in weight was born full term with good past health. One month ago, the child had a symptom of rapid heart rate. An electrocardiogram (ECG) showed atrial tachycardia. Holter monitoring showed the fastest heart rate (HR) was 188 beats/min and atrial tachycardia with varying degrees of atrioventricular conduction block. Digoxin was given to control the heart rate by adenosine triphosphate (ATP) and propafenone after cardioversion failure. The boy was then scheduled to undergo radiofrequency ablation. During the operation, the earliest stimulation point was marked in the anterior region of the left atrial appendage. Immediate termination of the atrial tachycardia and conversion to sinus rhythm was achieved by trial discharge at this point. Consolidation ablation was performed for 600 s (43 °C, 35 W, 1 2 mL/min). After the procedure, atrial pacing failed to induce atrial tachycardia with or without adding epinephrine. One week after the operation, the patient started to take propafenone, aspirin, furosemide, and spironolactone regularly. The boy was discharged 1 month later. ECG showed sinus rhythm + ectopic rhythm, a short burst of atrial tachycardia, and a short burst of atrial flutter.

Therefore, after stopping aspirin, furosemide, and spironolactone, the patient was admitted to

J. Zheng et al. (eds.), *Selected Pediatric Cardiovascular Surgery Anesthesia Cases*,
https://doi.org/10.1007/978-981-96-5614-1_59

the hospital for an elective left atrial appendectomy.

Physical examination: HR 110 beats/min, noninvasive blood pressure (BP) 95/70 mm Hg, irregular heart rhythm, strong heart sounds, no murmurs heard.

Laboratory test: No significant abnormalities in blood routine, coagulation, liver, and kidney function.

Electrocardiogram: Sinus rhythm + ectopic rhythm, short burst of atrial tachycardia, short burst of atrial flutter.

Holter monitoring: The average HR was 82 beats/min, the slowest 71 beats/ min, and the fastest 188 beats/min. The entire course showed atrial tachycardia with varying degrees of atrioventricular conduction block and intraventricular differential conduction defects.

Echocardiography: Arrhythmia, slight enlargement of the left ventricle (end-diastolic diameter of the left ventricle is 4.22 cm, normal value for 7 years is 3.99 cm), left ventricular wall contraction activity is acceptable, left ventricular systolic function is within normal range, aortic valve opening activity is acceptable, left and right coronary artery openings are visible, no obvious dilatation, no dilatation of the pulmonary artery, valve opening activity is acceptable, mild tricuspid regurgitation, regurgitation speed is 2.14 m/s.

Chest X-ray: Enlarged cardiac shadow, cardiothoracic ratio is 0.6, increased lung markings.

Preoperative diagnosis: Atrial tachycardia, elective left atrial appendage removal surgery.

59.2 Anesthetic Management

Basic vital signs: HR 78 beats/min, BP 105/65 mm Hg, pulse oxygen saturation (SpO_2) 100%. Anesthesia was induced with intravenous bolus doses of 0.5 mg midazolam, 6.0 mg etomidate, 50 μg sufentanil, and 15 mg rocuronium. An ID 5.5 mm cuffed endotracheal tube was intubated under a visual laryngoscope and fixed after verification of the appropriate position by bilateral auscultation of the lungs. Left radial artery and right internal jugular vein catheterization were performed under ultrasound guidance to continuously monitor invasive blood pressure (ABP) and central venous pressure (CVP). A 7 F endobronchial blocker tube (Hangzhou Tappa Medical Technology Co. Ltd.) was then placed in the left bronchus under the support of a bronchoscope. During the period of single lung ventilation, the boy was ventilated with PCV-VG mode: gas flow rate of 1.6 L/min, fraction of inspired oxygen (FiO_2) 50%, tidal volume (VT) of 120 mL, respiratory rate (RR) of 20 times/min, I:E ratio of 1:2, PEEP 6 cm H_2O. VT and RR were adjusted according to blood gas analysis results to maintain $SpO_2 \geq 90\%$ and $ETCO_2 \leq 60$ mm Hg; blood gas analysis results are shown in Table 59.1. General anesthesia was maintained by continuous intravenous infusion of 5.0 mg/(kg·h) propofol, 1.5 μg/(kg·h) sufentanil, 0.6 mg/(kg·h) rocuronium, and combined with 0.5 minimum alveolar concentration (MAC) sevoflurane.

After induction of anesthesia, atrial tachycardia occurred with HR 192 beats/min, ABP 51/32 mm Hg. Immediately, 13 mg of propafenone was slowly injected via the peripheral vein. The atrial tachycardia was successfully defibrillated with HR, and BP returned to normal. Then, 5.0 μg/(kg·min) amiodarone was continuously infused. Before the operation, atrial tachycardia recurred, 30 J synchronous defibrillation did not work, and then slow reinjection of 17 mg propafenone, the child returned to sinus rhythm. After recovery of the heart rhythm, the boy's BP was still at 60/48 mm Hg, 5.0 μg/(kg·min) dopamine, 0.05 μg/(kg·min) norepinephrine were administered to increase the blood pressure.

The operation was performed under video-assisted thoracoscopy. While the left atrial appendage was clamped with a 45 mm cutting suture clamp, the heart rate decreased from 162 bpm to 82 bpm. Subsequently, the left atrial appendage was transected (Fig. 59.1). After removing the left atrial appendage, the patient's hemodynamics were stable. Amiodarone was discontinued, and blood gases were rechecked. The alveolar recruitment maneuver consisting of a peak inspiratory pressure of 30 cm H_2O for 15 was performed to reopen the non-aerated lung

Table 59.1 Intraoperative blood gas test results

Time point	Hb (g/dL)	HCT (%)	pH	PaO_2 (mm Hg)	$PaCO_2$ (mm Hg)	BE (mmol/L)	Na^+ (mmol/L)	K^+ (mmol/L)	Cl^- (mmol/L)	Ca^{2+} (mmol/L)	Lac (mmol/L)
After induction	11.2	33.1	7.3	87.3	52.6	3.9	136	3.5	106	1.1	1.2
Chest closed	11.9	34.3	7.2	178.4	65.2	4.7	137	4.1	108	1.2	1.1

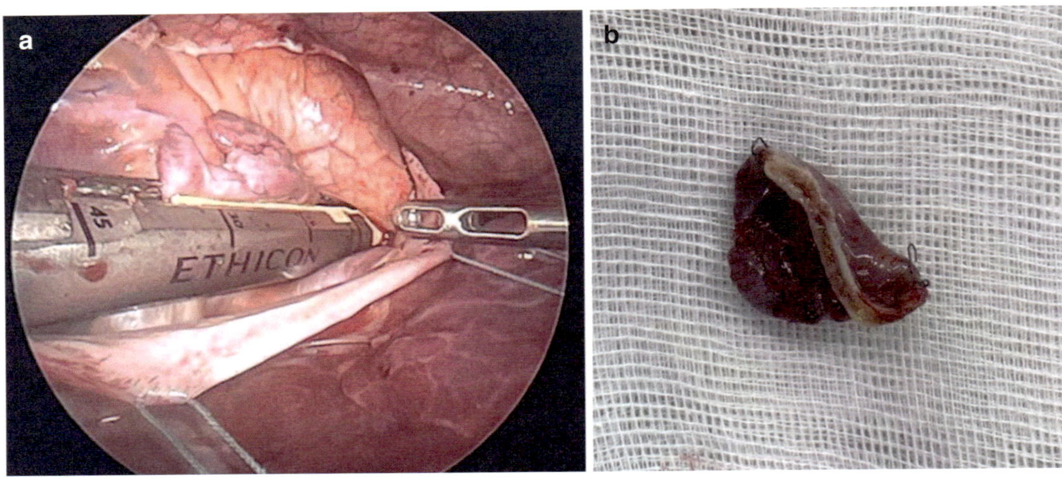

Fig. 59.1 Surgical diagram. (**a**) Thoracoscopic clamping of the left atrial appendage; (**b**) the excised left atrial appendage

regions. Then the chest wall was closed with satisfactory hemostasis.

The surgery lasted approximately 75 min in total. The patient was then transferred to the Cardiac Intensive Care Unit (CICU) for close monitoring with mechanical ventilation assistance. The tracheal tube was successfully removed on the next day. 9 days later, the ECG showed sinus rhythm. Holter showed sinus rhythm + ectopic rhythm, sinus node to atrial downstream wandering rhythm. The patient was discharged with medication.

59.3 Review of Knowledge Points

59.3.1 Clinical Manifestations of Atrial Tachycardia

In Europe, the incidence of asymptomatic atrial tachycardia in adults is about 0.34%, and symptomatic atrial tachycardia is about 0.46%. Most studies demonstrate that atrial tachycardia in children is higher than in adults. Therefore, early and accurate clinical diagnosis and management in children is very important. The symptoms of atrial tachycardia in children are usually atypical and may be asymptomatic. They could present with rapid heartbeat, abdominal pain, vomiting, poor appetite, pale complexion, palpitations, chest tightness, etc.

59.3.2 Treatments of Atrial Tachycardia

Antiarrhythmic drug treatment and radiofrequency ablation treatment are the two mainstream strategies for atrial tachycardia treatment in children. The first-line antiarrhythmic drugs in children are slightly different from those in adults, with an efficacy rate of only 54–75%. Amiodarone, a class III antiarrhythmic medication, is among the most effective medications for pediatric atrial tachycardia. Class Ic antiarrhythmic drugs are relatively effective in controlling pediatric atrial tachycardia. It is well known that calcium-channel blockers and class Ia antiarrhythmic drugs do not work well for the treatment of pediatric atrial tachycardia. However, amiodarone-induced hypotension, bradycardia, cardiovascular collapse, short-term side effects, and the potentially fatal toxicities of long-term use require vigilant monitoring and a low threshold for dose reduction or change in medication whenever possible. Therefore, amiodarone should be used with caution, especially in children. Radiofrequency ablation should be considered for children with atrial tachycardia that presents as continuous, unrelenting attacks for which drug therapy is not effective and may be associated with cardiac dysfunction. The left atrial appendage resection should be performed for pediatric atrial tachycardia relapsed after radiofrequency because most of the lesions related to atrial tachycardia come from the left atrial appendage.

59.3.3 Management of Single Lung Ventilation

One lung ventilation (OLV) is performed to provide a clearer surgical field of view. With the initiation of OLV in the lateral decubitus position, the nondependent lung collapses with atelectasis, decreases compliance, and shifts ventilation to the dependent lung. Furthermore, alveolar hypoxia in the nondependent lung can induce hypoxic pulmonary vasoconstriction (HPV) within seconds, directing blood away from poorly ventilated areas to well-ventilated areas. HPV in these segments will peak at 15–20 min, followed by a second delayed response. The infant thoracic cage is relatively soft and offers less resistance to the lung's inward recoil. Hence, the end-expiratory lung volume of infants is significantly reduced, resulting in the functional residual capacity closer to the residual volume and making the dependent lung's airway easily closed even during tidal breathing. The decreased hydrostatic pressure gradient between the nondependent and dependent lungs reduces the degree of redistribution of pulmonary blood flow. The high metabolic state of children and other factors can further aggravate hypoxemia during OLV.

59.4 Discussion

59.4.1 Preoperative Assessment and Preparation

In this case, the boy had a long history of persistent tachycardia, which was not well controlled by propafenone. Echocardiography showed a slightly enlarged left ventricle and normal left ventricular systolic function. Preoperative Holter monitoring showed persistent atrial tachycardia with varying degrees of atrioventricular conduction block and intraventricular differential conduction defects. Long-term persistent tachycardia can result in left ventricular dilation and dysfunction, which is known as tachycardia-induced cardiomyopathy. Once the atrial tachycardia is controlled, the left ventricular ejection fraction may significantly improve, but the structural abnormalities in cardiomyocytes and the ventricular diastolic dysfunction may persist. Preoperative echocardiography can fully assess the boy's cardiac function and left ventricular end-diastolic volume. Recurrent arrhythmias can cause the deterioration of cardiac function in a very short time and increase the risk of sudden death. Therefore, any risk factors causing the onset of atrium tachycardia should be avoided during the perioperative period. A detailed medical and medication history should also be obtained during preoperative assessment.

Before induction of anesthesia in the present case, an appropriate-sized defibrillation pad was placed in case of the onset of atrial tachycardia during induction of anesthesia. The antiarrhythmic drugs, including amiodarone and propafenone, were also prepared. After induction of anesthesia, a 7 F endobronchial blocker tube was placed down the tracheal lumen under fiberoptic bronchoscope (FOB) visualization for a better surgical field.

59.4.2 Intraoperative Anesthetic Management

The anesthetics with minimal myocardial suppression, including midazolam, etomidate, sufentanil, and rocuronium, were chosen for induction and maintenance of anesthesia. Furthermore, these anesthetics were intravenously titrated cautiously to maintain hemodynamic stability.

During the endobronchial blocker tube placement, it is necessary to maintain sufficient depth of anesthesia, fully lubricated, and gentle movements to avoid causing atrial tachycardia. However, the boy's atrial tachycardia was not well controlled during induction of anesthesia by synchronized electrical cardioversion, so intravenous propafenone was slowly given over 10 min; the total dosage should not exceed 1 mg/kg. Finally, the atrial tachycardia was successfully controlled. Although amiodarone has been widely used for pharmacological cardioversion, it can cause hypotension and toxic effects on the thyroid, liver, and nervous system. Furthermore, a loading dose of amiodarone with intravenous maintenance is required due to the long elimination half-life. Therefore, in this case, we first chose propafenone to treat the atrial tachycardia with significant hypotension; then, amiodarone was subsequently used for maintenance after successful cardioversion. We closely monitored the electrocardiogram changes during the surgery and maintained the sinus rhythm and hemodynamic stability. A low tidal volume ventilation strategy was used for OLV management. Studies have shown that a ventilation strategy of 4 mL/kg tidal volume combined with 6 cm H_2O PEEP can be better than 6 mL/kg tidal volume without PEEP in reducing the incidence of postoperative pulmonary complications. A certain degree of hypercapnia is allowed during the OLV period. Once bilateral lung ventilation is restored, high-end tidal carbon dioxide will quickly return to the normal range, but a blood gas test is still needed. Maintaining $SpO_2 \geq 90\%$ with FiO_2 30%–50% during the OLV period is better. If SpO_2 is <90%, proactive measures should be taken, such as increasing FiO_2, VT, and PEEP. If hypoxia persists, the surgery should be temporally stopped to restore bilateral lung ventilation. In this case, FiO_2 50% was sufficient to maintain $SpO_2 \geq 90\%$ during the OLV period.

59.5 Conclusion

In summary, the anesthetic management of video-assisted thoracoscopic left atrial appendage resection should be based on the pathophysiological characteristics of atrial tachycardia, correct selection of antiarrhythmic drugs, and appropriate ventricular rate control. The lung protective ventilation strategy and permissive hypercapnia during OLV should be used to reduce the incidence of postoperative respiratory complications (Yingying Ji).

60 Anesthetic Management of Atrial Septal Defect Repair in a Child with Short-Chain Acyl-coenzyme A Dehydrogenase Deficiency

Ying Sun

Abstract

A 19-month-old boy with short-chain acyl-CoA dehydrogenase deficiency underwent atrial septal defect repair surgery under general anesthesia. The anesthetic management of such patients should focus on preoperative fasting and perioperative blood glucose control. The intravenous anesthetic propofol contains high lipids, which cannot be fully metabolized in these patients. Therefore, the use of propofol is contraindicated in this patient population. Short-acting non-depolarizing muscle relaxants are the preferred choice. In addition, it is necessary to conduct symptomatic treatment once complications occur.

Short-chain acyl-coenzyme A dehydrogenase deficiency (SCADD) is an autosomal recessive genetic disease with an incidence of about 1/40,000 to 1/100,000, which is caused by mutations in the short-chain acyl-coenzyme A gene located on the long arm of the 12th chromosome (12q24.31) and manifests as an inability to use short-chain fatty acids. SCADD has been listed as a rare disease in our country. The corresponding acyl-coenzyme A dehydrogenase function is defective because of gene mutations and results in short-chain fatty acids β-oxidation impairment, which further causes the reduction of energy production and large accumulation of metabolic intermediates in the body. Clinically, SCADD is often accompanied by symptoms such as hypoglycemia, hypotonia, metabolic acidosis, central nervous system defects, epileptic seizures, and gastroesophageal reflux.

60.1 Case Presentation

A 19-month-old boy with 10 kg in weight and 85 cm in height was preoperatively diagnosed with atrial septal defect (ASD). The boy was scheduled to undergo ASD repair surgery under general anesthesia. Based on neonatal mass spectrometry screening (heel blood), he was diagnosed with short-chain acyl-coenzyme A dehydrogenase deficiency. The parents reported that his muscle strength was not significantly affected, while his growth and development were normal.

Preoperative laboratory tests were basically normal.

Echocardiography showed ASD (septum secundum).

Y. Sun (✉)
The National Children's Medical Center (Shanghai), Department of Anesthesiology of Shanghai Children's Medical Center, Shanghai Jiao Tong University School of Medicine, Shanghai, China
e-mail: sunying@scmc.com.cn

J. Zheng et al. (eds.), *Selected Pediatric Cardiovascular Surgery Anesthesia Cases*,
https://doi.org/10.1007/978-981-96-5614-1_60

Table 60.1 Intraoperative blood gas test results

Time point	pH	GLU (mmol/L)	LAC (mmol/L)	K^+ (mmol/L)	Na^+ (mmol/L)	CL^- (mmol/L)	Ca^{2+} (mmol/L)	BE (mmol/L)	AG	HCT (%)
After induction	7.37	4.8	1.4	3.8	133	106	1.18	−3.55	9.6	34.7
1 h after induction	7.46	4.2	1.6	3.5	137	103	1.21	−2.73	11.7	32.4
Aortic occlusion	7.32	6.8	1.2	3.3	143	105	1.01	−1.1	16.3	26.5
Before stopping extracorporeal	7.37	5.7	2.1	4	141	106	1.4	0	15.1	26.3
End of extracorporeal	7.37	6.1	2.5	4.1	138	103	1.11	−1.06	14.8	32.2
Admission to CICU	7.45	7.8	2.8	3.6	141	101	1.08	−1.6	13.5	37.9

60.2 Anesthetic Management

Considering the characteristics of the child's disease, the parents were instructed that the patient should fast for 6 h and not drink after feeding sugar water 2 h before surgery. After entering the operating room, 1.0 mg of midazolam, 10 mg of ketamine, 20 μg of sufentanil, and 6.0 mg of rocuronium were intravenously administered for the induction of anesthesia. An ID 4.0 mm cuffed endotracheal tube was intubated smoothly under the support of video laryngoscopy. The left radial artery and right internal jugular vein were catheterized under ultrasound guidance to continuously monitor invasive blood pressure (ABP) and central venous pressure (CVP). General anesthesia was maintained by continuous intravenous infusion of sufentanil 2.0 μg/(kg·h), dexmedetomidine 1.0 μg/(kg·h), and rocuronium 0.6 mg/(kg·h), combined with 1–2% sevoflurane inhalation. The operation went smoothly. Modified ultrafiltration and routine protamine neutralization were performed after separation from CPB. At the end of the operation, the patient was transferred to the Cardiac Intensive Care Unit (CICU) with endotracheal intubation. After induction, the basic blood gas analysis was performed (Table 60.1), and 10% glucose injection was intravenously infused at 20 mL/h by a syringe pump. The blood gas analysis was conducted every 1 hour to monitor blood glucose and potassium values closely. The perioperative blood glucose and blood potassium values are shown in Table 60.1.

60.3 Postoperative Outcome

The endotracheal tube was removed 5 h after surgery in the CICU, and then the formula was pumped into the stomach through a gastric tube, and blood glucose was maintained at a normal level. The patient was discharged from the CICU on the postoperative day 1. On postoperative day 4, the patient was discharged from the hospital.

60.4 Review of Knowledge Points

Short-chain acyl-CoA dehydrogenase (SCAD) is one of the mitochondrial enzymes that catalyzes short-chain fatty acids (four to six carbons in length) by dehydrogenation and initiates the β-oxidation cycle. SCAD deficiency is an autosomal recessive genetic disease with a complex inheritance pattern. Patients may present with a wide variety of clinical manifestations. Therefore, the preoperative, intraoperative, and postoperative management of patients with SCADD is complex, especially the patient with SCADD is accompanied by contraindications to conventional anesthetics.

60.4.1 Abnormal Metabolic Pathway of SCADD

Lipid metabolism is an important alternative energy source during fasting and stressful conditions. The first step of lipid metabolism is mitochondrial oxidation, which involves splitting long carbon chains of fatty acids into acetyl-CoA and then entering the tricarboxylic acid cycle. Mitochondrial oxidation involves three types of acyl-CoA dehydrogenases, including long-chain, medium-chain, and short-chain. Each has a specific chain length: long-chain acts on C20 C12, medium-chain acts on C12 C4, and short-chain acts on C6 C4 fatty acyl-CoA. Many genetic diseases are caused by errors in lipid metabolism, including deficiencies of long, medium, and short-chain acyl-CoA dehydrogenases.

Defects in long- and medium-chain acyl-coenzyme A dehydrogenase have been reported much more frequently than short-chain defects in those affected children. Short-chain acyl-CoA dehydrogenase is the first catalyst of short-chain fatty acid β-oxidation. The deficiency of this enzyme leads to the production of toxic intermediates, mainly butyryl-CoA. The accumulation of intermediates is subsequently broken down by other pathways and causes the accumulation of methylmalonic acid, methylsulfonyl-CoA, and butyryl carnitine 2, 5, 6, which finally results in the formation of aciduria (Fig. 60.1).

60.4.2 Common Complications of SCADD

SCAD metabolic disorder is characterized by the inability to use short-chain fatty acids, which is often accompanied by some clinical symptoms such as hypoglycemia, hypotonia, metabolic acidosis, central nervous system defects, epileptic seizures, and gastroesophageal reflux (Table 60.2). The clinical symptoms should attract the attention of both surgeons and anesthesia teams. Long- and medium-chain acyl Co-A dehydrogenase deficiency disorders have been well-studied in the past, whereas the short-chain acyl-coenzyme A dehydrogenase deficiency encountered in this case is relatively rare.

60.4.3 Issues Related to SCADD and Anesthesia

The impact of these excess metabolites on the skeletal muscle and central nervous system of children with SCADD is manifested through some clinical signs.

Fig. 60.1 The metabolism of fatty acid chains and the formation of organic acids in SCAD deficiency. *LCAD* long-chain acyl-CoA dehydrogenase, *MCAD* medium-chain acyl-CoA dehydrogenase, *SCAD* short-chain acyl-CoA dehydrogenase

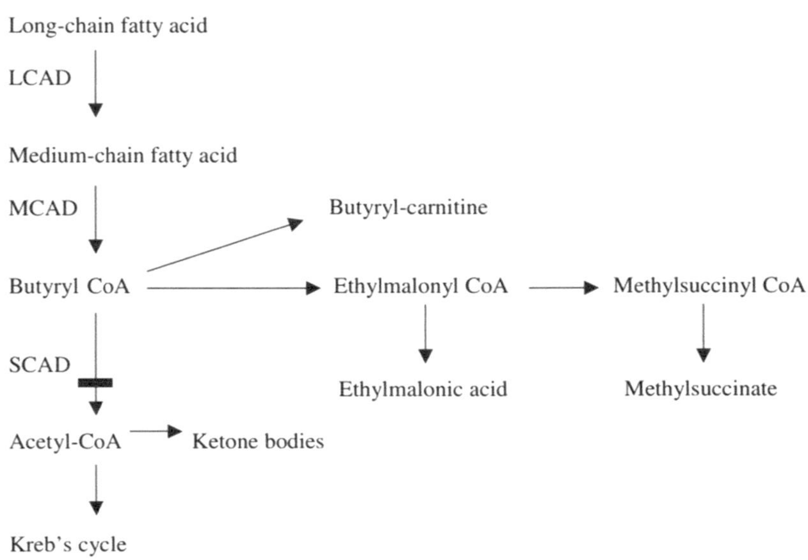

Table 60.2 Signs and symptoms of SCAD deficiency (from most common to least common)

Common	Rare
Acidic urine	Craniofacial deformity features
Metabolic acidosis	Hypoglycemia
Developmental delay	Convulsions
	Scoliosis
	Hyperactive muscle tone and reflexes
	Periodic vomiting
	Cardiac dysfunction

These clinical signs span a considerable range, varying from virtually no clinical manifestations to severe organ failure. These children require particular attention to blood glucose during fasting and adequate preoperative rehydration. Some children even need to be admitted to the hospital the day before surgery to prevent severe hypoglycemia during the fasting period. Propofol, a commonly used intravenous anesthetic, is contraindicated in this patient population due to its high lipid content and inability to be fully metabolized. At the same time, etomidate was chosen due to its rapid onset of action and low cardiovascular risk. Thiopental or methohexital may also be considered if this patient is not allergic to barbiturates. The most common symptom of SCAD defects is hypotonia. More than half of the patients in the literature were reported to have hypotonia ranging from mild weakness to alterations in muscle function that may result in patients with severe muscle atrophy. In the perioperative period, a number of potentially influential factors exist in patients with any myopathic disease. In particular, there is a need to avoid the use of depolarizing muscarinic agents, such as succinylcholine, which has been associated with rhabdomyolysis and hyperkalemia in some patients with myopathies. In addition, sensitivity to non-depolarizing neuromuscular blocking agents (NMBAs) may be increased. Therefore, non-depolarizing muscarinic agents with short onset and duration of action are clinically recommended for such children.

As the key enzyme for entering two carbon fragments into the tricarboxylic acid cycle, SCAD plays a key role in the energy production of short-chain fatty acids and the utilization of gluconeogenesis. For anesthesiologists, the most important thing about these children is metabolic disorders, including hypoglycemia and metabolic acidosis. In addition, respiratory muscle tension may be reduced. The central nervous system may be involved, manifesting seizures, airway management problems, gastroesophageal reflux, and the risk of hypoglycemia caused by long-term fasting. Furthermore, for those children with unexplained issues such as acidosis or hypoglycemia during the perioperative period, SCAD deficiency should be considered for screening.

60.5 Discussion

60.5.1 Preoperative Assessment and Preparation

SCADD is not common in clinical practice, but it has been gradually recognized in recent years with the popularization of mass spectrometry screening in newborns. In this case, a 19-month-old boy was diagnosed with SCADD by neonatal mass spectrometry screening. The parents informed the anesthesiologist that their child was diagnosed with SCADD without a special diet on ordinary days during the preoperative assessment. His growth and development were basically normal. There was no history of epilepsy or other disease-related clinical manifestations, such as changes in muscle tone.

It is necessary to make an appropriate preoperative fasting plan and prevent severe hypoglycemia before surgery. As the protagonist of the entire surgical team before surgery, the surgeon team should notify the anesthesiologists and postoperative cardiac intensive care physicians to make a plan for the child's disease-related issues. In addition to the 6-h preoperative fasting, glucose water feeding 2 h before surgery should be emphasized. No drinking was allowed after feeding the glucose water. In order to strictly implement the fasting and drinking plan, this patient was specifically arranged to be the first one to receive surgical treatment in the morning. The first blood gas analysis after the induction of anesthesia showed that the child's blood glucose value was 4.8 mmol/L.

Literature reports that such patients can take carnitine orally before surgery. Carnitine can promote the transport of fatty acids through the mitochondrial membrane, which increases the concentration of substrates for β-oxidation in the mitochondria. In addition, carnitine can combine with the excessive metabolites from fatty acid oxidation disorders to promote their excretion. Although there is no literature to support that the use of carnitine fully is beneficial to SCAD deficits, there is theoretical support for the use of carnitine in children with SCADD based on the few systemic adverse effects of carnitine application and the effectiveness of carnitine application in other β-oxidation disorders. However, carnitine was not used in our case.

60.5.2 Intraoperative Anesthetic Management

Propofol should be avoided for anesthesia induction and maintenance in these patients since propofol has a high lipid content and cannot be fully metabolized. Midazolam, esketamine, sufentanil, and rocuronium were used for anesthesia induction and intubation. The choice of muscle relaxants was still based on medium and short-acting non-depolarizing muscle relaxants. Well-equipped hospitals can perform muscle relaxation monitoring. Anesthesia maintenance is performed with sufentanil and dexmedetomidine intravenously infusion, supplemented by sevoflurane inhalation.

For intraoperative blood glycemic control, 10% dextrose solution was intravenously infused at the rate of 20 mL/h when the surgery started. The blood glycemic level was checked every hour after the dextrose infusion. The blood glucose value was in the normal range (4.2 mmol/L). It has also been suggested in the literature that the glucose infusion rate in these children should be maintained at 6–8 mg/(kg·min) while keeping the blood glucose above 5.3 mmol/L to inhibit lipolysis. The glucose control during the cardiopulmonary bypass and in the postoperative period was satisfactory when 10% glucose infusion was maintained at a rate of 20 mL/h throughout the procedure. In addition, appropriate potassium supplementation is required to avoid hypokalemia.

60.6 Conclusion

Although there were no complications, such as changes in muscle tone, epilepsy, and gastroesophageal reflux in this case, there was no corresponding symptomatic treatment. However, anesthesiologists need to be very vigilant about the occurrence of these complications in children with SCADD. As the understanding of rare diseases and metabolic disorders gradually gets deeper, anesthesiologists need to keep abreast of the times and understand the pathophysiological changes related to anesthesia and surgery so as to guide the implementation of clinical anesthesia more accurately (Ying Sun).

Anesthetic Management of Anaphylactic Shock Induced by Bioprotein Glue in a Child Undergoing Cardiac Tumor Resection

61

Ming Zhu

Abstract

A 2-year-old boy was found with a left ventricular tumor by echocardiography due to a heart murmur heard during a physical examination. The tumor was successfully removed under general anesthesia and cardiopulmonary bypass support. Biological protein glue (Beixiu glue) was applied to the surgical suture site during hemostasis. Blood pressure suddenly dropped to a minimum of 50/30 mm Hg after the sternum was closed, which was accompanied by an airway peak pressure increase and SpO_2 decrease. We suspected that acute anaphylactic shock induced by biological protein glue occurred. The treatment principles of this case include ventilation support, rapid fluid infusion, positive inotropic drug use, and avoidance of cardiac and other important organ dysfunctions.

Anaphylactic shock is an acute, multi-system, potentially fatal hypersensitive reaction that is caused by the sudden release of various immune mediators into the circulation by mast cells and basophils. It is usually characterized by widespread urticaria in the skin and mucous membranes, respiratory symptoms, a drop in blood pressure, etc. Biological protein glue is a synthetically produced biological preparation that has hemostasis, wound sealing, tissue adhesion prevention, and wound healing promotion effects. However, as a heterologous protein, it has certain antigenicity and can cause allergic reactions, arrhythmia, or even shock in severe cases.

61.1 Case Presentation

The patient was 2 year and 2-month-old boy with a height of 90 cm and weight of 11.5 kg. Basic blood pressure (BP) was 95/55 mm Hg, heart rate (HR) 125 beats/min, and respiratory rate (RR) of 25 breaths/min. A mass was detected in the left ventricle by fetal ultrasound. He was born full-term without any complications. Echocardiography showed a moderate echo mass in the left ventricular wall with a size of 6.8 cm × 3.42 cm, lobulation in morphology, and focal compression on the mitral annulus and left ventricle. The left atrium and left ventricle sizes are within the normal ranges. The left ventricular wall contraction was normal. Mild to moderate mitral regurgitation.

M. Zhu (✉)
The National Children's Medical Center (Shanghai), Department of Anesthesiology of Shanghai Children's Medical Center, Shanghai Jiao Tong University School of Medicine, Shanghai, China
e-mail: zhuming@scmc.com.cn

J. Zheng et al. (eds.), *Selected Pediatric Cardiovascular Surgery Anesthesia Cases*, https://doi.org/10.1007/978-981-96-5614-1_61

61.2 Anesthetic Management

The patient preoperatively took oral midazolam 5.0 mg syrup. He was calmly separated from his parents and brought into the operating room. Routine monitoring was established. The anesthesia was induced by peripheral venous injection of etomidate 2.0 mg, sufentanil 20 μg, and rocuronium 6.0 mg. The endotracheal intubation was performed for mechanical ventilation. Intraoperative arterial blood pressure (ABP) was 88/56 mm Hg, central venous pressure (CVP) was 10 cm H_2O, heart rate (HR) was 120 beats/min, and respiratory rate (RR) was 20 breaths/min. End-tidal carbon dioxide ($ETCO_2$) was maintained at about 38 mm Hg. The vital signs were stable during the operation.

The surgery was performed under cardiopulmonary bypass (CPB) support. During the operation, a large tumor was seen on the free wall of the left ventricle with a hard texture and fixed, measuring 9 cm × 5 cm. The tumor was completely removed. After the aortic cross-clamp was released, the heart automatically resumed beating with a sinus rhythm. No residual tumor was seen on transesophageal echocardiogram (TEE) and there was mild mitral regurgitation. After weaning off CPB, dopamine 5.0 μg/(kg·min) was used to maintain blood pressure at about 92/56 mm Hg. Then, heparin was neutralized with an intravenous infusion of protamine. Biological protein glue (Beixiu glue) was applied to the cardiac incision suture site for hemostasis. When the chest wall incision was sutured layer by layer, the patient suddenly experienced a significant drop in blood pressure, dropping to the lowest about 50/30 mm Hg while HR was 150 beats/min, SpO_2 was 90%, CVP was 5 cm H_2O, the peak airway pressure was increased to 20 cm H_2O with VT about 60 mL, which was preliminarily diagnosed as anaphylactic shock The chest wall was immediately reopened to remove the biological protein glue, manual ventilation was used to increase the ventilation volume per minute, a single dose of epinephrine 0.1 mg and calcium gluconate 300 mg were administered, but blood pressure was not significantly improved, then epinephrine 0.05–0.3 μg/(kg·min) combined with norepinephrine 0.02–0.3 μg/(kg·min) was intravenously infused, methylprednisolone 40 mg was also intravenously dripped. In contrast, Ringer's acetate solution of 200 mL was rapidly infused. Around minutes later, ABP recovered to 82/51 mm Hg, HR 130 beats/min, CVP 8 cm H_2O, and the patient's airway resistance was also reduced. Then, the dosages of epinephrine and norepinephrine were reduced, TEE reevaluated the blood volume level and TEE-guided fluid replacement. Arterial blood gas was rechecked. The total urine output at this time was 30 mL. After the vital signs stabilized, the sternum was closed layer by layer. After the operation, unevenly distributed red rashes all over the body were found when the surgical drape was removed. The patient was transferred to the Cardiac Intensive Care Unit (CICU) for further treatment, with vital signs monitored.

61.3 Postoperative Outcome

Epinephrine 0.05 μg/(kg·min) and dopamine 5.0 μg/(kg·min) were continuously infused in CICU until the vital signs were stabilized. The endotracheal tube was removed on the postoperative day 1. The patient was transferred to the general ward on postoperative day 2 and discharged from the hospital 1 week later.

61.4 Review of Knowledge Points

61.4.1 Anaphylactic Shock

Diagnostic Criteria for Anaphylactic Shock mainly include widespread rashes on the skin and mucous membranes, hypersensitivity reactions in the respiratory tract, and hemodynamic or end-organs dysfunction. However, it is sometimes very hard to early determine the occurrence of anaphylaxis under general anesthesia due to:

Clinical symptoms and signs such as difficulty breathing, abdominal pain, and anxiety cannot be detected.

1. Surgical drapes obstruct the observation of allergic skin changes, such as erythema and rashes.
2. It is sometimes difficult to distinguish the hypotension or tachycardia caused by anaphylaxis from other related factors during anesthesia.
3. Anesthesia affects the compensatory mechanism of awake patients when anaphylaxis occurs.

The incidence of allergic reactions during anesthesia is 1/10,000 to 1/20,000. The main allergic sources during anesthesia include muscle Relaxants (40–60%), latex (20%), antibiotics (18%), opioids (2–3%), and sedative-hypnotics (1%).

61.4.2 Immunoreaction of Biological Protein Glue

The main components of biological protein glue include fibrinogen, thrombin, activated coagulation factor VII, calcium ion, and fibrinolysis inhibitors, which are produced from the plasma of healthy pigs by separation, extraction, and virus inactivation. To slow down the degradation of fibrin clots, fibrinolysis inhibitors are added to the biological protein to extend the average survival period to 10–14 days. Biological protein glue is a kind of heterologous protein and can cause immunoreactions.

61.5 Discussion

61.5.1 Diagnosis of Anaphylactic Shock

It is very important to detect the occurrence of anaphylaxis during surgery early. Relatively speaking, anaphylaxis caused by muscle relaxants is more severe than those caused by latex. Early clinical manifestations of anaphylaxis that anesthesiologists can observe include pulse rate drop or disappearance, blood pressure drop, VT reduction, and widespread skin erythema. Skin manifestations are the most common (accounting for 66–70%), followed by cardiovascular failure and bronchospasm. In severe cases, cardiac arrest may occur even without any other symptoms. Sometimes, the airway spasm is very severe and difficult to correct, which poses a risk of brain hypoxia and death. Children with a history of bronchial asthma must be alert to allergic reactions. A retrospective study found that the symptoms of anaphylactic shock in children are more severe, of which the cardiovascular symptoms are more pronounced and the incidence of bronchospasm is higher. Severe allergic reactions mostly occur within 30 min of medication. In this case, the child showed early signs of anaphylactic shock about 10 min after using biological protein glue. The anaphylactic shock was quickly and effectively treated due to timely and correct diagnosis and management. Therefore, detecting such allergic reactions sometimes also depends on the anesthesiologist's rich experiences and timely diagnosis.

The diagnostic criteria for severe allergic reactions are shown in Table 61.1. Other possible atypical symptoms should also be noted.

The grading criteria for severe allergic reactions are shown in Table 61.2.

61.5.2 Management of Anaphylactic Shock

Once the children are diagnosed with grade II and above severe allergic reactions, epinephrine should be used. Epinephrine and fluid resuscitation are recommended as first-line treatment. Other measures of treating anaphylactic shock are shown in Table 61.3. In addition to routine medication treatment in this case, it was also very important to quickly remove the allergenic source of biological protein glue, which is different from other intravenous allergens.

Table 61.1 Diagnostic criteria for severe allergic reactions

When the symptoms meet any one of the following three criteria, the child is very likely to have an acute severe allergic reaction. 1. The disease has an acute onset (within a few minutes to several hours), with symptoms of the skin or mucosal system, such as rash, itching or flushing, red and swollen lips and tongue, and numbness, as well as any one of the following system symptoms (regardless of the history of allergen contact). 1. Respiratory symptoms include hoarseness, cough, chest tightness, shortness of breath, difficulty breathing, wheezing, bronchospasm, cyanosis, decreased peak expiratory flow, insufficient blood oxygen, etc. 2. Drop in blood pressure (see criterion 3) or related end-organ dysfunction, such as numbness, decreased muscle tone, fainting, and incontinence.
When the symptoms meet any one of the following three criteria, the child is very likely to have an acute severe allergic reaction. 2. The child has a rapid onset of two or more of the following symptoms within a few minutes to several hours after contact with a suspected allergen. 1. Skin and mucosal tissue symptoms include rashes, itching or flushing, red and swollen lips and tongue, numbness, etc. 2. Respiratory symptoms include chest tightness, shortness of breath, difficulty breathing, wheezing, bronchospasm, cyanosis, decreased peak expiratory flow, insufficient blood oxygen, etc. 3. Drop in blood pressure or end-organ function impairment, such as decreased muscle tone, fainting, and incontinence. 4. Persistent gastrointestinal symptoms, such as abdominal pain, nausea, and vomiting. 3. The child's blood pressure drops within a few minutes to several hours after contact with a known allergen. 1. Infants and children: Systolic pressure lower than the normal value for the corresponding age: <1 year old, systolic pressure < 70 mm Hg 1–10 years old, systolic pressure < (70 mm Hg + 2 × age) 11–17 years old, systolic pressure < 90 mm Hg or a drop >30% from the baseline 2. Adults: Systolic pressure lower than 90 mm Hg or a drop of 30% from the baseline.

Table 61.2 Grading standards for severe allergic reactions

Grade	Clinical manifestations
Grade I	Only symptoms of the skin and mucous membrane system and gastrointestinal system, stable hemodynamics, stable respiratory system function Skin and mucous membrane system symptoms: rash, itching or flushing, lip and tongue swelling and (or) numbness, etc. Gastrointestinal system symptoms: abdominal pain, nausea, vomiting, etc.
Grade II	Obvious respiratory system symptoms or drop in blood pressure Respiratory system symptoms: chest tightness, shortness of breath, wheezing, bronchospasm, cyanosis, decrease in peak expiratory flow rate, insufficient blood oxygen, etc. Drop in blood pressure: 1. Infants and children: systolic pressure lower than the normal value for the corresponding age: <1 year old, systolic pressure < 70 mm Hg 1–10 years old, systolic pressure < (70 mm Hg + 2 × age) 11–17 years old, systolic pressure < 90 mm Hg or a drop >30–40% from the baseline value 2. Adults: systolic pressure 80–90 mm Hg or a drop of 30–40% from the baseline value
Grade III	Any of the following symptoms: confusion, loss of consciousness, drowsiness, severe bronchospasm and (or) laryngeal edema, cyanosis, severe drop in blood pressure (systolic pressure < 80 mm hg or a drop >40% from the baseline value), incontinence, etc.
Grade IV	Occurrence of cardiac and (or) respiratory arrest

Table 61.3 Treatment plan for anaphylactic shock

Treatment method	Treatment measures
First-line treatment	1. Airway management and oxygenation 2. Epinephrine (1:100,000, 10 μg/mL): 0.75–1.5 μg/kg iv 3. Colloid 10–20 mL/kg IV
Second-line treatment	1. Diphenhydramine 25 mg IV. Cimetidine 300 mg IV. (slowly over 3–5 min) 2. Hydrocortisone 200 mg 3. Glucagon 1.0 mg IV. Can be repeated if necessary after 5 min; then 5.0–15 μg/min iv 4. Vasoconstrictor drugs: Norepinephrine 2.0–10 μg/min, dopamine 5.0–20 μg/(kg·min)
Empirical treatment	1. Naloxone 2. Anti-shock trousers 3. Thyrotropin-releasing hormone

61.6 Conclusion

Early detection and timely management is the key to successfully manage the allergic reactions. Once an allergic reaction or anaphylactic shock is suspected during surgery, any suspicious drug infusion should be immediately stopped. Epinephrine is the first choice of rescue drug for anaphylactic shock. Rapid infusion of crystalloids can effectively maintain circulatory blood volume. Intraoperative use of biological protein glue may cause serious allergic reactions. Therefore, anesthesiologists should keep sufficient vigilance when biological protein glues are used during surgery, especially for those of high-risk populations; comprehensive preparations should be made in advance (Ming Zhu).

62 Management of Severe Allergic Reaction During Cardiopulmonary Bypass in a Child Undergoing Arial Septal Defect Repair

Lu Wang

Abstract

A 2-year-old girl suddenly experienced difficulty in maintaining the safe level of blood in the reservoir, accompanied by a drop in blood pressure during the post-parallel circulation of cardiopulmonary bypass (CBP). After ruling out other potential causes, a severe allergic reaction was highly suspected, which was alleviated after the administration of a large volume of fluids, epinephrine, and methylprednisolone. For this particular type of allergic reaction, it is essential to administer standard treatment based on the pathophysiology of allergic reactions, while the unique situation of CBP should also be considered.

Allergic reactions are common complications during the perioperative period. Opioids, muscle relaxants, protamine, antibiotics, blood products, and hemostatic drugs used in CBP circulation cardiac surgery may all trigger allergic reactions in children. In severe cases, they can lead to respiratory and circulatory failure. This chapter reports a case of severe allergic reaction occurring during cardiopulmonary bypass (CPB) in a child undergoing atrial septal defect (ASD) repair surgery and its management.

62.1 Case Presentation

The patient was a 2-year-old girl with a weight of 10.5 kg and a height of 92 cm. Cardiac ultrasound at a local hospital showed ASD (type II). There was no noticeable decrease in physical endurance. There were no symptoms such as palpitations or fatigue. No history of drug or food allergies.

Physical examination: The child was conscious without apparent cyanosis. Slightly coarse breath sounds in both lungs at auscultation but no rales. Strong heart sounds, regular heart rhythm, and II/VI-grade systolic murmur in the second to third intercostal space along the left sternal border. There was no obvious liver and spleen enlargement. The extremities were warm, without edema.

Laboratory tests: Routine blood, liver, and kidney function tests revealed no abnormalities.

Cardiac ultrasound: ASD with a size of 0.60 cm, left-to-right shunt. The right atrium and right ventricle enlargement.

Chest X-ray: Plump cardiac shadow and left lower lung infiltration.

Electrocardiogram (ECG): Sinus rhythm with sinus tachycardia and incomplete right bundle branch block present.

L. Wang (✉)
The National Children's Medical Center (Shanghai), Department of Anesthesiology of Shanghai Children's Medical Center, Shanghai Jiao Tong University School of Medicine, Shanghai, China
e-mail: wanglu@scmc.com.cn

J. Zheng et al. (eds.), *Selected Pediatric Cardiovascular Surgery Anesthesia Cases*,
https://doi.org/10.1007/978-981-96-5614-1_62

Preoperative diagnosis: ASD. Elective lateral thoracotomy was scheduled for ASD repair surgery under general anesthesia.

62.2 Anesthetic Management

The patient orally took 0.5 mg/kg midazolam syrup 30 min prior to surgery. After she was brought into the operating room, ECG, noninvasive blood pressure (BP), and pulse oxygen saturation (SpO_2) were routinely monitored with basic BP 85/42 mm Hg, heart rate (HR) 133 beats/min, and SpO_2 96%. After the peripheral vein was accessed, the anesthesia was induced by intravenous bolus injection of midazolam 1.0 mg, etomidate 2.5 mg, sufentanil 20 μg, and rocuronium 7.5 mg. Once the eyelash reflex disappeared, an ID 4.5 mm cuffed endotracheal tube was intubated with the assistance of a video laryngoscope. The depth of the endotracheal tube was 13 cm. Mechanical ventilation with pressure-controlled ventilation (PCV) mode was conducted with an oxygen flow rate at 2 L/min, fraction of inspired oxygen (FiO_2) at 60%, peak inspiratory pressure (PIP) at 18 cm H_2O, and inspiratory to expiratory time ratio at (I:E) 1:2. The tidal volume was maintained at 90 to 100 mL. Adjusting RR maintained the end-tidal carbon dioxide pressure ($ETCO_2$) at 35 to 40 mm Hg. Intraoperative monitoring was initiated, which included the left radial artery catheterized for invasive arterial blood pressure (ABP) measurement. The right jugular vein was catheterized for central venous pressure (CVP) measurement and vasoactive drug infusion. Bispectral index (BIS) and regional cerebral tissue oxygen saturation (rSO_2) monitoring were also performed during surgery. General anesthesia was maintained by intravenous infusions of propofol at 4.0 mg/(kg·h), sufentanil at 2.0 μg/(kg·h), and rocuronium at 0.5 mg/(kg·h). Additionally, 1.0–2.0 MAC sevoflurane was intermittently inhaled to maintain the BIS value at 40–60. The intraoperative arterial blood gas analysis results are presented in Table 62.1.

After the aortic cross-clamp was released, the heart resumed spontaneously beating and sinus rhythm without defibrillation. Dopamine at 5.0 μg/(kg·min) was initiated to maintain blood pressure at 74/51 mm Hg, HR at 132 beats/min, and CVP at 10 cm H_2O. During the post-parallel circulation of CBP, the safe blood level in the oxygenator blood reservoir could not be sustained. Then, ABP suddenly dropped to 40–45/32–38 mm Hg, HR rose to 150–164 beats/min, SpO_2 transiently decreased to 89%, and airway pressure rose to 26 cm H_2O. Although VT could be maintained around 80 mL, there were no significant changes in ECG. The surgeon conducted intrathoracic suction, but no hemothorax was found. No surgical bleeding and venous drainage obstruction were confirmed after repetitive adjustment of tube position. A significant reduction in heart volume was found by direct observation. Furthermore, transesophageal echocardiography indicated insufficient blood volume and a high dynamic state in the left ventricle. The CBP team tried to solve this issue by adding 50 mL of crystalloid into the oxygenator blood reservoir, but normal blood levels could still not be maintained. At this time, large patches of flushing on both sides of the head and large patches of urticaria on both sides of the neck and shoulder were found, indicating a severe allergic reaction. Subsequently, 100 mL of Ringer's acetate was rapidly infused via the femoral vein. At the same time, phenylephrine 10 μg and 0.1 μg/(kg·min) of epinephrine, 10 μg/(kg·min) of dopamine were administered through the internal jugular vein. Additionally, methylprednisolone 40 mg was intravenously infused via the peripheral vein; calcium gluconate was also intermittently injected with a total of 500 mg. After the aforementioned treatments, the blood pressure was gradually increased to 60–78/42–59 mm Hg, HR was stabilized at 145–155 beats/min, and SpO_2 rose to 95–98%. Airway pressure was decreased to 18 cm H_2O. There were no significant abnormalities in ECG. The blood products in the CBP priming fluid as the allergen were suspected. The post-parallel circulation of CBP was promptly terminated after the vital signs became stabilized and the autologous blood salvage was discarded. Protamine 60 mg was slowly infused via the right jugular vein to neutralize heparin.

Table 62.1 Intraoperative blood gas test results

Time point	FiO_2 (%)	pH	PaO_2 (mm Hg)	$PaCO_2$ (mm Hg)	BE	HCT (%)	K^+ (mmol/L)	Ca^{2+} (mmol/L)	Lac (mmol/L)	Cl^- (mmol/L)	HCO_3^- (mmol/L)
After intubation	60	7.35	223.7	42.8	−2.53	32.3	3.50	1.17	1.6	103	28.1
After ultrafiltration	60	7.36	70.2	46.2	1.46	33.2	3.51	1.12	1.7	102	24.2

The arterial blood gas analysis result (refer to Table 62.1) showed the oxygen partial pressure was 70.2 mm Hg, which might be attributed to the airway edema and exudation caused by the allergic reaction. Therefore, the FiO_2 was increased. The positive end-expiratory pressure (PEEP) 6.0 cm H_2O was applied. The sternum was closed after an adequate hemostasis. Then, the child was transferred to the Cardiac Intensive Care Unit (CICU) with an intravenous infusion of epinephrine at 0.1 μg/(kg·min) and dopamine at 10 μg/(kg·min). Vital signs remained stable during the transfer.

62.3 Postoperative Outcome

The surgery lasted a total of 150 min, including 33 min of CBP and 4 min of aortic cross-clamp. The estimated blood loss was approximately 150 mL. The urine output was 120 mL. Transfusion included 350 mL of Ringer's acetate, 150 mL of red blood cell suspension, and 100 mL of fresh frozen plasma. Before leaving the operating room, the patient's vital signs were as follows: ABP 75/41 mm Hg, HR 152 beats/min, SpO_2 96%, CVP 11 cm H_2O, and rectal temperature 36.3 °C. After the patient was admitted to the CICU, crystalloid remained the primary fluid input and blood products were still avoided. The child's blood pressure remained stable, and the urine output was normal. There were no recurring symptoms, such as skin flushing or urticaria. Endotracheal intubation was successfully removed on the postoperative day 1. The patient was transferred to the general ward on postoperative day 3 and discharged from the hospital on postoperative day 5.

62.4 Review of Knowledge Points

62.4.1 Allergic Reactions

Allergic reactions are systemic hypersensitive responses triggered by some specific substances. They often occur suddenly and unpredictably, which can pose a life-threatening risk to children, particularly in those severe cases. According to literature reports, the incidence of allergic reactions ranges from 1:10,000 to 1:20,000, but perioperative allergic reactions in children are less common, which is estimated at around 1:37,000.

The mechanism of allergic reactions involves the breakdown of immune tolerance to allergens and leads to the subsequent immune responses mediated by IgE and/or non-IgE. In IgE-mediated allergy, the initial exposure to an allergen can activate B cells to produce specific IgE antibodies (sIgE), which then bind to mast cells and basophils and sensitize them. Once the allergen is exposed again, the bound allergen can trigger the degranulation of sensitized mast cells and basophils and cause the release of histamine and other inflammatory mediators. This cascade of events results in various allergic symptoms such as urticaria, angioedema, bronchospasm, and laryngospasm. The mechanism of non-IgE-mediated allergies is not yet fully understood, but it involves immune responses independent of IgE antibodies.

The clinical manifestations of perioperative allergic reactions mainly involve the cardiovascular, respiratory, and skin. Acute cardiopulmonary dysfunction is a hallmark of severe allergic reactions, which can present as bronchospasm, upper airway edema (angioedema), hypotension, and even cardiac arrest. Once a severe allergic reaction occurs, it is essential to stop the suspected allergen immediately, along with sufficient fluid volume and vasoactive drugs to stabilize the hemodynamics, the relief of bronchospasm, the effective ventilation, and intravenous administration of adrenal corticosteroids, which are often combined antihistamines.

62.4.2 Allergic Reactions During CBP

Levy and others reported that the incidence of allergic reactions in children undergoing CBP surgery was about 0.46%, which is notably higher than in children undergoing noncardiac surgery; among the allergens encountered during CBP cardiac surgery, antibiotics, colloidal fluids, muscle relaxants, protamine, blood products, and morphine rank in decreasing order of incidence for allergic reactions. According to Ford and others, in cases where children undergoing CBP surgery experience allergic reactions, skin manifestations constitute 70% of the cases, while bronchospasm occurs in 21%. Notably, all affected children experience severe hypotension. Additionally, 9% of children may experience cardiac arrest, which requires cardiac compression, defibrillation, and urgent establishment of CBP. It is crucial to differentiate between allergic reactions and venous drainage obstruction during CBP surgery. The rapid decrease in the oxygenator's blood reservoir level is an important indicator of allergic reaction. The decrease of mean arterial pressure without improvement event with an increased perfusion flow rate and the dynamic rise of hematocrit may be related to the capillary dilation and the increased permeability induced by allergic reactions, which results in fluid redistribution into the interstitial space. In those children with preexisting heart failure and compromised cardiopulmonary reserve, it is very challenging to differentiate cardiopulmonary failure from perioperative allergic reactions and the symptoms of underlying diseases during cardiac surgery. Therefore, diagnosing perioperative allergic reactions during cardiac surgery is very difficult.

62.5 Discussion

62.5.1 Preoperative Assessment and Preparation

It is very important to understand the history of allergy prior to surgery. Children with prior allergies to penicillin, barbiturates, protein drugs, fish, and seafood are at higher risk of experiencing allergic reactions during the perioperative period. In this particular case, the parents denied any history of drug or food allergies during the preoperative assessment. However, given the diverse array of medications utilized in CBP surgery, allergic reactions to various drugs and blood products remain inevitable. Hence, it is still necessary to make appropriate preparations for allergic reactions.

62.5.2 Diagnosis and Treatment of Allergic Reactions During CBP

During CBP surgery, it is easy to find that the blood level in the oxygenator reservoir decreases. In this particular pediatric case, the blood pressure decrease was also noted, indicating potential causes, such as absolute volume deficiency, insufficient cardiac output, or vasodilation/fluid leakage (relative volume deficiency). First, a cardiac surgeon should rule out the absolute volume deficiency due to blood loss or the poor venous return related to the blood level decrease in the oxygenator decrease. Second, the CBP perfusionist should exclude issues like poor venous return and inadequate perfusion flow. In addition, the ultrasound physician noted an inadequate heart filling without cardiac output. Therefore, it was concluded that vasodilation or fluid leakage might be the main reason causing low blood pressure. Considering the child's skin manifestations, increased airway pressure, and decreased oxygen saturation, it was very possible that an allergic reaction occurred. The blood products in the prefilled fluid were speculated to trigger the allergic reaction. Then, the CBP and ultrafiltration were stopped immediately to eliminate the suspected allergen. To prevent or avoid the great risk of aortic air embolism resulting from an insufficient blood level in the oxygenator reservoir, the CBP perfusionist immediately added the crystalloid fluid to raise the blood level of the oxygenator reservoir and replenish the child's blood volume. Simultaneously, epinephrine was administered via the venous pump to alleviate bronchial smooth muscle spasms by stimulating the epinephrine β_2 receptors. Stimulation of epinephrine α receptor can cause vasoconstriction, cardiac output increase by myocardial excitation, and inhibition of inflammatory mediator release. Adrenal cortex hormones exert potent anti-inflammatory effects. Despite the large dose of dexamethasone included in the prefilled fluid of the CBP system, the onset of action is slow. Therefore, methylprednisolone, which acts more rapidly, was administered during the procedure. The use of antihistamines during the operation was deemed to be controversial. Therefore, the antihistamines were omitted in his patient. Norepinephrine and dopamine were utilized to rapidly elevate the patient's blood pressure and minimize the duration of inadequate perfusion. Empirically, calcium gluconate was administered to alleviate the allergic reactions while enhancing the blood pressure.

62.6 Shortcomings and Limitations

Due to the conditions, the blood samples were not collected for further analysis to confirm the allergic reaction and identify the specific allergen in this case. Typically, the blood samples are collected at intervals of 1, 2, and 24 h following the onset of an allergic reaction to assess for the presence of tryptase, which can help confirm the occurrence of an allergic reaction. Additionally, a skin test is recommended after an allergic reaction occurs 4–6 weeks and the patient has returned to normal condition to pinpoint the specific allergen. In this scenario, the suspected allergen was presumed to be a blood product after excluding medications administered during the procedure based on clinical expertise, given the absence of blood samples for analysis during the operation.

62.7 Conclusion

In summary, a rapid decrease in the blood level of the oxygenator reservoir during CPB, along with the blood pressure drop and the increase in airway pressure, may indicate a severe allergic reaction after excluding causes such as bleeding. In such cases, the main methods to treat severe allergic reactions during CPB are eliminating the suspected allergen, replenishing volume, and administering epinephrine, bronchodilators, and adrenal cortex hormones (Lu Wang).

Part III

Discussion of Anesthesia Cases for Congenital Heart Disease Undergoing Non-cardiac Surgery

Anesthetic Management of Common Bile Duct Exploration in Infants with Tetralogy of Fallot

63

Zhezhe Peng

Abstract

A 2-month-old male infant with jaundice was admitted for common bile duct exploration under general anesthesia. The infant also had uncorrected tetralogy of Fallot (TOF). Preoperative laboratory tests showed elevated serum alanine aminotransferase, aspartate aminotransferase, direct bilirubin, and abnormal coagulation function. Due to the presence of intracardiac shunting and partial obstruction of the right ventricular outflow tract, extra attention should be paid to prevent hypoxic episodes and the effects of hepatic impairment and jaundice on drug metabolism and interaction when the patient with uncorrected TOF undergoes noncardiac surgeries.

Tetralogy of Fallot (TOF) is the most common form of cyanotic congenital heart disease combined with ventricular septal defect, obstruction of the right ventricular outflow tract, aortic straddle, and right ventricular hypertrophy. Although TOF is one of the first to successfully correct congenital heart diseases, the best timing to perform corrective cardiac surgery for TOF patients is still controversial. Therefore, more and more TOF patients have the possibility to receive noncardiac surgeries prior to TOF correction. Intracardiac shunt, partial obstruction of the right ventricular outflow tract, and "Tet spell" make the anesthesia of TOF patients for noncardiac surgeries very challenging. This chapter reports the anesthetic management of a TOF infant undergoing common bile duct exploration.

63.1 Case Presentation

The patient was a male, 2 months and 19 days old, weighing 6.1 kg, had a full-term cesarean section, and had no history of asphyxia. After birth, he gradually developed jaundice accompanied by clay-colored stools and progressively worsened. He was then brought to the local hospital for medical treatment, and magnetic resonance imaging showed that the common bile duct and gallbladder were unclear. Biliary atresia could not be ruled out. He was treated with hormone shock, anti-infection, liver protection, and cholagogic therapy. After treatment, his clay-colored stools were slightly better than before. Echocardiography suggested ① ventricular septal defect; ② pulmonary artery stenosis; ③ patent foramen ovale. For further diagnosis and treatment, he was admitted to our hospital with the

Z. Peng (✉)
The National Children's Medical Center (Shanghai), Department of Anesthesiology of Shanghai Children's Medical Center, Shanghai Jiao Tong University School of Medicine, Shanghai, China
e-mail: pengzhezhe@scmc.com.cn

J. Zheng et al. (eds.), *Selected Pediatric Cardiovascular Surgery Anesthesia Cases*,
https://doi.org/10.1007/978-981-96-5614-1_63

preliminary diagnosis of "jaundice, congenital heart disease," and symptomatic treatment such as liver protection and cholagogic therapy was given.

Physical examination: The patient was conscious, responsive, and well-nourished, with cyanotic lips, jaundiced skin, and sclera. A grade III/VI systolic murmur could be heard in the precordial area.

Laboratory tests: Hemoglobin 164 g/L, hematocrit 51.3%; liver function showed prealbumin 0.17 g/L, total protein 62.3 g/L, TBIL 287.1 μmol/L, DBIL 167.8 μmol/L, ALT 224 IU/L, AST 542 IU/L, GGT 37 U/L, ALKP 742 IU/L; PT 12.3 s, APTT 65.4 s, INR 1.14; kidney function was normal.

Electrocardiogram: Right axis deviation, right atrial hypertrophy, right ventricular hypertrophy.

Echocardiography: Right atrium and right ventricle enlargement, right ventricular wall thickening, good left ventricular systolic function (LVEF 74.3%, LVFS 40.7%). Ventricular septal defect 0.63 cm, malposition type, bidirectional shunt with right-to-left shunt predominance; aortic enlargement, annulus 1.1 cm, straddling the ventricular septum (less than 50%); pulmonary valve stenosis, main pulmonary artery trunk diameter 0.58 cm, flow rate 4.71 m/s, pressure difference 89 mm Hg; left pulmonary artery diameter 0.45 cm, right pulmonary artery diameter 0.62 cm. Normal atrioventricular valve. Patent ductus arteriosus, pulmonary artery end about 0.18 cm, left-to-right shunt velocity 2.75 m/s.

Abdominal ultrasound: Small gallbladder, enlarged liver, dense parenchymal echo.

Hepatobiliary scintigraphy: General radioactive uptake in the liver, no obvious imaging of the gallbladder and intestines (up to 24 h after the tracer injection).

Preoperative diagnosis: Jaundice, tetralogy of Fallot, and elective common bile duct exploration were proposed.

63.2 Anesthetic Management

No preoperative medications were administrated. Routine monitoring was performed before anesthesia. Noninvasive blood pressure (BP) was 96/55 mm Hg, heart rate (HR) was 146 beats/min, and pulse oxygen saturation (SpO_2) was 89%. Anesthesia induction was conducted with etomidate 2.0 mg, fentanyl 10 μg, and cisatracurium 0.6 mg intravenously. After the eyelash reflex disappeared, an ID 3.5 mm cuffed endotracheal tube was intubated under direct laryngoscopy. The depth of intubation was 11 cm. Pressure-controlled ventilation-volume guaranteed (PCV-VG) mode was adopted with 1 L/min oxygen flow, 50% inhaled oxygen concentration (FiO_2), 60 mL tidal volume (VT), 24 breaths/min respiratory rate (RR), 1:2 inhalation to exhalation ratio (I:E), and about 35 mm Hg end-tidal carbon dioxide pressure ($ETCO_2$). Ultrasound-guided left radial artery catheterization was performed for continuous invasive arterial monitoring and arterial blood gas analysis. Based on the blood gas test result (Table 63.1), 12 mL 5% $NaHCO_3$ was intravenously administered to correct acidosis. The left external jugular vein catheterization was established for rapid fluid infusion. The duration of the operation was 30 min, 1–2 MAC of sevoflurane was inhaled for anesthesia maintenance, and the Bispectral Index (BIS) varied between 40 and 60. The patient's initial BP was 91/52 mm Hg, HR was 133 beats/min, and SpO_2 was 97%. The patient's vital signs were stable during the operation.

Table 63.1 Intraoperative blood gas test results

Time point	pH	PaO_2 (mm Hg)	$PaCO_2$ (mm Hg)	BE (mmol/L)	HCT (%)	K^+ (mmol/L)	Ca^{2+} (mmol/L)	Cl^- (mmol/L)	Lac (mmol/L)	HCO_3^- (mmol/L)
Admission	7.35	98	35.2	−4.2	43.2	3.9	1.15	108	0.4	22.3
Discharge	7.42	94	32.1	−2.2	39.3	3.6	1.11	112	1.0	24.7

After the operation, arterial blood gas was rechecked (Table 63.1) to assess the patient's internal environment.

63.3 Postoperative Outcome

The operation lasted a total of 30 min. During the operation, the liver showed obvious cholestasis and small nodules, and a liver biopsy was performed. The gallbladder was shrunken with a small amount of pale-yellow bile. Cholangiography showed that the contrast agent could enter the duodenum, but the common hepatic duct and left and right hepatic ducts were not visible, confirming biliary atresia. The intraoperative blood loss was small. Fifty milliliter acetate Ringer's solution was infused in total. The ventilation mode was switched to synchronized intermittent mandatory ventilation with pressure-controlled ventilation-volume guaranteed (SIMV PCV-VG) at the end of surgery after cleaning up tracheal and oral secretions. The respiratory rate was gradually reduced to four times/minute. When SpO_2 was over 92% with air inhalation, $ETCO_2$ was 42 mm Hg, and the child could open his eyes by calling his name; the endotracheal tube was then removed, and the child was transferred to the anesthesia recovery room. One hour later, the child's Aldrete score reached 9 points, and then he was transferred back to the ward. The child was discharged smoothly on the third day after surgery.

63.4 Review of Knowledge Points

63.4.1 Congenital Biliary Atresia

Congenital biliary atresia is the main cause of long-term obstructive jaundice in newborns, leading to cholestatic cirrhosis and, ultimately, liver failure. It is the most common indication for pediatric liver transplantation. Typical cases of biliary atresia are full-term infants with normal stool color at birth, and jaundice generally appears gradually in the next 2–3 weeks. Once jaundice appears, it usually deepens day by day. In some cases, clubbing or cyanosis may occur. The liver of the affected child is enlarged, but in the early stages, a hard spleen is rarely palpable. If the spleen is palpable in the first few weeks, it may be due to portal hypertension caused by the progression of intrahepatic disease. In the early stages of the disease, the overall condition of the infant is still good, but with varying degrees of malnutrition. The chief complaint of the infant is excitable and restless with the complications of being underweight and undergrown. In children with congenital biliary atresia, the disease progresses rapidly after birth due to the complete failure to drain bile, causing progressive liver damage and leading to irreversible biliary cirrhosis after 3 months, so surgery should be performed as soon as possible after birth to drain the bile.

63.4.2 Pathophysiology of TOF

TOF is a common cyanotic congenital heart disease, accounting for 10% of congenital heart diseases in newborns and 30% of cyanotic congenital heart diseases. The main lesions of TOF are ventricular septal defect, obstruction of the right ventricular outflow tract, aortic override, and right ventricular hypertrophy. Hypoxia is the main basis for the pathophysiological changes of TOF. Cases of TOF that show severe cyanosis shortly after birth may be due to underdevelopment of the pulmonary valve ring, causing outflow tract obstruction. The earlier systemic hypoxemia occurs, the greater the possibility of the right ventricular outflow tract obstruction or atresia. The key factors determining whether TOF can be surgically corrected are the anatomical condition of the patient's right ventricular outflow tract and the development of the pulmonary artery, not the age and weight of the patient.

63.5 Discussion

63.5.1 Preoperative Assessment and Preparation

For children with TOF undergoing noncardiac surgery, it is necessary to fully understand the medical history, assess the risk of surgical anesthesia, and adjust the function of important organs before surgery. In this case, the child was suspected of having obstructive jaundice, with severely abnormal preoperative liver function indicators and prolonged coagulation indicators, posing a risk of bleeding. The infant was treated with liver protection and cholagogic therapy before surgery. Since the child can maintain an oxygen saturation of SpO_2 over 85% without oxygen therapy, no special treatment has been given to his heart disease for the time being. On the day of the surgery, the child was given intravenous rehydration after fasting to avoid exacerbating cyanosis due to metabolic acidosis.

63.5.2 Choices of Anesthetics

Since the child's preoperative test indicated abnormal liver function, the situation might be further worse by the choice of anesthesia methods and drugs. The liver is the main site of drug biotransformation, and liver dysfunction will affect the distribution and elimination of drugs. The degree of liver dysfunction and the binding force of drugs to plasma proteins are the main factors determining the pharmacokinetic parameters in children with liver disease. In addition to minimal impact on respiratory and cardiovascular systems, good sedation and analgesic effects with fewer types of anesthetic drugs should also be considered. Furthermore, hypoxia and liver ischemia should be avoided or reduced since they can aggravate liver damage. Anesthetics primarily metabolized in the liver may have a prolonged half-life in patients with liver dysfunction. Therefore, it is better to choose the anesthetics that are less or not metabolized or easily excreted by the liver and have little impact on the circulatory system. Cisatracurium is a non-depolarizing neuromuscular blocking agent of the benzylisoquinolinium class with an intermediate duration of action. Cisatracurium is metabolized organ independently, mainly through Hofmann elimination, and is suitable for patients with liver dysfunction. Sevoflurane is a relatively potent inhalational anesthetic with a lower blood/gas partition coefficient and less irritating odor, making it the preferred inhalational agent for pediatric anesthesia due to its faster induction of anesthesia and lesser complications. The depth of anesthesia can be easily adjusted by turning the sevoflurane vaporizer. Most sevoflurane is excreted through the respiratory tract without metabolism, and only 3% of sevoflurane is metabolized by the liver and kidney. It should be noted that some scholars have pointed out that the expression and function of P450 enzymes in children with obstructive jaundice may be impaired, the activity of CYP3A4 isoenzymes decreases, and the minimum alveolar concentration (MAC) also decreases; however, other studies suggest that the recovery time of pure sevoflurane inhalational anesthesia in children with obstructive jaundice is prolonged, but without clinical significance.

63.5.3 Intraoperative Anesthetic Management

The principles of TOF anesthetic management are to maintain vascular volume and avoid the decrease of SVR with/without the increase of PVR (such as acidosis or excessive airway pressure). Increasing the PVR/SVR ratio for any reason can increase the right to left shunt, reduce pulmonary blood flow, and exacerbate cyanosis. For children with small TOF shunts, inhalation anesthesia induction can be tolerated, but the uptake time of inhalation anesthesia is relatively slow, while the onset of intravenous anesthetics is relatively fast, but transient high blood drug concentrations should be avoided. Volume expansion can be achieved through intravenous fluid infusion to prevent hemoconcentration. If hypoxia occurs during surgery, a relatively large dose of phenylephrine 5.0–10 μg/kg can be administered intravenously or infused at 2–5 μg/(kg·min) to increase systemic vascular resistance and reduce right-to-left shunting; subcutaneous injection morphine 0.1 mg/kg can effectively relieve infundibular spasm and improve hypoxemia; sodium bicarbonate can correct metabolic acidosis, restore normal SVR, and help alleviate the severity and duration of hypoxemia; respiratory management is also helpful to control PVR. About 100% oxygen inhalation is recommended as soon as a hypoxic spell. Lower peak inspiratory pressure, slower respiratory rate, and lower intrathoracic pressure, etc., can increase venous return.

63.6 Conclusion

In summary, the anesthetic management of children with TOF combined with extracardiac malformations should be based on the pathophysiology of TOF itself. Choose anesthetics with the least impact on cardiac function, minimize right-to-left shunting, and prevent hypoxic episodes. The principle of organ protection should be followed as far as possible when using drugs, and precise management should be implemented based on intraoperative monitoring (Zhezhe Peng).

64 Anesthetic Management of Palatopharyngoplasty in a Child with Ventricular Septal Defect

Zhezhe Peng

Abstract

A one-year-old boy was diagnosed with a cleft palate and ventricular septal defect after birth and was scheduled for cleft palate repair under general anesthesia. The child also has microtia and mandibular retrognathia. The key points of perioperative anesthetic management, in this case, are the control of the difficult airway and hemodynamic changes related to intracardiac shunting in congenital heart disease.

Cleft palate is a common maxillofacial deformity in infants and young children, with an incidence of 1/2000 in live births. Among them, the incidence of cleft palate deformity accompanied by congenital heart disease is as high as 3–5%. Ventricular septal defect (VSD) causes right ventricular volume overload and increased pulmonary blood flow due to left-to-right shunting at the ventricular level. This article introduces the anesthetic management of palatopharyngoplasty in a child with ventricular septal defect.

Z. Peng (✉)
The National Children's Medical Center (Shanghai), Department of Anesthesiology of Shanghai Children's Medical Center, Shanghai Jiao Tong University School of Medicine, Shanghai, China
e-mail: pengzhezhe@scmc.com.cn

J. Zheng et al. (eds.), *Selected Pediatric Cardiovascular Surgery Anesthesia Cases*,
https://doi.org/10.1007/978-981-96-5614-1_64

64.1 Case Presentation

The boy was 1 year and 4 days old, weighing 9.18 kg. He was delivered by cesarean section at 36 weeks, with no history of asphyxia. The child was found to have a cleft palate and ventricular septal defect after birth and has been followed up to date. The child's weight and age now meet the surgical requirements, so he was admitted to the hospital for elective palatopharyngoplasty.

Physical examination: The child is conscious, mentally normal, and moderately nourished. Appearance shows microtia, and no obvious abnormalities in the upper lip and external nose; the oral cavity shows a cleft palate and the widest part of the cleft is about 1.5 cm. Neck mobility is normal; thyromental distance is short, mandibular retrognathia, and the width of incisors with mouth open maximally is three fingers. Auscultation reveals a systolic heart murmur at the left sternal border 3–4 intercostal spaces.

Laboratory tests: Hemoglobin 127 g/L, white blood cell count 12.87 × 10^9/L, lymphocytes 50.8% in blood routine test. Liver and kidney functions are normal; coagulation function is also normal.

Electrocardiogram: Sinus tachycardia, T wave notch at the top.

Echocardiography: LVEF 66.51%, pulmonary artery enlargement, total trunk inner diameter 1.54 cm, valve movement is good, tricuspid valve has mild regurgitation, maximum regurgitation pressure difference 32 mm Hg, pulmonary artery systolic pressure 37 mm Hg, ventricular septal defect 0.5 cm (muscular outflow tract, near the ventricular crest), left to right shunt, shunt speed 4.37 m/s, left aortic arch.

Chest X-ray: Increased and blurred lung markings in both lungs.

Neck CT: Fissure-like changes are seen in the middle of the soft and hard palate, the trachea is normal in shape, no obvious abnormalities are seen in the attachments of the cervical vertebrae, fluid accumulation in the mastoid on both sides, thickening of the sinus mucosa.

Preoperative diagnosis: Palatal cleft, ventricular septal defect. Planned to undergo palatopharyngoplasty.

64.2 Anesthetic Management

The child had no preoperative medication. and the vital signs were routinely monitored before anesthesia with noninvasive blood pressure (BP) 108/68 mm Hg, heart rate (HR) 148 beats/min, and pulse oxygen saturation (SpO_2) 98%. Midazolam 0.5 mg and etomidate 2.5 mg were injected intravenously. After the child fell asleep, the mask ventilation was given to confirm that there was no difficulty in mask ventilation. Then, fentanyl 20 μg and rocuronium 5.5 mg were continuously injected intravenously. After the child's eyelash reflex disappeared, a direct laryngoscope was inserted. It was difficult to expose the glottis, Cormack–Lehane grade IV. A visual laryngoscope was changed to expose the glottis with cricoid pressure. The epiglottis and the glottic notch could be seen. After two attempts, an ID 4.0 mm cuffed reinforced endotracheal tube was inserted with a tube depth of 13 cm. Pressure-controlled ventilation-volume guaranteed (PCV-VG) ventilation mode was used with oxygen flow rate 1 L/min, inhaled oxygen concentration (FiO_2) 50%, tidal volume (VT) 90 mL, respiratory rate (RR) 20 times/min, inhalation to exhalation ratio (I:E) 1:2, positive end-expiratory pressure (PEEP) 4 cm H_2O, end-tidal carbon dioxide partial pressure ($ETCO_2$) 35–40 mm Hg.

Invasive arterial pressure (ABP) and arterial blood gas analysis (Table 64.1) were established after the left radial artery catheterization. The left great saphenous vein was catheterized for rapid fluid replacement. Anesthesia was maintained by intravenous infusion of propofol 4.0 mg/(kg·h), remifentanil 0.3 μg/(kg·min), and sevoflurane inhalation. The child's initial ABP was 86/52 mm Hg, HR 117 beats/min, and SpO_2 99%. Before the skin incision, tranexamic acid 10 mg/kg was injected intravenously. After the surgeon used lidocaine combined with epinephrine for a palatal plate separation block, the major blood vessels and nerve bundles of the palate were stripped and loosened, the muscle layer was separated, and layered sutures were performed. During the palatopharyngoplasty, the amount of bleeding was closely monitored. Arterial blood gas was rechecked during the operation (Table 64.1), and corrections were made based on the results.

Table 64.1 Intraoperative blood gas test results

Time point	pH	PaO_2 (mm Hg)	$PaCO_2$ (mm Hg)	BE (mmol/L)	HCT (%)	K^+ (mmol/L)	Ca^{2+} (mmol/L)	Cl^- (mmol/L)	Lac (mmol/L)	HCO_3^- (mmol/L)
After intubation	7.38	226	37.3	−3.6	35.6	3.7	1.15	105	0.6	23.2
During surgery	7.37	194	38.1	−3.9	33.5	3.6	1.10	110	0.9	22.6

64.3 Postoperative Outcome

The operation lasted 50 min with an estimated blood loss of about 20 mL, urine output of 30 mL, and a total infusion of 150 mL of acetate Ringer's solution. The ventilation mode was switched to synchronized intermittent mandatory ventilation with pressure-controlled ventilation-volume guaranteed (SIMV PCV-VG) at the end of surgery and cleaning up tracheal and oral secretions. The respiratory rate was gradually reduced to four times per minute. When SpO_2 was over 95% with air inhalation, $ETCO_2$ was 42 mm Hg. The child could open his eyes in response to calling; the endotracheal tube was then removed, and the child was transferred to the anesthesia recovery room. About 70minutes later, the child was fully awake, the Aldrete score reached 10 points, and he was escorted back to the ward. The child recovered well and was discharged on the third day after surgery.

64.4 Review of Knowledge Points

64.4.1 Cleft Palate

The cleft palate is one of the most common maxillofacial deformities in infants and young children. Surgical repair is recommended before the development of normal language function, usually at 9–18 months of age. It has been reported that cleft palate deformity is related to nearly 150 syndromes, among which craniofacial syndromes are more common, and the child may have difficult airway manifestations. Cleft lip and palate may be associated with congenital heart disease, more common with atrial septal defects and ventricular septal defects. Cardiac malformations may not be easily recognized in the absence of cyanosis. Since most children with cleft palate have feeding difficulty, their overall nutritional status, growth, and development often lag behind their peers. Furthermore, these children are prone to reflux after feeding and cause chronic rhinorrhea, which is sometimes difficult to distinguish from symptoms of respiratory tract infection.

64.4.2 Ventricular Septal Defect

A ventricular septal defect is caused by incomplete development of the embryonic ventricular septum (inflow tract, trabecular part, and outflow tract) and is the most common congenital heart disease. The clinical manifestations of children with VSD are related to the size of the defect, the amount of left-to-right shunt, and pulmonary vascular resistance. Children with a shunt index (Qp/Qs) less than 1.5 and normal pulmonary artery pressure usually have no symptoms, normal activity and growth development, and an extremely low possibility of bacterial endocarditis. Therefore, surgery can be appropriately delayed, and follow-up can be carried out. For VSD patients with accompanying symptoms, such as Qp/Qs greater than 2, increased pulmonary artery pressure, and slightly increased pulmonary vascular resistance, early surgery should be considered to prevent irreversible changes in the pulmonary vessels.

64.5 Discussion

64.5.1 Preoperative Assessment and Preparation

The medical history and physical examination should be fully obtained during the preoperative assessment of children with cleft palate and VSD. The medical history should focus on the types and complications of cardiovascular disease, drug treatment history, previous hospitalizations, surgical operations or other interventions, allergy history, anesthesia experience, complications, etc. Anesthesiologists should observe whether the child has symptoms such as shortness of breath, tachycardia, and easy fatigue. Infants are characterized by feeding difficulty and sweating, while older children mainly show decreased activity levels or exercise intolerance. Recent respiratory infections or lung diseases in the child can increase the possibility of perioperative complications. Echocardiography, electrocardiogram, and neck CT are helpful to understand the size and location of the child's intracardiac defect, the degree of shunting, pulmonary artery pressure, and airway development. The preoperative visit found that the child had a small lower jaw and small ear deformity, indicating the possibility of a difficult airway. It was often impossible to assess the Mallampati airway classification due to the child's noncooperation.

64.5.2 Difficult Tracheal Intubation

To ensure the anesthesia safety of children with cleft palate, it is critical for anesthesiologists to predict the possibility of difficult tracheal intubation accurately. The laryngoscopy's convex edge is often embedded in the cleft, making it difficult for the laryngoscopy to move in the throat and possibly cause tissue damage and bleeding in children with cleft palate. Using a curved laryngoscope with a low convex edge, such as a Robert–Shaw or Oxford laryngoscope, is attributed to ease this problem. However, in most cases, a standard straight Miller laryngoscope can meet the needs of children with enough space in the oropharynx, and this can also be solved by padding with gauze. During the preoperative assessment, it was found that the child might have difficulty in intubation, and the anesthesiologist decided to use a visual laryngoscope in case of intubation failure by direct laryngoscope. After two attempts of glottis exposure with cricoid pressure, the endotracheal tube was finally intubated and properly fixed. Although the child's head was covered with a surgical towel during the operation, carefully monitoring the changes in end-tidal carbon dioxide waveform can indicate the possibilities of tracheal tube twisting, bending, and slippage.

64.5.3 Anesthetic Management During Surgery

Children with VSD often have right ventricular volume overload and increased pulmonary blood flow due to the existence of the left-to-right shunt. Therefore, SVR increase and PVR decrease during anesthesia should be avoided in order to prevent the reduction of effective systemic circulation blood volume and increment of the pulmonary blood flow, and exacerbate the anterior and posterior loads of the right ventricle. Adequate application of opioids such as fentanyl can effectively decrease stress reactions with stable hemodynamics during intravenous induction. Adjusting ventilation parameters is also an effective method to regulate pulmonary vascular resistance. During the operation, we adjust the ventilation parameters by monitoring arterial blood gas and end-tidal carbon dioxide, avoiding hyperventilation to prevent an increase in left-to-right shunt.

Oropharyngeal suction through the nose should be avoided for cleaning the child's secretions and blood at the end of the surgery. Oropharyngeal airway placement is also not advocated after extubation to avoid damaging the surgical incision. For children with moderate to severe airway obstruction symptoms before surgery, tongue suspension surgery can be considered to prevent postoperative airway obstruction.

64.6 Conclusion

The anesthetic management of children with VSD combined with cleft palate should be based on the pathophysiology of VSD and airway condition. Anesthesiologists should choose anesthetics with the least impact on heart function. Maintaining heart rate, myocardial contractility, and preload to ensure cardiac output is important. Avoiding a decrease in the PVR: SVR ratio to maintain effective systemic circulation is also critical. Volume management should be guided by intraoperative monitoring indicators. It is essential to fully assess the child's airway condition and formulate an effective airway management plan to ensure the child's safety (Zhezhe Peng).

Anesthetic Management of Exploratory Laparotomy Due to Intestinal Perforation in a Child with Persistent Truncus Arteriosus

65

Yong Bian

Abstract

A 4-month-old male infant was admitted to our hospital due to recurrent lung infections and fever. He was diagnosed with persistent truncus arteriosus (type AIII) and pulmonary infection based on echocardiography. During the anti-infection treatment, bile-like fluid and feces were drained out from the abdominal cavity, indicating the occurrence of intestinal obstruction and perforation caused by abdominal infection. Emergency exploratory laparotomy was performed under general anesthesia. The risk of heart failure and multiple organ dysfunction is significantly increased during emergency surgery for children with persistent truncus arteriosus. In treating these patients, it is imperative to maintain a balance in systemic pulmonary circulation, ensure adequate fluid resuscitation, and optimally utilize positive inotropic agents to prevent the onset of sepsis-induced shock.

Persistent truncus arteriosus (TA) is a rare congenital heart disease characterized by a single arterial trunk at the base of the heart supplying the systemic, pulmonary, and coronary circulation with a series of cardiac anatomical malformations. If the anatomical issues of these children are not corrected in time after birth, the 1-year mortality rate can be as high as 90%. Due to the significant increase in pulmonary blood flow, the probability of severe pneumonia in TA patients during the early time is very high, and a few patients may even develop septic shock. Shock accompanied by intestinal necrosis and perforation is a very severe complication that requires emergency surgery once it occurs. This chapter reports the anesthetic management of a case of intestinal perforation undergoing exploratory laparotomy complicated by persistent truncus arteriosus.

65.1 Case Presentation

The patient was a 4-month-old and 26-day-old boy with a weight of 6.0 kg. He was born full-term without asphyxia. The boy was found to have a heart murmur when he was diagnosed with pneumonia at a local hospital more than a month ago. Echocardiography indicated persistent truncus arteriosus (TA, type AIII), atrial septal defect (ASD, II), patent ductus arteriosus (PDA, left side), right aortic arch, and left pulmonary artery flow speed increase. CT scan showed persistent TA (type AIII), ventricular septal defect (VSD), ASD, PDA, stenosis of the left pul-

Y. Bian (✉)
The National Children's Medical Center (Shanghai), Department of Anesthesiology of Shanghai Children's Medical Center, Shanghai Jiao Tong University School of Medicine, Shanghai, China
e-mail: bianyong@scmc.com.cn

J. Zheng et al. (eds.), *Selected Pediatric Cardiovascular Surgery Anesthesia Cases*,
https://doi.org/10.1007/978-981-96-5614-1_65

monary artery origin, right arch, and right lung infection.

Physical examination: Auscultation of wet rales in the right middle and lower lungs, 2–3 intercostal II/VI systolic murmurs were heard, and the second heart sound of the pulmonary valve was accentuated.

Chest X-ray: Pulmonary blood flow increases. Electrocardiogram (ECG): Sinus rhythm, biatrial hypertrophy, first-degree atrioventricular block, T wave notch at the top.

The boy had repeated high fever after admission due to a lung infection. The white blood cell count was 17.13×10^9/L, with a neutrophil count of 29.0. The C-reactive protein was 29.8 mg/L. The respiratory syncytial V-RNA test was positive. Blood culture showed G^+ cocci infection. The anti-infection treatment with cefotaxime sodium and vancomycin was not effective. Furthermore, antibiotics-related adverse effects such as infectious rash and increased dyspnea occurred. He was then transferred to the intensive care unit (ICU). The child's condition became worse at night. The pulse oxygen saturation (SpO_2) was about 85% at room air. Rapid breathing, cyanosis of the face and extremities, and oliguria were also present. Invasive arterial blood pressure (ABP) dropped to 52/25 mm Hg. Considering the septic shock might occur, tracheal intubation and positive pressure ventilation with pressure control-assist control ventilation (PC-AC) mode were given. The ventilator parameters were set as follows: Fraction of inspired oxygen (FiO_2) 60%, peak airway pressure (PIP) 25 cm H_2O, positive end-expiratory pressure (PEEP) 6 cm H_2O, and respiratory rate (RR) 35 times/min. Norepinephrine 0.1 μg/(kg·min) and epinephrine 0.1 μg/(kg·min) were intravenously infused. The arterial blood gas analysis results effectively rectified the child's fluid, electrolyte, and acid–base balance disorders. ABP and SpO_2 were maintained at about 100/40 mm Hg and 79–90%, respectively. On the seventh day after entering the ICU, the child's abdomen was found to be bulging, and abdominal B-ultrasound suggested abdominal pelvic effusion, free anechoic area seen from the inter-intestinal space to the pelvis, about 50 mm at the deeper part. After the symptomatic treatment, bile-like fluid and feces were drained out from the abdominal cavity. The occurrence of intestinal obstruction and intestinal perforation caused by infection was suspected, and an emergency laparotomy was scheduled. The laboratory test showed PT 71.0 s, APTT 82.6 s, and FDP 42.3 μg/mL. Prothrombin 300 IU, fibrinogen 500 mg, and frozen plasma 1 U were intravenously infused before surgery.

65.2 Anesthetic Management

The patient was transferred to the operating room with endotracheal intubation and positive inotropic agents, including norepinephrine 0.05 μg/(kg·min) and epinephrine 0.05 μg/(kg·min). ECG, SpO_2, ABP, body temperature, and bispectral index (BIS) were routinely monitored. The primary vital signs are ABP 100/42 mm Hg, HR 138 beats/min, and SpO_2 90%. INVOS regional (renal area) tissue oxygen saturation (rSO_2) was also monitored to ensure sufficient perfusion of vital organs. Anesthesia was induced by intravenous bolus injection of midazolam 0.5 mg, etomidate 1.5 mg, sufentanil 6.0 μg, and rocuronium 4.0 mg. During the operation, propofol 4.0 mg/(kg·h) combined with sevoflurane inhalation was used for the maintenance of anesthesia with BIS at 40–60. The pressure-controlled ventilation-volume guaranteed (PCV-VG) mode was adopted with an oxygen flow rate of 1 L/min, FiO_2 50%, tidal volume (VT) 50 mL, RR 24 times/min, inspiratory-to-expiratory ratio (I:E) 1:2, PEEP 4 cm H_2O. Blood gas analysis was rechecked every 30 minutes to 1 hour during the operation (Table 65.1). The respiratory parameters were adjusted according to the blood gas analysis results to maintain SpO_2 at 85–90% and the partial pressure of end-tidal carbon dioxide ($ETCO_2$) at 40–45 mm Hg.

The right internal jugular was catheterized for intraoperative fluid replacement, central venous pressure (CVP) monitoring, and postoperative parenteral nutrition. During the operation, 5% albumin, red blood cell suspension, 5% sodium bicarbonate, and vasoactive drugs, etc. were

Table 65.1 Intraoperative blood gas test results

Time point	pH	Hb (g/dL)	HCT (%)	PaO_2 (mm Hg)	$PaCO_2$ (mm Hg)	BE (mmol/L)	Na^+ (mmol/L)	K^+ (mmol/L)	Cl^- (mmol/L)	Ca^{2+} (mmol/L)	Lac (mmol/L)
Upon admission	7.264	8.5	26.4	47	51.2	−3.9	133	3.9	103	1.32	0.9
30 min after admission	7.327	8.4	26.2	46.8	53.6	−5.4	134	4.2	107	1.28	1
60 min after admission	7.314	14	41	56.1	45.1	−2.9	131	4.4	104	1.27	1.4
90 min after admission	7.396	13.8	39.2	57.4	44.4	−3.4	130	3.9	105	1.23	2.9

intravenously infused to maintain CVP at 6–12 cm H_2O and rSO_2 (renal area) at 55–75%.

The necrosis at the descending colon, sigmoid colon, rectal wall, and a large perforation at the mesentery margin were found. The surgeon removed the necrotic intestine, and the splenic area of the colon was pulled out from the left end of the incision for a single-cavity ostomy. The entire operation went smoothly.

65.3 Postoperative Outcome

The operation lasted 110 min with blood loss of 20 mL, total infusion of Ringer's acetate solution of 60 mL, red blood cell suspension of 50 mL, and urine output of 10 mL. The child's postoperative BP was 98/42 mm Hg, HR 125 beats/min, SpO_2 88%, rectal temperature 36.5 °C, CVP 9 cm H_2O, BIS 48, and rSO_2 (renal area) 55%. The child was transferred to the intensive care unit with endotracheal intubation after the operation. Anti-infection and nutritional support was given. The endotracheal tube was removed on the 14th day after surgery. On the 28th day after surgery, the child underwent a surgery repair for persistent truncus arteriosus. The child's heart surgery went smoothly, and the postoperative recovery was good. The child was discharged from the hospital on the 27th day after heart surgery.

65.4 Review of Knowledge Points

65.4.1 Persistent Truncus Arteriosus

The anatomical basis of persistent truncus arteriosus is that the pulmonary artery and its branches, the coronary arteries, and the aorta all come from the same large artery originating from the base of the heart. At the same time, the single arterial trunk also manifests as a single semilunar valve and the corresponding ventricular septal defect at the conal septum. The underdevelopment of the semilunar valve can lead to valve regurgitation and stenosis. The malformation of the arterial trunk valve can sometimes lead to anatomical abnormalities of the coronary arteries. The incomplete separation of the arterial trunk and valve disease is closely related to increased pulmonary blood flow and ventricular dysfunction in the later stage of persistent truncus arteriosus. In addition, 30–40% of cases of persistent truncus arteriosus have a deletion of chromosome 22q11, and organs related to this chromosome, such as the thymus, parathyroid, and maxillofacial area, may also be abnormal. This chromosomal abnormality can also increase the incidence of aortic arch dysplasia, thereby increasing the pulmonary blood flow in the common trunk and further exacerbating pulmonary circulation overload in children with this cardiac anomaly.

With the reduction of pulmonary circulation resistance after birth, a large amount of arterial trunk blood flow enters the pulmonary circulation. It causes pulmonary circulation overload and heart failure in children with persistent truncus arteriosus, which is accompanied by bidirectional shunting at the ventricular level and leads to varying degrees of hypoxia. In addition, the increased pulmonary circulation blood flow increases the end-diastolic ventricular pressure and atrial pressure, making children with persistent truncus arteriosus with underdeveloped arterial valves more prone to congestive heart failure in the early stage. The pulse is usually bounding, caused by increased pulse pressure due to aortic blood flow into the pulmonary artery during diastole. High SpO_2 in these children often indicates the possibility of heart failure. It is worth noting that there may not be a significant difference in preductal or postductal SpO_2, even in cases accompanied by aortic arch stenosis or interruption, because the same artery trunk supplies both systemic and pulmonary circulation. Therefore, clinically, there is not always a significant difference in SpO_2 between the upper and lower limbs.

65.4.2 Septic Shock

The 2005 International Pediatric Consensus Conference defined septic shock as acute circulatory failure in children with sepsis, characterized by persistent hypotension (specific age < 2 standard deviations) that is difficult to resuscitate

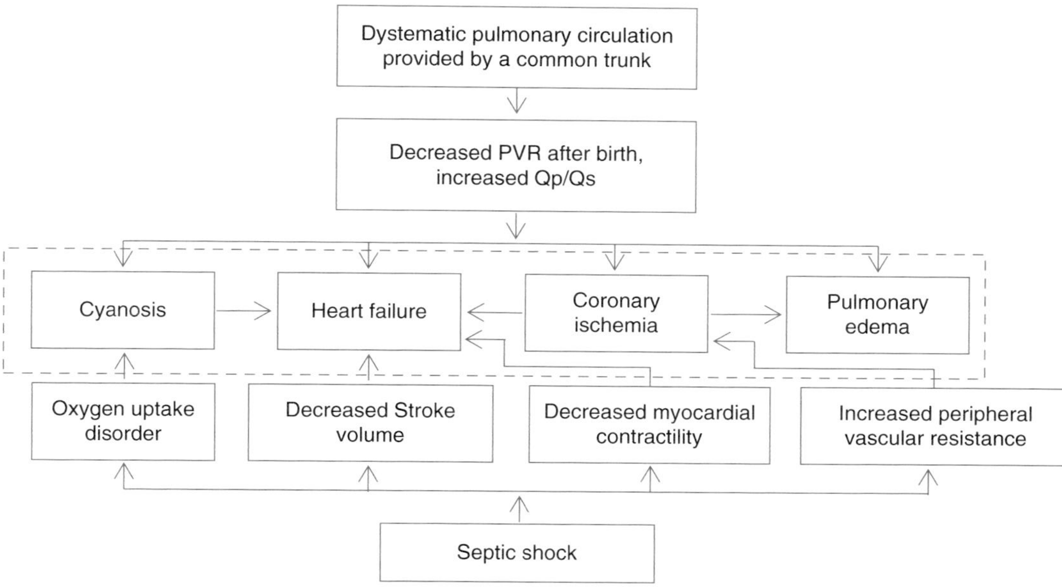

Fig. 65.1 Interaction of pathophysiology between persistent truncus arteriosus and septic shock

fully and cannot be explained by other reasons. Severe septic shock may cause intestinal complications, such as necrotizing enterocolitis, chronic pseudo-obstruction of the small intestine, intestinal fistula, and acute paralytic ileus. However, sometimes, due to the combination of other diseases, the clinical manifestations are diverse. The main manifestations are lethargy and poor peripheral circulation. Early manifestations are predominantly heat shock, while late manifestations are cold shock.

It may be accompanied by tachycardia, high fever, or low fever. Unlike adult shock, pediatric septic shock usually manifests as a decrease in cardiac output and an increase in peripheral resistance. Shock in adults is characterized by increased oxygen consumption, while shock in children shows oxygen uptake disorders and affects peripheral perfusion. This difference is fatal to children with persistent truncus arteriosus because they already have adverse factors such as tissue hypoxia and elevated lactate levels. If oxygen uptake disorder occurs, it may rapidly worsen the condition. The treatment principles include fluid resuscitation (>20 mL/kg), active anti-infection, and using vasoactive drugs and hormones. Norepinephrine is recommended for treating heat shock, and epinephrine is recommended in the guidelines for cold or indistinguishable shock. The pathophysiologic relationship between persistent truncus arteriosus and septic shock is shown in Fig. 65.1.

65.5 Discussion

65.5.1 Preoperative Assessment and Preparation

Preoperative cardiotonic, diuresis, and mechanical ventilation interventions improve the systematic-pulmonary circulation ratio to reduce pulmonary circulation overload and heart failure. Adjusting the systematic-pulmonary circulation ratio (Qp: Qs) is the key to such patients' survival. In order to balance the systematic-pulmonary circulation ratio, it is necessary to adjust the respiratory parameters to avoid over-ventilation and high oxygen concentration and maintain SpO_2 at 80–90%. Otherwise, it may aggravate pulmonary hypertension and coronary artery ischemia. The preoperative examination showed no signs of valve regurgitation and insufficiency in this patient, which benefits the coronary blood supply. This property also explains why the patient did not experience refractory arrhythmia and myocardial ischemia during the process of diagnosis and treatment. The septic shock in this patient was treated with fluid resuscitation, broad-spectrum antibiotics, and albumin. In addition, the patient had coagulation dysfunction before surgery, which may be related to tissue oxygen uptake disorder, increased lactate, liver function injury caused by protein loss due to septic shock, and tissue hypoxia exacerbated by persistent truncus arteriosus.

65.5.2 Intraoperative Anesthetic Management

The key to anesthetic management in persistent truncus arteriosus accompanied by septic shock is maintaining the systemic circulation perfusion pressure, reducing the pulmonary circulation overload, and actively treating the refractory hypotension. In the early stage of septic shock, due to peripheral vasodilation, transient warm shock symptoms may appear (warm extremities, decreased blood pressure, decreased peripheral vascular resistance, etc.). Hence, the guidelines recommend using norepinephrine to increase peripheral resistance, reduce the loss of vascular content to improve circulation, and reduce organ damage. However, for children with persistent truncus arteriosus, high doses of norepinephrine may increase the pulmonary artery shunt of the arterial trunk, exacerbate pulmonary artery hypertension, and thus induce heart failure. Some literature shows that norepinephrine can constrict both systemic and pulmonary arteries. However, its ability to constrict the aortic system is more significant than its effect on the pulmonary artery. So, the possibility of a relative increase in pulmonary blood cannot be ruled out. Therefore, in this case, titration administration was adopted when using norepinephrine and other positive inotropic agents. If it is possible, the systematic-pulmonary circulation ratio can be indirectly assessed based on SpO_2, arterial oxygen partial pressure (PaO_2), mixed venous oxygen saturation ($ScvO_2$), and bedside ultrasound technology (including cardiac and pulmonary ultrasound) to guide the use of positive inotropic agents. Due to the increase of peripheral resistance in the late stage of pediatric septic shock, capillary leakage syndrome is present with volume loss in the third space. It manifests as refractory hypotension and multiple organ failure. For children with unstable circulation due to persistent truncus arteriosus, this may further exacerbate cardiac ischemia and hypoxia and affect coronary circulation. This case showed oliguria and coagulation dysfunction symptoms, which reflected vital organ dysfunction. Secondly, patients with persistent truncus arteriosus always have poor oxygenation due to mixed arterial and venous blood, and septic shock decreases tissue oxygen utilization and exacerbates vital organ damage. Furthermore, in the late stage of septic shock, the increase of peripheral systemic circulation resistance may increase the pulmonary blood, thereby accelerating the heart failure process. Although epinephrine can maintain heart function and ensure the perfusion of vital organs such as the heart and kidneys to avoid further tissue hypoxia, we need to be alert to the increase in myocardial oxygen consumption and heart rate caused by epinephrine, which may exacerbate coronary ischemia. Therefore, on the basis of sufficient fluid resuscitation, administering epinephrine and norepinephrine can effectively maintain systemic circulation perfusion pressure, avoid excessive heart rate, improve heart function, and enhance tissue oxygenation. However, it is undeniable that the process of surgical removal of the necrotic intestinal cavity may cause inflammatory factors and toxins to re-enter the blood, which possibly exacerbate the symptoms of septic shock and tissue hypoxia. The intraoperative blood gas results of this case showed a gradual increase in lactate levels, which also indicated a significant impact of septic shock.

65.5.3 Postoperative Anesthetic Management

Routine treatment after intestinal perforation repair surgery includes the use of broad-spectrum antibiotics, nutritional support, vasoactive drugs, and fluid therapy. The focus of persistent arterial trunk treatment is to maintain the balance of systemic and pulmonary circulation and coronary perfusion, avoid the decrease of Pulmonary vascular resistance/Systemic vascular resistance (PVR/SVR), and ensure adequate systemic circulation perfusion.

65.6 Shortcomings and Limitations

Previous studies have shown that stroke volume variation (SVV) can indicate fluid responsiveness in children with sepsis. Although there is no standard reference value for SVV in children of different ages, assessing the volume responsiveness and quality of fluid resuscitation in children through the dynamic changes of SVV is still valuable. Unfortunately, SVV monitoring equipment was not used in this case, and no practical volume resuscitation judgment was made for this particular case.

65.7 Conclusion

The primary treatment principle for intestinal necrosis caused by septic shock associated with persistent truncus arteriosus is to maintain the stability of the systemic-pulmonary circulation ratio, sufficient fluid resuscitation, and positive inotropic agents to delay the progression of septic shock. If conditions permit, methods such as $ScvO_2$ and SVV can dynamically monitor tissue oxygen supply–demand balance and the effect of fluid resuscitation (Yong Bian).

Anesthetic Management of Emergency Exploratory Laparotomy in a Neonate with Transposition of the Great Arteries

66

Yang Shen

Abstract

A 7-day-old female infant with transposition of the great arteries underwent emergency laparotomy for intestinal perforation and septic shock under general anesthesia. The anesthesia for this case was extremely challenging. It is necessary to make a detailed anesthetic plan in advance based on the physiological characteristics of the newborn period, the pathophysiology of transposition of the great arteries, and the principles of septic shock treatment. Among them, the key points of perioperative anesthetic management are adjusting the systemic and pulmonary vascular resistance to improve tissue organ perfusion, rational use of vasoactive drugs, and optimal fluid management.

Transposition of the great arteries (TGA) is a congenital heart disease caused by abnormal twisting, separation, and absorption of the conus during embryonic development, resulting in the transposition of the aorta and pulmonary artery. Newborns with TGA are prone to necrotizing enterocolitis (NEC) due to long-term hypoxia, ischemia, and low perfusion of the intestinal mucosa. Once NEC occurs, intestinal perforation and septic shock can easily happen, which requires emergency surgery. This chapter reports the anesthetic management of an emergency laparotomy for intestinal perforation and septic shock in a newborn with TGA.

66.1 Case Presentation

A 7-day-old female infant 50 cm in height and 3.8 kg in weight was diagnosed with complete transposition of the great arteries by hearing a heart murmur during a postnatal physical examination and echocardiographic examination. The infant was born full-term via cesarean section without a history of asphyxia at birth. She was admitted to our hospital for further treatment, and relevant examinations (echocardiography, chest radiography, routine blood tests, etc.) were promptly completed. Echocardiography demonstrated complete TGA, ventricular septal defect (VSD), atrial septal defect (ASD), patent ductus arteriosus (PDA), slightly reduced left ventricular systolic function, pulmonary hypertension, and slightly underdeveloped aorta. The patient was strictly forbidden to inhale oxygen before surgery. Prostaglandin E_1 was intravenously administrated to maintain PDA. During the preparation

Y. Shen (✉)
The National Children's Medical Center (Shanghai), Department of Anesthesiology of Shanghai Children's Medical Center, Shanghai Jiao Tong University School of Medicine, Shanghai, China
e-mail: shenyang@scmc.com.cn

J. Zheng et al. (eds.), *Selected Pediatric Cardiovascular Surgery Anesthesia Cases*,
https://doi.org/10.1007/978-981-96-5614-1_66

for surgery, the patient began to have abdominal distension, increased abdominal wall tension, and yellow-green stools without blood, all of which indicated the possibility of neonatal necrotizing enterocolitis (NEC). Then, the enteral nutrition was temporarily stopped, but the parenteral nutrition was initiated immediately. Cefotaxime was also administrated for anti-infection treatment. The patient's axillary temperature was 37.8 °C, heart rate (HR) was 145 beats/min, respiratory rate (RR) was 35 breaths/min, percutaneous pulse oxygen saturation (SpO_2) 75–80%, blood pressure (BP) 64/37 mm Hg. The patient's SpO_2 and abdominal oxygen saturation (rSO_2) were low, skin mottling, difficulty breathing, and ventilation support. Considering neonatal intestinal perforation and septic shock, an emergency laparotomy was performed.

Physical examination: The patient was sedated and intubated with mechanical ventilation. Bilateral lung breath sounds were symmetrical without rales by auscultation. Pulse oxygen saturation (SpO_2) was 81%, heart rate (HR) was 180–190 beats/min, regular heart rhythm, systolic murmur in the 2–3 intercostal space on the left edge of the sternum, accentuation of second heart sound, drum-like abdomen, the increased abdominal wall tension. The liver was not palpable under the ribs. The extremities were warm without edema.

Laboratory test: White blood cell count 8.03×10^9/L, platelet count 165×10^9/L, hemoglobin 113.0 g/L, lymphocytes 7.7%, monocytes 10.3%, neutrophils 80.7%; C-reactive protein 112.0 mg/L. N-terminal pro-brain natriuretic peptide (NT-proBNP) 29,992 pg/mL, procalcitonin (PCT) 23.48 ng/mL. Arterial blood gas: pH 7.5, $PaCO_2$ 40.6 mm Hg, PaO_2 37.8 mm Hg, Na^+ 135 mmol/L, K^+ 3.9 mmol/L, Ca^{2+} 1.0 mmol/L, GLU 74.0 mg/dL, Lac 1.9 mmol/L, HCT 33.8%, SO_2 79.3%, THb 10.9 g/dL. The abdominal plain film demonstrated pneumoperitoneum, uneven intestinal gas filling, and blurred intestinal space.

66.2 Anesthetic Management

The child was transferred to the operating room (OR) under electrocardiographic (ECG) monitoring and intravenous infusion of norepinephrine at 0.03 μg/(kg·min). The femoral artery, femoral vein, and right internal jugular vein were catheterized in the Neonatal Intensive Care Unit (NICU). Upon entering the operating room, ECG, SpO_2, invasive arterial blood pressure (ABP), central venous pressure (CVP), abdominal oxygen saturation (rSO_2, and body temperature were quickly connected to OR monitors. Basic vital signs: HR 141–158 beats/min, ABP 58/32 mm Hg, CVP 9 cm H_2O, SpO_2 85%, and abdominal rSO_2 47%. Pressure control ventilation was used with respiratory parameters set as 21% fraction of inspired oxygen(FiO_2), 16 cm H_2O peak inspiratory pressure (PIP), 30–40 mL tidal volume (VT),30 breaths/min respiratory rate (RR),and 1:2 inspiratory time to expiratory time (I:E) ratio. Anesthesia was induced with intravenous injection of etomidate 1.2 mg, sufentanil 5.0 μg, and rocuronium 2.5 mg. General anesthesia was maintained by continuous infusion of sufentanil 2.0 μg/(kg·h), rocuronium 0.5 mg/(kg·h) combined with 1–2% sevoflurane intermittent inhalation. Calcium gluconate 100 mg was supplemented based on blood gas analysis results. Packed red blood cells were transfused. During the operation, ABP dropped to the lowest ABP at 43/26 mm Hg, HR rose to 149 beats/min, CVP was 7 cm H_2O, and abdominal rSO_2 was 35%. After a fast infusion of Ringer's acetate solution and packed red blood cells, ABP recovered to 60/38 mm Hg, HR dropped to 135 beats/min, and CVP was 10 cm H_2O. Considering that norepinephrine might exacerbate intestinal ischemia and hypoxia, the dose of norepinephrine was not increased during the operation. Body temperature was monitored during the operation and active warming measures such as warm air blankets and fluid warming were used. The body temperature was maintained at 36.4–36.7 °C (Table 66.1).

Table 66.1 Intraoperative blood gas analysis results

Time point	pH	PaO_2 (mm Hg)	$PaCO_2$ (mm Hg)	BE (mmol/L)	HCT (%)	Hb (g/dL)	K^+ (mmol/L)	Ca^{2+} (mmol/L)	Cl^- (mmol/L)	Lac (mmol/L)
Admission	7.4	49.4	46.3	5.5	26.8	8.7	4.0	0.98	103	1.9
Discharge	7.4	48.4	45.1	5.6	30.8	9.5	4.3	1.2	103	2.1

66.3 Postoperative Outcome

The surgery lasted approximately 65 min in total, with an estimated blood loss of 10 mL and urine output of 5 mL. About 80 mL of sodium acetate Ringer's solution and 40 mL of packed red blood cells were transfused during the operation. The abdominal area rSO_2 was maintained at around 50%. At the end of the operation, ABP was 66/39 mm Hg, HR was 141 beats/min, SpO_2 was 79%, CVP was 10 cm H_2O, and rectal temperature was 36.5 °C. After the operation, the patient was transferred to the pediatric Cardiac Intensive Care Unit under invasive blood pressure monitoring and manual ventilation with a simple respiratory bag. The endotracheal tube was successfully removed on the postoperative day 6. Arterial switch operation was conducted 2 weeks later. The patient was discharged from hospital 1 month later.

66.4 Review of Knowledge Points

66.4.1 Pathophysiology of TGA

TGA is a relatively common cyanotic congenital heart disease, second only to Tetralogy of Fallot in incidence, accounting for 5–7% of congenital heart diseases. TGA is defined as a concordant atrioventricular (AV) connection but discordant ventriculo-arterial (VA) connection, which means that the aorta originates from the right ventricle, and the pulmonary artery originates from the left ventricle. The aorta receives deoxygenated venous blood from the systemic circulation, while the pulmonary artery receives oxygenated arterial blood from the pulmonary circulation. Cyanosis and severe hypoxemia occur immediately after birth. The child's survival depends on one or more communications between the systemic and pulmonary circulations to allow blood mixing.

66.4.2 Necrotizing Enterocolitis

Necrotizing enterocolitis is one of the most common gastrointestinal emergencies in newborns. Intestinal wall hypoxia and ischemia are the two main factors resulting in necrotizing enterocolitis in newborns. When a newborn is in a hypoxic state, blood in the body will be redistributed by reducing the blood supply to the gastrointestinal tract and increasing the blood supply to the heart, brain, kidney, etc., vital organs, which cause hypoxia, ischemia, and low perfusion in the intestinal mucosa. Furthermore, the metabolic activity of the intestinal mucosa is relatively active. Once hypoxia and ischemia occur, it will cause acidosis, causing metabolic disorders in the intestinal wall cells and damage the intestinal mucosal tissue. In addition, the speed of mesenteric blood flow will decrease after hypoxia, thereby reducing oxygen consumption and increasing intestinal wall permeability.

66.5 Discussion

66.5.1 Preoperative Assessment and Preparation

Gastrointestinal decompression was preoperatively conducted via a gastric tube in this case. Therefore, a negative pressure suction device should be prepared before anesthesia. Various warming measures (warm air blanket, blood warmer) should be prepared since newborns are prone to hypothermia during anesthesia. It is necessary to use an incubator with a covering to transport the newborn patients. The operating room temperature should be maintained at 26–30 °C. Since the neonate's body weight and total blood volume is low, it is necessary to precisely estimate the possible intraoperative bleeding situation and reserve enough blood in advance for timely replenishment of blood loss during surgery. This child was preoperatively on mechanical ventilation and infusion of norepinephrine 0.03 μg/(kg·min). Blood pressure was maintained within an acceptable range matched for the age with a mild increase in lactate levels. To prevent further deterioration of systemic circulation, drugs such as epinephrine, norepinephrine, dopamine, lidocaine, and atropine should also be prepared in advance.

66.5.2 Anesthetic Induction and Maintenance

For the anesthetic management of emergency exploratory laparotomy in a neonate with TGA, it is necessary to maintain HR, myocardial contractility, and preload to maintain cardiac output. The myocardium of a newborn is not yet mature and is sensitive to myocardial inhibition caused by anesthetic drugs. For TGA patients, the decrease in cardiac output will lower the oxygen saturation of systemic venous blood, ultimately resulting in a decrease in arterial blood oxygen saturation. The increase in pulmonary vascular resistance (PVR) will reduce the pulmonary blood flow and the mixing of blood flow between the systemic and pulmonary circulation. The decrease in systemic vascular resistance (SVR) will cause an increase in systemic venous blood recirculation and a decrease in arterial blood oxygen saturation. Therefore, it is better to choose those anesthetics that have minimal impact on myocardial inhibition and do not increase PVR or decrease SVR. Etomidate and sufentanil can meet these requirements. Therefore, etomidate and sufentanil were chosen for the induction of anesthesia in this case. In addition, a low concentration of sevoflurane inhalation was intraoperatively used to help maintain appropriate sedation and analgesia. Adequate muscle relaxation is required for an exploratory laparotomy. Rocuronium was used for intravenous infusion maintenance during surgery since postoperative mechanical ventilation support was still needed.

For those patients with TGA dependent on PDA, prostaglandin E_1 0.01–0.05 μg/(kg·min) continuous infusion is necessary to keep the ductus arteriosus open to ensure sufficient mixing of blood flow between the systemic and pulmonary circulation. In this case, prostaglandin E_1 was not infused during surgery since the patient had a large VSD and did not depend on PDA.

66.5.3 Intraoperative Anesthetic Management

1. Ventilation management. Pressure control ventilation mode with PIP, RR, and FiO_2 adjustment is usually chosen in neonate patients. It is better to use the lung protective ventilation strategy with (PIP) at 14–18 cm H_2O, relatively fast RR, and $ETCO_2$ maintained at 35–40 mm Hg, which can prevent lung injury (barotrauma) caused by increased airway resistance and excessive airway pressure and also avoid insufficient effective ventilation due to the leak of anesthetic breathing circle in volume control mode. For children with TGA, it is necessary to avoid the increase of pulmonary vascular resistance, especially in children combined with pulmonary hypertension. Ventilation interventions can effectively reduce PVR. Neonates, especially preterm infants, have very small VT, and the flow sensor cannot accurately measure $ETCO_2$. So blood gas analysis is usually required for ventilation parameter adjustment. The preoperative PCV ventilation mode was continuously sued during the operation in this case. pH, PaO_2, and $PaCO_2$ were controlled within satisfactory ranges to avoid hypercapnia, acidosis, and unacceptable hypoxemia. In order to maintain the patency of the arterial duct, mechanical ventilation with air was used during the operation.
2. Fluid management. Neonates and low birth weight infants are prone to fluid underload and fluid overload. Preoperative electrolyte disorders should be corrected as much as possible. The preoperative lost fluid and physiological maintenance volume should be reasonably supplemented during the operation. The infusion rate and volume in neonates should be precisely controlled. It is better to use an infusion pump to manage the fluid infusion. During the operation, crystalloid fluid is usually infused and adjusted at 10–20 mL/(kg·h) based on the change of HR, BP, and urine output [not less than 0.5–1.0 mL/(kg·h)]. Neonates have less glycogen reserves, and children who are fasting and under stress are prone to hypoglycemia frequently in neonates with long fasting and stress due to the less glycogen reserve. Blood glucose should be routinely monitored during neonatal surgery. The amount of blood transfusion should be supplemented according to the estimate of

blood lost. Neonates can tolerate a loss of 10% of the total blood volume without blood transfusion, but crystalloid fluid must be replenished. If intraoperative blood loss exceeds 10% of the blood volume and the hematocrit is less than 30%, whole blood or red blood cells should be timely supplemented. The fluid infusion in this patient was managed according to the above principles and the hemodynamic was well maintained during the operation.

3. Regional tissue oxygen saturation monitoring. In this case, the drop in blood pressure abdominal rSO_2 may be related to intraoperative bleeding and insufficient volume. If intraoperative fluid and blood loss cannot replenish in time, cardiac output will decrease. On the contrary, if the blood volume is overloaded, it will not only fail to increase cardiac output but will worsen cardiac function.

Infection increases the overall metabolic level and cardiac burden. Severe infection can further cause septic shock and reduce myocardial perfusion and cardiac function. Inflammatory mediators induced by infection directly inhibit myocardial contractility. rSO_2 is an important indicator of reflecting regional tissue perfusion. In the early shock stage, non-vital organs or tissues show signs of low perfusion. Therefore, it is of great help for anesthesiologists to assess the regional tissue perfusion situation via monitoring rSO_2 and guide the septic shock treatments. Near-infrared spectroscopy (NIRS) is a noninvasive method for assessing tissue oxygen metabolism, which can nondestructively monitor the oxygenation parameters of local tissues. Lactate, an important metabolic indicator of the body, can also be used to assess the body's tissue perfusion and oxygen metabolism.

4. Postoperative Management. The child was transferred to the Cardiac Intensive Care Unit with endotracheal intubation after surgery. She received continued ventilation support treatment. Hyperglycemia is common during the recovery period after surgery. The incidence of intracranial hemorrhage and mortality in neonates with hyperglycemia is high and needs to be closely monitored.

66.6 Shortcomings and Limitations

For newborns with congenital heart disease, intraoperative hemodynamic monitoring is crucial, but there is still a lack of effective hemodynamic monitoring techniques and devices for neonates or infants. The direct pulse contour recording analysis method (Most Care® monitor) can monitor hemodynamic indicators such as stroke volume, peripheral vascular resistance, and cardiac circulation efficiency. Studies have shown that those parameters measured by Most Care® monitor during cardiac surgeries are very reliable in children with congenital heart disease. Comprehensive analysis of ABP, CVP, rSO_2, cardiac output, etc. and their trends is of great significance to guide the precise circulatory management and fluid therapy during surgery for such patients.

66.7 Conclusion

The anesthetic management of noncardiac surgery in children with congenital heart disease should be based on the understanding of the anatomical structure and pathophysiology of related diseases. In order to effectively reduce the incidence of complications and perioperative mortality rate, intensive hemodynamic monitoring, optimal use of vasoactive drugs, and satisfied tissue perfusion are required (Yang Shen).

67 Anesthetic Management of Tonsillectomy and Adenoidectomy in a Child with Noonan Syndrome

Jing Jiang

Abstract

A 9-year-old boy with unusual facies, wide-slanting forehead, hypertelorism, ptosis, and mandibular retrusion was diagnosed with Noonan syndrome through a genetic test. Echocardiography showed left ventricular hypertrophy. The activity of the coagulation factor was reduced. He was brought to our hospital to see a doctor due to snoring and mouth breathing during night sleep. A polysomnogram indicated severe obstructive sleep apnea–hypopnea syndrome (OSAHS). He was scheduled for an elective tonsillectomy and adenoidectomy under general anesthesia. The key point of anesthetic management for this patient includes the management of difficult airway, hemodynamics, and coagulation abnormalities.

Noonan syndrome (NS) is typically a genetically inherited autosomal dominant disorder that can affect multiple systems, including facial features, circulation, and coagulation. NS occurs in approximately 1/1000 to 1/2500 live births. The distinctive facial features can manifest as a wide-slanting forehead, hypertelorism, ptosis, low-set ears, down-slanting palpebral fissures, epicanthic folds, mild neck webbing, and torticollis. NS can also be accompanied by various congenital heart diseases, such as pulmonary artery stenosis (PS), hypertrophic obstructive cardiomyopathy (HOCM), atrial septal defect (ASD), and ventricular septal defect (VSD). Coagulation abnormalities in NS are often manifested as a deficiency in coagulation factors and platelets, which may be accompanied by a tendency for spontaneous bleeding. This chapter reports the anesthetic management of tonsillectomy and adenoidectomy in a child with Noonan syndrome.

67.1 Case Presentation

The patient was a 9-year-old boy with 118 cm in height and 19.9 kg in weight. Transcatheter closure of ASD was conducted in 2013 year at another hospital. Genetic testing in the 2020 year indicated NS. He had been treated with growth hormone for 1 year. There was no relevant family history. He was brought to our hospital to see a doctor due to snoring and mouth breathing during night sleep for 8 years and worsening in the past 6 months.

Physical examination: Wide-slanting forehead, hypertelorism, ptosis, mandibular retrusion, and mild neck webbing. Mouth breathing with maximal mouth opening at a scale of 2–3.

J. Jiang (✉)
The National Children's Medical Center (Shanghai), Department of Anesthesiology of Shanghai Children's Medical Center, Shanghai Jiao Tong University School of Medicine, Shanghai, China
e-mail: jiangjing@scmc.com.cn

J. Zheng et al. (eds.), *Selected Pediatric Cardiovascular Surgery Anesthesia Cases*,
https://doi.org/10.1007/978-981-96-5614-1_67

Modified Mallampati classification was class II. Cervical extension was slightly limited. He could only walk up one flight of stairs due to his poor physical activity.

Laboratory tests: Normal complete blood count test. NT-proBNP 494 pg/mL (0–125 pg/mL), coagulation factor activity test at another hospital: IX 53.6% (70–120%), XII 24.2% (70–150%). PT, APTT was normal after preoperative supplementation of 100 mL fresh frozen plasma.

Electrocardiogram (ECG): Sinus arrhythmia, hyperacute T waves, high QRS voltage in the left ventricle.

Chest X-ray: Enlarged heart shadow, increased lung markings.

Head MRI: Small posterior cranial fossa, low position of the cerebellar tonsils, thickened adenoids, airway compression.

Echocardiography: Post-intervention of ASD, no residual shunt, ejection fraction (EF) 65%, left ventricular hypertrophy (LVH), left ventricular outflow tract obstruction (LVOTO) with pressure difference 39 mm Hg.

Polysomnogram (PSG): OAHI index 100 times/h, lowest nocturnal pulse oxygen saturation (SpO_2) 59%, indicating severe OSAHS.

Preoperative diagnosis: Noonan syndrome with severe OSAHS and HOCM.

Preoperative preparation: Nocturnal hypoxemia was treated by continuous positive airway pressure (CPAP) assistant ventilation for 1 week before surgery. PT and APTT were improved to the normal range by intravenous supplementing 100 mL of fresh frozen plasma 2 days before surgery, and another 100 mL of fresh frozen plasma was supplemented again 2 h before surgery to improve coagulation function and supplement blood volume.

67.2 Anesthetic Management

After entering the operating room, ECG, blood pressure (BP), and SpO_2 were routinely monitored. Basic vital signs: BP 107/82 mm Hg, heart rate (HR) 102 beats/min, SpO_2 97%. Anesthesia was induced through intravenous bolus injection of Midazolam 1.5 mg, sufentanil 5.0 μg, etomidate 6.0 mg, and rocuronium 13 mg. After the eyelash reflex disappeared, an ID 5.0 mm cuffed endotracheal tube was intubated with the assistance of a video laryngoscope. The depth of intubation was 15 cm. Pressure-controlled ventilation-volume guaranteed (PCV-VG) mode was adopted with a 2 L/min oxygen flow rate, 50% fraction of inspired oxygen (FiO_2), 150 mL tidal volume (VT), 1:2 inspiratory to expiratory (I:E) time ratio. Adjustment of respiratory rate (RR) was done to maintain end-tidal carbon dioxide ($ETCO_2$) at 35–40 mm Hg. After intubation, the left radial artery was catheterized to measure invasive arterial pressure (ABP). During surgery, propofol 4.0 mg/(kg·h) and remifentanil 0.3–0.5 μg/(kg·min) were intravenously infused for the maintenance of anesthesia, while 0.5–1.0 MAC sevoflurane was intermittently inhaled to maintain BIS at 40–60. Intraoperative arterial blood gas analysis results in pH 7.34, $PaCO_2$ 49 mm Hg, PaO_2 485 mm Hg, K^+ 3.40 mmol/L, BE -0.71, HCT 38.80%. Tranexamic acid 190 mg was intravenously infused before surgery. The hemostatic effect of electrocoagulation at the surgical view was not good. Therefore, the coagulation and platelet function tests were conducted with Sonoclot, which showed that activated clotting time (ACT) was 129 (100–155), coagulation rate (CR) was 13.3 (9–35), platelet function (PF) 0.4 (>1.5). So, 300 U of prothrombin complex was given to assist hemostasis. No platelet products were transfused during the operation due to unavailability.

67.3 Postoperative Outcome

The operation lasted 70 min in total. After the operation, 40 mg of sugammadex was given to antagonize the residual muscle relaxation. Once the spontaneous breathing was restored, the tracheal tube was successfully removed, and the child was transferred to the intensive care unit. The child was discharged from the intensive care unit on postoperative day 2 and was discharged from the hospital a week later.

67.4 Review of Knowledge Points

67.4.1 Noonan Syndrome

NS is characterized by a mutation on the PTPN11 gene on chromosome 12, which encodes the tyrosine phosphatase in nearly half of the cases of NS. Tyrosine phosphatase is responsible for many enzymatic reactions involving the interactions of various growth factors and hormones in various physical and mental developmental processes. Anesthesia-related issues mainly include distinctive facial features, congenital heart disease, and coagulation dysfunction.

In addition to facial abnormalities, children with NS may also have mild neck webbing and torticollis, which can affect neck mobility and lead to difficult intubation. Congenital heart disease (CHD) accounts for about 80% of NS-related heart diseases, with PS being the most common type of CHD. Other CHDs include ASD, VSD, and atrioventricular septal defect. Hypertrophic cardiomyopathy (HCM) accounts for about 20%. Almost 25% of patients with NS and HCM die within the first year after birth because of heart failure.

The congenital coagulation dysfunction in children with NS includes prolonged APTT due to a lack of coagulation factors XI, FVIII, and FXII in the endogenous coagulation pathway. Platelet dysfunction or von Willebrand factor abnormalities occur in some children with NS.

67.4.2 Obstructive Sleep Apnea–Hypopnea Syndrome

OSAHS is a disease characterized by recurrent episodes of apnea during sleep, each lasting ≥10 s. Enlarged tonsils and adenoids are the main causes of OSAHS in children. Clinically, it can manifest as recurrent nocturnal awakenings, increased sympathetic tension, excessive daytime sleepiness, memory loss, and psychomotor dysfunction. Children with OSAS may also develop adenoid facies, developmental delay, and serious cardiovascular diseases such as pulmonary hypertension and hypertension.

67.4.3 Hypertrophic Cardiomyopathy

HCM is characterized by asymmetric myocardial hypertrophy, which often involves the interventricular septum and leads to the reduction of ventricular cavities, the restriction of left ventricular blood filling, and the decrease of diastolic compliance. Anesthesia and surgical stress can exacerbate LVOTO in children with HCM. Complications such as congestive heart failure, myocardial ischemia, and diastolic dysfunction are prone to occur during the perioperative period. Anesthetic management should be based on the pathophysiological characteristics of HCM to prevent complications. The pathophysiological characteristics of HCM are shown in Table 67.1.

Table 67.1 Pathophysiological characteristics of HCM

Diastolic function and atrial blood flow function	Left ventricular diastolic dysfunction Decreased left ventricular compliance Left atrial dilation Increased left atrial pressure
Ventricular contraction function	Left ventricular contractility is preserved or enhanced Right ventricular contractility is normal
Pulmonary vascular bed	Chronic elevation of LAP leads to a reversible increase in PVR, followed by an irreversible increase
Impact of preload changes on hemodynamics	Decreased LV compliance leads to increased LAP when preload increases Obstructive patients with reduced LV volume will increase obstruction
Heart rate changes	Avoid tachycardia: LV filling is limited, subendocardial perfusion is impaired Can tolerate bradycardia
Afterload changes	Avoid reduction in SVR, especially in obstructive patients; reduction in left ventricular end-systolic volume will exacerbate obstruction Can tolerate increased SVR

67.5 Discussion

67.5.1 Preoperative Assessment and Preparation

1. Airway assessment. The risk of a difficult airway is increased in children with NS. So, conducting a comprehensive and careful preoperative airway assessment is necessary, which includes maximal mouth opening capacity, head and neck mobility, thyromental distance, modified Mallampati classification, etc. In this case, the child had mandibular retrusion, maximal mouth opening at scale 2–3, Mallampati classification at class II, and slightly limited cervical extension. In addition, severe OSAHS and tonsillar hypertrophy can also cause difficult mask ventilation and tracheal intubation. Therefore, emergency airway management tools such as video laryngoscope, flexible fiberoptic bronchoscopy, tracheal tubes, laryngeal masks, and oropharyngeal airways should be well prepared. Rocuronium and its antagonist, sugammadex, should also be prepared before the induction of anesthesia.
2. Coagulation function assessment. Twenty percent of children with NS have a tendency for spontaneous bleeding. Therefore, it is necessary to assess the coagulation function based on the patient's bleeding history and coagulation and platelet function tests. If necessary, supplementation of related blood products should be given based on the coagulation and platelet function test results. In this case, the coagulation factors IX and XII were reduced before surgery. The coagulation function returned to a normal level after the transfusion of fresh frozen plasma.
3. Cardiovascular system assessment. The presence and degree of LVOTO should be determined in Children with HCM. LVOTO not only affects the hemodynamics of children with HCM, but it is also an independent risk factor for heart failure and sudden cardiac death. Previous studies showed that the risk of death from HCM or progression to congestive heart failure in children with LVOT (defined as a baseline gradient of at least 30 mm Hg) is increased, which is four times more than those children without obstruction. Therefore, these children with HCM should be carefully assessed for the related risk factors, such as a history of syncope, myocardial ischemia (dyspnea, chest pain), and arrhythmias before surgery.

The preoperative exertion tolerance was significantly reduced in this case. He could only walk up one flight of stairs with NYHA heart function classification II–III, but there was no history of syncope, dyspnea, or other symptoms. Furthermore, echocardiography showed EF was 65% with a left ventricular outflow tract pressure difference of 39 mm Hg. Based on these preoperative assessments, it was speculated that the reduced exertion tolerance might be mainly caused by chronic hypoxia. After a week of nighttime CPAP preoperative treatment, the preoperative oxygenation and exertion tolerance significantly improved, further confirming our speculation.

Blood volume should be supplemented before anesthesia to reduce LVOTO associated with preload reduction caused by positive pressure ventilation and vasodilation from anesthesia. In this case, the child was preoperatively supplemented with fresh frozen plasma based on the low coagulation factor activity of IX and XII. The supplementation of fresh frozen plasma can not only enhance the activity of coagulation factors and reduce perioperative bleeding, but it can also replenish the blood volume insufficiency caused by preoperative fasting and fluid restriction.

67.5.2 Intraoperative Anesthetic Management

1. Induction of anesthesia. The goal of anesthetic management in patients with HCM is to maintain a relatively high preload and afterload while reducing heart rate and myocardial contractility. Therefore, an appropriate depth of anesthesia should be maintained during surgery to avoid being too deep or too light. It

is beneficial to use the anesthetics with minimal hemodynamic impact. The anesthesia should be induced with a slow titration strategy to maintain hemodynamic stability. Compared to propofol, etomidate causes less hemodynamic fluctuation and is more suitable for patients with HCM. For those patients without venous access, sevoflurane can be used for inhalational induction of anesthesia, but there is a risk of hypotension. Monitoring the depth of anesthesia using BIS for precise anesthetic management is necessary. In this case, sedatives and analgesics are intravenously given by slow titration during induction; mask ventilation was checked to ensure the ventilation was not obstructed, and then the muscle relaxant rocuronium was given. The glottis was well exposed under video laryngoscopy and the endotracheal intubation was successfully completed.

2. Hemodynamic management.
   (a) Avoid hypotension: To maintain hemodynamic stability, it is necessary to conduct invasive arterial pressure monitoring during the perioperative period. If hypotension occurs, a small dosage of α-adrenergic agonists such as norepinephrine and phenylephrine can be considered after the blood volume deficiency and deep anesthesia is ruled out.
   (b) Avoid the increase of HR and myocardial contractility: The increase in myocardial contractility and HR can exacerbate LVOTO. During anesthesia, β-receptor blockers (esmolol), non-dihydropyridine calcium channel blockers (diltiazem), and other negative inotropic drugs can be used to moderately inhibit myocardial contractility without causing significant peripheral vascular resistance reduction and reflex tachycardia. The use of β-adrenergic agonists such as ephedrine, dopamine, dobutamine, and epinephrine are contraindicated and should be avoided during surgery.
   (c) Maintain adequate preload: It is very important to prevent the exacerbation of LVOTO and stroke volume reduction by maintaining adequate preload. Intraoperative volume therapy is often guided by monitoring central venous pressure measurement and cardiac ultrasound. Tonsillectomy and adenoidectomy in children usually take a short time with a small amount of blood loss. Therefore, the central venous access was not established in this case. Preoperative fresh frozen plasma infusion replenishes the blood volume deficiency from fasting and fluid restriction.
   (d) Maintain an appropriate depth of anesthesia: It is necessary to maintain an appropriate depth of anesthesia to avoid the increase of HR and BP due to strong perioperative stimulations. The postoperative pain of tonsillectomy and adenoidectomy is usually very strong, and the patient's desire to relieve postoperative pain is also very strong. However, the poor tolerance to opioids in children with OSAHS can easily cause complications such as respiratory depression after opioid analgesia due to the increased μ receptors caused by long-term repeated hypoxia. Therefore, postoperative pain management should be emphasized. The dosage of long-acting opioids for postoperative analgesia should be reduced to reduce the risk of respiratory depression, which can be supplemented with nonsteroidal drugs and local anesthetic infiltration.

67.6 Shortcomings and Limitations

The child's coagulation function had temporarily returned to normal after preoperative supplementation with fresh frozen plasma, but the platelet function might still be abnormal. The poor hemostasis effect during surgery indicated low platelet function. The Sonoclot test subsequently confirmed the low platelet function. Unfortunately, the platelet reserve was prepared on the surgery day, so the child was not supplemented with platelets.

67.7 Conclusion

Anesthetic management in NS poses many challenges to anesthesiologists, especially those related to airway management, maintenance of cardiovascular stability, and coagulation function. It is necessary to optimize the blood volume through the regulation of fluid supplements, to maintain an appropriate depth of anesthesia to inhibit sympathetic excitation, and to reduce LVOTO during anesthesia, especially for those children with HCM. Postoperative pain should be fully relieved to avoid sympathetic excitement caused by pain (Jing Jiang).

Anesthetic Management of Giant Retroperitoneal Teratoma Resection in a Child with Left Cardiac Insufficiency

68

Jianwei Zhang

Abstract

A 4-month-old female infant was admitted to our hospital due to a large tumor found in the abdominal cavity. Preoperative echocardiography indicated spherical dilation of the left ventricle, left atrium enlargement, left ventricular myocardial tissue decrease, and left ventricular contractility reduction, suggesting dilated cardiomyopathy. Retroperitoneal tumor resection under general anesthesia was scheduled. The key of anesthetic management is to maintain stable hemodynamics, improve cardiac contractility, maintain stroke volume and cardiac output, and ensure appropriate volume load to maintain organ function.

Teratomas are common retroperitoneum tumors in children, accounting for about 1/3 of retroperitoneal tumors in children under 1 year old, second only to Wilms' tumor and neuroblastoma, ranking third in pediatric tumors. The cause of this disease is unclear, but it may be related to abnormal differentiation of germ cells during embryonic development. Pediatric dilated cardiomyopathy (DCM) is a type of myocardial disease characterized by dilation of the left ventricle or both ventricles and cardiac contractility decrease, with or without congestive heart failure. Therefore, anesthetic management for DCM patients undergoing large tumor resection is challenging. This chapter reports the anesthetic management of huge retroperitoneal teratoma resection in a patient with DCM and heart failure.

J. Zhang (✉)
The National Children's Medical Center (Shanghai), Department of Anesthesiology of Shanghai Children's Medical Center, Shanghai Jiao Tong University School of Medicine, Shanghai, China
e-mail: zhangjianwei@scmc.com.cn

68.1 Case Presentation

The patient was a 4-month-old girl with a weight of 4.88 kg. She was born full-term without asphyxia. In the later stages of her mother's pregnancy, a large tumor was found in the fetus's abdominal cavity. After birth, an abdominal CT scan at another hospital suggested a teratoma in the abdominal cavity. Echocardiography showed the cardiac ejection fraction was 27%. She was admitted to our hospital with an abdominal tumor at the outpatient clinic. After admission, she received nutritional support and oral digoxin 20 μg every 12 h to improve cardiac function for elective surgery.

Physical examination: Malnourished, shortness of breath, and excessive sweating. Obvious bulging in the abdomen. The large tumor could be palpated in the left abdomen, which extended from the diaphragm to the pelvis and crossed the midline of the abdomen by 5 cm on the right side. In addition, the tumor texture was firm.

J. Zheng et al. (eds.), *Selected Pediatric Cardiovascular Surgery Anesthesia Cases*,
https://doi.org/10.1007/978-981-96-5614-1_68

Laboratory tests: Hemoglobin 91 g/L, hematocrit 38.5%, albumin 29.4 g/L, total protein 44.3 g/L, no abnormalities in liver and kidney function, normal coagulation function, carcinoembryonic antigen 6.36 ng/mL, alpha-fetoprotein (AFP) 1970.16 ng/mL, human chorionic gonadotropin (HCG) is normal.

N-terminal pro-brain natriuretic peptide (NT-ProBNP) 16,506 pg/mL, troponin I 0.13 ng/mL, lactate dehydrogenase 696 U/L, creatine kinase is normal.

Electrocardiogram (ECG): Left axis deviation, left atrial enlargement (possible?), incomplete right bundle branch block, T wave inversion on leads I, V5, V6, and flat T wave on lead avF.

Echocardiography: The left ventricle was spherically dilated, left ventricular end-diastolic diameter (LVDd) 3.22 cm, left ventricular end-systolic diameter (LVDs) of 2.65 cm, mild left atrium enlargement, mild to moderate mitral regurgitation, right ventricular outflow tract flow velocity increase, slight left ventricular myocardial tissue lose (loose layer/dense layer = 2.1), left heart contractility reduction, left ventricular ejection fraction (LVEF) 37.97%, left ventricular short-axis shortening rate (LVFS) 17.7%.

Abdominal CT: A large mass in the abdominal cavity with clear boundaries, measuring 143.7 mm × 122.8 mm × 154.1 mm, which was mainly cystic components, coexisted with fat density shadows and calcification spots inside. The abdominal aorta was compressed and shifted to the right. The left kidney was significantly anterior due to pressure, and the right kidney was rotated, suggesting the possibility of a teratoma.

Preoperative diagnosis: Retroperitoneal teratoma, cardiomyopathy (to be investigated), heart failure, severe malnutrition.

68.2 Anesthetic Management

The patient was not premeditated. After entering the operating room, routine monitoring was established. Noninvasive blood pressure (NIBP) was 107/52 mm Hg, heart rate (HR) was 158 beats/min, and pulse oxygen saturation (SpO_2) was 98%. After the peripheral vein was accessed, 0.5 mg of midazolam, 1 mg of etomidate, 2.5 μg of sufentanil, and 2.5 mg of rocuronium were given intravenously for the induction of anesthesia. After the eyelash reflex disappeared, an ID 4.0 mm cuffed endotracheal tube was intubated under direct laryngoscopy with a tube depth of 10 cm. Pressure-controlled ventilation-volume guaranteed (PCV-VG) mode was used for mechanical ventilation with an oxygen flow rate of 1 L/min, fraction of inspired oxygen (FiO_2) of 50%, tidal volume (VT) of 35 mL, respiratory rate (RR) of 24 breaths/min, inspiratory time to expiratory time (I:E) ratio of 1:2, and positive end-expiratory pressure (PEEP) of 4 cm H_2O. The respiratory rate was adjusted during the operation to maintain the end-tidal carbon dioxide pressure ($ETCO_2$) at 35–40 mm Hg.

Invasive arterial blood pressure (ABP, left radial artery), Most Care® hemodynamics (left femoral artery), central venous pressure (CVP, right internal jugular vein), and INVOS local (renal area) tissue oxygen saturation (rSO_2) was established and monitored. An external jugular vein was also accessed for rapid fluid replacement. During the operation, propofol 4.0 mg/(kg·h), sufentanil 2.0 μg/(kg·h), and rocuronium 0.5 mg/(kg·h) were intravenously infused, combined with sevoflurane inhalation for anesthesia maintenance. The initial BP was 113/58 mm Hg, HR was 117 beats/min, CVP was 7 cm H_2O, cardiac index (CI) was 3.10 L/(min·m^2), the maximum rate of left ventricular pressure rise during isovolumic contraction (dp/dt max) was 0.79, stroke volume variation (SVV) was 10.8%, and renal area rSO_2 was 82%. During the operation, when the CI dropped to 2.08 L/(min·m^2), the maximum dp/dt dropped to 0.27, and when BP dropped to 72/43 mm Hg, both dopamine and dobutamine was started at 5.0 μg/(kg·min) via intravenous infusion respectively. When SVV increased to 14.1% with a drop in CVP, fluid resuscitation was accelerated. Blood gases were rechecked every 30 min to 1 h during surgery (Table 68.1). When hemoglobin dropped below 8 g/dL, packed red cells were transfused. Electrolytes were supplemented based on blood gas analysis results (10% KCL 1 mL was infused with fluid replacement. Acidosis was corrected

Table 68.1 Intraoperative blood gas test results

Time point	Admission	Exit room
Hb (g/dL)	8.1	10.1
HCT (%)	25.2	31.2
PH	7.36	7.41
PaO_2 (mm Hg)	202	186
$PaCO_2$ (mm Hg)	43.2	33.8
BE (mmol/L)	−0.9	−2.4
Na^+ (mmol/L)	136	134
K^+ (mmol/L)	2.9	3.3
Cl^- (mmol/L)	104	103
Ca^{2+} (mmol/L)	1.31	1.24
Lac (mmol/L)	0.6	0.7

by sodium bicarbonate infusion. Body temperature was monitored during surgery by active warming measures such as warm air blankets and fluid warming. Tranexamic acid 10 mg/kg was intravenously injected before surgery, and 100 mL of fresh-frozen plasma was transfused during surgery.

68.3 Postoperative Outcome

The operation lasted a total of 125 min. The estimated blood loss was about 250 mL. The urine output was 10 mL. About 150 mL of acetate Ringer's solution, 200 mL of packed red blood cells, and 100 mL of fresh-frozen plasma were transfused. Renal area rSO_2 was maintained at 73–80%. The lactate levels remained within the normal range during the operation. Postoperative BP was 99/61 mm Hg, HR was 123 beats/min, SpO_2 was 99%, CVP was 8 cm H_2O, and rectal temperature was 36.5 °C. After the operation, the patient was transferred to the intensive care unit (ICU) under ABP, ECG, and SpO_2 monitoring with an endotracheal tube in place. The endotracheal tube was removed on the postoperative day 2. The patient was discharged from the ICU on postoperative day 4 and discharged from the hospital 1 week later. The tumor pathology result was immature teratoma (malignant).

A 3-month postoperative echocardiogram follow-up suggested left ventricular spherical dilation, possible dilated cardiomyopathy, and left ventricular systolic function decrease with LVEF of 49.2%. The 6-month postoperative echocardiogram follow-up suggested slight left ventricle enlargement and normal left ventricular systolic function with LVEF of 68.1%.

68.4 Review of Knowledge Points

68.4.1 Retroperitoneal Teratoma

Teratomas are common retroperitoneal tumors in children. There was no difference in the incidence between boys and girls. Teratomas are usually benign and relatively large; only 25–30% of patients were malignant. Most children with teratomas have atypical clinical symptoms and often seek medical attention due to the discovery of an abdominal mass during a physical examination. The patients with malignant teratomas have a higher AFP positive rate (up to 80%), while those with benign teratomas only have a 50% positive rate. AFP and HCG can serve as biological markers for malignant teratomas. Currently, surgical removal is considered the only effective treatment. Postoperative pathological examination of the maturity of the tumor tissue can serve as an effective indicator for prognosis.

68.4.2 Dilated Cardiomyopathy

Pediatric DCM is a type of left ventricular dilation and systolic dysfunction that hemodynamic reasons cannot explain. It must exclude physiological (such as sepsis) or anatomical reasons (such as aortic stenosis) that cause abnormal cardiac load states or myocardial ischemia caused by coronary artery abnormalities. It can be divided into primary and secondary DCM. Primary DCM includes familial/genetic DCM and idiopathic DCM. There are many causes of secondary DCM, including inflammatory cardiomyopathy, toxic cardiomyopathy, and cardiomyopathy caused by metabolic diseases, structural heart diseases, and nutritional disorders.

68.4.3 Pediatric Heart Failure

Pediatric heart failure is referred to as a complex clinical syndrome caused by abnormal changes in cardiac structure and/or function, which further results in ventricular contraction and/or relaxation dysfunction, neuroendocrine regulatory disorders, and the cardiac output cannot meet the body's needs. Ultimately, the heart's and other organs' functions throughout the body were all affected. The diagnosis and assessment of pediatric heart failure mainly depend on the cause, medical history, clinical manifestations, and auxiliary examinations. In laboratory tests, B-type natriuretic peptide (BNP) or N-terminal pro-B-type natriuretic peptide (NT-proBNP) are important markers of heart failure, while troponin I or T are often used for the etiological diagnosis of acute heart failure (such as determining acute myocardial injury) and prognosis assessment. Ejection fraction (EF) and fractional shortening (FS) are commonly used indicators in echocardiography to reflect ventricular contractile function. Left ventricular EF less than 55% and/or FS less than 25% usually suggests left ventricular systolic dysfunction.

68.5 Discussion

68.5.1 Preoperative Assessment and Preparation

Before the operation, we focused on the child's echocardiogram, ECG, and related laboratory tests to assess the child's cardiac function status and anesthesia risk. The Pediatric Risk Assessment Score (PRAm) is a useful tool for predicting the perioperative mortality risk for pediatric noncardiac surgery, developed by Boston Children's Hospital. The PRAm score in this case was ≥9 points, indicating that the child was at extremely high anesthesia risk, perioperative mortality rate may be as high as 35% or more. In addition, the child's overall nutritional and cardiac status was optimized by clinical nutritionists and cardiologists before the operation. The child began to take 20 μg of digoxin orally every 12 h a week before the operation. It is better to test the blood concentration of digoxin before anesthesia since the safe drug concentration is narrow. Unfortunately, we did not measure the blood concentration of digoxin before anesthesia. So, we closely monitored the heart rate and rhythm and maintained the heart rate over 100 beats/min. The child did not show any premature beats, conduction block, or changes in the ST segment during the operation.

68.5.2 Intraoperative Anesthetic Management

(a) The induction and maintenance of general anesthesia in this child referred to the anesthesia plan for pediatric cardiac surgery, which can maintain stable vital signs such as heart rate and blood pressure while satisfying the depth of anesthesia by choosing the anesthetics with minimal impact on cardiac function.
(b) The giant retroperitoneal teratoma can elevate the diaphragm and restrict the respiratory movement of the thorax, which may further lead to airway pressure increase and blood return reduction. This child experienced a transient increase in airway pressure, $ETCO_2$ increases, and VT reduction after intubation. The child's oxygenation was barely maintained by adjustment of ventilator parameters. The airway pressure decreased after the abdomen was opened and returned to normal after the tumor was removed.
(c) The preload increase cannot significantly increase the stroke volume in children with DCM due to the exhausted preload reserves, which makes the stroke volume relatively fixed. Once bradycardia occurs, the cardiac output will be reduced. Tachycardia cannot reduce the left ventricular filling but may impair subendocardial perfusion. Appropriately enhancing the myocardial contractility and reducing systemic vascular resistance may help increase the stroke volume and cardiac output. In addition to rou-

tine monitoring, invasive blood pressure, central venous pressure, and renal area tissue oxygen saturation monitoring during the operation was recommended for this child. Most care monitors can be used in neonates and infants to continuously monitor the stroke volume, peripheral vascular resistance, cardiac circulation efficiency, maximum pressure gradient, stroke volume variability, and pulse pressure variability via invasive artery pressure wave analysis. We also recommend using the Most Care® monitor to guide the application of inotropic drugs, vasoactive drugs, and fluid replacement. Due to the large size of the tumor, tissue adhesion, and wrapping around large blood vessels, dissection of tumor tissue may cause traction, compression, and bleeding, which further exacerbates intraoperative hemodynamic fluctuations. When intraoperative blood pressure, CI, dp/dt index, and other hemodynamic fluctuations occur, the cardiac function status and surgical operations related to abdominal aorta, renal artery traction, and compression factors should be considered. When the cardiac index is significantly reduced and accompanied by a drop in blood pressure, small doses of dopamine and dobutamine can be combined to increase myocardial contractility and improve cardiac output without increasing systemic vascular resistance.

(d) Although children can tolerate hypokalemia relatively well, low potassium levels may lead to arrhythmia for those children taking digoxin. Therefore, blood gases and electrolytes should be repeatedly checked, and hypokalemia and metabolic acidosis should be corrected promptly during surgery.

68.6 Conclusion

The anesthetic management of children with giant retroperitoneal teratoma combined with heart failure should be based on the pathophysiology of the disease itself, rational selection of anesthetic drugs, monitoring indicators as guidance, effective volume supplementation, and optimal use of positive inotropic drugs, continuous monitoring and assessment of tissue perfusion. These precise implementations can effectively maintain the function of important organs and reduce perioperative mortality (Jianwei Zhang).

Part IV

Discussion of Sedation/Anesthesia Cases for Cardiovascular Disease Outside the Operating Room

69 Anesthetic Management in Pediatric Patients Undergoing Cardiac Catheterization Examination for Transitional Atrioventricular Septal Defect

Wei Ji

Abstract

A 4-year-old girl was diagnosed with transitional atrioventricular septal defect, severe mitral regurgitation, moderate-to-severe tricuspid regurgitation, and pulmonary hypertension (moderate) by echocardiography due to heart murmurs. She was scheduled for cardiac catheterization examination under general anesthesia. The left-to-right intracardiac shunt increased pulmonary blood flow, recurrent episodes of upper respiratory tract infections, and suboptimal pulmonary development. The key to anesthetic management in this should focus on the hemodynamic changes caused by mitral regurgitation and pulmonary hypertension and the cardiac catheterization-related complications such as arrhythmias and hypotension.

Atrioventricular septal defect (AVSD), also known as endocardial cushion defect, accounts for 4–5% of all congenital heart diseases, which can be classified as partial, transitional, or complete AVSD. The clinical severity of transitional atrioventricular septal defect is predominantly determined by the degree of impairment of the left atrioventricular valve function. For those older children who have not yet shown obvious symptoms of congestive heart failure and cyanosis, preoperative cardiac catheterization is needed to directly measure pulmonary vascular resistance and provide a basis for subsequent diagnosis and treatment. This chapter reports the anesthetic management of a child with transitional AVSD undergoing cardiac catheterization.

69.1 Case Presentation

A 4-year-old girl with a height of 110.5 cm and a weight of 15 kg was brought to a local hospital due to coughing. A heart murmur was heard during the physical examination. Her medical history revealed frequent upper respiratory infections, excessive sweating, breathlessness, and fatigue after activities. Cardiac ultrasound indicated AVSD, pulmonary hypertension, severe mitral regurgitation (MR), and moderate-to-severe tricuspid regurgitation (TR). Consequently, she was scheduled for a diagnostic cardiac catheterization examination under general anesthesia.

Physical examination: Consciousness, rapid breathing, about 30 breaths per minute, wet rales in both lungs, grade III/VI systolic murmur in the precordial area. Pulse oxygen saturation (SpO_2) is 98% on room air.

W. Ji (✉)
The National Children's Medical Center (Shanghai), Department of Anesthesiology of Shanghai Children's Medical Center, Shanghai Jiao Tong University School of Medicine, Shanghai, China
e-mail: jiwei@scmc.com.cn

J. Zheng et al. (eds.), *Selected Pediatric Cardiovascular Surgery Anesthesia Cases*, https://doi.org/10.1007/978-981-96-5614-1_69

Laboratory tests: Hemoglobin is reported at 98.0 g/L, Elevated Troponin I at 0.06 μg/L, and Creatine kinase-MB subtype at 5.6 μg/L. Liver and kidney functions are within normal limits, as is coagulation function. N-terminal pro-brain natriuretic peptide levels are significantly elevated at 16,104 pg/mL.

Electrocardiogram (ECG): Sinus rhythm, incomplete right bundle branch block (IRBBB), and bi-atrial hypertrophy.

Chest X-ray: Cardiac silhouette enlargement and lung markings increase.

Echocardiography: AVSD (Transitional type), patent foramen ovale (PFO), severe MR, moderate-to-severe TR, slightly increased forward flow velocity of the mitral valve, increased flow velocity of the main pulmonary artery, pulmonary hypertension (pressure difference 54 mm Hg), and a small amount of pericardial effusion.

Preoperative diagnosis: Transitional AVSD, severe MR, moderate-to-severe TR, pulmonary hypertension, upper respiratory tract infection.

69.2 Anesthetic Management

The child did not receive any preoperative medication. After entering the operating room, ECG, noninvasive blood pressure (BP), and SpO_2 were monitored: heart rate (HR) 110 beats/minute, BP 82/45 mm Hg, SpO_2 98%. Anesthesia was induced by titrated administration of midazolam 1.5 mg, etomidate 4.5 mg, sufentanil 15 μg, and rocuronium 9.0 mg. After sufficient preoxygenation with a face mask and the disappearance of the eyelash reflex, an ID 5.0 mm cuffed endotracheal tube was intubated orally under direct video laryngoscopy with a tube depth of 14 cm (from the incisors). The left external jugular vein was accessed to infusion sodium acetate Ringer's solution. Anesthesia was maintained with sevoflurane at a minimum alveolar concentration (MAC) of 1.0 throughout the procedure. Ventilation was managed in pressure-controlled ventilation-volume guaranteed (PCV-VG) mode with the setting as the oxygen flow rate 1 L/min, fraction of inspirited oxygen (FiO_2) 30%, tidal volume (VT) 120 mL, and inspiratory time to expiratory time (I:E) ratio 1:2. Ventilation frequency was adjusted to maintain end-tidal CO_2 ($ETCO_2$) between 35 and 40 mm Hg. Following routine disinfection and draping, a downward trend in BP was observed during the cannulation of the right femoral artery and vein. Dopamine infusion was initiated at 5.0 μg/(kg·min) to maintain BP around 75/50(58) mm Hg. After successful cannulation, heparin was administered intravenously at 100 IU/kg for anticoagulation and followed by routine monitoring of pressures and oxygen saturation in various parts of the heart. During the process of the catheter entering the right atrium, the child suddenly developed supraventricular tachycardia, ST segment depression, and a continuous drop in BP to 54/30 mm Hg. The operation was then stopped, the ventilator was adjusted to pure oxygen ventilation, the fluid replacement speed was increased, and the dopamine was increased to 10 μg/(kg·min). The child's HR returned to normal and the hemodynamics was stabilized. When the procedure was finished, sevoflurane inhalation was discontinued, and the airway was suctioned under deep anesthesia. Sugammadex sodium at 2.0 mg/kg was administered to reverse the residual muscle relaxation. Spontaneous breathing was restored 2 min later, and the ventilation mode was switched to PSV-Pro mode. With pressure support reduced to 8.0 cm H_2O, VT reached approximately 100 mL, SpO_2 96%, and $ETCO_2$ 50 mm Hg, the endotracheal tube was then removed.

69.3 Postoperative Outcome

The cardiac catheterization examination showed transitional AVSD, congenital mitral valve insufficiency, congenital tricuspid valve insufficiency, and moderate pulmonary hypertension. The child was transferred to the Department of Cardiothoracic Surgery for surgical treatment.

69.4 Review of Knowledge Points

69.4.1 Pathophysiology

Pediatric endocardial cushion dysplasia can result in abnormal morphology and function of the atrioventricular valve, as well as atrial septal defect (ASD) and ventricular septal defect (VSD). The transitional AVSD is composed of ostium primum defect, common atrioventricular (AV) valve, and functionally independent mitral and tricuspid valves formed by common anterior superior and posterior inferior bridge valve leaf attached to the ventricular septum (IVS) through dense tendinous cords. In addition, there may be a very small inlet-type VSD or non-inlet-type VSD. The shunt volume in children with transitional AVSD is small at the ventricular level, which is physiologically similar to the partial AVSD, but the incidence of AV valve morphology and functional abnormalities is higher. The child usually has mild symptoms when there is no obvious valve dysfunction. When the child has severe left atrial ventricular valve dysfunction, the left-to-right shunt increased by ASD will cause severe pulmonary blood flow, and such children often have symptoms of poor lung development, rapid breathing, and recurrent respiratory infections in infancy. The left-to-right shunt eventually leads to volume overload and ventricular dilation, which leads to a vicious cycle of atrioventricular valve dysfunction and congestive heart failure (CHF).

69.4.2 Diagnosis and Treatment

Echocardiography assessment mainly focuses on the morphological features of ASD, VSD, and AV valves. It can also assess the size and function of both ventricles. For older children with AVSD without obvious symptoms of congestive heart failure, the feasibility of surgical treatment needs to be determined through preoperative cardiac catheterization to assess pulmonary vascular resistance (PVR), pulmonary-to-systemic flow ratio, etc. The timing of surgical treatment depends on the severity of symptoms and response to drug treatment. The treatment plan for AVSD repair surgery mainly includes the closure of ASD and VSD and the division of common AV valve tissue into independent, non-narrowed, and well-functioning mitral and tricuspid valves. For those children with obvious pulmonary circulation overload and contraindications to early complete repair, pulmonary artery banding can be first performed to prevent irreversible pulmonary vascular disease.

69.5 Discussion

69.5.1 Preoperative Evaluation and Preparation

Due to the complicated conditions of AVSD in children, the preoperative assessment includes a review of medical history, complications, current medications, preoperative examination, and detailed physical examination, especially the signs and symptoms of the child's CHF and pulmonary hypertension. Preoperative manifestations of CHF include shortness of breath, respiratory work increase, rales, growth retardation, hepatomegaly, tachycardia, cold extremities, weak pulse, delayed capillary refill, and mottled skin. Cyanotic children must carefully search for the cause of decreased blood oxygen saturation, such as right ventricular outflow tract obstruction, pulmonary hypertension, or right-to-left shunt caused by CHF.

Preoperative evaluation should encompass recent echocardiography for assessing ventricular function, atrioventricular valve regurgitation severity, and intracardiac shunt direction. Electrocardiography should be used to detect arrhythmias. The chest radiography to identify pulmonary edema or pneumonia. Routine preoperative laboratory tests should cover complete blood count (for polycythemia due to cyanosis or anemia from malnutrition) and electrolytes (to check for hypokalemia caused by vomiting or diuretic use).

69.5.2 Intraoperative Anesthetic Management

Despite preoperative anti-infection treatment, this child still had increased reactivity of the pulmonary vascular bed and poor pulmonary compliance before surgery. For children with high reactivity of the pulmonary vascular bed, large doses of fentanyl can effectively alleviate the increase in PVR and SVR caused by surgical stimulation, and the increase in SVR will exacerbate mitral regurgitation. Inhalation induction can be used for children with small defects, no mitral regurgitation, and pulmonary hypertension. However, for children with large shunts and increased pulmonary blood flow, their cardiac reserve function is limited or exhausted; Mitral regurgitation increases left ventricular volume load, further reducing the cardiac reserve. Thus, combining inhalation anesthesia with opioids is preferred. Anesthesia induction should be carefully titrated to avoid significant hemodynamic fluctuations. For those children with high pulmonary blood flow and decreased pulmonary compliance, peak inspiratory pressure during mask ventilation may need to be increased. Intubation should be performed as soon as possible once the child is fully relaxed to reduce gas insufflation into the stomach.

The ventilation mode, PaO_2, and $PaCO_2$ levels regulate PVR. It is very important to maintain lower FiO_2, avoid hyperventilation, and keep low peak inspiratory pressure can minimize the hemodynamic fluctuations during the diagnostic cardiac catheterization examination. Positive pressure ventilation, particularly with high peak inspiratory pressure, can reduce the preload of the right and left atria, increase the afterload of the right ventricle, and decrease the afterload of the left ventricle.

69.5.3 Perioperative Adverse Events and Management Principles

During pediatric cardiac catheterization examination, respiratory complications such as respiratory depression, coughing, bronchospasm, laryngospasm, increased respiratory secretions, and airway obstruction are the most commonly occurring anesthesia-related issues. The incidence rate is about 3.88%. In this case, preoperative respiratory infection symptoms such as coughing, expectoration, and lung rales existed. Therefore, it was necessary to maintain deep anesthesia to minimize airway irritation and reduce adverse respiratory events during airway suctioning. Arrhythmias occur in 12.14% of pediatric cardiac catheterization examinations, with being the most common complication, followed by hypotension. Before femoral artery or vein cannulations, anesthesia depth should be increased, and 1% lidocaine is recommended for local anesthesia at the puncture site. Transient arrhythmias, such as premature ventricular contractions, ventricular tachycardia, supraventricular tachycardia, atrioventricular block, and bradycardia, commonly occur during catheter advancement, usually due to catheter-induced atrial or ventricular wall stimulation. Most arrhythmias resolve upon immediate catheter withdrawal. If an arrhythmia persists, antiarrhythmic drugs like lidocaine, atropine, or propafenone may be considered.

In addition to the peripheral vasodilation caused by general anesthesia, femoral artery and vein cannulation-related blood loss may further increase the risk of intraoperative hypotension in pediatric patients. Systemic hypotension or systemic vascular resistance reduction can decrease the coronary blood flow and cause potential biventricular ischemia, which may trigger compensatory right ventricular hypertrophy or dilation, further compress the left ventricular septum, impair the left ventricular filling, and lower cardiac output. Hypoxemia caused by inadequate ventilation, lung disease, or diminished pulmonary blood flow can further compromise the ventricular function. Volume replenishment is essential during treatment, and vasoactive drugs should be administered as needed. Furthermore, considering the child's moderate pulmonary hypertension, perioperative factors increasing pulmonary vascular resistance, such as hypercapnia, hypoxia, acidosis, pain, and airway irritation, should be avoided to prevent a rapid rise in PVR, potentially triggering a pulmonary hypertension crisis and/or right heart failure.

69.6 Conclusion

Prior to undergoing cardiac catheterization surgery for a transitional atrioventricular septal defect, it is imperative for the anesthesiologist to conduct a comprehensive preoperative evaluation of the pediatric patient's clinical severity, comprehend the underlying pathophysiological features specific to the condition, and ensure thorough preoperative preparation. During the surgery, it's essential to maintain the child's optimal heart rate, myocardial contractility, and preload to preserve cardiac output. Additionally, any arrhythmias, hypotension, or related complications should be quickly detected and addressed (Wei Ji).

70 Anesthetic Management of Cardiac Catheterization in a Child with Idiopathic Pulmonary Arterial Hypertension

Bin Xue

Abstract

A 5-year-old boy suspected of idiopathic pulmonary arterial hypertension due to a significant decrease in exercise tolerance was scheduled for cardiac catheterization under general anesthesia. Young age, general anesthesia, pulmonary artery pressure higher than aortic pressure, and heart failure can all trigger intraoperative pulmonary hypertension crisis. Preoperative thorough assessment and avoidance of intraoperative hypoxia, acidosis, and hypotension are key to the successful anesthetic management of cardiac catheterization for this kind of case.

Idiopathic pulmonary arterial hypertension (IPAH) manifests as unexplained progressive pulmonary vascular remodeling with both pulmonary vascular resistance (PVR) and pulmonary artery pressure (PAP) gradually increasing, ultimately leading to right heart failure and even death. The pathogenesis of the disease has not yet been fully understood. Right heart catheterization is the golden standard for the hemodynamic diagnosis of PAH. For those young children who are difficult to cooperate with, heart catheterization must be performed under general anesthesia. This chapter reports the anesthetic management of a child with idiopathic pulmonary hypertension undergoing heart catheterization.

70.1 Case Presentation

The patient was 5 years and 11 months old boy with a weight of 22.8 kg. Full-term cesarean section, no history of asphyxia. Due to a significant decrease in exercise tolerance, echocardiography indicated pulmonary hypertension (PH, severe), tricuspid valve mild-to-moderate regurgitation, pulmonary valve mild regurgitation, decreased right ventricular systolic function, and normal left heart systolic function. The boy was admitted with a diagnosis of "pulmonary hypertension and heart failure."

Physical examination: The child is conscious, with no abnormal mental reactions. No cyanosis in the lips and limbs, no eyelid edema, steady breathing, clear lung sounds, strong heart sounds, regular heart rhythm, and no obvious murmurs in the precordial area. The liver and spleen are not palpable below the ribs.

Laboratory tests: CRP 36.2, NT-proBNP 3059 pg/mL, normal liver, kidney, and coagulation function.

B. Xue (✉)
The National Children's Medical Center (Shanghai), Department of Anesthesiology of Shanghai Children's Medical Center, Shanghai Jiao Tong University School of Medicine, Shanghai, China
e-mail: xuebin@scmc.com.cn

J. Zheng et al. (eds.), *Selected Pediatric Cardiovascular Surgery Anesthesia Cases*,
https://doi.org/10.1007/978-981-96-5614-1_70

Electrocardiogram(ECG): Right ventricular hypertrophy(possible), ST segment depression 0.05 mV in leads II, aVF, T wave changes.

Echocardiography: Severe pulmonary hypertension, mild-to-moderate tricuspid regurgitation, regurgitation width 0.32 cm, tricuspid flow velocity 5.13 m/s, pressure difference 105 mm Hg, mild pulmonary valve regurgitation, regurgitation width 3.84 cm, pressure difference 59 mm Hg, decreased right ventricular systolic function, normal left ventricular systolic function.

Cardiac magnetic resonance: Pulmonary artery enlargement, right ventricular enlargement, and hypertrophy, tricuspid regurgitation (mild to moderate), a small amount of pericardial effusion.

Preoperative diagnosis: Pulmonary hypertension, heart failure. Elective heart catheterization under general anesthesia.

70.2 Anesthetic Management

The patient did not take any preoperative medication. After entering the catheterization room, ECG, noninvasive blood pressure (BP), and pulse oxygen saturation (SpO_2) were monitored: BP 98/65 mm Hg, heart rate (HR) 101 beats/min, SpO_2 99%. After the peripheral vein was accessed, 1.0 mg midazolam, 30 μg fentanyl, and 60 mg propofol were intravenously administered for induction of anesthesia. After the eyelash reflex disappeared, a 2.5 laryngeal mask was inserted, the spontaneous breathing was maintained. The oxygen flow rate was 3 L/min, the fraction of inspired oxygen (FiO_2) was 21%, the tidal volume (VT) was 160 mL, and the respiratory rate (RR) was 28 times/min. During the operation, the end-tidal carbon dioxide partial pressure ($ETCO_2$) was 45–48 mm Hg, and the SpO_2 was maintained above 98%. The depth of anesthesia was maintained by 1.0 MAC of sevoflurane inhalation. After the surgeon disinfected and draped, the right femoral artery and vein were catheterized to measure the pressures and oxygen levels in each chamber, and then the pulmonary vasodilation test was performed. Before iloprost (PGI_2)was inhaled, the main pulmonary artery (MPA) pressure was 89/57 (71) mm Hg, the descending aorta (DAO) pressure was 85/54 (67) mm Hg, the calculated pulmonary blood flow (Qp)/systemic blood flow (Qs) was 0.49, and the pulmonary vascular resistance index (PVRI) was 15 WU/m^2. After PGI_2 was inhaled for 15 min, the MPA was re-measured at 93/52 (69) mm Hg, DAO at 87/55 (69) mm Hg, Qp/Qs was calculated to be 0.85, and PVRI was 20.8 WU/m^2. The lowest blood pressure during the operation was 92/54 mm Hg, and the highest was 105/69 mm Hg. The operation lasted a total of 55 min, with an estimated blood loss of about 3 mL. About 200 mL of Ringer's acetate solution was intravenously infused. At the end of the operation, BP was 92/54 mm Hg, HR was 113 beats/min, and SpO_2 was 99%. The laryngeal mask was removed when the MAC value dropped to 0.4 after turning off the sevoflurane vaporizer. Oxygen was administered via a face mask for 5 min, and then the patient was returned to the ward when the Aldrete score reached 9. Upon leaving the room, BP was 102/68 mm Hg, HR was 105 beats/min, and SpO_2 was 98%.

70.3 Review of Knowledge Points

70.3.1 Definition and Classification of Pulmonary Hypertension

Pulmonary hypertension is a clinical syndrome associated with a variety of cardiovascular and respiratory diseases. According to the latest guidelines for the diagnosis and treatment of pulmonary hypertension published by the European Society of Cardiology (ESC) and the European Respiratory Society (ERS) in 2022, PH is defined as a mean pulmonary artery pressure > 20 mm Hg at rest based on hemodynamic evaluation by right heart catheterization.

The clinical classification of PH includes Idiopathic pulmonary arterial hypertension (IPAH), PH related to left heart disease, PH related to lung disease and/or hypoxia, PH related to pulmonary artery obstructive disease, PH of unknown and/or multifactorial etiology.

70.3.2 Pulmonary Hypertension Crisis

Pulmonary hypertension crisis (PHC) refers to the severe contraction of pulmonary vessels caused by various factors, such as hypoxia on the basis of pulmonary hypertension, with the pulmonary artery contraction pressure rapidly rising ≥20 mm Hg. The increase of pulmonary vascular resistance leads to a sudden increase in right heart load and right ventricular ejection obstruction, which may cause acute right heart failure and venous system congestion, while the left ventricle shows symptoms of low cardiac output, and insufficient systemic perfusion leads to tissue hypoxia due to a sudden decrease in oxygenated blood returning to the heart.

70.3.3 Pulmonary Vasodilation Test

During the test, patients are given air inhalation for more than 10 min while waiting for PAP and other indicators to return to baseline levels, then PGI_2 inhalation is initiated. PAP, systolic aortic pressure (SAP), and SpO_2 are continuously monitored during PGI_2 inhalation. If the mean pulmonary artery pressure (mPAP) drops by more than 10 mm Hg, the absolute value is ≤40 mm Hg, and the cardiac output increases or at least does not change, the test result is positive with both criteria met. Its significance lies as follows: ① It can be used to judge the prognosis of children with PH, and those with a positive response often have a better prognosis; ② it can be used to guide the use of calcium channel blockers (CCBs) and those with a positive response often have better effects from oral CCBs, thus saving treatment costs, while those with a negative response cannot benefit from long-term treatment with CCBs, and may even exacerbate their conditions. Therefore, in diagnosing and treating pediatric IPAH, all children who may take CCBs for the long term must undergo an acute pulmonary vasodilation test. For children who cannot take CCBs for long term, such as those with obvious right heart failure or hemodynamically unstable, there is no need for an acute pulmonary vasodilation test.

70.4 Discussion

70.4.1 Preoperative Assessment and Preparation

Before surgery, it is necessary to understand the degree of PH, cardiac valve regurgitation, and myocardial contractibility in children with PH through echocardiography. For children with IPAH who have pulmonary artery pressure exceeding systemic artery pressure and have not received any medicine treatment, the risk of anesthesia is particularly high. General anesthesia in children with idiopathic pulmonary arterial hypertension can easily induce PHC; the incidence of cardiac arrest and mortality are higher than other types of PAH. PHC has a rapid onset and progression. Without proper treatment, it can quickly deteriorate and cause death. Hypoxemia, acidosis, and coronary perfusion insufficiency caused by hypotension and other factors that increase pulmonary vascular resistance can all induce PHC. Therefore, systemic vasoconstrictors such as norepinephrine and phenylephrine or positive inotropic drugs such as epinephrine and dopamine should be prepared in advance. In order to prevent PHC, inhaled pulmonary vasodilators such as PGI_2 should also be simultaneously prepared. If cardiac arrest occurs, immediate resuscitation should be conducted according to the advanced life support guidelines, and extracorporeal membrane oxygenation (ECMO) can be used if it is necessary.

70.4.2 Intraoperative Anesthetic Management

1. Anesthetic drugs.
   The ideal anesthetics for children with PH should have specific pulmonary vasodilatory effects, but there are no or minimal effects on systemic vasodilation and myocardial contractility. However, existing anesthetics cannot satisfy these requirements. Most anesthetics change the heart rate or rhythm, cardiac contractility, systemic vascular resistance, and pulmonary vascular resistance to varying degrees (depending on the dose and

speed of administration). For this case, midazolam and fentanyl, which have little effect on systemic and pulmonary circulation, were chosen for induction of anesthesia. Supplementing a small dose of propofol can help reduce pulmonary artery and pulmonary vascular resistance, which may prevent drastic fluctuations in blood pressure. Since the pain stimulus during catheter examination is not severe, only a certain depth of sedation is needed. We chose to maintain anesthesia with about 1.0 MAC of sevoflurane during the operation.

2. Perioperative management.
Normally, the anesthesiologist keeps away from children's heads. If airway problems occur, it is difficult to find in time. It is better to equip the catheter lab with comprehensive monitoring equipment. The femoral artery is usually catheterized, and the operation may cause interruption of pressure monitoring or changes in the waveform, so noninvasive blood pressure of the upper limb should be considered for additional measurement. Peripheral veins are usually accessed in the upper limbs for easy administration of drugs. Because the catheter physician needs to wear protective clothing during the operation, a lower temperature in the catheter lab is often set, so special attention should be paid to maintaining the child's body temperature to prevent recovery delay.

The insertion of a laryngeal mask causes less stimulation to the child. This technique is suitable for short-term cardiac catheter examination. Since this case required a pulmonary vasodilation test, spontaneous breathing was maintained, which is similar to the child's physiological state. However, under spontaneous breathing, it is required to monitor $ETCO_2$ changes closely. Otherwise, a higher arterial carbon dioxide pressure ($PaCO_2$) can cause an increase in pulmonary artery pressure and even induce PHC. Studies have shown that PVR will not increase when the arterial pH exceeds 7.40 with the arterial oxygen partial pressure (PaO_2) greater than 60 mm Hg. Therefore, hypoxia and respiratory acidosis should be avoided during surgery. If PHC occurs, early use of systemic vasoconstrictors or positive inotropic drugs can improve coronary perfusion and cardiac function and prevent cardiac arrest. Since hypotension may be related to acute intravenous injection of vasodilators, it is better to administer pulmonary vasodilators by inhalation in emergencies, such as nitric oxide and PGI_2. If PVR increases while ventricular function decreases, cardiac arrest may be difficult to avoid. ECMO can be considered for cardiac assistance at this time.

At the end of the surgery, all preventive measures must be taken to avoid hypoxemia, hypotension, and hypovolemia and control postoperative pain. If possible, try not to suction sputum or maintain a certain depth of anesthesia to remove secretions. Any treatment that reduces PVR, such as nitric oxide, should be carefully discontinued to avoid PVR rebound.

70.5 Conclusion

Children with IPAH have an increased risk of perioperative complications during cardiac catheterization treatment. Although many factors can cause the progression of PAH, PAP increase is the most common cause. Since all of the current anesthetics impact the cardiovascular system, it is better for anesthesiologists to optimize the use of these anesthetics reasonably. It is also necessary to avoid factors that induce PHC. Once PHC occurs, immediate and correct treatment must be initiated (Bin Xue).

71 Anesthetic Management of Cardiac Catheterization in Children with Dilated Cardiomyopathy and Pulmonary Arterial Hypertension

Huiyan Hou

Abstract

A 4-year-old girl was diagnosed with incomplete myocardial densification and pulmonary arterial hypertension (PAH) at a local hospital 3 years ago, which was not alleviated by treatment with internal medicines. She was diagnosed with dilated cardiomyopathy (DCM) and severe PAH at our hospital 8 months ago. Targeted drugs, including tadalafil and bosentan treated the PAH. Metoprolol was used to control heart rate. Furosemide and spironolactone were used for symptomatic treatments. Recently, she experienced recurrent syncope with the New York Heart Association (NYHA) classification of heart failure class III. She was scheduled to undergo cardiac catheterization under general anesthesia. The key point of anesthetic management is to maintain heart function and avoid the increase of pulmonary vascular resistance.

DCM is characterized by widespread heart dilation accompanied by systolic dysfunction, of which the left ventricular enlargement is more significant. The cause of DCM is unknown in most pediatric patients, which may relate to infection, genetics, metabolic disorders, and endocrine disorders. DCM can occur at any age. The onset of DCM is usually very insidious, with irritability, anorexia, fatigue, abdominal pain, cough, and dyspnea being the most common symptoms. It can suddenly develop heart failure sometimes. In the late stage of disease progression, left ventricular dysfunction can occur and lead to pulmonary congestion and post-capillary PAH. Other factors may also cause the PAH. This chapter reports the anesthetic management of cardiac catheterization in children with DCM and PAH.

71.1 Case Presentation

The patient was a 4-year-old girl with a weight of 13.3 kg. She was born full-term without a history of asphyxia. Three years ago, she was diagnosed with incomplete myocardial densification and PAH by echocardiography due to dyspnea, wheezing, and coughing. Despite the treatment with digoxin, captopril, and diuretics, she still experienced recurrent symptoms of dyspnea, coughing, and reduced exercise tolerance. Echocardiography at the local hospital showed that the whole heart was enlarged (the left atrium and ventricle were more obvious). The movement in the middle and lower segments of the interventricular septum was uncoordinated. The forward flow speed of the mitral valve was

H. Hou (✉)
The National Children's Medical Center (Shanghai), Department of Anesthesiology of Shanghai Children's Medical Center, Shanghai Jiao Tong University School of Medicine, Shanghai, China
e-mail: houhuiyan@scmc.com.cn

J. Zheng et al. (eds.), *Selected Pediatric Cardiovascular Surgery Anesthesia Cases*,
https://doi.org/10.1007/978-981-96-5614-1_71

slightly faster, with mild to moderate regurgitation of the tricuspid valve. The compliance of the left and right ventricular walls was poor with left ventricular noncompaction. The left ventricular systolic function was within the lower limit of normal range. A cardiac MRI at the local hospital indicated the left and right ventricular noncompaction. The movement in the middle segment of the interventricular septum was uncoordinated. Genetic testing suggested variation in the SCN5A gene. Therefore, SCN5A gene variation-related cardiomyopathy was considered. After 15 days of treatment with bosentan and tadalafil to reduce pulmonary artery pressure, metoprolol to control heart rate, furosemide and spironolactone for diuresis, and captopril to protect heart function, the patient became better and was discharged from the hospital. Two months ago, the child suddenly fell into a faint after crying, manifesting as cyanosis of the lips, loss of consciousness, cold sweat, but no convulsions, no incontinence. She got relief after a few seconds with a total of four to five episodes. Outpatient echocardiography suggested whole heart enlargement, double-chambered left ventricle, moderate tricuspid valve regurgitation, PAH, poor left and right ventricular compliance, and normal left and right ventricular contractibility.

Physical examination: The child's growth and development were slightly behind her peers, her general activity was poor, and any slightly intense activity could lead to fainting. Special examination found that the precordial area was significantly raised, the heart rate was 85 beats/min, the rhythm was regular, the heart sounds were strong, and a III/VI grade systolic murmur could be heard in the precordial area.

Laboratory tests: Complete cell count with differential was normal. Liver and kidney function were normal. N-terminal pro-brain natriuretic peptide (NT-proBNP) 4513 pg/mL.

Electrocardiogram (ECG): Sinus rhythm, upright T wave in the right chest leads, right atrial and ventricular enlargement (possible), left atrial enlargement. Total amplitude in V3 lead >60 mm, T wave changes.

24-h dynamic ECG: The average heart rate was 87 beats/min, the slowest heart rate was 59 beats/min, and the fastest was 148 beats/min. A total of 123,572 heartbeats were analyzed, and no pauses greater than 2.0 s were observed. Sinus arrhythmia with nocturnal sinus bradycardia and ST-T changes.

Chest CT: left and right atrial enlargement, right ventricular enlargement, double-chambered left ventricle. Infection in the right lower lung, possible congenital airway malformation in the left lower lung.

Echocardiography: The whole heart was enlarged, with the left atrial enlargement being the most obvious. The atrial septum bulged towards the right atrium; the interventricular septum bulged towards the left ventricle during systole. Left ventricular wall and apex noncompaction, the noncompaction layer/compaction layer>2, acceptable left ventricular wall contractibility. The left ventricle was separated into two chambers by the hypertrophic noncompaction muscle bundles in the inner posterior part of the left ventricle with a muscle layer thickness of 1.52 cm and a flow speed of 1.9 m/s at this area. The right ventricle was slightly hypertrophic with messed trabeculae. Aortic tricuspid valve with acceptable opening activity. The openings of left and right coronary arteries could be seen with inside forward blood flow signals. The pulmonary artery was widened with a main trunk inner diameter of 1.97 cm and acceptable valve opening activity, mild pulmonary valve regurgitation with a speed of 3.66 m/s, and a pressure difference of 54 mm Hg. The diameter of the mitral valve annulus was 2.6 cm with mild regurgitation. The diameter of the tricuspid valve annulus was 2.45 cm with anterior valve tip thickening, curling, slightly prolapsed, closure point misplaced, moderate regurgitation, regurgitation bundle width 0.44 cm, regurgitation speed 5.81 m/s, pressure difference 135 mm Hg. The atrial septum and ventricular septum were intact. The movement in the middle and lower segments of the ventricular septum was uncoordinated with contradictory movement. Left aortic arch. No pericardial effusion was seen. PAH (severe), noncompaction left and right ventricles, double-chambered left ventricle without obstruction.

Moderate tricuspid regurgitation, normal range of left and right ventricular contractibility.

Cardiac MRI: Enlargement of the right ventricle with decreased right ventricular systolic function, obvious noncompaction of left and right ventricles, and abnormal left ventricular muscle bundles.

Preoperative diagnosis: DCM, incomplete myocardial densification of the left ventricle, PAH (severe). Cardiac catheterization surgery was scheduled for this patient.

71.2 Anesthetic Management

The patient did not take any preoperative medications. Upon entering the operating room, basic vital signs were closely monitored with cuff blood pressure (BP) at 102/58 mm Hg, heart rate (HR) was 102 beats/min (atrial flutter rate), and pulse oxygen saturation (SpO_2) was 97%. General anesthesia was induced by intravenous bolus injection of midazolam 1.0 mg, etomidate 4.0 mg, fentanyl 40 μg, and rocuronium 10 mg. Once the eyelash reflex disappeared, an ID 5.0 mm cuffed endotracheal tube was intubated under direct laryngoscopy. The tube depth was fixed after verification of the appropriate position by bilateral auscultation of the lungs. The patient was ventilated with pressure-controlled ventilation-volume guaranteed (PCV-VG) mode with oxygen flow rate 2 L/min, fraction of inspired oxygen (FiO_2) of 60%, tidal volume (VT) 140 mL, respiratory rate (RR) 20 times/min, inspiratory to expiratory (I:E) time ratio of 1:2. The end-tidal carbon dioxide ($ETCO_2$) was maintained around 35–45 mm Hg during surgery. After the induction of anesthesia, the left radial artery was catheterized for continuous invasive arterial pressure (ABP) monitoring. At the same time, the left external jugular vein was catheterized for vasoactive drugs administered as a backup route. Anesthesia was maintained with sevoflurane inhalation, with the minimum alveolar concentration (MAC) maintained at 0.8–1.0. About 100 mL of sodium acetate Ringer's solution was intravenously infused.

71.3 Postoperative Outcome

The operation lasted for 20 min in total. The pulmonary artery pressure measured by cardiac catheterization was 105/47 mm Hg, the aortic pressure was simultaneously measured at 106/59 mm Hg, the left pulmonary artery wedge pressure was 33 mm Hg, and the left ventricular end-diastolic pressure was 40 mm Hg. After cardiac catheterization examination, the inhalation of anesthetic drugs was turned off. Airway and oral secretions were first suctioned under deep anesthesia, and then 30 mg of Sugammadex was intravenously administered to antagonize residual muscle relaxation. After the patient's spontaneous breathing resumed, the tracheal tube was successfully removed from the operating room. This patient was transferred to the general ward from the post-anesthesia care unit (PACU) 35 min after surgery.

71.4 Review of Knowledge Points

71.4.1 DCM

It is necessary to effectively control heart failure and arrhythmia, prevent sudden death and embolism, and improve the quality of life and survival rate for children with DCM. By using small doses of dopamine and dobutamine, the myocardial contractility and cardiac output are usually increased without increasing the systemic vascular resistance. The management of preload in DCM patients is very critical. Preload increase does not significantly increase the stroke volume. Excessive blood volume overload does not increase cardiac output; on the contrary, it can aggravate heart failure. However, insufficient blood volume may lead to cardiac output decrease. Therefore, it is better to use blood volume monitoring methods such as central venous pressure (CVP) and stroke volume variation (SVV) to ensure effective preload maintenance.

71.4.2 Pulmonary Hypertension Crisis

It should be very cautious for children with DCM and PAH to avoid the occurrence of pulmonary hypertension crisis (PHC), which refers to the severe contraction of pulmonary vessels caused by factors such as hypoxia on the basis of PAH, the rapid rise of pulmonary artery contraction pressure $\geq$ 20 mm Hg. The increase in pulmonary vascular resistance can cause a sudden increase in right heart afterload and acute right heart failure caused by right ventricular ejection obstruction and venous system congestion. While the left ventricle shows symptoms of low cardiac output due to a sudden decrease in cardiac return, insufficient systemic perfusion leads to tissue hypoxia, which can be life-threatening in severe cases. Therefore, the inducing factors during the perioperative period should be avoided to prevent the occurrence of PHC.

71.5 Discussion

71.5.1 Preoperative Evaluation and Preparation

It is necessary to fully understand the medical history, evaluate the cardiac function, and improve the cardiac function before surgery since the severity of children with DCM varies dramatically from mild to severe, and severe cases may experience heart failure, arrhythmia, or even sudden death during the perioperative period. For this patient, we made a comprehensive preoperative evaluation of anesthetic risk and focused on preoperative echocardiography, ECG, and cardiac MRI examination. The patient has been ill for over 3 years with symptoms of shortness of breath, fatigue after activity, and recent recurrent syncope. Despite the long-term treatment of PAH by targeted drugs, it was still progressively exacerbated with heart function at class III. Therefore, we made full preparations during the perioperative period. In addition to the basic monitoring such as ECG, SpO_2, $ETCO_2$, body temperature, and urine output, ABP monitoring was also conducted to help accurately regulate the depth of anesthesia and maintain hemodynamic stability.

71.5.2 Intraoperative Anesthetic Management

Children with DCM are mainly characterized by left ventricular enlargement or both ventricular enlargements and myocardial contractile dysfunction. The goal of anesthesia for children with DCM and heart failure should focus on stabilizing hemodynamics, improving cardiac pump function, and maintaining vital organ perfusion and function, which should be carried throughout the entire perioperative period. The preload reserves are usually exhausted and fixed in children with DCM. Therefore, stroke volume cannot be significantly increased by preload increase. Furthermore, bradycardia will reduce cardiac output. On the contrary, tachycardia may cause damage to the subendocardial perfusion without left ventricular filling reduction. Stroke volume and cardiac output may be improved by enhancing myocardial contractility and decreasing systemic circulation resistance.

In this case, the induction and maintenance of anesthesia followed the anesthesia strategies for pediatric cardiac surgery. The anesthetic with minimal impact on cardiac function, such as midazolam, etomidate, fentanyl, and rocuronium, was intravenously administered for the induction of anesthesia. The anesthesia was maintained by sevoflurane inhalation with a MAC value above 0.6 to keep hemodynamic stability and maintain the satisfactory depth of general anesthesia by adjustment of sevoflurane concentration.

Emergency treatment plans for pulmonary hypertension crisis (PHC) should be fully prepared for patients with DCM and PAH. The PHC treatment plans are as follows:

1. Pure oxygen ventilation.
2. Deepen anesthesia/sedation and administer analgesics.
3. Use pulmonary vasodilators, inhale iloprost, or intravenous administration of milrinone.
4. Use muscle relaxants.

5. Use the lowest level of PEEP during ventilation to maintain oxygenation, prolong the exhalation phase, and maintain low airway pressure.
6. Use sodium bicarbonate to correct acidosis.
7. Ensure good coronary perfusion.
8. Maintain sinus rhythm.
9. Maintain normal body temperature.
10. Consider using extra-corporeal membrane oxygenation (ECMO) support if it is necessary.

71.6 Shortcomings and Limitations

CVP, SVV, and other volume load monitoring methods were not used in this case, which would be more beneficial for maintaining the patient's blood volume load and cardiac function.

71.7 Conclusion

Maintaining stroke volume and cardiac output and ensuring appropriate volume load for the anesthetic management of children with DCM is necessary. The perioperative complications and mortality rate can only be effectively prevented and reduced by precise perioperative management (Huiyan Hou).

72 Anesthetic Management of Balloon Dilatation in a Neonate with Aortic Stenosis

Liping Sun

Abstract

During a postnatal examination, an 11-day-old full-term male infant was diagnosed to have a heart murmur. Upon echocardiographic evaluation, it was discovered that he had aortic valve stenosis, showing a transvalvular flow velocity of 5.62 m/s and a pressure gradient of 75 mm Hg, coupled with an atrial septal defect (type II). Given the critical nature of the aortic valve stenosis and the presence of heart failure, early intervention was deemed crucial. Percutaneous balloon aortic valvuloplasty emerged as a viable treatment option for congenital aortic valve stenosis in children, offering the benefit of avoiding invasive open-heart surgery in neonates. The anesthetic management for this procedure was centered on maintaining cardiac output and coronary perfusion to ensure a successful surgical outcome.

Aortic stenosis (AS) encompasses a range of conditions, including aortic valve stenosis, supravalvular stenosis, and subvalvular stenosis. Congenital aortic valve stenosis is a relatively common congenital heart disease, occurring in approximately 0.30–0.34 per 10,000 births. Males are disproportionately affected by AS, male-to-female ratio of 4:1. Infants with AS often present with smaller left ventricles and aortic valve rings, indicative of a mild form of left heart hypoplasia syndrome. Notably, about 10% of infants with severe AS experience symptoms of heart failure or even cardiogenic shock during the neonatal or infant period, necessitating urgent therapeutic intervention. Surgical procedures in these patients pose heightened anesthesia risks. This chapter highlights the anesthetic management considerations for a neonate with aortic valve stenosis undergoing balloon valvuloplasty.

72.1 Case Presentation

An 11-day-old boy, weighing 3.27 kg and standing at 50 cm tall, was born full-term through natural delivery but with a history of intrauterine distress. Shortly after birth, a heart murmur was detected, raising suspicions of congenital heart disease. Throughout his illness, he experienced a single episode of non-projectile vomiting, discharging a significant amount of milky fluid without any traces of bile or coffee-ground material. No cyanosis was evident, and there was no reported event of recurrent respiratory infections. An echocardiography subsequently revealed AS and an atrial septal defect (type II), prompting his hospitalization.

L. Sun (✉)
The National Children's Medical Center (Shanghai), Department of Anesthesiology of Shanghai Children's Medical Center, Shanghai Jiao Tong University School of Medicine, Shanghai, China
e-mail: sunliping@scmc.com.cn

J. Zheng et al. (eds.), *Selected Pediatric Cardiovascular Surgery Anesthesia Cases*,
https://doi.org/10.1007/978-981-96-5614-1_72

Physical examination: The baby exhibited consciousness, maintained relatively stable breathing, and a pulse oxygen saturation (SpO_2) of 96%. Auscultation of the lungs revealed coarse breath sounds with no audible rales. The heart rate (HR) was 157 beats/min, regular rhythm. A grade III/VI rough regurgitant murmur was audible at the 1–2 intercostal space along the right margin of the sternum. Upon examination, the liver was not palpable below the ribs, and the extremities were warm, devoid of any signs of edema.

Laboratory test (several abnormal and meaningful negative indicators were observed): The blood routine and coagulation function tests were normal, NT-proBNP levels at 255 pg/mL and CK-MB levels at 3.90 μg/L.

Chest X-ray: Enlarged heart shadow, multiple lung markings. Additionally, there is a possible right clavicle fracture.

Electrocardiogram: Paroxysmal supraventricular tachycardia.

Chest CT: Aortic valve stenosis, atrial septal defect.

Echocardiography: Aortic valve stenosis with mild regurgitation (pressure gradient 75 mm Hg), atrial septal defect (II).

Preoperative diagnosis: Aortic valve stenosis, paroxysmal supraventricular tachycardia, and an atrial septal defect. As a result, it is planned to proceed with an elective percutaneous balloon aortic valvuloplasty as the treatment strategy.

72.2 Anesthetic Management

The child was transferred to the operating theater with blood pressure (BP) at 65/35 mm Hg, HR 160 beats/min, and SpO_2 96%. A peripheral vein was accessed, followed by the induction of anesthesia using intravenous bolus doses consisting of 0.3 mg midazolam, 1.0 mg etomidate, 2.5 μg fentanyl, and 2.0 mg rocuronium. After the disappearance of the eyelash reflex, a cuffed endotracheal tube with an inner diameter of 3.5 was intubated under a visible laryngoscope and fixed after verification of the appropriate position by bilateral auscultation of the lungs. Pressure control with volume guarantee was used, with the following respiratory parameters set: 50% inhaled oxygen concentration, 16 cm H_2O inspiratory pressure, 30 mL tidal volume (VT), 26 breaths/min respiratory rate (RR), 1:2 inspiratory to expiratory ratio (I:E). End-tidal carbon dioxide ($ETCO_2$) was maintained within the range of 38–40 mm Hg. Anesthesia was maintained with sevoflurane inhalation, with the minimum alveolar concentration (MAC) maintained at 0.8–1.0. Atropine 0.1 mg and dexamethasone 2.0 mg were intravenously administered before aortic valve dilation.

Following standard disinfection and draping procedures, a 4F pigtail catheter and a 4F sheath were inserted via the right femoral artery. Subsequently, the pressures and oxygen saturation of each chamber were accurately measured. Selective angiography revealed thickening of the aortic valve, with a valve annulus diameter approximately measuring 8.5 mm. The aortic arch appeared morphologically normal, with no evident patent ductus arteriosus or significant aortic valve regurgitation. An 8 × 40 mm balloon was successfully navigated to the valve annulus via the right femoral artery, and the aortic valve was dilated twice with the balloon. Initially, the narrowed section was visible, but it subsequently disappeared upon completion of the dilation. Notably, hypotension and bradycardia occurred during the balloon dilation procedure but gradually returned to normal upon deflation of the balloon. Postoperative bedside ultrasound revealed a flow velocity across the aortic valve of approximately 2.5 m/s. After the operation, the child was transferred to the Neonatal Intensive Care Unit for close monitoring with mechanical ventilation assistance.

72.3 Postoperative Outcome

The operation lasted 35 min with 5 mL blood loss, and 30 mL Ringer's acetate solution was infused. At the end of the surgery, the patient's BP was 62/30 mm Hg, HR 155 beats/min, and SpO_2 95%. Subsequently, the patient was transferred to the NICU, where mechanical ventilation was administered. The patient was extubated on the next day and left the NICU on the tenth day after surgery.

72.4 Review of Knowledge Points

72.4.1 Pathophysiology of Aortic Stenosis

Aortic stenosis can occur in multiple locations, including the valve, subvalvular, or supravalvular regions. The most prevalent cause of aortic valve stenosis is a fused bicuspid aortic valve. While nonobstructive bicuspid aortic values may not present with overt clinical symptoms, symptomatic newborns often have severe aortic valve stenosis. Additionally, these patients frequently show underdevelopment of the aortic valve ring, ascending aorta, mitral valve, and left ventricular cavity. There are two distinct types of subaortic stenosis. One type involves a localized septum located 1–2 cm beneath the aortic valve ring. The other type arises from the overgrowth of fibromuscular tissue within the left ventricular outflow tract, resulting in a tunnel-like stenosis. In contrast, supravalvular aortic stenosis is primarily attributed to a microdeletion of the elastin gene at the 7q11.23 locus on chromosome 7. A characteristic feature of supravalvular aortic stenosis is the presence of an hourglass-shaped stenosis at the junction of the aortic sinus and the duct. In approximately 30% of cases, significant tubular stenosis extends throughout the ascending aorta, often reaching the aortic arch and the origin of the brachiocephalic trunk. Notably, approximately 40% of children with supravalvular aortic stenosis also exhibit severe pulmonary artery stenosis and right ventricular pressure overload.

72.4.2 Clinical Manifestations of Aortic Stenosis

Children with mild to moderate aortic typically remain asymptomatic, while severe stenosis can manifest as exertional chest pain or syncope, rapidly progressing to congestive heart failure. Most patients maintain normal blood pressure. However, those with severe aortic stenosis have a narrowed pulse pressure. In patients with supravalvular AS, it is possible to observe a higher systolic pressure in the right arm compared to the left. Mild stenosis may show a normal electrocardiogram, whereas severe stenosis can reveal left ventricular hypertrophy. Chest radiographs are generally normal, but in the case of valvular stenosis, an enlarged ascending aorta may occasionally be observed, and heart failure can result in significant cardiac enlargement.

72.4.3 Surgical Methods for Aortic Stenosis

Aortic stenosis can be effectively managed through catheter intervention or surgical procedures. Ideally, aortic valve balloon dilation can significantly reduce both the peak pressure gradient and average pressure gradient across the aortic valve without causing hemodynamically significant aortic regurgitation. Surgical treatment involves a transverse incision or opening of the ascending aorta to address isolated aortic valve stenosis, followed by a decision on whether to repair or replace the aortic valve. For children with aortic valve stenosis accompanied by hypoplasia of the left ventricular outflow tract, it may be necessary to employ a patch to enlarge the outflow tract and replace the aortic valve during repair of the aorta or subaortic stenosis. In certain instances, surgical correction of the narrowing at the coronary artery ostium may also be warranted.

72.5 Discussion

72.5.1 Preoperative Evaluation and Preparation

Severe aortic valve stenosis in newborns and small infants exhibits notable differences in pathophysiology, clinical manifestations, and treatment principles compared to older children and adult patients. In newborns with critical AS, the systemic circulation often relies heavily on the patency of the arterial duct. Signs of inadequate perfusion, cyanosis, and lethargy may emerge as the duct begins to close, resulting in decreased systemic blood flow that can lead to circulatory failure and, ultimately, death. Prompt diagnosis and management are crucial in these vulnerable patients to prevent such dire consequences. The administration of prostaglandin E_1 to reopen the arterial duct can be lifesaving for the child. In this particular case, the child exhibited systemic cyanosis coupled with respiratory distress. Cardiac imaging via two-dimensional pulsed color Doppler ultrasound revealed aortic valve stenosis with mild regurgitation (pressure gradient of 75 mm Hg), an atrial septal defect (II), and ultrasound findings indicative of severe aortic valve stenosis. Given the anesthesia risk involved, it is crucial to conduct a comprehensive and meticulous preoperative assessment for newborns with congenital heart disease. This evaluation should include an assessment of whether the child has any additional malformations or is part of a congenital disease syndrome, as approximately 8% of children with congenital heart disease also have other malformations. Additionally, as newborns have immature glycogen storage capabilities and limited glycogen decomposition and gluconeogenesis functions, minimizing the preoperative fasting time is essential to maintain their physiological status.

72.5.2 Anesthetic Management

In this case, the anesthesia induction and maintenance were administered using etomidate, sufentanil, and sevoflurane, anesthetics that exert minimal hemodynamic effects. A more controllable intravenous induction method was selected to ensure maximum hemodynamic stability, involving the gradual titration of the anesthetics to minimize any potential hemodynamic fluctuations.

The primary objective of intraoperative anesthetic management is to sustain cardiac output and coronary perfusion. During the process of aortic valve balloon dilation, there is a surge in left ventricular pressure load, which can lead to compromised left heart function, a sharp decrease in cardiac output, and potentially cardiac arrest. Therefore, anesthesiologists must vigilantly monitor hemodynamic indicators and maintain close communication with the interventional physician to promptly address any adverse cardiovascular events. Additionally, it is crucial to ensure the availability of emergency drugs and defibrillation equipment and to initiate cardiopulmonary resuscitation promptly in the event of cardiac arrest. In this particular case of balloon aortic valvopathy, although there were significant fluctuations in hemodynamics, these returned to normal promptly following balloon withdrawal and with the administration of appropriate drugs.

If a child with AS experiences tachycardia, it can be fatal. Even though there is sufficient time during systole for blood to traverse the narrowed aortic valve, the diastolic period and subendocardial perfusion are significantly shortened, leading to compromised cardiac function. Bradycardia is also disadvantageous as the transvalvular pressure gradient is directly proportional to the square of the transvalvular flow. In the case of bradycardia, to maintain cardiac output, it becomes necessary to increase the transvalvular flow, which unfortunately results in an elevation of the transvalvular pressure gradient, effectively increasing the stroke output. This pressure gradient increase can negatively affect the heart's function and hemodynamic stability. During the operation, it is crucial to avoid any elevation in systemic circulation resistance, as this would lead to an increased left ventricular pressure load and, consequently, a significant reduction in left heart output. Fortunately, in this case, the child's aortic valve stenosis was successfully corrected through interventional balloon dilation treatment, thus obviating the need for neonatal open-heart surgery.

72.6 Shortcomings and Limitations

This case was successfully carried out in the cardiac catheterization room outside the operating room. However, due to certain limitations, monitoring the child's body temperature and cerebral and renal perfusion was impossible.

72.7 Conclusion

In conclusion, anesthesiologists must possess extensive experience in pediatric cardiac anesthesia and excel in communicating with team members to guarantee the safety of children throughout the perioperative period. Given the diverse nature of congenital heart diseases and catheterization procedures, it is imperative to comprehensively consider the child's underlying condition and interventional treatment methods and make individualized anesthesia plans accordingly (Liping Sun).

73 Anesthetic Management of Interventional Balloon Valvuloplasty for a Child with Pulmonary Valve Stenosis

Liping Sun

Abstract

A heart murmur was heard in a 5-month-old female infant during a postnatal physical examination, and echocardiography showed pulmonary valve stenosis with a pressure gradient of 51 mm Hg and bilateral ventricular wall hypertrophy. This case involved an infant with isolated pulmonary valve stenosis and a history of subarachnoid hemorrhage after birth. She was scheduled to undergo balloon pulmonary valvuloplasty under general anesthesia. Interventional balloon pulmonary valvuloplasty will lead to a transient reduction in pulmonary blood flow, end-tidal carbon dioxide, and blood oxygen saturation. Bradycardia may even happen, which requires vasoactive agents to treat if it is necessary.

Pulmonary stenosis (PS) is predominantly caused by isolated pulmonary valve stenosis, accounting for approximately 90% of PS, followed by infundibular stenosis. Children with mild PS can normally grow and develop without surgical intervention. Those children with moderate PS may experience palpitations and shortness of breath after physical exertion around the age of 20. Those children with severe PS often present with noticeable symptoms in early childhood, which can result in early childhood mortality if left untreated. Prior to the 1980s, open heart surgical relief under cardiopulmonary bypass was the only treatment for PS. With the advancements in medicine, percutaneous balloon pulmonary valvuloplasty has emerged as the preferred treatment for isolated PS. This chapter discusses the anesthetic management of interventional balloon pulmonary valvuloplasty in a child with PS.

73.1 Case Presentation

The patient was a 5-month-old girl with a weight of 5 kg and a height of 60.5 cm. She was born full-term without a history of asphyxia during delivery. One month after birth, a heart murmur was heard during a physical examination, which raised suspicions of congenital heart disease (CHD). No cyanosis in her lips and extremities was found. She experienced limited physical exertion and significant delay in growth and development. There was no record of recurrent respiratory infection. She had a history of subarachnoid hemorrhage and she was under a close follow-up.

Physical examination: The patient was conscious with regular breathing. No cyanosis in her lips and extremities was found. Auscultation revealed symmetrical lung sounds without rales.

L. Sun (✉)
The National Children's Medical Center (Shanghai), Department of Anesthesiology of Shanghai Children's Medical Center, Shanghai Jiao Tong University School of Medicine, Shanghai, China
e-mail: sunliping@scmc.com.cn

J. Zheng et al. (eds.), *Selected Pediatric Cardiovascular Surgery Anesthesia Cases*,
https://doi.org/10.1007/978-981-96-5614-1_73

Heart rate (HR) was 142 beats/min with regular rhythm and accentuated P2 sound. The liver was not palpable below the ribs. Extremities were warm without edema.

Laboratory tests: C-reactive protein <0.8 mg/L, white blood cell count 15.14 × 10^9/L, platelet count 213 × 10^9/L, hemoglobin 116.0 g/L, neutrophils 2.38 × 10^9/L, PT 12.4 s, APTT 41.2 s, TT 19.5 s. CK 21 U/L, LDH 553 U/L. NT-proBNP 255 pg/mL.

Chest X-ray: Enlarged cardiac Silhouette, increased lung markings and blur in both lungs.

Electrocardiogram (ECG): Sinus tachycardia, left axis deviation, deep Q wave in I, aVL, right ventricular enlargement.

Echocardiography: PS (pressure gradient 51 mm Hg), bilateral ventricular wall hypertrophy.

Preoperative diagnosis: PS, myocardial hypertrophy. She was scheduled to undergo elective interventional balloon pulmonary valvuloplasty under general anesthesia.

73.2 Anesthetic Management

The patient did not take any preoperative medications. After entering the room, routine vital signs were monitored with baseline blood pressure (BP) 85/46 mm Hg, HR 150 beats/min, and pulse oxygen saturation (SpO_2) 99%. After the peripheral vein was accessed, anesthesia was induced by intravenous bolus injection of etomidate 1.5 mg, sufentanil 1.0 μg, and rocuronium 2.5 mg. After the eyelash reflex disappeared, a cuffed endotracheal tube with an inner diameter of 3.5 mm was intubated with video laryngoscopy assistance and fixed after verifying the appropriate position by bilateral lung auscultation. Pressure-controlled ventilation with volume guarantee mode was used with the following respiratory parameter settings: Oxygen flow rate 2 L/min, fraction of inspired oxygen (FiO_2) 50%, peak of inspiratory pressure (PIP) 15 cm H_2O, respiratory rate (RR) 20 breaths/min, inspiratory to expiratory (I:E) time ratio 1:2, and end-tidal carbon dioxide ($ETCO_2$) were maintained at 40–45 mm Hg during procedure. Anesthesia was maintained with sevoflurane inhalation, with the minimum alveolar concentration (MAC) maintained at 0.8–1.0. Atropine 0.1 mg and dexamethasone 2.0 mg were intravenously administered.

Following standard disinfection and draping procedures, a 4F pigtail catheter and a vertebral catheter were cannulated via the right femoral vein. The pulmonary artery and right ventricular pressures before balloon dilation were 30/19 mm Hg and 55/5 mm Hg, respectively. Right ventriculography showed valvular and subvalvular stenosis, jet sign, and dome sign were observable. The pulmonary valve annulus was about 9.5 mm. A 12 mm × 20 mm balloon was inserted into the narrow part via the catheter and expanded twice. Waist sign was visible during the first expansion but less prominent after the second expansion. During balloon expansion, the patient's $ETCO_2$ gradually decreased from 38 mm Hg to 21 mm Hg, and the waveform of $ETCO_2$ disappeared. The patient's SpO_2 dropped to a minimum of 65% but gradually returned to normal levels after the balloon was deflated. Bedside echocardiography revealed a transvalvular flow rate of approximately 2.25 m/s. Pulmonary artery and right ventricular pressures after balloon dilation were 40/14 mm Hg and 50/5 mm Hg, respectively. The endotracheal intubation was successfully removed at the end of the procedure, and the patient was safely transferred back to the ward.

73.3 Postoperative Outcome

The operation lasted 55 min in total. The blood loss was about 5 mL. About 80 mL of Ringer's acetate solution was infused. The patient smoothly recovered after surgery and the endotracheal tube was removed in the cardiac catheterization lab. Before leaving the cardiac catheterization lab, the vital signs with nasal cannula oxygen inhalation are BP 82/48 mm Hg, HR 140 beats/min, and SpO_2 98%. The patient was transferred to the cardiology ward and was discharged from the hospital on the postoperative day.

73.4 Review of Knowledge Points

73.4.1 Pathophysiology of Pulmonary Stenosis

Pulmonary stenosis in children is characterized by pulmonary valve thickness with fusion or absence at the junction and small valve opening. Pulmonary artery dilation often occurs due to pulmonary valve stenosis. Pulmonary valve hypoplasia, such as valve leaflets thickness and curl, often occurs in patients with Noonan syndrome. Subvalvular stenosis is typically associated with a large ventricular septal defect (VSD), which is similar to tetralogy of Fallot. The presence of cyanosis is dependent on the severity of pulmonary valve stenosis, particularly in newborns with severe pulmonary artery stenosis. Severe obstruction of right ventricular output can lead to right ventricular hypertrophy, right ventricular compliance reduction, and subsequent tricuspid regurgitation, which then results in right-to-left shunting at the atrial level (patent foramen ovale or atrial septal defect) and varying degrees of cyanosis.

73.4.2 Clinical Manifestations of Pulmonary Stenosis

Clinical manifestations depend on the severity of pulmonary artery obstruction. Children with mild or moderate PS are usually asymptomatic; heart murmurs may be the only sign found during physical examination. Severe stenosis can lead to symptoms of right heart failure, such as dyspnea, fatigue, exertion intolerance, abdominal distension, and lower limb edema. Chest radiographs may reveal right atrial and ventricular enlargement and post-stenotic dilation, which is thought to be caused by the high-speed jet of blood hitting the pulmonary artery wall. ECG typically shows right ventricular hypertrophy with right ventricular axis deviation. Echocardiography with Doppler imaging is often used to assess the morphology of the pulmonary valve, determine the presence of right ventricular hypertrophy, and accurately measure the pressure gradient before and after the stenosis.

73.4.3 iFlow Technology

SyngoiFlow technology involves real-time processing and color coding of conventional DSA's DICOM (Digital Imaging and Communications in Medicine) format data and analyzing the blood flow peak time and other blood flow change parameters. As a quantitative blood flow evaluation tool, iFlow technology reflects changes in the blood flow speed and perfusion volume through local peak time (TTP) and area under the curve (AUC) parameters. It is commonly used in peripheral vascular interventional treatment and is based on DSA angiography. SyngoiFlow technology can overcome the interference of heartbeat and respiratory movement on pulmonary artery blood flow, which can provide an instant quantitative evaluation tool for pulmonary artery hemodynamics and perform radiological analysis at the same time as angiography without increasing additional interventional operations, radiation dose, and contrast agent usage, thus providing a noninvasive hemodynamic quantitative evaluation method for balloon pulmonary valvuloplasty.

73.5 Discussion

73.5.1 Preoperative Assessment and Preparation

The clinical manifestations of children with PS vary dramatically depending on the severity of PS. Children with mild or moderate PS may present without symptoms. In contrast, those with severe PS can experience cyanosis, dyspnea, lower limb edema, and other symptoms and signs of right heart failure. In this case, a significant delay in growth and development happened, physical exertion was limited, and echocardiography revealed PS with a transvalvular pressure difference of 51 mm Hg and bilateral ventricular wall hypertrophy, indicating moderate PS and increased anesthetic risk.

For children presenting with cyanosis, polycythemia, and outflow tract obstruction, the preoperative fasting period should be appropriately reduced to minimize the degree of dehydration and decrease the likelihood of hypoglycemia. This is particularly crucial for infants under 6 months old since their glycogen breakdown and gluconeogenesis abilities are limited, and their glycogen storage function is not fully developed. Therefore, physiological rehydration prior to the surgery had already commenced in this case.

73.5.2 Anesthetic Management During Surgery

In this case, the child was induced and maintained by anesthetics with minimal impact on hemodynamics, such as etomidate, sufentanil, and sevoflurane. In addition, intravenous induction of anesthesia with better controllability and slower titration of anesthetics was adopted to minimize hemodynamic fluctuations as much as possible.

During the anesthetic management, it is important to know that elevated blood CO_2 can cause respiratory acidosis, disturb homeostasis, and potentially compromise hemodynamic stability. Therefore, it is better to maintain $ETCO_2$ level at 45–50 mm Hg by adjustment of ventilation parameters during surgery. As the balloon dilates the pulmonary valve, pulmonary blood flow will be decreased until it disappears, resulting in a gradual decrease in $ETCO_2$, transient reduction in SpO_2, and even bradycardia. Once the balloon is deflated, these parameters will gradually return to normal. Effective communication between an anesthesiologist and an interventional cardiologist is essential to prevent complications by knowing the extent and timing of balloon dilation to. Once severe arrhythmia or cardiac arrest happens, immediate release of the balloon should be conducted. Cardiac resuscitation should be initiated according to the real situation. The absence of the "waist sign" in the angiogram confirms the success of pulmonary valve balloon valvuloplasty. The increases in postoperative pulmonary blood flow and SpO_2 also indicate the effectiveness of pulmonary valve balloon valvuloplasty. Intraoperative arrhythmia may be associated with changes in sympathetic excitability, which necessitates timely adjustment of anesthesia depth based on the procedure's progression. The vasoactive drugs can be used if it is required. Furthermore, the potential allergic reaction to the contrast agent should be considered in cases of persistent hypotension.

73.6 Conclusion

Interventional balloon pulmonary valvuloplasty offers advantages such as reduced trauma, favorable outcomes, and fewer complications, making it the preferred treatment for children with PS. Given the rapid hemodynamic changes during the procedure, the anesthesiologist must closely monitor the child's condition and take proactive measures to prevent complications (Liping Sun).

74 Anesthetic Management of Transcatheter Closure of Ventricular Septal Defect in a Child with Recent Upper Respiratory Tract Infection

Kan Zhang

Abstract

A 2-year-old boy was diagnosed with perimembranous ventricular septal defect (VSD) by cardiac ultrasound and scheduled for transcatheter closure of VSD (nonsurgical) under general anesthesia. He had an upper respiratory tract infection (URI) with symptoms of fever, sneezing, runny nose, and coughing 1 week ago. Recent URIs can significantly increase the risk of perioperative respiratory adverse events (PRAE) and put a great challenge on anesthetic management during the perioperative period. The anesthetic management for children with recent URI should focus on the prevention and treatment of PRAE, including preoperative intranasal dexmedetomidine or/and aerosolized budesonide inhalation to reduce airway hyperreactivity, using laryngeal mask airway instead of endotracheal intubation as much as possible, endotracheal extubation under deep anesthesia.

Upper respiratory tract infection (URI) is more common in children with congenital heart disease (CHD) than general pediatric population. The incidence of URI in infants can be even as high as six to seven times per year. Children with CHD are vulnerable to URI, which is usually attributed to increased pulmonary blood flow, young age, and weaker immunity. Although elective surgeries can be postponed due to the obvious URI symptoms during the active period, the airway reactivity to stimuli remains very high even after the disappearance of URI symptoms, which can significantly increase the risk of perioperative respiratory adverse events (PRAE) and affect the patient's outcome.

For children with mild CHD lesions such as small atrial septal defect (ASD), and VSD, the cardiac and pulmonary function reserve is usually preserved, and most of them are usually present without obvious cardiac and pulmonary symptoms at rest. However, concurrent URI or

K. Zhang (✉)
The National Children's Medical Center (Shanghai), Department of Anesthesiology of Shanghai Children's Medical Center, Shanghai Jiao Tong University School of Medicine, Shanghai, China
e-mail: zhangkan@scmc.com.cn

J. Zheng et al. (eds.), *Selected Pediatric Cardiovascular Surgery Anesthesia Cases*,
https://doi.org/10.1007/978-981-96-5614-1_74

PRAE might worsen the cardiac function reserve and result in insufficient oxygen supply, which challenges the anesthetic management no matter whether the patients with CHD were treated by open-heart surgery or therapeutic cardiac catheterization. This chapter reports the anesthetic management of transcatheter closure of the ventricular septal defect in a child with a recent upper respiratory tract infection.

74.1 Case Presentation

This patient was a 2-year-old boy with 80 cm in height and 12 kg in weight. He was diagnosed with VSD by cardiac ultrasound and scheduled for transcatheter closure of VS. He had a fever 1 week ago; the highest temperature was 38.6 °C. URI symptoms such as sneezing, clear nasal discharge, and coughing appeared as the fever subsided after taking ibuprofen. The coughing was more severe in the morning and night, but no sputum was present. The growth and development were normal.

Physical examination: The patient was conscious without cyanosis in the lips and extremities. The breathing sounds were coarse without rales in both lungs. Temperature 37.5 °C, heart rate (HR) 118 beats/min, blood pressure (BP) 89/45 mm Hg, respiratory rate (RR) 25 times/min. The heart sound was dull, with an enlarged range. III/VI grade murmurs in the precordial area. No peripheral edema.

Laboratory tests: No obvious abnormalities were seen in the complete blood count, liver, and kidney function tests.

Chest X-ray: Enlarged cardiac silhouette, increased lung markings in both lungs.

Electrocardiogram (ECG): Sinus rhythm.

Echocardiography: Left atrial enlargement, stronger left ventricular contractibility with left ventricular ejection fraction (LVEF) at 55%, perimembranous VSD with left-to-right shunting and mild mitral regurgitation.

74.2 Anesthetic Management

The patient was fasted for 6 h for solid food and 2 h for clear liquid before surgery. Considering the preoperative cough, especially in the morning and at night, aerosolized budesonide inhalation and intranasal dexmedetomidine 2.0 μg/kg were conducted 30 min before surgery. Routine monitoring, including BP, ECG, and pulse oxygen saturation (SpO_2), was conducted upon entering the catheterization lab. Baseline HR was 126 beats/min, BP 92/50 mm Hg, and SpO_2 98%. Anesthesia was induced by intravenous bolus injection of propofol 3.0 mg/kg, sufentanil 0.3 μg/kg, atropine 0.01 mg/kg, and dexamethasone 2.5 mg. After the disappearance of the eyelash reflex, size 2 laryngeal mask airways (LMA) were placed for intraoperative ventilation. Anesthesia was maintained with sevoflurane inhalation at 1.0–1.2 MAC and 50% fraction of inspired oxygen. The whole procedure lasted for approximately 60 min in total. The spontaneous breathing returned after the procedure. After SpO_2 was maintained above 96% with room air for 5 min, the LMA was successfully removed under deep anesthesia. However, airway obstruction secondary to glossoptosis occurred, which was quickly relieved by the placement of the oropharyngeal airway. The patient was transferred to the ward for recovery when the modified Aldrete score was beyond 8. The patient was calm, with a Wong–Baker score of 2 during the next day's follow-up. His parents reported neither discomfort nor vomiting.

74.3 Review of Knowledge Points

74.3.1 Pediatric Upper Respiratory Tract Infection

The upper respiratory tract includes the nose, paranasal sinuses, pharynx, Eustachian tube, epiglottis, and larynx. The most common URI pathogens are influenza, parainfluenza, respiratory syncytial, coronavirus, rhinovirus, etc., which can induce secondary bacterial infections. URI is common in children, especially infants and preschool children, with six to eight times per year on average. Children, especially those with CHD, were vulnerable to URI. Recent URI referred to URI occurred within the latest 2 weeks. The patients can be diagnosed as active URIs if they present at least two of the following symptoms: runny nose, sore throat, sneezing, nasal congestion, discomfort, coughing, and fever. The initial symptoms of URI were sore or itchy throat and hoarseness, followed by a runny nose, sneezing, and coughing. The nasal secretion at the beginning is always watery and can turn purulent. After nasal congestion, mouth breathing is usually required. Unlike adults, children with URI often have a fever accompanied by fatigue, headache, muscle pain, and loss of appetite. Generally speaking, URI is a self-limiting disease. Most children with URI can recover within 7–10 days; it can last for 3 weeks in some children.

The tracheal diameters of children under 5 years old are significantly narrower than those of adults. Furthermore, the cartilage rings in children are soft with a poor supporting role, and exudation and edema more easily occur due to the loose respiratory mucosa. Therefore, a small amount of secretion, mild respiratory mucosal edema, or weak bronchial contract can cause a significant increase in airway resistance, which is clinically manifested as difficulty breathing during spontaneous respiration or higher airway pressure during mechanical ventilation. Of note, airway hyperreactivity secondary to URI is very common and can even last for 4–6 weeks after URI symptoms disappear, which can significantly increase the risks of serious perioperative complications such as laryngospasm and bronchospasm. Furthermore, this functional obstruction of the upper and lower airways can also cause fatal hypoxemia. Although URIs usually affect the upper respiratory tract in children, lung ventilation and gas exchange may also be affected and cause the mismatch of ventilation–perfusion ratio, the increase of lung closing volume, and the decrease of diffusion capacity, forced vital capacity, forced expiratory volume in 1 s, and peak expiratory flow (PEF).

74.3.2 Complications of Transcatheter Closure of VSD

For perimembranous VSD, the defect is very close to the atrioventricular conduction bundle of His. Thus, left bundle branch block and cardiac arrest may occur during and after the placement of closure devices. A conduction block at any time clearly indicates removing the closure devices. The ventricular outflow tract obstruction should be ruled out by echocardiography and ventricular/aortic angiography after the placement of the VSD closure device. In addition, it is also necessary to confirm the function of aortic valves. If aortic valve dysfunction or aortic valve regurgitation occurs after the placement of the VSD closure device, it is recommended to remove or change the VSD closure device or even abandon therapeutic cardiac catheterization. Other complications include hemodynamic fluctuations, thrombosis, and hemolysis caused by cardiac catheter sheath placement.

74.4 Discussion

74.4.1 Preoperative Assessment and Preparation

Preoperative visits for children with recent URIs should focus on symptoms (runny nose, itchy throat, sneezing, nasal congestion, general fatigue, cough, sputum and fever, etc.) and medications for treatment. It is important for parents to provide disease-related medical history. It is more important and reliable for anesthesiologists to predict the possibility of laryngospasm and bronchospasm during the perioperative period. If the parents can confirm the diagnosis of URIs instead of speculation based on chief complaints by anesthesiologists. In addition to URI, several other factors can also increase the risk of PRAE, which include history of asthma/wheezing, persistent dry cough at night for more than 2 weeks in the past year, allergic rhinitis, allergies, eczema, and passive smoking.

The timing of elective surgeries for children with recent URIs has been the most challenging and controversial issue. Actually, the airway remains hyperreactivity within 6 weeks after URI. During this period, general anesthesia with endotracheal intubation or LMA placement will significantly increase the risk of PRAE, including laryngospasm and bronchospasm. Furthermore, for those pediatric patients with recent URIs undergoing open heart surgery, the time of postoperative mechanical ventilation and stay in the ICU and hospital are prolonged. PRAE is obviously associated with delayed endotracheal extubation, prolonged stay in hospital/ICU, and an increase in anesthesia-related death. Therefore, it is previously recommended that it is better to postpone elective pediatric open-heart surgery over 4 weeks. However, it seems unnecessary for those undergoing therapeutic cardiac catheterization to postpone the procedure until 4 weeks after URI since therapeutic cardiac catheterization has less impact on the respiratory system, and the anesthetic management has been significantly improved. Our study showed that the highest incidence of PRAE occurred within 2 weeks after URI. The incidence of PRAE in patients with recent URI and undergoing therapeutic cardiac catheterization drops significantly 2 weeks after URI. Furthermore, The PRAE we observed mainly included upper airway obstruction, oxygen desaturation, coughing, and oral and/or airway secretions, which were all well handled with appropriate treatment. No serious adverse events, such as laryngospasm and bronchospasm, occurred.

74.4.2 Intraoperative Management

For those children with URI undergoing therapeutic cardiac catheterization, PRAE mainly includes transient desaturation, coughing, and airway obstruction, which may be associated with URI-induced airway secretion and hyperreactivity. Preoperative intranasal dexmedetomidine can not only significantly reduce preoperative anxiety and nervousness, but it can also significantly reduce the incidence of PRAE. Similarly, preoperative aerosolized budesonide or salbutamol inhalation can also protect children from postoperative strider and coughing. Unlike the endotracheal tubes, LMA and face masks have less airway irritation. Of note, it is necessary to clean airway secretions and remove LMA under deep anesthesia to avoid the occurrence of laryngospasm and bronchospasm. Early nasal/oral airway placement at the end of the procedure is also very useful. Once laryngospasm occurs, effective treatment strategies include mask-assisted ventilation with 100% oxygen, deepening sedation using intravenous propofol, and endotracheal intubation with muscle relaxants.

74.5 Conclusion

For children with recent URI undergoing elective therapeutic cardiac catheterization, the anesthetic management should focus on the hemodynamic changes and the timing of anesthesia and perioperative airway management to avoid PRAE. It is better to use LMA instead of endotracheal intubation if it is possible. Preoperative intranasal dexmedetomidine and/or aerosolized budesonide inhalation can help to reduce PRAE significantly. It is better to clean oral sections and remove LMA or endotracheal intubation under deep anesthesia (Kan Zhang).

Anesthetic Management of Radiofrequency Ablation in a Child with Atrial Flutter After Complex Congenital Heart Surgery

75

Huiyan Hou

Abstract

A 9-year-old boy with a history of complex congenital heart disease, diagnosed at birth, experienced frequent atrial flutter following multiple surgeries, including bidirectional cavopulmonary shunt, total anomalous pulmonary venous return correction, and common atrioventricular valvuloplasty. Recently, the episodes of atrial flutter increased significantly, and the patient was unresponsive to medication. The boy also reported fatigue and a notable decline in exercise tolerance. He was scheduled for radiofrequency ablation under general anesthesia. It is very important to maintain sinus rhythm, control the ventricular rate effectively, and avoid the occurrence of tachycardia during anesthetic management.

Atrial flutter is characterized by rapid and regular atrial electrical activity, representing a transitional state between supraventricular tachycardia and atrial fibrillation. It often exhibits an unstable pattern, typically occurring in paroxysms lasting from several minutes to hours or longer, eventually reverting to sinus rhythm or progressing to atrial fibrillation. Although less common, persistent atrial flutter can last months to years and cause significant hemodynamic fluctuations during episodes. Therefore, prior to surgery, medications such as propafenone, amiodarone, and norepinephrine should be prepared for symptomatic support. This chapter discusses the anesthetic management strategies employed during the radiofrequency ablation procedure in a child with frequent atrial flutter following complex congenital heart surgeries.

75.1 Case Presentation

The patient was a 9-year-old boy with 19.8 kg in weight and 125 cm in height. He was born full-term without a history of asphyxia, but his growth and development were significantly delayed. He was diagnosed with complex congenital heart disease (dextrocardia, single ventricle, single atrium, pulmonary valve stenosis, total anomalous pulmonary venous return, right aortic arch with right descending aorta, common atrioventricular valve) at a local hospital due to heart murmur after birth. He underwent a series of surgeries, including bidirectional cavopulmonary shunt surgery (modified BT shunt), bilateral bidirectional superior vena cava–pulmonary artery anastomosis (Glenn procedure) + total anomalous pulmonary venous return correction common

H. Hou (✉)
The National Children's Medical Center (Shanghai), Department of Anesthesiology of Shanghai Children's Medical Center, Shanghai Jiao Tong University School of Medicine, Shanghai, China
e-mail: houhuiyan@scmc.com.cn

J. Zheng et al. (eds.), *Selected Pediatric Cardiovascular Surgery Anesthesia Cases*,
https://doi.org/10.1007/978-981-96-5614-1_75

atrioventricular valvuloplasty. The symptoms of chest tightness occurred 1 month after surgery. An electrocardiogram (ECG) showed atrial flutter and right ventricular hypertrophy. The chest tightness was improved after the treatment with digoxin and amiodarone. The child often felt fatigued after physical exertion, which was accompanied by excessive sweating and irritability. The growth and development were significantly delayed. No recurrent respiratory infections, no obvious dyspnea, no cough, and no edema in both lower limbs. He was admitted to our hospital for further treatment with the primary diagnosis of postoperative congenital heart disease, atrial flutter.

Physical examination: The child was conscious with pulse oxygen saturation (SpO_2) of 80%, heart rate (HR) of 82 beats/min, regular rhythm, strong heart sounds, and grade III/VI systolic murmurs in the second to third intercostal spaces on the right side of the sternum. Surgical scar on the midline of the sternum and clubbed fingers/toes.

Laboratory tests: Complete blood count test results with white blood cell count 7.00×10^9/L, platelet count 384×10^9/L, hemoglobin 160.0 g/L, red blood cell counts 5.11×10^{12}/L. The liver, kidney, and coagulation functions are within the normal ranges.

Echocardiography: Most of the heart was located in the right thoracic cavity; the abdominal aorta and inferior vena cava were both located on the left side of the spine, indicating bilateral right atrial structure. Single atrium, single ventricle, and residual heart chamber were located at the right rear. The aorta and pulmonary artery both originate from the main heart chamber. The aorta was located at the right front with a valve ring diameter of 2.33 cm. The left and right coronary artery openings were not clearly displayed. The pulmonary artery was located at the left rear with valve and subvalvular stenosis. The diameter of the pulmonary valve ring was 0.59 cm. The inner diameter of the main pulmonary trunk was 0.66 cm with a flow speed of 3.92 m/s. The pulmonary artery valve pressure difference was 62 mm Hg. Common atrioventricular valve, forward flow speed 1.0 m/s, mild to moderate regurgitation, multiple regurgitation jets with the wider jet of 0.32 cm. Pulmonary vein flow speed was 0.8 m/s. Right-sided aortic arch, no significant shunting at the level of the aorta. The left pulmonary artery anastomosis diameter was 0.89 cm, the flow speed across the anastomosis was 0.48 m/s, and the blood flow fluctuated with respiratory movement. The right pulmonary artery anastomosis diameter was 0.93 cm, the flow speed across the anastomosis was 0.37 m/s, and the blood flow fluctuated with respiratory movement. The left pulmonary artery diameter was 0.79 cm, and the right pulmonary artery diameter was 0.99 cm.

Cardiac CT: Dextrocardia, single ventricle, single atrium, bilateral right atrial structure, pulmonary artery stenosis, postoperative total anomalous pulmonary venous return, and bilateral Glenn procedure.

Chest X-ray: Postoperative congenital heart disease, dextrocardia, right-sided aortic arch, heart shadow enlargement, multiple lung markings.

ECG: Ectopic rhythm, atrial flutter with 2:1 conduction, right-sided heart, possible right ventricular hypertrophy.

Twenty-four-hour Holter ECG: Sinus rhythm was the dominant rhythm with an average heart rate of 56 beats/min and slowest heart rate of 37 beats/min, sinus rhythm with second-degree atrioventricular block 2:1 conduction. The fastest heart rate was 72 beats/min with a second-degree atrioventricular block and no pause greater than 2 s. The longest RR interval was the second-degree type I atrioventricular block. ST segment horizontal displacement 0.075 mV with T wave biphasic on CH1 and CH3 channels.

Preoperative diagnosis: Atrial flutter, dextrocardia, single ventricle, single atrium, postoperative complex congenital heart disease.

75.2 Anesthetic Management

The patient did not take any preoperative medications before anesthesia. Upon entering the operating room, basic vital signs were closely monitored with cuff blood pressure (BP) at

102/56 mm Hg, HR was 210 beats/min (atrial flutter rate), and SpO_2 at 72%. The left radial artery was catheterized under local anesthesia for continuous invasive arterial pressure (ABP) monitoring. The basic ABP was 98/55 mm Hg. General anesthesia was induced by intravenous bolus injection of midazolam 2.0 mg, etomidate 6.0 mg, fentanyl 40 μg, and rocuronium 12 mg. Once the eyelash reflex disappeared, an ID 6.0 mm cuffed endotracheal tube was intubated under direct laryngoscopy. The tube depth was fixed at 18 cm after verification of the appropriate position by bilateral auscultation of the lungs. The patient was ventilated with pressure-controlled ventilation-volume guaranteed (PCV-VG) mode with oxygen flow rate 2 L/min, fraction of inspired oxygen (FiO_2) 50%, tidal volume (VT) 200 mL, respiratory rate (RR) 18 times/min, inspiratory to expiratory (I:E) time ratio 1:2. The end-tidal carbon dioxide ($ETCO_2$) was maintained around 35–45 mmHg during surgery. General anesthesia was maintained by intravenous infusion of remifentanil 0.1 μg/(kg·min), rocuronium 0.5 mg/(kg·h), and intermittent inhalation of 1–2% sevoflurane.

ECG monitoring upon entering the operating room showed atrial flutter. The induction of anesthesia was initiated after the establishment of invasive arterial blood pressure monitoring and hemodynamic stability. ABP decreased from 98/55 mmHg to 62/40 mmHg about 5 min after the endotracheal intubation. At the same time, SpO_2 dropped from 77% to 55%. Therefore, norepinephrine was used to increase the blood pressure with the initial dose of 0.05 μg/(kg·min), which was gradually increased to 0.08 μg/(kg·min). Then, ABP gradually increased to 105/62 mm Hg, while SpO_2 gradually increased to about 78%. Norepinephrine was used throughout surgery to maintain blood pressure to ensure sufficient perfusion.

75.3 Postoperative Outcome

The radiofrequency ablation started from the left lower pulmonary vein to the anterior wall of the common valve. After activation sequence mapping, the atrial flutter was terminated, but the ECG showed a junctional rhythm. Atrial flutter was induced again after atrial stimulation, but the morphology differed. The inferior vena cava–common valve isthmus-dependent atrial flutter was considered, so the ablation started from the common valve ring to the inferior vena cava. The atrial flutter was terminated, but ECG still showed a junctional rhythm. Anyway, atrial flutter could not be induced by repeated atrial stimulation later. The radiofrequency ablation surgery lasted for 135 min in total.

The endotracheal and oral secretion were cleaned under deep anesthesia after surgery. Then, sugammadex 40 mg was intravenously given to antagonize residual muscle relaxation. The patient's spontaneous breathing recovered well with stable hemodynamics and SpO_2 at room air. The endotracheal tube was successfully removed and norepinephrine was also discontinued. The patient was safely transferred to the ward with stable vital signs.

75.4 Review of Knowledge Points

75.4.1 Surgical Treatment of Functional Single Ventricle

Functional single ventricle is a broad category of complex congenital heart diseases that require staged surgical treatment. The modified BT shunt is a commonly used procedure for the first stage of systematic pulmonary shunt surgery, aiming to improve oxygen supply, promote pulmonary artery development, and provide an appropriate condition for later surgery. The advantages of the modified BT shunt include: the blood circulation of the affected arm being preserved, the shunt blood volume being adjusted based on the size of the systematic artery (subclavian or anonymous artery), the early patency rate of the artificial arterial blood vessel by PTFE is high, the shunt length can be guaranteed, and the shunt is easy to be removed. During the second stage of surgery, the superior vena cava is anastomosed with the ipsilateral pulmonary artery (i.e., bidirectional Glenn surgery), and the pulmonary blood flow will be increased after vena cava–pulmonary anastomosis, which can further increase the blood oxygen saturation of systematic artery without the increase of blood volume load in the systematic circulatory ventricle.

75.4.2 Atrial Flutter

Organic heart diseases such as cardiomyopathy, myocarditis, sick sinus syndrome, and postoperative congenital heart disease are the main causes of atrial flutter in children. The mechanism of atrial flutter is the circular motion caused by a single macro-reentry circuit around the inferior vena cava and adjacent slow conduction area in the right atrium. Atrial overdrive pacing can induce and terminate atrial flutter, and the entrainment phenomenon of atrial flutter suggests that a reentry mechanism causes atrial flutter. The ECG of atrial flutter shows that the P wave disappears and is replaced by a series of identical, sawtooth-like regular flutter waves, which are F waves. The QRS complex morphology is the same as the sinus rhythm; if it is accompanied by intraventricular differential conduction, it can be wide and deformed. The ventricular rhythm can be regular (the atrioventricular conduction ratio is mostly 2:1–4:1) or irregular (the atrioventricular conduction ratio is uneven).

The treatment measures for atrial flutter include ① direct current cardioversion, trans-esophageal cardiac pacing, antiarrhythmic drugs such as amiodarone and propafenone can be chosen to terminate the attack; ② when the drug or electric cardioversion turns into sinus rhythm, amiodarone, propafenone, and other drugs need to be taken to maintain this effect; and ③ radical cure can be achieved by catheter radiofrequency ablation or surgery.

75.5 Discussion

75.5.1 Preoperative Evaluation and Preparation

The anesthesiologist should have a full understanding of medical history and medication history to avoid sustained atrial tachycardia during the perioperative period, which may have further damage to the heart function. We prepared amiodarone and other antiarrhythmic drugs for the child before surgery. To avoid the child's nervous and fearful feelings, an appropriate dose of oral midazolam 0.5–1 mg/kg can be given for preoperative sedation to reduce stress response.

75.5.2 Intraoperative Anesthetic Management

The anesthetic management focuses on controlling the ventricular rate if atrial flutter occurs during the perioperative period. Digitalis drugs can be used to effectively control the ventricular rate, improve hemodynamics, and prevent heart failure. Hypoxia, carbon dioxide accumulation, anemia, hypokalemia, and hypomagnesemia, etc. should be ruled out during the perioperative period. For example, if the ventricular rate is <100 beats/min and the heart function is well compensated, it may not be necessary to manage atrial flutter. If heart failure occurs with the ventricular rate is >100 beats/min, cedilanid 0.4–0.8 mg can be used for slow intravenous injection after dilution. If it is necessary, half of the dose can be added 2 h later. If the ventricular rate is <180 beats/min and there is no obvious heart failure, propafenone, esmolol, and verapamil can be given in addition to digoxin. If the ventricular rate is >180 beats/min, there is severe hemodynamic disorder, and drug treatment is ineffective, synchronized electric shock defibrillation can be chosen.

The key points of anesthetic management for children after the Glenn procedure are to ensure sufficient cardiac output by maintaining heart rate, myocardial contractility, and preload. If it is necessary, vasoactive drugs (such as dopamine and norepinephrine) can be used. After the Glenn procedure, the key points of respiratory management for children are maintaining a normal level of $PaCO_2$, avoiding excessive airway pressure, and appropriately increasing inhaled oxygen concentration to improve oxygenation.

75.6 Conclusion

Regrettably, we did not place external defibrillation electrode pads on this patient before surgery in case of atrial flutter.

In summary, the key to successful anesthetic management in this kind of case is to ensure sufficient blood volume load and myocardial contractility, effectively control the ventricular rate, and maintain sufficient cardiac output. In addition, it is also very important to provide defibrillation treatment when it is necessary (Huiyan Hou).

Anesthetic Management of Fiberoptic Bronchoscopy in a Child with Tachycardia-Induced Cardiomyopathy

76

Siyi Zhou

Abstract

A 7-month-old female infant was diagnosed with tachycardia-induced cardiomyopathy due to coughing, wheezing, and shortness of breath. She still had intermittent coughing, wheezing, and sweating after symptomatic treatment. The child also had a significant choking cough after eating. In order to rule out the possibility of foreign bodies in the airway, elective fiberoptic bronchoscopy under intravenous anesthesia was scheduled. In addition to the shared airway issue during fiberoptic bronchoscopy, it was also very important to control the ventricular rate and prevent heart failure through medication in this child with tachycardia-induced cardiomyopathy.

Tachycardia-induced cardiomyopathy (TIC) is a special type of cardiomyopathy caused by persistent or recurrent tachycardia. TIC can be secondary to various types of rapid arrhythmias, which are mainly characterized by cardiac enlargement and heart failure. This disease can occur at all ages, and it is a reversible, generally good prognosis, acquired cardiomyopathy. A few children may relapse and have the possibility of sudden cardiac death. Therefore, the risk of anesthesia is relatively high. This chapter reports the anesthetic management of fiberoptic bronchoscopy in a child with tachycardia-induced cardiomyopathy.

76.1 Case Presentation

The patient was a 7-month-old girl with 73 cm in height and 7.5 kg in weight. She was born full-term without asphyxia. She was brought to a local hospital due to coughing, wheezing, and shortness of breath 2 months ago. Local echocardiography indicated that endocardial fibroelastosis could not be ruled out, diastolic cardiomyopathy was pending, severe mitral regurgitation, and left ventricular systolic function reduction (EF 42%). The dynamic electrocardiogram (ECG) showed atrial tachycardia (99.9%), with an average heart rate (HR) of 155 beats/min; the fastest heart rate was 207 beats/min with T wave changes. Chest CT showed mild ground-glass opacities in both lungs and a few patchy shadows in the lower fields of both lungs, considering heart failure and severe pneumonia. The symptom was improved after treatment with

S. Zhou (✉)
The National Children's Medical Center (Shanghai), Department of Anesthesiology of Shanghai Children's Medical Center, Shanghai Jiao Tong University School of Medicine, Shanghai, China
e-mail: zhousiyi@scmc.com.cn

J. Zheng et al. (eds.), *Selected Pediatric Cardiovascular Surgery Anesthesia Cases*,
https://doi.org/10.1007/978-981-96-5614-1_76

noninvasive ventilator-assisted hypoventilation, anti-infection, nebulization, diuresis, digoxin, and milrinone. The child still had intermittent coughing, wheezing, and sweating after discharge. Furthermore, the child had a significant choking cough after eating. So, the foreign bodies in the airway could not be ruled out.

Physical examination: HR 180 beats/min, irregular rhythm, strong heart sounds, and grade III/VI murmur in the precordial area. Coarse breath sounds in both lungs, along with dry rales. The pulse oxygen saturation (SpO_2) was 85% when breathing air. The abdomen was soft, and the liver and spleen were not palpable below the ribs.

Laboratory tests: No significant abnormalities were found in routine blood tests, liver, and kidney function.

Chest X-ray: Heart shadow enlargement, lung infiltration on both sides, consolidation in the lower lobe of the left lung, pleura thickening on both sides and increased transparency in the upper lobe of the left lung.

Electrocardiogram: Paroxysmal junctional tachycardia, high voltage in the left ventricle, ST-T changes.

Echocardiography: Whole heart enlargement (left heart dominated), spherically dilated left ventricle, moderate to severe regurgitation of the mitral valve, pulmonary hypertension, left heart contraction function decrease (EF 40.61%), a small amount of pericardial effusion.

Preoperative diagnosis: Tachycardia-induced cardiomyopathy, bronchial foreign body was pending. The child was scheduled for an emergency fiberoptic bronchoscopy.

76.2 Anesthetic Management

The child did not take any preoperative medications. After entering the operating room, routine vital signs were monitored; noninvasive blood pressure (BP) was 98/65 mm Hg, HR was 144 beats/min, sinus rhythm, and SpO_2 was 98%. After the peripheral vein was accessed, a loading dose of dexmedetomidine 2.0 μg/(kg·h) was intravenously infusion within 15 minutes. Then, sufentanil 0.1 μg/kg, ketamine 0.3 mg/kg, and propofol 1.0 mg/kg were slowly administered to induce anesthesia via the peripheral vein. Furthermore, dexmedetomidine 1.0 μg/(kg·h) was continuously infused during fiberoptic bronchoscopy. Before the insertion of fiberoptic bronchoscopy, 2% lidocaine was sprayed to the pharynx and larynx for local anesthesia. Oxygen was supplied at 2 L/min through the side hole of the bronchoscope during bronchoscopy. The child maintained spontaneous breathing during fiberoptic bronchoscopy without coughing and hemodynamic fluctuations. The child was safely transferred to the ward after the operation.

76.3 Postoperative Outcome

The operation lasted a total of 15 min. There was no bleeding during the operation. About 30 mL of Ringer's acetate solution was infused. After the operation, the child was transferred into post anesthesia care unit with BP 85/45 mm Hg, HR 118 beats/min, and SpO_2 98%. After recovery, the patient was safely transferred to the ward. The child was discharged on the postoperative day 7. Bronchoscopy results: No airway foreign body was found, left main bronchus softening (moderate), potential external compression.

76.4 Review of Knowledge Points

76.4.1 Tachycardia-Induced Cardiomyopathy

Tachycardia-induced cardiomyopathy (TIC) refers to a type of cardiomyopathy that results in heart enlargement and heart failure due to persistent or recurrent rapid arrhythmias. In 2006, TIC was listed in the acquired cardiomyopathy by the American Heart Association. The pathogenesis of TIC still remains unclear. Various mechanisms have been used to explain TIC arrhythmias' different types and clinical symptoms. The severity of the disease mainly depends on the speed of the ventricular rate and the duration. Long-time and persistent tachycardia in children can lead to increased left ventricular filling pressure, peripheral resistance increase, decreased ejection fraction, decreased left ventricular volume enlargement without weight changes, secondary mitral regurgitation, and chronic heart failure. The treatment strategy of TIC is to control the ventricular rate, improve heart failure symptoms, restore sinus rhythm, reverse cardiac remodeling, and prevent recurrence. Drug treatment is preferred. For those children who are ineffective or intolerant to drug treatment, radiofrequency ablation is recommended.

76.4.2 Airway Foreign Body

Airway foreign bodies usually refer to objects located below the glottis, in the trachea or bronchi. It is more common in infants and toddlers under 3 years old. It is a common pediatric emergency and a major cause of accidental death in children. Most airway foreign bodies are located in the bronchus, a few are located below the glottis and the main airway, and very few foreign bodies may be located in multiple parts of the child's airway. Inhalation of foreign bodies can cause mucosal damage, bleeding, or mechanical obstruction. The foreign body can be lodged in the bronchi at various levels in the lung, causing changes such as atelectasis and emphysema in the lung lobe or lung segment below the obstruction site. If the foreign body remains long, it may also cause indirect damage, such as inflammation, infection, and granuloma formation.

76.5 Discussion

76.5.1 Preoperative Assessment and Preparation

For children undergoing emergency bronchoscopy for airway foreign bodies, the first step is to quickly assess whether there are critical conditions that require emergency treatment, such as suffocation, respiratory distress, cyanosis, and loss of consciousness. The location, size, type, and retention time of airway foreign bodies can be determined through a comprehensive assessment of medical history, symptoms, signs, and imaging examinations if the child's condition is relatively stable. The anesthesiologists should make a detailed plan based on the preoperative assessment, including the methods and drugs of anesthesia induction and maintenance, intraoperative ventilation and postoperative airway maintenance methods, and preparation for various accidents and complications. For this case, our team also assessed the anesthesia risk based on the child's electrocardiogram and echocardiogram. Premature beats, conduction block, and ST segment changes should be detected early and managed symptomatically due to the suffering of tachycardia cardiomyopathy. If the children took amiodarone for tachycardia control before surgery, blood potassium should be monitored to prevent hypokalemia. In addition, myocardial ischemia, arrhythmia, or even cardiac arrest may occur during the fiberoptic bronchoscopy due to hypoxia. Before the operation, it is necessary to fully communicate with the family and prepare cardiovascular active drugs, antiarrhythmic drugs, and defibrillators.

76.5.2 Anesthetic Management

The difficulty of anesthesia for fiberoptic bronchoscopy lies in the shared airway between the anesthesiologist and the otolaryngologist. It is necessary to maintain sufficient anesthesia depth and ensure adequate ventilation and oxygenation during anesthesia. Retaining the child's spontaneous breathing after anesthesia can avoid the difficulty of bronchoscope insertion and operation caused by using jet ventilation devices and reduce the risk of complete obstruction of the distal bronchus due to positive pressure ventilation-related movement of an unstable foreign body. During the fiberoptic bronchoscopy, the child's SpO_2 was maintained at 98–100% by supplying oxygen through the side hole of the bronchoscope. Thus, the child's oxygen supply was ensured.

The pathophysiological characteristics of TIC are similar to those of dilated cardiomyopathy. The anesthetic management of such patients should aim to control HR, stabilize hemodynamics, improve cardiac ejection function, and maintain organ perfusion and function, all of which should be followed throughout the perioperative period. This child had rapid arrhythmia combined with moderate to severe mitral regurgitation. Therefore, sinus rhythm should be maintained as much as possible. Dexmedetomidine can reduce the child's HR, but there is no direct inhibitory effect on the sinus node and myocardium. Previous studies have shown that dexmedetomidine can stimulate the dorsal nucleus and the ambiguous nucleus of the vagus nerve and α_2 receptor to enhance the vagal nerve's activity and negatively affect the cardiovascular system. Dexmedetomidine can effectively reduce the occurrence of ventricular and supraventricular tachyarrhythmias after cardiac surgery in children. Moreover, for refractory rapid arrhythmias that are ineffective with antiarrhythmic drugs such as amiodarone, dexmedetomidine also has a therapeutic effect. However, it is worth noting that the patient also had moderate to severe mitral regurgitation. Therefore, tachyarrhythmias should be prevented and treated during surgery, but an appropriately faster sinus rhythm should be maintained to ensure sufficient cardiac output. The heart rate should not be allowed to slow down too much. In addition to dexmedetomidine, small doses of ketamine, sufentanil, and propofol are also used to maintain intraoperative hemodynamic stability as much as possible. In addition, the child is supplemented with lidocaine spray for endotracheal surface anesthesia to enhance the anesthetic effect, but it should be noted that surface anesthesia should be performed after a certain depth of anesthesia is reached. Otherwise, it can cause adverse events such as breath-holding and laryngospasm. The child had preoperative pulmonary hypertension, hypercapnia, hypoxemia, and acidosis should be avoided during the operation since these factors may exacerbate pulmonary hypertension and cause acute heart failure.

76.6 Shortcomings and Limitations

In this case, the control of HR and the resulting changes in hemodynamics are the key points of anesthetic management. Unfortunately, we did not perform invasive arterial pressure monitoring on the child, so we could not timely detect and deal with the hemodynamic changes caused by arrhythmias.

76.7 Conclusion

When a child with TIC undergoes fiberoptic bronchoscopy, the goals of anesthetic management should focus on controlling HR, stabilizing hemodynamics, improving cardiac ejection function, and maintaining organ perfusion and function while ensuring sufficient ventilation and oxygenation and avoiding the occurrence of cardiovascular adverse events (Siyi Zhou).

77 Procedural Sedation Management of an Infant with Kawasaki Disease Undergoing Cardiac Magnetic Resonance Examination

Bin Xue

Abstract

A 10-month-old female infant was diagnosed with Kawasaki disease due to fever for 1 week. She was admitted to our hospital for cardiac magnetic resonance (CMR) examination under sedation. Kawasaki disease is characterized by acute systemic vasculitis, including coronary artery lesions (15–25%), which can cause coronary artery dilation and aneurysm formation. The patients may die from coronary aneurysm rupture, thrombosis, myocardial infarction, or myocarditis. CMR evaluation of coronary arteries and myocardial perfusion is an appropriate noninvasive evaluation method. Optimization of sedative drugs and methods to improve the rate of successful sedation with fewer complications has now become an important link in the diagnosis of Kawasaki disease.

Kawasaki disease (KD), also known as mucocutaneous lymph node syndrome, is an acute febrile disease of unknown etiology, which often occurs in children under 5 years old and involves the coronary arteries of the heart. It is necessary to diagnose KD and the degree of coronary artery damage as early as possible in order to take effective treatment measures to control the progression of KD. Currently, cardiovascular magnetic resonance (CMR) is a suitable noninvasive method for examining the degree of coronary artery damage. Sedation must be performed for awake children who cannot cooperate with the CMR examination. This chapter reports the sedation management of a 10-month-old patient with KD undergoing a CMR examination.

77.1 Case Presentation

The patient was a 10-month-old girl with a weight of 9 kg. She was born full-term without asphyxia. She was admitted to our hospital with Kawasaki disease due to a fever for 1 week, and echocardiography indicated that the right coronary artery was dilated. After treatment with gamma globulin, the patient's body temperature returned to normal.

Physical examination: Axillary temperature 36.8 °C, pulse 118 beats/min, blood pressure (BP) 98/60 mm Hg. The patient had dry, cracked lips, a strawberry tongue, and scattered rashes in the perineal area. No abnormalities were found on the auscultation of the heart and lungs.

B. Xue (✉)
The National Children's Medical Center (Shanghai), Department of Anesthesiology of Shanghai Children's Medical Center, Shanghai Jiao Tong University School of Medicine, Shanghai, China
e-mail: xuebin@scmc.com.cn

J. Zheng et al. (eds.), *Selected Pediatric Cardiovascular Surgery Anesthesia Cases*,
https://doi.org/10.1007/978-981-96-5614-1_77

Laboratory tests: White blood cell 16.42 × 10^9/L, lymphocytes 35%, neutrophils 52.2%, red blood cell 3.48 × 10^{12}/L, hemoglobin 86 g/L, platelet 493 × 10^9/L, C-reactive protein 92 mg/L, serum amyloid A > 320 mg/L, erythrocyte sedimentation rate 79 mm/hour, NT-proBNP 1863 pg/mL, C-TNI quantitative <0.03 μg/L. Liver, kidney, and coagulation function parameters were not significantly abnormal.

Electrocardiogram (ECG): Incomplete right bundle branch block (IRBBB), first-degree atrioventricular block (AVB), T wave notch at the peak.

Echocardiography: The inner diameter of the proximal right coronary artery was 0.2 cm. The inner diameter of the distal part from the opening was 1.36 cm, and the widest inner diameter was 0.3 cm; mini mitral regurgitation, mild tricuspid regurgitation, flow velocity of 2.27 m/s, left ventricular systolic function within the normal range.

77.2 Sedation Management

After the peripheral vein was accessed, the patient was brought into the MRI examination room. Heart rate (HR) and pulse oxygen saturation (SpO_2) were monitored by using an MRI-compatible vital signs monitor. The patient's HR before sedation was 110 beats/min, SpO_2 was 97%. After 1.0 mg midazolam and 30 mg propofol were slowly infused intravenously, the patient quickly lost consciousness, and Ramsay's score reached ≥5. Then, the CMR examination began with continuous vital sign monitoring. Initially, the patient's HR gradually slowed to a minimum of 93 beats/min, while SpO_2 showed no significant changes. The examination lasted for a total of 34 minutes, during which the child did not move, and the vital signs were stable. After the examination, the child was transferred to the recovery room for further observation. A modified Aldrete score was taken every 5 min after sedation. The child woke up 10 min later with the modified Aldrete score of 10 points. HR was 106 beats/min, and SpO_2 was 97%. The child was instructed to drink a small amount of water without choking. Then the child was safely returned to the ward.

77.3 Review of Knowledge Points

77.3.1 Kawasaki Disease

The diagnosis of KD mainly depends on symptoms such as fever, red and cracked lips, rash, conjunctival congestion, hard swelling of hands and feet, and enlargement of cervical lymph nodes. The diagnosis of complete KD requires at least five to six items of the clinical manifestations, including fever, non-purulent bilateral conjunctival congestion, rash, acute phase palmoplantar erythema, hand and foot hard swelling, recovery phase finger (toe) end membranous desquamation, lip congestion, cracking, strawberry tongue, and non-purulent cervical lymphadenopathy, and no matter coronary artery injury occurs or not. If the child only meets four of the above clinical manifestations, the diagnosis of complete KD needs to be confirmed by ultrasound, which indicates coronary artery injury. The diagnostic criteria for coronary artery lesions (CAL) refer to the presence of enhanced echogenicity of the coronary artery intima including coronary artery dilation (inner diameter ≥ 2.5 mm for children aged 0–3 years old, ≥3 mm for children aged 4–9 years old, ≥3.5 mm for children aged 10–14 years old), coronary artery aneurysm (coronary artery inner diameter 4–7 mm) and giant coronary artery aneurysm (coronary artery inner diameter ≥ 8 mm).

Aspirin and intravenous human immunoglobulin (IVIG) injections are still the main therapeutic methods for KD. Clinically, most children's body temperature will gradually return to normal after receiving sufficient IVIG treatment, while other clinical symptoms will also gradually disappear. However, 10–20% of the patients are still not relieved even after sufficient IVIG treatment. If the fever persists over 36 hours after sufficient IVIG treatment or reappears after the fever subsides, the phenomenon is known as "IVIG-resistant KD." Reusing IVIG combined with glucocorticoids may be an effective therapy for IVIG-resistant KD. In addition, TNF-α blockers can also be used as an alternative treatment for IVIG-resistant KD.

77.3.2 Deep Sedation in Children

Pediatric procedural sedation should be conducted by anesthesiologists or pediatricians who have received special training. The requirements for fasting food and drink before sedation are shown in Table 77.1. The place of sedation must be equipped with negative pressure suction devices, oxygen, and airway opening devices, including endotracheal intubation, laryngeal mask, oropharyngeal airway, monitors, rescue drugs, and equipment. Commonly used drugs include chloral hydrate, dexmedetomidine, barbiturates, sevoflurane, midazolam, ketamine, propofol, etc. Medication can be administered orally, by enema, nasal drops, inhalation, muscle, and intravenous injection. After the child falls asleep, the depth of sedation is assessed according to the Ramsay Sedation Score (Table 77.2). Different types of examinations have different requirements for the depth of sedation. Sedative drugs should be used reasonably to meet various examination requirements.

Table 77.1 Pre-sedation fasting time

Type of food	Minimum fasting time (h)
Clear liquids	2
Breast milk	4
Formula milk	6
Cow's milk and other liquid dairy products	6
Light meal	6
Fried, fatty, and meat foods	May require longer time

Table 77.2 Ramsay sedation score

Rating	Status	Description
1	Awake	Anxious, agitated, or irritable
2		Quiet, cooperative, oriented
3		Only responsive to commands
4	Asleep	Agile response to light tap between eyebrows or loud auditory stimulus
5		Sluggish response to light tap between eyebrows or loud auditory stimulus
6		No response to light tap between eyebrows or loud auditory stimulus

77.4 Discussion

77.4.1 Pre-sedation Assessment and Preparation

The inflammation during the acute febrile phase of KD can involve medium-sized arteries and multiple organs throughout the body, specifically affecting the coronary arteries and resulting in CAL. Therefore, before sedation, we need to assess the child's cardiac function and the degree of cardiovascular disease damage based on echocardiography and electrocardiogram, which includes cardiac perfusion, contractility, valve damage, and the severity of coronary damage. For children with coronary aneurysms, MRI examination under anesthesia sedation is currently not considered. In this case, the child's ECG showed CRBBB and I° AVB. Echocardiography showed mini mitral regurgitation and mild tricuspid regurgitation. The inner diameter of the widest part of the right coronary artery was 0.3 cm, which was diagnosed as coronary artery dilation according to the CAL diagnostic criteria. Therefore, we thought that the child could tolerate the procedural sedation after the assessment. In addition, we also prepared positive inotropic drugs before implementing sedation.

77.4.2 Selection of Sedative Methods and Drugs

For children with a history of heart disease, sedatives with mild inhibitory effects on myocardial contraction and hemodynamics are the top priority to choose. Currently, the most commonly used non-intravenous sedatives include chloral hydrate, barbiturates, and dexmedetomidine. It is not good for children to orally take chloral hydrate for procedural sedation due to the poor taste, low bioavailability, and high risk of nausea and vomiting. In addition, a large chloral hydrate dosage can cause myocardial contractility inhibition. Repeated use of chloral hydrate can cause drug resistance and delayed recovery or sedation after recovery. Barbiturates cause significant irritation when administered intramuscularly. The sedative effect is not satisfactory when it is used alone, and large doses can cause severe respiratory depression. Although intranasal dexmedetomidine does not cause respiratory depression, it can cause hypotension and dose-dependent bradycardia. So, it is unsuitable for children with sinus bradycardia and atrioventricular block (AVB). Since the child, in this case, has normal heart function and good tolerance, we chose to use propofol combined with midazolam for sedation. The main reason is that propofol has a fast onset, short recovery time, and high rate of sedation success. The combined use of midazolam can extend the sedation duration of propofol, avoiding the need for repeated drug administration due to the child's movement during the examination. It should be noted that propofol and midazolam have a certain degree of myocardial inhibitory effect, and their combined use may decrease HR and BP. Vital signs should be continuously monitored during sedation, and resuscitation drugs should also be prepared.

77.4.3 Recovery After Sedation

The child, in this case, woke up quickly after the examination. There was no choking after drinking water, and the child resumed eating early. Intravenous sedation is different from general anesthesia. There is no need for a long period of fasting after the sedation, which is more conducive to the child's recovery. If nausea and vomiting occur, the fasting period can be appropriately extended. Feeding can be resumed after the symptoms disappear.

77.5 Shortcomings and Limitations

The child's HR slowed down after the administration of sedatives. However, due to the limitations of the monitoring equipment, BP was not monitored throughout. If insufficient tissue perfusion occurs, it might not be found in time.

77.6 Conclusion

In this case, the child was fully evaluated before the examination, and contraindications were ruled out. Intravenous propofol–midazolam combination was used for sedation. The success rate of the examination was high, and the vital signs were also stable during the examination. The recovery was quick after the examination with no other adverse reactions. This proves that intravenous propofol combined with midazolam sedation is a safe and effective sedative method for KD patients without significant cardiac function impairment (Bin Xue).

78 Procedural Sedation Management for Cardiac Magnetic Resonance Imaging in a Child After Pulmonary Atresia Surgery

Yingying Ji

Abstract

A 3-year-old boy underwent right ventricular outflow tract reconstruction and arterial duct closure due to pulmonary artery atresia (PA) 3 years ago. Postoperative cardiac CT showed the main pulmonary artery stenosis. He was scheduled to undergo cardiac magnetic resonance imaging (MRI) to clarify the diagnosis. Due to the long duration and loud noise during the MRI examination, oral chloral hydrate and intranasal dexmedetomidine were given to facilitate procedural sedation for the MRI examination.

Cardiac magnetic resonance imaging (MRI) examination usually takes a long time and makes a large noise. Moderate to deep sedation is usually required for pediatric MRI examination. Chloral hydrate, dexmedetomidine, pentobarbital sodium, and midazolam are the most currently used sedatives. Concomitant sedatives can increase the success rate of sedation, but they also can increase the side effects and prolong the recovery time. Both the success rate and the safety of the sedation must be considered in children with cyanotic congenital heart diseases due to their complicated pathophysiological changes. This case report focuses on the sedative management of cardiac MRI examination in a child after pulmonary atresia surgery. The child was sedated with oral chloral hydrate and intranasal dexmedetomidine.

78.1 Case Presentation

A 3-year-old boy with 15 kg in weight was diagnosed with pulmonary atresia (PS) due to cyanosis in the lips and fingertips after birth. He was born full-term without a history of asphyxia. Echocardiography at the age of 5 months demonstrated atresia at the pulmonary valve and pulmonary artery trunk, atrial septal defect (ASD) 0.3 cm, ventricular septal defect (VSD) 1.57 cm, and a patent ductus arteriosus (PDA). He underwent right ventricular outflow tract reconstruction (transvalvular patch) and surgical PDA ligation under general anesthesia 3 years ago. The surgery appeared to be effective for his hypoxia symptoms. During follow-up, restenosis at the main pulmonary artery and thickening of the right ventricular outflow tract muscle bundle was detected by cardiac CT examination. The child was scheduled to undergo an MRI examination under sedation for a definitive diagnosis.

Y. Ji (✉)
The National Children's Medical Center (Shanghai), Department of Anesthesiology of Shanghai Children's Medical Center, Shanghai Jiao Tong University School of Medicine, Shanghai, China
e-mail: jiyingying@scmc.com.cn

J. Zheng et al. (eds.), *Selected Pediatric Cardiovascular Surgery Anesthesia Cases*,
https://doi.org/10.1007/978-981-96-5614-1_78

Physical examination: The child was conscious with pulse oxygen saturation (SpO_2) of 95%, heart rate (HR), 93 beats/min, regular rhythm, and grade III/VI systolic murmur in the precordial area.

Electrocardiogram: Right ventricular hypertrophy.

Echocardiography: No significant residual shunt at the patch level, slight shunt at the atrial level, residual pulmonary artery obstruction, left pulmonary artery stenosis, normal left ventricular systolic function.

Cardiac CT: Main pulmonary artery stenosis at the end of right ventricular, left pulmonary artery stenosis, right ventricular outflow tract muscle bundle thickening.

78.2 Sedative Management

A 6-h fast for solids and a 2-h fast for liquid prior to examination were required. On the examination day, the anesthesiologist first assessed the patient and then informed his parents about the risks of sedation. The child's baseline SpO_2 was 96%, and HR was 84 beats/min. After the parents signed the informed consent form, 10% chloral hydrate 50 mg/kg was orally taken, and 2.0 μg/kg dexmedetomidine was intranasally administered for sedation. SpO_2 and HR were monitored every 5 min. The patient fell asleep 15 min after sedative administration with a Ramsay sedation score of 5. SpO_2 and HR were maintained at approximately 96% and 80 beats/min during the MRI examination. The MRI examination lasted 35 min in total. After the examination, the patient was brought back to the recovery room. The child woke up 30 min later with SpO_2 96%, HR, 85 beats/min, and Aldrete score of 10. Then, the patient was discharged from the hospital.

78.3 Review of Knowledge Points

78.3.1 Pulmonary Atresia

PS accounts for 1–2% of all congenital heart diseases and is classified into ductus arteriosus-dependent pulmonary circulation and non-ductus arteriosus-dependent pulmonary circulation based on the source of pulmonary blood supply. Approximately 35–70% of patients have ductus arteriosus-dependent pulmonary circulation, which means the pulmonary blood supply depends entirely on the ductus arteriosus supply. In the remaining patients, all or most of the pulmonary blood flow is derived from large main pulmonary collateral arteries. The severity of cyanosis depends on the amount of collateral supply of pulmonary blood and the distribution of pulmonary vessels in the lung parenchyma. A patient may have only mild cyanosis if the collateral supply is large and there is no stenosis at the junction with the pulmonary artery.

Due to the differences in the PS spectrum, surgical procedures are based on the pulmonary blood source and the pulmonary artery's thickness, origin, course, and obstruction. Radical surgery (i.e., reconstruction of the right ventricular outflow tract) is preferred in children with ductus arteriosus-dependent large pulmonary arteries where the pulmonary artery can connect to all bronchopulmonary segments and the branches are normal. The method of right ventricular outflow tract reconstruction depends on the type of PS. An outflow tract patch and atresia valve incision can be used in membranous atresia. In long-segment atresia, reconstruction or conduit implantation is usually required. As the child is still growing, even if stable hemodynamics can be maintained after surgery, regular follow-up is required, and the conduit may need to be replaced to maintain right ventricular function. Children who are dependent on collateral arteries may need to have the independent pulmonary arteries and collaterals combined into a single source due to large variations and may require multiple surgeries to bring the patient's pulmonary blood supply closer to normal.

78.3.2 Moderate to Deep Sedation

Moderate to deep sedation is defined as the child being unconscious, normal spontaneous breathing during sedation without mechanical ventilation support, and stable hemodynamics. In the 2018 American Society of Anesthesiologists guidelines for moderate sedation and analgesia, sedatives include benzodiazepines and dexmedetomidine, and analgesics mainly include opioids. The administration is divided into intravenous sedatives and non-intravenous sedatives. Intravenous sedation has the advantage of a high success rate of sedation and rapid recovery. However, it is more expensive and requires specialists and special monitoring equipment. Non-intravenous sedation may be considered when equipment and manpower are limited.

78.4 Discussion

78.4.1 Pre-sedation Assessment and Preparation

The child with PS has undergone right ventricular outflow tract reconstruction. The baseline value of SpO_2 and HR was 96% and 84 beats/min, respectively with air breathing. NYHA cardiac function classification was II–III. Although the cardiac CT showed the main pulmonary artery restenosis and the left pulmonary artery stenosis, the echocardiogram showed that the systolic function of the left heart was still normal. Therefore, sedation was conducted after a comprehensive assessment of the patient's cardiac function based on the clinical symptoms, the echocardiogram results, and the cardiac CT examination.

78.4.2 Sedative Medication

Children with PS often undergo several anesthesia and sedation during the treatment and follow-up. The child is usually required to stay still for over 30 min during an MRI examination, and the success rate of sedation with a single sedative has been reported to be less than 50%. Chloral hydrate was once the most commonly used sedative in pediatric sedation. However, its clinical use is declining due to its cardiotoxicity, neurotoxicity, gastrointestinal reactions, and potential carcinogenicity. The success rate of sedation increases with the higher dose of chloral hydrate. However, the adverse effects are also increased. Dexmedetomidine is becoming widely used in pediatric sedation due to its low nasal irritation and high bioavailability. Many studies have shown that it is feasible to use dexmedetomidine for sedation in children with cyanotic congenital heart diseases. According to the statistics from the author's hospital, the successful rate of cardiac MRI sedation by oral chloral hydrate and nasal dexmedetomidine combination in children with congenital heart disease is over 90%. The respiratory depression in children is usually mild. If sedation fails, an appropriate amount of dexmedetomidine can be added for rescue, or intravenous anesthesia can be used for the cardiac MRI sedation. Therefore, it is recommended that two sedatives be used for cardiac MRI sedation in older children who have had multiple sedations in the past.

78.5 Shortcomings and Limitations

Children tend to cry and resist when noninvasive blood pressure is measured, which can affect the sedative effect. Therefore, blood pressure was not measured in children after sedation.

78.6 Conclusion

For children with PA undergoing MRI examination under sedation, the combined use of oral chloral hydrate and nasal dexmedetomidine may increase the success rate of sedation. However, the increase in adverse effects should also be considered (Yingying Ji).

Sedation Management of Cardiac CT Scan in a Child with Mucopolysaccharidosis and Severe Aortic Valve Regurgitation

79

Pan He

Abstract

A 15-year-old boy was diagnosed with mucopolysaccharidosis (MPS) type II and severe aortic valve regurgitation at a local hospital. He was brought to our hospital for further treatment of aortic valve regurgitation. A preoperative cardiac CT scan was ordered to make a definitive diagnosis. Pre-sedation assessment demonstrated that the boy had a difficult airway and severe heart failure, which increased the risk of sedation for the cardiac CT scan. The keys to sedation management during a cardiac CT scan in a child with MPS II include managing the difficult airway and maintaining stable hemodynamics.

Mucopolysaccharidosis (MPS), also known as mucopolysaccharide disease, is a rare congenital genetic disease caused by a decrease or lack of hydrolase activity that degrades mucopolysaccharides in lysosomes, leading to the accumulation of mucopolysaccharides in various organs of the body, ultimately resulting in genetic metabolic disorders that impair the function of multiple tissues and organs. The clinical manifestations are diverse, including varying degrees of skeletal deformities, distinctive facial features, intellectual disabilities, short stature, hepatosplenomegaly, heart valve disease, and corneal opacities. These clinical manifestations are mainly related to different gene mutations. Genetic testing is the most reliable method for the diagnose of MPS. Children with MPS often have complications such as difficult airways and severe heart and lung dysfunction, which significantly increase the risks of sedation during preoperative examination. This chapter reports a case of sedation management in a child with MPS and severe aortic valve regurgitation for a cardiac CT scan.

79.1 Case Presentation

A 15-year-old boy of 121 cm in height and 34 kg in weight was born full-term without a history of asphyxia. At the age of 2, he was diagnosed with MPS II at a local hospital and had been taking idursulfase to control the progression of the disease. Seven years ago, he underwent uvulopalatopharyngoplasty at a local hospital. It was difficult to expose the glottis after induction of general anesthesia using a standard laryngoscope. The endotracheal tube was successfully intubated with the assistance of a video laryngoscope combined with the head and neck position adjustment and pressure on the cricoid cartilage. A local hospital

P. He (✉)
The National Children's Medical Center (Shanghai), Department of Anesthesiology of Shanghai Children's Medical Center, Shanghai Jiao Tong University School of Medicine, Shanghai, China
e-mail: hepan@scmc.com.cn

J. Zheng et al. (eds.), *Selected Pediatric Cardiovascular Surgery Anesthesia Cases*,
https://doi.org/10.1007/978-981-96-5614-1_79

echocardiogram indicated severe aortic valve regurgitation. He was scheduled to undergo a pre-operative cardiac CT scan for the treatment of aortic valve regurgitation in our hospital.

Physical examination: The child appeared indifferent with slow reactions, low intelligence, short stature, large head, short neck, protruding forehead, boat-shaped skull, wide-set eyes, flat nasal bridge, enlarged nostrils, thick and everted lip, large tongue, stiff temporomandibular joint, contracted phalangeal joints, hirsutism, and enlarged liver and spleen. A blowing murmur can be heard during diastole in the auscultation area of the aortic valve between the third and fourth ribs along the left margin of the sternum.

Laboratory tests: Routine blood tests, liver function, kidney function, and coagulation function were all within normal ranges.

Echocardiography: Severe aortic valve regurgitation with an ultrasound beam width of 0.82 cm, left ventricle enlargement. Left ventricular systolic function was slightly reduced.

Pre-sedation diagnosis: MPS II with severe aortic valve regurgitation.

79.2 Sedation Management

The child was routinely fasted for 6 h and no drinking for 2 h. Prior to sedation, thorough communication was conducted with his family members, informing them of the risks of sedation, and an informed consent form was signed. Upon the child entering the sedation room, basic vital signs were closely monitored with non-invasive blood pressure (BP) at 128/63 mm Hg, heart rate (HR) at 55 beats/min, and pulse oximetry (SpO_2) at 96%. Oxygen was administered via a face mask. End-tidal carbon dioxide pressure ($ETCO_2$) was continuously monitored via a side stream sampling tube placed in the nose. Esketamine 0.5% was intravenously titrated until the child lost consciousness and the Ramsay sedation score was beyond 4. The total dose of esketamine was 35 mg. Before the initiation of the cardiac CT scan, the child's position was first adjusted to ensure airway patency and avoid excessive head extension to prevent cervical dislocation and spinal cord injury. During the CT scan, BP was 133/66 mm Hg, HR was 93 beats/min, SpO_2 was 99%, and $ETCO_2$ was 42 mmHg. The CT scan lasted for 5 min. After the CT scan, the boy was transferred to the post-anesthesia care unit (PACU) for recovery. After the boy fully awakened, Aldrete scored 10 and could walk independently; he was discharged from PACU under the parent's accompany.

79.3 Review of Knowledge Points

79.3.1 MPS Classification

MPS can be classified into seven types and multiple subtypes, including I, II, III, IV, VI, VII, and IX, based on clinical manifestations, type of mucopolysaccharides in urine, and genetic characteristics. Type II is the most common MPS type, accounting for approximately half of all MPS cases. Except for type II, which is X-linked inheritance, the other types are autosomal recessive inheritance. Children with type I, II, IV, VI, and VII may have difficult airways. In addition, those children with type I, II, III, IV, VI, and VII may also have cardiovascular diseases, including ventricular hypertrophy, valvular disease, coronary heart disease, and congestive heart failure.

79.3.2 MPS and Difficult Airways

Children with MPS may have difficult airways, including ① Difficulty in mask ventilation. Due to the thickening of the oropharyngeal soft tissues, large tongue, narrow nasal cavity, thickened nasal mucosa, and enlarged adenoids, children with MPS may have difficulty in mask ventilation. ② Difficulty in intubation. Children with MPS may have a short and fixed neck, limited cervical spine mobility, increased oral contents, accumulation of glycosaminoglycans obstructing the exposure of the glottis, and glycosaminoglycan accumulation on the tracheal mucosal surface resulting in tracheal stenosis or even twisting and deformation, all of which can contribute to difficulty in intubation.

79.3.3 MPS and Valvular Heart Disease

Children with MPS often present with heart diseases primarily characterized by valvular lesions, mainly manifesting as leaflet thickening and deformation and leading to valve stenosis or insufficiency. The mitral valve is the most commonly affected valve, followed by the aortic valve. When the aortic insufficiency occurs, the left ventricle receives more blood input from both the left atrium and the aorta during the diastolic phase and causes an increase in end-diastolic volume, which further causes the compensatory dilation and hypertrophy of the left ventricle. Once the left ventricle fails to compensate, the end-diastolic pressure of the left ventricle will increase, the amount of aortic valve regurgitation will decrease, eventually resulting in left heart failure, increased left atrial pressure, pulmonary congestion, and pulmonary arterial hypertension, and eventually right heart failure. Most children with MPS show cardiovascular symptoms around the age of 10 (median age), and some severe patients already have valvular lesions around the age of 3 months. Regular echocardiography can detect heart valve and myocardial lesions earlier. Antibiotics can be routinely used to prevent bacterial endocarditis when the heart valves are involved. Valve replacement can be performed to prevent heart failure due to significant cardiac regurgitation when the valve lesion is severe.

79.4 Discussion

79.4.1 Pre-sedation Assessment and Preparation

The key to pre-sedation assessment in children with MPS should focus on evaluating difficult airways. Although we were unable to assess the boy's mouth opening conditions, mandibular protrusion ability, pharyngeal structure (modified Mallampati classification), etc., before sedation due to his intellectual disability and uncooperating, he had a short neck, large tongue, temporomandibular joint stiffness, and a history of difficult intubation during previous uvulopalatopharyngoplasty, all of which indicate a difficult airway.

According to previous reports, the incidence of difficult mask ventilation, difficult intubation, and failed intubation in children with MPS are 12–14%, 25–43%, and 2–12%, respectively. The incidence of airway difficulties in children with MPS II increases with age and disease progression, leading to increasingly severe airway obstruction. For this child with MPS, the most important thing is to maintain the child's spontaneous breathing and avoid emergency tracheal intubation. We have prepared an appropriate sedation plan in advance, prepared various emergency airway management tools (such as laryngeal mask, oral/nasopharyngeal airway, fiberoptic bronchoscopes, and cricothyroid membrane puncture kit), and emergency drugs (such as rocuronium, sugammadex, atropine, and epinephrine).

79.4.2 Sedative Drugs

The commonly used sedative drugs for pediatric procedural sedation include chloral hydrate, phenobarbital, dexmedetomidine, midazolam, propofol, ketamine, etc. Previous retrospective studies demonstrated that the failure rate of moderate and deep sedation with chloral hydrate and/or phenobarbital increases with age. Therefore, it is better not to choose chloral hydrate and phenobarbital for moderate and deep sedation in older children. Propofol can dose-dependently inhibit respiration and increase the risk of airway obstruction. Studies have shown that dexmedetomidine has an advantage over propofol in maintaining airway patency, which reduces the percentage of airway intervention by 37% in children with MPS II for MRI scan sedation. However, the boy's pre-sedation HR was 55 beats/min, and the aortic valve regurgitation was severe. Therefore, dexmedetomidine-based procedural sedation protocol was not appropriate for this boy. Considering his intellectual disability and the bitter taste and uncomfortable mouth feel of midazolam, we also did not choose midazolam for sedation in this case.

Esketamine is the pure S-enantiomer of ketamine with a higher affinity for N-methyl-D-aspartic acid receptors (NMDA) and μ-opioid receptors. It can provide strong sedative, amnestic, and analgesic effects with half a dose of ketamine. Esketamine produces rapid-onset sedation with mild respiratory depression and a high safety profile in children. Esketamine also offers a faster recovery time compared to ketamine, making it a safer and more suitable choice for pediatric sedation examinations. In addition, ketamine can increase sympathetic activity, heart rate, and blood pressure and increase cardiac output and cardiac output. Increasing heart rate can reduce regurgitation time and increase aortic forward blood flow for children with severe aortic valve regurgitation. The increase in blood pressure, especially diastolic pressure, can improve myocardial blood supply, but the increase in heart rate and blood pressure also increases oxygen consumption, so a balance must be struck.

After careful consideration, we decided to choose esketamine as a sedative drug in this case because esketamine can produce not only satisfactory sedation but also mild respiratory and circulatory depression and increase the sympathetic excitatory effects on the circulatory system. In order to reduce esketamine induced hemodynamics changes and individual differences, intravenous titration of 0.5% esketamine for sedation in this case was opted. This method involves slow administration of esketamine while assessing the drug's effects until the child falls asleep to a certain level of sedation that meets the requirements for enhanced CT scan examination. Compared with the traditional dosing method based on body weight, the titration method has a clear endpoint, which avoids sedation failure due to individual differences in patients, avoids excessive sedation, and maintains stable hemodynamics.

79.4.3 Recovery and Discharge After Sedation

This child was an outpatient, so it was crucial to strictly follow the discharge criteria and provide detailed instructions to his parents. After the examination was completed, the child was transferred to the PACU for recovery. Considering the difficult airway and an American Society of Anesthesiologists (ASA) classification of level III, the boy was discharged from PACU under the parent's accompany after being fully awake with an Aldrete score 10 and able to walk independently.

79.5 Shortcomings and Limitations

Even though the child had met the discharge criteria, the residual effects of the medication may still exist. Therefore, it is necessary for us to provide a phone follow-up 48 h after sedation.

79.6 Conclusion

In conclusion, esketamine intravenous titration is an appropriate sedation option for children with difficult airways and severe aortic valve regurgitation (Pan He).

Sedative Management of Enhanced Cardiac CT Scan in a Child with Tetralogy of Fallot

80

Pan He

Abstract

A 7-month-old female infant was diagnosed with Tetralogy of Fallot (TOF) after birth. She was scheduled for a preoperative enhanced cardiac CT scan. She experienced two hypoxic episodes, and her pulse oxygen saturation (SpO_2) was 78% with air breathing. CT scan was successfully finished after intranasal administration of 20 μg dexmedetomidine and 10 mg ketamine. The key point of sedative management in children with TOF is to avoid or prevent the occurrence of hypoxic episodes.

Tetralogy of Fallot (TOF) is the most common cyanotic congenital heart disease, representing about 5–7% of all congenital heart defects. TOF is mainly characterized by ventricular septal defect (VSD), pulmonary stenosis (PS), aortic overriding, and right ventricular hypertrophy. Children with TOF may present with cyanosis, dyspnea, and even hypoxic episodes. Sedation of children with TOF is very challenging for anesthesiologists. This chapter reports the sedative management of enhanced cardiac CT scan in a child with TOF.

80.1 Case Presentation

The infant was a 7-month-old female infant, 70 cm in height and 10.2 kg in weight. He was born full-term by cesarean section without asphyxia, and the birth weight was 2700 g. Due to the detection of an abnormal heart structure during prenatal routine examination, the infant was diagnosed with TOF after birth in a local hospital. Her lips appeared cyanotic in room air and worsened when crying. She experienced two hypoxic episodes. A preoperative cardiac enhanced CT scan was planned.

Physical examination: The infant presented with cyanosis in the lips. SpO_2 was 82% in room air. Cardiac auscultation demonstrated a regular heart rhythm with a grade III/IV systolic murmur in the third to fourth intercostal space along the left margin of the sternum. Auscultation of the lungs revealed coarse breath sounds without dry or moist rales.

Laboratory tests: Hemoglobin 154 g/L, hematocrit 46.1%, normal liver function, kidney function, and coagulation function.

Chest X-ray: Heart shadow enlargement, multiple lung markings.

Echocardiography: Right atrium and right ventricle enlargement, right ventricular wall

P. He (✉)
The National Children's Medical Center (Shanghai), Department of Anesthesiology of Shanghai Children's Medical Center, Shanghai Jiao Tong University School of Medicine, Shanghai, China
e-mail: hepan@scmc.com.cn

J. Zheng et al. (eds.), *Selected Pediatric Cardiovascular Surgery Anesthesia Cases*,
https://doi.org/10.1007/978-981-96-5614-1_80

thickening. Aorta enlargement, straddling 50% of the ventricular septum. Pulmonary artery and subvalvular stenosis, flow rate 3.42 m/s, pressure difference 47 mmHg. Pulmonary valve annulus 0.51 cm, main pulmonary artery trunk diameter 0.92 cm, flow rate 5.15 m/s, pressure difference 106 mm Hg. Tricuspid valve thickness and curliness with mild to moderate regurgitation, regurgitant velocity 4.58 m/s, pressure difference 84 mm Hg, VSD with bidirectional shunt small collateral vessels formation.

Diagnosis: TOF.

80.2 Sedative Management

The infant was fasted food and drink for 4 h before sedation. The anesthesiologist first assessed the infant and then communicated with the parents about the risks of sedation and obtained informed consent. Upon the infant entering the sedation room, basic vital signs were closely monitored: heart rate (HR) at 165 beats/min, SpO_2 at 78%, and respiratory rate (RR) at 36 times/min. During the establishment of the peripheral venous catheterization for injection of contrast agent of enhanced CT scan, the infant became agitated with worsening cyanosis. The anesthesiologist decided to suspend the venipuncture temporarily. The infant's mood was stabilized after oxygen inhalation and pacifier consolidation. Subsequently, dexmedetomidine 20 μg and ketamine 10 mg were slowly dripped into the infant's bilateral nostrils. Ramsay sedation score was conducted every 5 min. HR and SpO_2 were also measured every 5 min. Around 15 min after administration, the infant's Ramsay sedation score was 4. The peripheral venous access was successfully established again. Then the infant was transferred to the examination room for an enhanced CT scan. Supplemental oxygen was continued. The infant's HR was 93 beats/min, SpO_2 95%, RR 22 times/min. The CT scan lasted 5 min, and then the child was transferred to the recovery room for further observation. About 40 min later, the child was fully awake with a modified Aldrete score of 10, HR of 116 beats/min, and SpO_2 of 80%. The infant ate a small amount of food without choking cough and was discharged from the hospital.

80.3 Review of Knowledge Points

80.3.1 Moderate to Deep Sedation

Children often need moderate to deep sedation to complete related pediatric outpatient examinations. Moderate sedation refers to the sedative level at which the child can consciously respond to targeted verbal instructions or tactile stimuli without airway intervention. At the same time, spontaneous breathing and hemodynamic stability are maintained. Deep sedation refers to the sedative level at which the child can consciously respond to repetitive and harmful stimuli with the possibility of airway and spontaneous breathing intervention. At the same time, hemodynamic stability can still be maintained.

80.3.2 Hypoxic Episodes

Hypoxic episodes are characterized by pulmonary infundibular stenosis and sudden spasms of infundibular muscle, which results in the exacerbation of right ventricular outflow obstruction and cerebral hypoxia. Hypoxic episode more commonly occurs in infants and can be triggered by breastfeeding, coughing, crying, anemia, pain stimuli, etc. The first symptom is often paroxysmal tachypnea with deepened and accelerated breathing and worsening cyanosis. The child may suddenly faint, convulse, or even die. During the hypoxic episode, it is necessary to alleviate the child's anxiety, reduce the overall oxygen consumption, increase systemic resistance, and reduce pulmonary resistance to reduce right-to-left shunting. In addition to providing oxygen inhalation, fluid supplementation, and correcting acidosis, α-receptor agonists (such as phenylephrine or norepinephrine) can be used to increase peripheral vascular resistance. β-Receptor blockers can also be used to relieve muscle spasms in the infundibular region.

80.4 Discussion

80.4.1 Pre-sedation Assessment and Preparation

During pre-sedation assessment, it is necessary to know the detailed timing and severity of cyanosis in children with TOF, whether there is a history of squatting, fainting, or hypoxic episodes. Feeding difficulty and growth and development delay also indicate cardiac reserve function insufficiency. Various preparations for preventing hypoxic episodes should be made in advance before sedation, including oxygen supply, endotracheal intubation devices, and various emergency drugs such as phenylephrine, esmolol, dopamine, and sodium bicarbonate.

80.4.2 Sedation Methods and Sedatives

Currently, there is no consensus on the sedative choice for children with cyanotic congenital heart disease. In addition to the rapid onset of action and minimal adverse reactions, the ideal sedation protocol should have a high sedation success rate and no respiratory and circulatory function suppression.

Ketamine can be used for pediatric sedation due to its strong sedative and analgesic effects, good controllability, quick onset, and mild respiratory suppression in children. Furthermore, ketamine can increase sympathetic nerve tension and peripheral vascular resistance, reduce right-to-left shunting, and improve hypoxemia, but with minimal impact on pulmonary vascular resistance. Therefore, it is a suitable sedative drug choice for children with TOF. Ketamine can be administered through various clinical routes, mainly including intravenous injection, intramuscular injection, oral administration, nasal administration, rectal administration, etc. Although the intravenous injection route has the fastest onset and highest bioavailability, it may not be immediately available for this infant. The intramuscular injection route stimulates the infant greatly. The oral and rectal administration routes have low bioavailability, so the nasal administration route is adopted, which has the advantages of rapid onset, no liver first-pass effect, no irritation to the gastrointestinal tract, low coordination requirements, and easy tolerance for children.

Dexmedetomidine is a highly selective α_2-adrenergic receptor agonist. Dexmedetomidine can be effectively used for pediatric sedation due to its sedative, analgesic, and anti-anxiety effects. The activation of α_2-adrenergic receptors can cause peripheral vasoconstriction and increase systemic resistance. So far, insufficient evidence shows its impact on the pulmonary vascular bed. This feature makes dexmedetomidine a preferred choice for sedation in children with TOF. The recommended dexmedetomidine intranasal dosage for moderate to deep sedation in children is 1.0–4.0 μg/kg. The two major adverse reactions of dexmedetomidine include hypotension and bradycardia, which need to be noted. When dexmedetomidine is combined with ketamine, the sympathetic inhibitory effect of the former balances the sympathetic excitatory effect of the latter, which is beneficial for maintaining hemodynamic stability. Intranasal administration of dexmedetomidine combined with ketamine can shorten the onset time of sedation, increase the sedation success rate, prevent the occurrence of adverse airway events, and reduce the adverse reactions of both medications. It has been reported that the sedation success rate of dexmedetomidine 2.0 μg/kg and ketamine 1.0 mg/kg nasal administration in children can reach 93%.

80.5 Shortcomings and Limitations

Prolonged preoperative fasting time for children with TOF can easily lead to many adverse consequences, such as restlessness, hypoxia, dehydration, and hypoglycemia. Therefore, it is necessary to appropriately shorten the fast food and drink time before sedation in children, such as drinking Outfast® (≤5 mL/kg) 2 h before sedation.

80.6 Conclusion

In conclusion, the combination of dexmedetomidine and ketamine intranasal administration is a safe and effective sedation protocol for cardiac CT scan in children with TOF. However, attention should still be paid to prevent hypoxic episodes after administration (Pan He).

Management of Cardiac Arrest in a Child with Complex Congenital Heart Disease During Cardiac Catheterization

81

Liping Sun

Abstract

A 6-year-old boy with cyanosis shortly after birth was initially suspected of congenital heart disease based on local echocardiography findings, but the precise diagnosis remained elusive. Recently, his cyanosis progressively became worse, and his activity level was severely limited, prompting him to seek medical attention. Cardiac ultrasound examination showed multiple complex abnormalities, including the functional single atrium, complete atrioventricular septal defect, total anomalous pulmonary venous connection (supracardiac type), pulmonary artery atresia, and collateral vessel formation. To further clarify the diagnosis and develop an effective treatment plan, diagnostic cardiac catheterization under general anesthesia was needed. The child's red blood cells were significantly increased with hematocrit level reaching 70% due to long-term hypoxia. To reduce the risks of thrombosis, embolism, and coagulation dysfunction, acute normovolemic hemodilution with plasma was performed before the cardiac catheterization procedure, which was carried out by blood withdrawal of 20 mL from the femoral artery and simultaneous administration of an equivalent volume of homologous frozen plasma through the femoral vein. When the 180 mL volume of blood was replaced, the end-tidal carbon dioxide waveform was significantly altered with a partial pressure drop from 40 mm Hg to about 23 mm Hg, SpO_2 decreased markedly, and the heartbeat gradually slowed, leading to cardiac arrest. Prompt cardiopulmonary resuscitation was initiated, the heartbeat resumed shortly after cardiopulmonary resuscitation, and the vital signs were also back to baseline. In the end, this cardiac catheterization procedure was postponed, and the child was transferred to the intensive care unit with mechanical ventilation for further monitoring.

With the development of cardiac interventional technology, more and more pediatric complex congenital heart diseases can now be precisely diagnosed or averted from open-heart surgery to cardiac interventional procedures through therapeutic cardiac catheterization. Although cardiac interventional procedures are generally less traumatic and less adverse events, the occurrence of perioperative cardiac arrest (CA) remains significantly higher compared to routine pediatric surgeries under general anesthesia, which is close to or slightly higher than those of cardiac surgery,

L. Sun (✉)
The National Children's Medical Center (Shanghai), Department of Anesthesiology of Shanghai Children's Medical Center, Shanghai Jiao Tong University School of Medicine, Shanghai, China
e-mail: sunliping@scmc.com.cn

J. Zheng et al. (eds.), *Selected Pediatric Cardiovascular Surgery Anesthesia Cases*, https://doi.org/10.1007/978-981-96-5614-1_81

about 0.96% and 0.79% respectively. Given that the successful rate of resuscitation in children with congenital heart disease experiencing CA is relatively low, it is necessary to prioritize the prevention and prompt management of CA during cardiac catheterization. Multiple factors, ranging from the child's underlying conditions to the doctor's techniques and the anesthetic management, can cause intraoperative cardiac arrest during cardiac catheterization. The possibility of successfully resuscitating a patient experiencing CA is influenced by the resuscitation measures employed in each setting, including the prediction and preparation for an unexpected or accidental event and the effectiveness of the adopted strategies. This chapter reports a case of successful resuscitation in a child with complex congenital heart disease who experienced a sudden cardiac arrest in the catheterization laboratory.

81.1 Case Presentation

The patient was a 6-year-old boy with 18.2 kg in weight and 110 cm in height. He was born full-term without asphyxia by cesarean. Shortly after birth, the boy was brought to a local hospital because of blue lips. A local echocardiography examination indicated that the boy had a congenital heart disease. As the boy grew, his blue lips and extremities gradually worsened, his physical activity was significantly limited, and his growth and development were delayed. There is no history of recurrent upper respiratory infections and easy sweating.

Physical examination: Central cyanosis and clubbing of the fingers and toes were seen. Pulse oxygen saturation (SpO_2) was about 69% with air breathing. Normal lung sounds were heard during auscultation. No lung rales or tactile fremitus existed. Heart rate (HR) 101 beats/min, regular rhythm, L II–IV/VI systolic murmur. The abdomen was soft, and neither the liver nor the spleen was palpable beneath the ribs.

Laboratory tests: C-reactive protein 1.0 mg/L, hematocrit (HCT) 70.0%, hemoglobin 231.0 g/L, white blood cell counts 9.85×10^9/L, neutrophils 2.51×10^9/L, platelet count 137×10^9/L; PT 18.9 seconds, APTT 78.3 seconds, TT 13.3 seconds, INR 1.75, FIB 1.93 g/L; NT-proBNP 1319 pg/mL, cardiac troponin I (cTnI) 0.03 μg/L.

Chest X-ray: Increased lung markings and enlarged cardiac silhouette.

Electrocardiogram: Sinus rhythm, first-degree atrioventricular block, incomplete right bundle branch block (IRBBB) with enlarged right ventricular, left atrial enlargement.

Echocardiography: Bilateral right atrial structure, pulmonary artery atresia, functional single atrium, aorta from the right ventricle, complete atrioventricular septal defect with moderate regurgitation of a common atrioventricular valve, bilateral superior vena cava, total anomalous pulmonary venous connection (supra cardiac type), collateral vessel formation.

Cardiac CT: Right-sided atrial isomerism, discordant ventriculoarterial connection, right pulmonary artery absence in the mediastinum, of the proximal and middle segments of left pulmonary artery atresia, atrioventricular septal defect, bilateral superior vena cava, supracardiac total anomalous pulmonary venous drainage, right coronary artery, and circumflex branch from the right posterior sinus, anterior descending branch from the left anterior sinus, rich collaterals.

Preoperative diagnosis: Right-sided atrial isomerism, discordant ventriculoarterial connection, pulmonary artery atresia, atrioventricular septal defect, total anomalous pulmonary venous drainage, single atrium, and bilateral superior vena cava. Given the complexity of this boy's heart disease, an elective cardiac catheterization is scheduled for further evaluation and potential therapeutic intervention.

81.2 Anesthetic Management

No preoperative medications were given to the boy before anesthesia. Upon entering the cardiac catheterization laboratory, basic vital signs were closely monitored with cuff blood pressure (BP) at 85/36 mm Hg, HR at 90 beats/min and at SpO_2 66%. The boy was intravenously administered midazolam 2.0 mg, propofol 40 mg, fentanyl 40 μg, and rocuronium 12.5 mg for anesthetic

Table 81.1 Intraoperative blood gas analysis result

Time point	Hb (g/dL)	HCT (%)	pH	PaO_2 (mm Hg)	$PaCO_2$ (mm Hg)	BE	Na^+ (mmol/L)	K^+ (mmol/L)	Cl^- (mmol/L)	Ca^{2+} (mmol/L)	Lac (mmol/L)
Admission	19.6	59.7	7.41	39.9	26.4	−7.3	140	3.0	122	0.9	6.6

induction after the peripheral vein was accessed. Once the eyelash reflex disappeared, an ID 5.5 mm cuffed endotracheal tube was intubated under direct laryngoscopy. The tube depth was fixed at 16 cm after verification of the appropriate position by bilateral auscultation of the lungs. The boy was ventilated with pressure-controlled ventilation-volume guaranteed (PCV-VG) mode, total oxygen flow rate of 2 L/min, inspired oxygen fraction (FiO_2) of 30%, tidal volume (VT) of 130 mL, respiratory rate (RR) of 18 times/min, inspiratory to expiratory ratio (I:E) of 1:2. The end-tidal carbon dioxide ($ETCO_2$) was maintained around 40 mm Hg during surgery. Sevoflurane inhalation with 0.8 to 1.0 minimal alveolar concentration (MAC) value was used for anesthetic maintenance.

Due to the high preoperative hemoglobin levels (231 g/L) and hematocrit (70.0%), acute normovolemic hemodilution with plasma was conducted before cardiac catheterization examination. According to the preoperative plan, the boy's hematocrit will be decreased to approximately 56.0% after acute normovolemic replacement of 300 mL of homologous plasma.

After routine disinfection and draping, the right femoral artery and vein catheterization were performed. Acute normovolemic hemodilution was initially conducted by blood withdrawal of 20 mL from the femoral artery and simultaneous administration of an equivalent volume of homologous frozen plasma through the femoral vein each time. When the 180 mL blood volume was replaced, the $ETCO_2$ waveform was significantly altered, with an $ETCO_2$ value dropping from 40 mm Hg to about 23 mm Hg. The tracheal tube position and respiratory parameter settings were confirmed correct after a quick check. However, SpO_2 quickly dropped below 50%, and HR dropped to approximately 30 beats/min; cuff BP could not be measured, and the femoral artery systolic pressure was 40 mm Hg. The cardiologist was immediately notified to stop the hemodilution procedure, and the sevoflurane vaporizer was also turned off. FiO_2 was adjusted to 100% pure oxygen. X-ray fluoroscopy showed that the heartbeat was very weak. Prompt chest compressions were initiated with 2.0 mL of 1:10,000 epinephrine intravenously injected. The heart rate did not recover even after 2 min of resuscitation. Therefore, it is necessary to inject epinephrine again intravenously. Subsequently, the heart rate was increased to 90 beats/min, and the chest compressions were stopped. Epinephrine (0.8 μg/(kg·min)) and 0.4 μg/(kg·min) norepinephrine were infused intravenously to maintain hemodynamics stability. According to the result of blood gas analysis (Table 81.1), 18 mL sodium bicarbonate was intravenously administered to correct acidosis. Ringers' acetate solution was fast-infused to replenish blood volume and electrolytes. Fifteen minutes later, the boy's HR and arterial blood pressure began to be stabilized with HR 140 beats/min, BP 120/98 mm Hg, SpO_2 approximately 60%, and $ETCO_2$ 48 mm Hg. After careful discussion, the scheduled cardiac catheterization was canceled, and the boy was transferred to the pediatric intensive care unit (PICU) for further treatment, including mechanical ventilation and vasoactive drugs.

81.3 Postoperative Outcome

The entire procedure lasted for 60 min, during which 200 mL of Ringer's acetate solution and 180 mL of homologous plasma were infused. In addition, 180 mL of blood was withdrawn. The infusion of epinephrine and norepinephrine was gradually tapered off after admission to the PICU according to the hemodynamic stability. Simultaneously, the boy received anti-infection treatment and mannitol to reduce intracranial pressure. Additional therapeutic measures include Piracetam for myocardial nourishment and omeprazole to protect the stomach. Levetiracetam, valproate, and clonazepam were given as anti-epileptic due to the occurrence of on and off convulsions. The boy had been on ventilator assistance for 20 days in the PICU. On PICU day 22, the boy was transferred to the cardiology general ward and discharged 5 days later.

81.4 Review of Knowledge Points

81.4.1 Right Atrial Isomerism

Right atrial isomerism (RAI), also called right atrial appendage isomerism, is a subset of heterotaxy syndrome characterized by two right sides with bilateral right atria and atrial appendages and without left-sided structures (such as coronary sinus). Specifically, the connection with the right atrium is wide, and the shape is short and blunt, resembling Snoopy's nose. Furthermore, the right atrial appendage is distinct from the smooth atrial wall due to the presence of pectinate muscles. The right isomerism frequently manifests as asplenia, also known as Ivemark syndrome. Beyond the isomerism of the right atrium, this condition is characterized by the presence of bilateral trilobed lungs accompanied by bilateral eparterial bronchi. Cardiac defects that often coexist include transposition of the great arteries, single ventricle physiology, and pulmonary atresia. Notably, nearly half of all cases exhibit total anomalous pulmonary venous drainage. These anomalies are typically more severe than those observed in polysplenia, leading to severe cyanosis and respiratory distress in patients. The prognosis for this syndrome is poor, with a high mortality rate ranging from 80% to 90% within the first year of life. Additionally, abdominal examinations may reveal abnormalities such as a midline liver, microgastria, and malrotation.

81.4.2 Normovolemic Hemodilution

Normovolemic hemodilution is not only a widely used blood conservation strategy during the perioperative period, but it is also an effective method of erythrocytosis management and reducing the risks of thrombosis, embolism, and coagulation dysfunction. Typically, a certain amount of whole blood is first drawn from the patient, either reserving it for intraoperative transfusion or discarding it, then or simultaneously, the same amount of plasma substitutes such as fresh plasma, albumin solution, or balanced solution is infused back to the patient at a corresponding rate. This approach can effectively reduce the hematocrit and blood viscosity and the need for allogeneic blood transfusion during major surgeries. It can also reduce the risks of thrombosis, embolism, and coagulation dysfunction.

81.4.3 Cardiac Arrest

Cardiac arrest is referred to as the abrupt cessation of the heart's ejection function triggered by various risk factors. The occurrence of intraoperative cardiac arrest is usually unpredictable except for a few critically ill patients. Therefore, it is necessary to immediately terminate the surgery and initiate cardiopulmonary resuscitation (CPR). The underlying causes should also be eliminated as early as possible. In addition, CPR should be initiated whenever there is a loss of pulse or blood pressure or when cardiac output is insufficient to maintain organ perfusion, such as in cases of bradycardia (infant heart rate < 60 beats/min). The absence of a pulse oximetry waveform, a sudden disappearance or decrease in the amplitude of the end-tidal carbon dioxide waveform, and the inability to measure blood pressure are all indicators of an impending cardiac arrest. To ensure successful CPR, it is crucial to perform high-quality chest compression, rapid defibrillation, and early elimination of the underlying causes. Particular attention should be paid to cerebral protection during CPR since it can significantly affect a patient's long-term outcome. Moreover, the anesthesiologist must keep close communication and cooperation with the surgical and nursing teams to maintain circulatory stability, ensure effective ventilation, and eliminate the causes of cardiac arrest as soon as possible.

81.5 Discussion

81.5.1 Preoperative Evaluation and Preparation

Due to the chronic hypoxia in children with cyanotic congenital heart diseases, the development of organs and weight gain is significantly delayed compared to their healthy peers. The preoperative medication should be cautiously administrated and in small dosages to prevent the hypoxic attacks triggered by overdose-related respiratory depression and intracardiac shunt changes. Preexisting severe hypoxemia (SpO_2 66%), heart failure [NT-proBNP 1319 pg/mL, cardiac troponin I (cTnI) 0.03 μg/L], NYHA class IV status, and a poor cardiac reserve can result in a dramatic reduction in cardiac output even with minor physiological fluctuations, which can compromise the coronary artery blood supply, aggravate myocardial ischemia and hypoxia, and cause cardiac arrest. Once hypotension occurs, dopamine and/or epinephrine should be administrated as soon as possible. Fluid replacement should also be properly expedited.

81.5.2 Anesthetic Management

For children with cyanotic congenital heart diseases, it is very important to prevent the aggravation of hypoxia and hypotension and reasonably adjust the dosage of medicines and the depth of anesthesia during induction of anesthesia. In the present case, anesthesia was induced and maintained by etomidate, fentanyl, sevoflurane, and other anesthetics with minimal hemodynamic effects. Additionally, a more controllable intravenous induction method involving gradual titration of the anesthetic agents was used to prevent any sudden hemodynamic fluctuations. During the surgical procedure, we first observed the changes in the $ETCO_2$ waveform, then the dramatic drops of HR, BP, and SpO_2, and finally, cardiac arrest. Subsequently, we immediately initiated advanced life support (ALS) measures for cardiopulmonary resuscitation. Due to the timely and effective resuscitation, the boy's spontaneous heartbeat resumed within 5 min, and his hemodynamic parameters were stabilized within 15 min.

The incidence of intraoperative cardiac arrest in children with complex congenital heart diseases is significantly higher than in those without congenital heart diseases. The reason for intraoperative cardiac arrest is very complicated and mainly includes three factors: patient-related factors, surgery-related factors, and anesthesia-related factors. In the present case, poor cardiac reserve, general anesthesia, and acute normovolemic hemodilution might contribute to the hemodynamic fluctuations, compromising both the coronary artery blood supply and the collateral blood flow supply to the pulmonary artery, aggravate myocardial ischemia and hypoxia, and cause cardiac arrest. These factors aggravated the boy's hypoxemia, which further caused cardiac arrest due to myocardial ischemia and hypoxia.

Regardless of the location or the reason for cardiac arrest, immediate and correct cardiopulmonary resuscitation is paramount. In March 2021, the European Resuscitation Council (ERC) released the 2021 Cardiopulmonary Resuscitation Guidelines, drawing upon the 2020 International Consensus on Cardiopulmonary Resuscitation Science and Treatment Recommendations. The resuscitation protocol specific to the cardiac catheterization laboratory is outlined in Fig. 81.1.

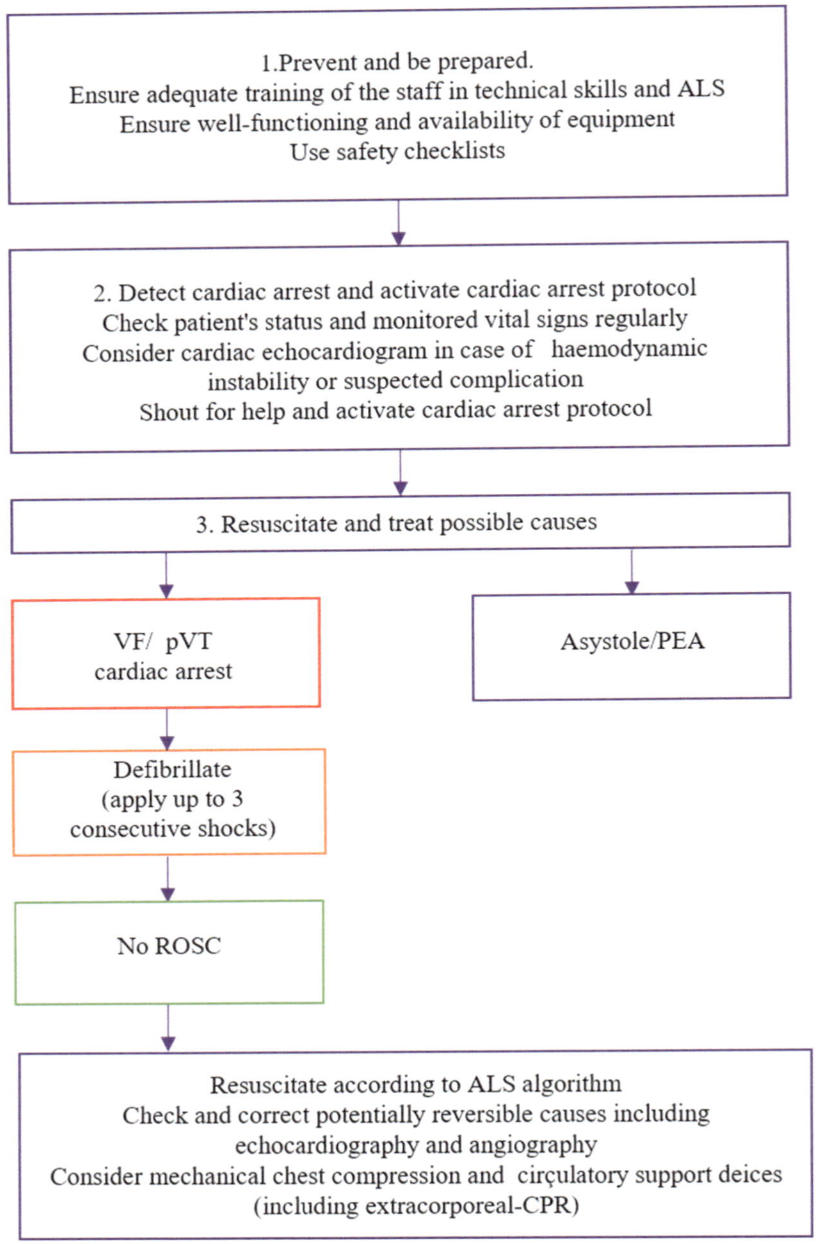

Fig. 81.1 Cardiac catheterization room resuscitation process. Management of cardiac arrest in the catheterization laboratory. *ALS* advanced life support, *VF* ventricular fibrillation, *pVT* pulseless ventricular tachycardia, *CPR* cardiopulmonary resuscitation, *ROSC* return of spontaneous circulation, *PEA* pulseless electrical activity

81.6 Shortcomings and Limitations

This case involves a child with complex cyanotic congenital heart disease for diagnostic cardiac catheterization examination. Therefore, it is very possible for this patient to have exacerbated hypoxia and cardiac arrest during the perioperative period. Preparing the external defibrillation electrodes and keeping them on standby is reasonable, which can ensure immediate defibrillation and enhance the overall quality of cardiopulmonary resuscitation.

81.7 Conclusion

For patients with cyanotic congenital heart disease, it is crucial to develop personalized anesthetic management plans tailored to their unique pathophysiological changes and anatomical features. These plans aim to regulate shunt volume and direction while maintaining oxygenation and circulation stability. Moreover, proficiency in managing complications such as hypoxia, low cardiac output syndrome, and cardiac arrest is paramount to ensure the safety and favorable outcomes of these patients' surgical procedures (Liping Sun).

Anesthetic Management of Pulmonary Hypertension Crisis in a Child with Pulmonary Hypertension After Right Heart Catheterization

82

Huiyan Hou

Abstract

A 4-year-old boy was diagnosed with pulmonary hypertension by echocardiography at a local hospital. To clarify the cause of pulmonary hypertension, the right heart catheterization examination under general anesthesia was scheduled at our hospital. The pulmonary artery pressures before and after pure oxygen inhalation during the operation were 56/17(34) mm Hg and 60/20(35) mm Hg, respectively, while the aortic pressures were 90/58(65) mm Hg and 94/51(72) mm Hg, respectively. When the patient woke up, he was restless, coughing, and intolerant to tracheal intubation. Then severe cyanosis and hypotension occurred. Emergency bedside cardiac ultrasound: the right ventricle was significantly enlarged, and the left ventricle shrank sharply with decreased myocardial contractility, indicating that a pulmonary hypertension crisis might have occurred. The child's spontaneous breathing recovered, and vital signs were gradually stabilized after treatment with epinephrine, milrinone, sodium bicarbonate, and hyperventilation. Then, the tracheal tube was successfully removed under deep anesthesia, and the patient was returned to the ward.

Pulmonary hypertension (PH): PH is also known as pulmonary artery high pressure, which is a relatively rare disease with poor outcomes. PH is a clinical and pathophysiological syndrome characterized by changes in pulmonary vessel structure or function caused by different causes and/or mechanisms. This further leads to increased pulmonary vascular resistance and pulmonary arterial pressure. Clinically, it mainly manifests as progressive right heart dysfunction-related symptoms, which can further develop into right heart failure, even death. Hypoxia, carbon dioxide accumulation, some medications, and harmful stimuli can cause a sharp increase in pulmonary artery pressure and trigger pulmonary hypertensive crisis (PHC) in children with PH, which can significantly increase the rate of cardiac arrest and mortality. Right heart catheterization is currently the gold standard for PH diagnosis. Unlike adult patients who can undergo right heart catheterization under local anesthesia, general anesthesia is required for children with PH to undergo right heart catheterization. Improper perioperative anesthetic management can trigger PHC. This chapter reports the diagnosis and treatment process of an episode of PHC in a child with PH after right heart catheterization.

H. Hou (✉)
The National Children's Medical Center (Shanghai), Department of Anesthesiology of Shanghai Children's Medical Center, Shanghai Jiao Tong University School of Medicine, Shanghai, China
e-mail: houhuiyan@scmc.com.cn

J. Zheng et al. (eds.), *Selected Pediatric Cardiovascular Surgery Anesthesia Cases*,
https://doi.org/10.1007/978-981-96-5614-1_82

82.1 Case Presentation

The patient was a 4.5-year-old boy with 17 kg in weight and 108 cm in height. He was born full-term without a history of asphyxia. A heart murmur was once found during the diagnosis and treatment of cold. Echocardiography at a local hospital showed: normal heart position and connection, right atrium and right ventricle enlargement, mild left ventricle enlargement with left ventricle diastolic diameter (LVDD) 3.62 cm (the upper limit of LVDD normal range for 4 years old child is 3.41 cm), normal left ventricular systolic activity. Pulmonary artery widening with the inner diameter of main trunk 2.72 cm, no aorta widening. Normal aortic and pulmonary artery valve opening activity, mild pulmonary artery valve regurgitation with regurgitation speed 3.81 m/s, pressure difference 57.9 mm Hg, mild tricuspid valve regurgitation with regurgitation speed 4.19 m/s, pressure difference 70.2 mm Hg. Atrial septal defect (ASD) with size 0.24 cm × 0.26 cm. For further diagnosis and treatment, the patient was admitted to our hospital with a primary diagnosis of ASD with PH (severe).

Physical examination: The child was conscious, tolerable to general activities, no cyanosis of the lips, clear lung sounds, no obvious rales, heart rate (HR) 100 beats/min, regular rhythm, strong heart sounds, no obvious murmurs, heart sound P2 > A2, pulse oxygen saturation (SpO_2) 98% under room air.

Laboratory tests: Complete blood count test, coagulation function, liver and kidney function were all normal.

Echocardiography: Normal heart position and connection, LVDD 3.91 cm, slight right ventricular wall thickening, normal left ventricular systolic activity. Left-sided aortic arch without widening, mild pulmonary artery widening, normal aortic valve, and atrioventricular valve opening activity, mild tricuspid valve regurgitation with regurgitation speed 3.53 m/s, pressure difference 50 mm Hg. ASD(II) at the lower part of the atrial septum with a defect range of 0.4 cm and 2 defect bundles; the wider defect bundle was 0.27 cm. Left-to-right shunt at the atrial level, patent foramen ovale, intact ventricular septum.

Cardiac CT: ASD, pulmonary artery dilation.

Electrocardiogram (ECG): Sinus bradycardia, complete right bundle branch block with right ventricular enlargement.

Preoperative diagnosis: ASD (II), PH.

82.2 Anesthetic Management

The patient did not take any preoperative medications. Upon entering the operating room, basic vital signs were closely monitored with cuff blood pressure (BP) 102/56 mm Hg, heart rate (HR) 106 beats/min, and pulse oxygen saturation (SpO_2) 97%. General anesthesia was induced by intravenous bolus injection of midazolam 1.0 mg, etomidate 6.0 mg, fentanyl 35 μg, and rocuronium 10 mg. Once the eyelash reflex disappeared, an ID 5.0 mm cuffed endotracheal tube was intubated under direct laryngoscopy. The tube depth was fixed at 15 cm after verification of the appropriate position by bilateral auscultation of the lungs. The patient was ventilated with pressure-controlled ventilation-volume guaranteed (PCV-VG) mode, oxygen flow rate 2 L/min, fraction of inspired oxygen (FiO_2) 50%, tidal volume (VT) 160 mL, respiratory rate (RR) 18 times/min, inspiratory to expiratory (I:E) time ratio 1:2. The end-tidal carbon dioxide ($ETCO_2$) was maintained around 35–45 mm Hg during surgery. Sevoflurane 0.5–1.0 MAC was inhaled to maintain anesthesia during the operation. The arterial blood gas analysis result after anesthesia induction is shown in Table 82.1.

Table 82.1 Artery blood gas analysis results after anesthesia induction

Hb g/dL	HCT %	pH	PaO_2 mm Hg	$PaCO_2$ mm Hg	BE mmol/L	Na^+ mmol/L	K^+ mmol/L	Ca^{2+} mmol/L	Cl^- mmol/L	Lac mmol/L
10.9	33.5	7.42	113	39.1	−4.0	134	3.9	1.2	104	0.8

82.3 Postoperative Outcome

The right heart catheterization examination went smoothly. The left ventricular end-diastolic pressure was 18 mm Hg, the aortic pressure was 90/58 mm Hg, and the pulmonary artery pressure was 56/17 mm Hg. After 100% oxygen ventilation, the aorta and pulmonary artery pressures were 94/51 mm Hg and 60/20 mm Hg, respectively.

Sevoflurane inhalation was turned off after the heart catheterization examination was finished. The airway and oral secretions were first suctioned under deep anesthesia. The child's spontaneous breathing recovered 5 min later, but spontaneous breathing was irregular with body movements, breath-holding, coughing, etc. The child could not tolerate the tracheal tube. Then, manual-assisted ventilation was initiated. At this time, the child's HR suddenly increased from 95 beats/min to 135 beats/min with cyanosis of lips, SpO_2 also progressively decreased, and $ETCO_2$ waveform became flat and gradually disappeared. FiO_2 was adjusted to 100% and manual assisted breathing continued. Two minutes later, SpO_2 dropped from 98% to 65%, HR rose to 185 beats/min, and the right upper limb BP dropped from 68/35 mm Hg to 52/30 mm Hg. Emergency bedside echocardiography showed significant right ventricle enlargement, sharp left ventricle reduction, and myocardial contractility decrease, indicating that PHC occurred. Anesthesia was immediately deepened with sevoflurane. Epinephrine 10 μg and furosemide 20 mg were intravenously injected. The child's HR suddenly dropped to 45 beats/min, SpO_2 dropped to around 30%, and the right upper limb BP was 47/28 mm Hg. Epinephrine 10 μg was intravenously injected one more time. About 5% sodium bicarbonate 50 mL and milrinone at 0.5 μg/(kg·min) were intravenously infused, respectively. HR rose to 80 beats/min about 2 min later, but there was no significant improvement in BP and SpO_2. Another 20 μg of epinephrine was intravenously administered. HR rose to 105 beats/min, BP rose to 115/62 mm Hg, and SpO_2 gradually rose to 98% about 1 min later. The child's spontaneous breathing recovered about 15 min later. Milrinone at 0.5 μg/(kg·min) continued to be used to maintain vital signs stable, and the endotracheal tube was successfully removed.

82.4 Review of Knowledge Points

82.4.1 Pulmonary Hypertension Crisis

PHC refers to a clinical crisis state where the rapid increase of pulmonary vascular resistance and pulmonary artery pressure on the basis of PH in a short time occurs, which can approach or exceed the systemic circulation pressure and further lead to severe low cardiac output, hypoxemia, hypotension, and acidosis. Various factors, such as hypoxia, carbon dioxide accumulation, and harmful stimuli, can trigger the occurrence of PHC. Once PHC occurs, the right ventricular afterload will dramatically increase, leading to significant right ventricle enlargement and myocardial contractibility reduction. Furthermore, PHC can cause a significant reduction of left heart blood return and preload and result in significant hypotension. In addition, the increased pressure in the right ventricle can push the interventricular septum toward the left ventricle with insufficient preload due to the relatively high ventricular compliance, which further reduces the output of the left ventricle and leads to severe hypotension and insufficient myocardial perfusion.

82.4.2 Right Heart Catheterization

Right heart catheterization can accurately measure the pressure of the right atrium, right ventricle, and pulmonary artery. Furthermore, it can also measure cardiac output and mixed venous oxygen saturation. It is the gold standard for diagnosing PH. Right heart catheterization combined with an acute pulmonary vasodilation test can be used to assess pulmonary vascular reactivity and determine the diagnosis and guide treatment in children with PH.

Acute vasoreactivity test (AVT): AVT can be conducted by inhaling nitric oxide (NO), iloprost, 100% oxygen, or intravenous injection of epoprostenol and adenosine. If the absolute value of mean pulmonary artery pressure (mPAP) is ≤40 mm Hg, the decrease of mPAP beyond 10 mm Hg, and the cardiac output remains the same or increases after using the above medications, it is a positive response, indicating that the pulmonary arterioles are in a state of spasm, belonging to reactive PH or dynamic PH. These kinds of children with PH usually respond well to calcium channel blockers and often have good prognoses. Otherwise, it is a negative response, indicating that PH is not caused by pulmonary arteriole spasm and is more likely caused by severe vascular structural changes or a number decrease in the pulmonary artery, belonging to organic PH.

The positive criteria for AVT experiments in children differ from those in adults. Furthermore, they are related to the type of diseases. In children with idiopathic pulmonary arterial hypertension (IPAH)/hereditary pulmonary arterial hypertension (HPAH): A decrease in the ratio of mPAP and pulmonary vascular resistance index to systemic vascular resistance index (PVRI/SVRI) to >20% before and after medication without cardiac output decrease indicates a positive response. Calcium channel blockers can be used for treatment, and the prognosis is generally good. In children with pulmonary arterial hypertension related to shunt caused by congenital heart disease (APAH-CHD shunt, Qp:Qs > 1.5:1): A decrease in PVRI and PVRI/SVRI >20% and absolute values of <6 WU/m^2 and < 0.3 respectively, indicates a positive response and surgical correction is safe. In addition, PVRI 6–8 WU/m^2 and PVRI/SVRI ratio 0.3–0.5 are usually thought of as a gray area, and the safety of surgery cannot be guaranteed.

82.5 Discussion

82.5.1 Preoperative Evaluation and Preparation

The risk of cardiac catheterization under general anesthesia in children with PH is relatively high. The incidence of PHC was about 20.5%, and the mortality rate was about 1.4%. Preoperative evaluation should include the child's condition of growth and development, exertion tolerance, symptoms of right heart failure, and history of PHC attacks, etc. Furthermore, preoperative echocardiographic examination is also very important. All of the above preoperative evaluation and preparation should be comprehensively conducted to prevent the occurrence of PHC actively. Our preoperative preparation for this case included ① oral intake of carbohydrate drink 5.0 mL/kg (Outfast®, Renfu Farewell Pharmaceutical Company, China) 2 h before surgery to avoid the discomfort from prolonged fasting; ② oral administration of midazolam syrup 0.5 mg/kg (maximum dose 15 mg) for sedation 20–30 min before surgery to reduce anxiety and crying (the patient in this case did not take any preoperative medications); and ③ close monitoring: In addition to monitoring ECG, SpO_2, $ETCO_2$, body temperature, urine output, etc., it is also necessary to conduct ABP and CVP monitoring. It is also very important to avoid hypoxia, carbon dioxide accumulation, and harmful stimuli during the whole perioperative period to prevent the occurrence of PHC. Furthermore, it is also necessary to prepare for rescue.

82.5.2 Intraoperative Anesthetic Management

The anesthesia process should be smooth to achieve good sedation and analgesia without causing circulatory suppression. It is better to choose anesthetics with little effect on systemic vascular resistance (SVR), such as etomidate, fentanyl, and rocuronium, for the induction of anesthesia. Children with PH are very sensitive to the decrease of SVR, which can easily lead to significant hypotension. Although ketamine can increase SVR, it can also potentially increase pulmonary vascular resistance (PVR), especially in cases of poor ventilation. There are some controversies about whether ketamine can be used in children with PH. High concentrations of inhaled anesthetics should be avoided due to the significant suppression of SVR. The inhaled anesthetic concentration should be adjusted according to the changes in HR and BP.

In this case, the patient experienced apnea and choking during the awakening period, which caused the potential occurrence of PHC, and the condition progressed rapidly. Bedside ultrasound revealed significant right ventricle enlargement and significant left ventricle reduction, which further confirmed the diagnosis of PHC. The child's vital signs gradually stabilized after symptomatic treatment, such as deepening anesthesia, increasing FiO_2, hyperventilation, epinephrine, and milrinone, and correcting acidosis. The tracheal tube was successfully removed under deep anesthesia in the end, and the patient was transferred to the ward. PHC usually occurs suddenly and progresses rapidly. The mortality rate is usually very high if PHC is not effectively controlled. Therefore, it is necessary to make a detailed PHC rescue plan for such kind of children before surgery. The PHC rescue plan can be referred to as follows: Pure oxygen ventilation. Deepen anesthesia with sedative/analgesic drug administration. Pulmonary artery dilation with prostacyclin inhalation or intravenous infusion of milrinone. Avoid patient-ventilator asynchrony by use of neuromuscular blocking agents. Maintain sufficient VT to avoid atelectasis. Maintain satisfactory oxygenation via low airway pressure, low PEEP, and prolonged exhalation. Avoid hypercapnia via appropriate hyperventilation. Be cautious with fluid resuscitation, consider using sodium bicarbonate to correct acidosis, use medications such as norepinephrine and vasopressin to maintain coronary perfusion, and consider pulmonary vasodilators such as treprostinil if it is necessary. Maintain sinus rhythm and atrioventricular synchrony. Maintain normal body temperature. Consider extracorporeal membrane oxygenation (ECMO) support if cardiac arrest occurs.

82.6 Shortcomings and Limitations

In this case, the patient was relatively stable before the completion of cardiac catheterization examination; the depth of anesthesia during the awakening process was relatively light because the patient could not tolerate the endotracheal intubation, showing choking, body movement, and apnea, which led to the occurrence of PHC and rapid exacerbation. Although the rescue was relatively successful, the perioperative management process should be more meticulous to ensure that the patient could tolerate the endotracheal intubation and avoid apnea and choking during the waking period. It is necessary to remove the endotracheal tube under deep anesthesia and sufficient spontaneous breathing for this kind of patient.

82.7 Conclusion

In summary, for the anesthetic management of children with congenital heart disease accompanied by PH, preoperative measures should be taken to avoid hypoxia, respiratory depression, and harmful stimuli. The depth of anesthesia during induction should be appropriately controlled, and endotracheal intubation should be avoided under light anesthesia or insufficient muscle relaxation. Hypotension during anesthesia induction and maintenance should be avoided. It is better to maintain relatively high concentrations of oxygen and appropriate hyperventilation. The awakening process should be stable. It is necessary to remove the endotracheal tube under deep anesthesia and sufficient spontaneous breathing. A detailed PHC prevention plan should be prepared during the whole perioperative period (Huiyan Hou).

83 Anesthetic Management of Pericardial Tamponade During Radiofrequency Catheter Ablation in a Child with Supraventricular Tachycardia

Yingying Tao

Abstract

A 6-year-old girl with supraventricular tachycardia was scheduled for radiofrequency catheter ablation. During the procedure, she developed pericardial tamponade, which showed a significant reduction in heart rate and blood pressure. The patient's hemodynamics were stabilized after the timely treatment of inotropic medicines and fluid replacement. Pericardial tamponade is a serious complication of radiofrequency catheter ablation. Early detection and timely relief of pericardial tamponade are the key to determining the patient's outcomes.

Supraventricular tachycardia, abbreviated as SVT, is a relatively common type of rapid arrhythmia in children, affecting their growth and development if it persists for a long time. In some severe cases, SVT can even threaten the children's life. Radiofrequency catheter ablation (RFCA) should be considered for patients whose drug treatment is not effective or who want to avoid adverse reactions related to antiarrhythmic drugs. Although RFCA has significant advantages, such as minor trauma and a high cure rate, intraoperative procedures and other factors may result in pericardial tamponade due to mechanical injury and perforation of the wall of the cardiac chambers. The incidence of pericardial tamponade is about 0.3–0.9%. This case report focuses on the anesthetic management of a 6-year-old child who developed pericardial tamponade during elective RFCA for SVT.

83.1 Case Presentation

A 6-year-old girl was delivered full term without any complications. Her weight was 30.4 kg. In the past 2 years, she had experienced intermittent rapid heart rates and was diagnosed with SVT. Physical examination addressed normal growth and development. When breathing calmly, the patient's lips showed no obvious cyanosis, lung sounds were coarse, and no obvious rales were heard. Her heart sounds were strong, and no murmurs were heard in the precordial area. The heart rhythm was regular, with a heart rate (HR) of 104 beats/min. Her abdomen was soft. Her extremities were warm, and her pulse oxygen saturation (SpO_2) was 99% when breathing air.

Laboratory tests: Normal blood routine test and normal liver, kidney, and coagulation function.

Y. Tao (✉)
The National Children's Medical Center (Shanghai), Department of Anesthesiology of Shanghai Children's Medical Center, Shanghai Jiao Tong University School of Medicine, Shanghai, China
e-mail: taoyingying@scmc.com.cn

J. Zheng et al. (eds.), *Selected Pediatric Cardiovascular Surgery Anesthesia Cases*,
https://doi.org/10.1007/978-981-96-5614-1_83

Electrocardiography (ECG): SVT (atrioventricular reentry tachycardia, AVRT).

Echocardiography: No abnormal heart structure was found.

Chest X-ray: No active lesions were found in both lungs.

Preoperative diagnosis: AVRT. The patient was scheduled for elective RFCA.

83.2 Anesthetic Management

The patient did not receive any sedative medication before surgery. After entering the cardiac catheterization lab, ECG, noninvasive blood pressure (BP), and SpO_2 were routinely monitored. Anesthesia was induced with intravenous bolus doses of 3.0 mg midazolam, 50 mg propofol, 6 μg sufentanil, and 20 mg rocuronium. After the patient's eyelash reflex disappeared, an ID 5.5 mm cuffed endotracheal tube was intubated under a visual laryngoscopy with an endotracheal tube depth of 16 cm. Pressure control ventilation (PCV) mode was used with the following respiratory parameters set: 2 L/min oxygen flow rate, 50% fraction of inspiration O_2 (FiO_2), 15 cm H_2O inspiratory peak pressure, 20 times/min respiratory rate (RR), and 1:2 inspiratory time to expiratory time (I:E) ratio, to maintain intraoperative tidal volume (VT) between 200 and 240 mL and end-tidal carbon dioxide ($ETCO_2$) between 35 and 40 mm Hg. General anesthesia was maintained by continuous inhalation of 2–3% sevoflurane.

After surgical sterilization and draping, the cardiologists inserted catheters into the patient's left and right femoral veins for intracardiac electrophysiological examination and the RFCA. When the surgery was performed for about 20 min, ECG showed that HR and BP gradually dropped to 72 beats/min(from 145 beats/min) and 70/33 mm Hg (from 88/40 mm Hg), respectively. The surgery was stopped immediately after careful communication with the cardiologists. X-ray fluoroscopy showed slight enlargement of the cardiac shadow and weakened cardiac contractions of the patient. An emergency bedside transthoracic echocardiogram demonstrated a 0.5–1.0 cm dark area in the pericardium, suggesting pericardial effusion. Immediate pericardiocentesis under ultrasound guidance was conducted by the cardiologists 50 mL of fresh, non-coagulated blood was drawn out, and a pericardial drainage tube was placed. At the same time, 300 mL of Ringer's acetate solution was rapidly infused, and dopamine was continuously pumped at 5.0 μg/(kg·min) to maintain the patient's HR and BP. The patient's arterial blood gas analysis showed pH 7.37, PaO_2 145.1 mm Hg, $PaCO_2$ 40.4 mm Hg, BE -1.6, HCT 30.8%, Hb 9.6 g/dL, K^+ 4.0 mmol/L, Ca^{2+} 1.10 mmol/L, Cl^- 103 mmol/L, Lac 2.0 mmol/L. The patient was observed for 30 min with 100 mL of red blood cell transfusion. Meanwhile, a total of 50 mL of drainage fluid was collected from the pericardial cavity. Then, the patient's HR was maintained at around 90 beats/min, and BP was maintained at around 85/40 mm Hg. The cardiologists decided to terminate the RFCA and transferred the patient to the Cardiac Intensive Care Unit (CICU) for further treatment without extubation.

83.3 Postoperative Outcome

The surgery lasted a total of 50 min. After the patient was transferred to CICU, the pericardial drainage volume was 30 mL in 24 h. On the second day after the surgery, the echocardiography did not show significant pericardial effusion. On the third day after the surgery, the 24-h pericardial drainage volume was less than 5.0 mL, and the pericardial drainage tube was removed. On the seventh day after the surgery, the patient returned to the general ward and was discharged from the hospital on the 15th day.

83.4 Review of Knowledge Points

83.4.1 Supraventricular Tachycardia

Supraventricular tachycardia, which is abbreviated as SVT, refers to a condition where the atrial and/or ventricular rate exceeds 100 beats per minute at rest due to any disease of the His bundle and its upstream conduction system. SVT is the most common type of rapid arrhythmia in children, with an incidence rate of about 1.03/1000. The main types include atrioventricular reciprocating tachycardia (AVRT), atrioventricular nodal reentrant tachycardia (AVNRT), etc. Repeated or persistent SVT can damage heart function and may lead to tachycardia-induced cardiomyopathy, which needs to be treated as soon as possible.

RFCA is an interventional technique that involves inserting an electrode catheter into a specific part of the heart chambers via a vein or artery to release radiofrequency current and cause local endocardial and subendocardial myocardial coagulative necrosis. Ultimately, the tachyarrhythmia's abnormal conduction bundles and point of origin were blocked. It has been used in clinics for over 30 years since pediatric pre-excitation syndrome was successfully treated by RFCA in 1991.

83.4.2 Complications of RFCA

Common complications associated with RFCA include acute pericardial tamponade, complete atrioventricular block, and coronary artery injury. Acute pericardial tamponade refers to the series of hemodynamic abnormalities caused by the rapid accumulation of blood in the pericardial cavity, which results in cardiac compression and ventricular filling obstruction. Severe hemodynamic abnormality with a rapid onset and progression can be potentially life-threatening. Acute pericardial tamponade during RFCA is commonly caused by violent operations and incorrect electrode placement in the cardiac chambers, which results in cardiac perforation and rupture. The common perforation sites are usually located at the left atrium and ventricle wall, coronary venous sinus, and the left atrium and pulmonary veins. On the other hand, excessive ablation power during catheter discharge can also cause cardiac perforation due to burst injury. Acute pericardial tamponade is usually characterized by sudden dyspnea, agitation, confusion or loss of consciousness. A sudden drop in BP and HR, with a subsequent increase in HR, can be observed in children under general anesthesia. Enlarged heart shadow and disappearance of pulsation can be seen during X-ray examination. Some patients in the early stage of pericardial tamponade may have symptoms similar to vasovagal reflexes, such as slow heart rate, pallor, and sweating. Therefore, the imaging examinations should promptly clarify the disease's cause. Pericardial tamponade should be highly suspected if the symptoms cannot be improved after treatment with atropine dopamine. Emergency bedside echocardiography can be used to facilitate diagnosis and track the dynamic changes after pericardiocentesis.

83.5 Discussion

83.5.1 Diagnosis of Pericardial Tamponade

The procedures of RFCA in pediatric patients are usually performed under general anesthesia with endotracheal intubation, so it is impossible to obtain the early subjective feelings of chest tightness, shortness of breath, dyspnea, and indifference when pericardial tamponade occurs. Anesthesiologists should closely monitor the patient's vital signs and observe the surgical details and progress. Pericardial effusion and/or acute pericardial tamponade should be highly suspected in the absence of vagal reflex when the following conditions occur: weakened cardiac contractions, enlarged cardiac shadow, increased transparency of medial cardiac shadow under X-ray fluoroscopy, systolic blood pressure drop with pulse pressure less than 30 mm Hg and cannot be corrected by rapid fluid infusion. X-ray fluoroscopy and/or bedside ultrasound can help confirm the diagnosis. It is important to know that children have smaller size of hearts and narrower Koch's triangle areas than adults, so the ablation target is closer to the conduction bundle. Therefore, the risk of atrioventricular block caused by ablation is also higher. When a third-degree atrioventricular block occurs, it also clinically manifests as a slowed heart rate and a drop in blood pressure, which requires to be differentially diagnosed from pericardial tamponade.

83.5.2 Management of Pericardial Tamponade

Pericardiocentesis is the first choice for the rescue of pericardial tamponade. Once confirmed, it should be performed as quickly as possible. The procedure can be performed blindly according to the anatomical position or under ultrasound or X-ray fluoroscopy guidance. During the puncture, the patient's vital signs should be closely observed. The volume, color, and characteristics of the drainage should be recorded. The patient's symptoms will usually be relieved after pericardiocentesis. Surgical intervention should be conducted immediately if the blood is continuously drained out or the symptoms cannot be significantly improved or even worsened after effective drainage. It has been shown that 13% of atrial perforations and 55% of ventricular perforations complicated by pericardial tamponade require surgical intervention. Complications that occur immediately after pericardiocentesis include myocardial puncture or laceration, vascular (coronary artery, intercostal vessels, intrathoracic artery or intra-abdominal vessels) injury, pneumothorax, air embolism, and arrhythmias (such as ventricular and supraventricular). Therefore, vigilance must be kept during pericardiocentesis. In preparation for pericardiocentesis, multiple venous accesses should be first accessed for rapid fluids and blood product replacement, and vasoactive drugs should be administrated to maintain the patient's hemodynamic stability. When it is available, uncontaminated autologous blood could be infused back to the patient.

83.5.3 Postoperative Management

After the occurrence of pericardial tamponade, the RFCA surgery should be terminated immediately. After initial medical treatment, the patient should be sent to the intensive care unit. More attention should be paid to the changes in the patient's blood pressure, pulse, heart rhythm, and urine output. Myocardial and coronary artery punctures that occur during pericardiocentesis may be initially asymptomatic and may manifest as a delayed pericardial effusion or poor catheter suction effect. Studies have shown that the incidence of pericarditis, sepsis, infection, and post-myocardial injury syndrome significantly increases after pericardiocentesis or surgical repair. Bedside echocardiography examination can clarify the disease's progression and assess the patient's cardiac function and circulatory volume status.

83.6 Shortcomings and Limitations

In this case, the noninvasive blood pressure monitoring monitored the hemodynamic fluctuation, which could not timely find the occurrence of serious complications, such as pericardial tamponade. Therefore, it is recommended that invasive arterial blood pressure should be adopted during long-term RFCA surgery, which can reflect the patient's circulatory function in real-time and rapidly detect serious complications.

83.7 Conclusion

Anesthesiologists should pay attention to the potential occurrence of serious complications such as pericardial tamponade and cardiac rupture during the process of RFCA. The possibility of pericardial tamponade should be considered when there is an unexplained drop in BP and changes in HR during the procedure. Pericardiocentesis is an effective measure to rescue pericardial tamponade. Bedside ultrasound can quickly, conveniently, and accurately diagnose pericardial tamponade and guide pericardiocentesis. If the patient's hemodynamics cannot be stabilized after pericardiocentesis, immediate surgical intervention should be considered (Yingying Tao).

Anesthetic Management of Intraoperative Arrhythmia During Transcatheter Closure of Ventricular Septal Defect

84

Yingying Tao

Abstract

A 2-year-old girl with ventricular septal defect (VSD) was scheduled for cardiac catheterization therapy. Supraventricular tachycardia suddenly occurred during the procedure, which was relieved by stopping the procedure and treated with medications. Once the supraventricular tachycardia was controlled, the surgery went on again until completion eventually. It is well-recognized that transcatheter closure of VSD in pediatric patients is safe and effective. However, severe arrhythmias such as ventricular arrhythmia and supraventricular arrhythmia might occur due to stimulation from surgical procedures or other reasons during the procedure. Timely symptomatic treatment and effective elimination of the cause of induced arrhythmia are the key points of anesthetic management for such patients.

Ventricular septal defect (VSD) is the most common congenital heart disease with interventricular blood flow communication through the tissue defects on the ventricular septum. VSD accounts for about 40% of all congenital heart diseases. It has been explored for nearly 30 years by using interventional cardiac catheterization to repair VSD. More and more clinical centers have started to use this technique due to the advantages of minimal vascular injury and simple procedures. The incidence of complications during cardiac catheterization procedure is 4.1–19%, of which arrhythmia is the most common complication caused by violent operations, anatomical abnormalities, etc. The arrhythmias can be manifested as transient intraoperative or postoperative attacks in mild injured cases or permanent postoperative arrhythmia in severe injured cases, which can affect the patient's postoperative recovery to varying degrees. This case report focuses on the anesthetic management of pediatric intraoperative supraventricular tachycardia during transcatheter closure of VSD.

84.1 Case Presentation

A2-year-old girl with 12 kg in weight was naturally delivered at full term without any history of asphyxia. A murmur in the precordial region was detected on auscultation after birth. He was diagnosed with VSD (perimembranous) by echocardiography at the local hospital. Normal feeding and growth development history.

Y. Tao (✉)
The National Children's Medical Center (Shanghai), Department of Anesthesiology of Shanghai Children's Medical Center, Shanghai Jiao Tong University School of Medicine, Shanghai, China
e-mail: taoyingying@scmc.com.cn

J. Zheng et al. (eds.), *Selected Pediatric Cardiovascular Surgery Anesthesia Cases*,
https://doi.org/10.1007/978-981-96-5614-1_84

Physical examination: Consciousness, body temperature 37 °C, heart rate (HR) 110 beats/min, blood pressure (BP) 96/55 mm Hg, respiratory rate (RR) 23 times/min, pulse oxygen saturation (SpO_2) 99% at room air, soft abdomen, warm extremities.

Specialized examination: Coarse breath sounds in both lungs without obvious rales, strong heart sounds, regular rhythm, grade III/VI systolic murmur in the precordial area. There is no obvious cyanosis of the lips when breathing air calmly and no cyanosis or clubbing of the extremities.

Laboratory tests: Routine blood tests within normal ranges, normal liver, kidney, and coagulation function.

Electrocardiogram (ECG): Sinus rhythm, HR within normal range.

Echocardiography: VSD (perimembranous type) with a diameter of 11 mm, patent foramen ovale with a diameter of 2.3 mm.

Preoperative diagnosis: VSD (perimembranous type), patent foramen ovale. Elective transcatheter closure of VSD was scheduled.

84.2 Anesthetic Management

The patient did not take any preoperative oral sedatives. After entering the cardiac catheterization lab, a 12-lead ECG, noninvasive BP, and SpO_2 were monitored. BP 95/54 mm Hg, HR 120 beats/min, SpO_2 98%. Anesthesia was induced with intravenous bolus doses of 1.0 mg midazolam, 30 mg propofol, and 3.0 μg sufentanil. After the patient's eyelash reflex disappeared, an Ambu® AuraFlex™ disposable laryngeal mask sized 2.5 was inserted. Pressure control ventilation (PCV) mode was used with the following respiratory parameters set: 2 L/min oxygen flow rate, 50% fraction of inspiration O_2 (FiO_2), 15 cm H_2O peak inspiratory pressure, 20 times/min RR, and 1:2 inspiratory time to expiratory time (I:E) ratio. Tidal volume (VT) and end-tidal carbon dioxide ($ETCO_2$) were maintained at 80–100 mL and 35–40 mmHg, respectively. General anesthesia was maintained by 1–2% sevoflurane inhalation. The patient's vital signs were continuously monitored during the procedure. After laryngeal mask insertion, the patient's vital signs were: BP 94/46 mm Hg, HR 125 beats/min, SpO_2 97%. After routine surgical disinfection, draping in the right inguinal region, and 100 IU/kg heparin intravenous injection for anticoagulation, the femoral vein and artery were cannulated. When cardiologists prepared to remove the sheath from the guide wire already located in the superior vena cava through the femoral vein via the end-hole catheter, the patient's ECG showed a sudden onset of paroxysmal supraventricular tachycardia with HR up to 200 beats/min, SpO_2 91%, and BP 80/40 mm Hg measured immediately. The cardiologist stopped the procedure, and FiO_2 was increased to 100%. The supraventricular tachycardia disappeared after half a minute of observation and returned to sinus rhythm with HR 118 beats/min, SpO_2 99%, BP 90/40 mm Hg. The supraventricular tachycardia did not occur within 5 min of observation. The patient's BP and SpO_2 were also stable, so the cardiologist continued the clinical procedure. Another paroxysmal supraventricular tachycardia occurred again with HR up to 195 beats/min, SpO_2 90%, BP 82/36 mm Hg. The cardiologists immediately stopped the procedure, administering 5 mg dexamethasone and 2.0 mg/kg propafenone intravenously. BP was measured every 1 min. Ten minutes after symptomatic treatment, the patient's HR returned to around 110 beats/min, and BP was stabilized at around 92/50 mmHg. The cardiologists tried one more time, but no more tachyarrhythmias occurred afterward. FiO_2 was readjusted downward to 50% and VSD occlude was successfully placed by the cardiologist. Bedside echocardiography showed no residual shunt around the original VSD and normal atrioventricular valve activity.

84.3 Postoperative Outcome

The operation lasted 55 min. The estimated blood loss was about 5 mL. About 100 mL of Ringer's acetate solution was transfused. BP was 90/49 mm Hg, HR was 110 beats/min, and SpO_2 was 98% at the end of the procedure. After sevoflurane inhalation was stopped at the end of the procedure, the patient's spontaneous breathing soon recovered, and the laryngeal mask was quickly removed. Once the Aldrete score reached 9 or above and hemodynamics became stable, the patient was transferred to the cardiology ward for further observation. On the postoperative day 2, ECG showed sinus rhythm with notched T waves in some leads. After the procedure, the patient's BP and SpO_2 were within the normal range. She was conscious without adverse events such as blackouts, palpitations, and fainting. The patient was discharged from the hospital on postoperative day 6 with a post-discharge prescription of daily oral aspirin.

84.4 Review of Knowledge Points

Arrhythmia is the most common adverse event of the cardiac catheterization procedure, including various types of ventricular arrhythmias, sinus arrest, complete left bundle branch block (CLBBB), complete right bundle branch block, CRBBB), etc. 12-Lead ECG monitoring is usually used to detect the occurrence of arrhythmias early. Once arrhythmias occur, the first step is to determine the arrhythmic types and their impacts on the hemodynamics, then to treat them with appropriate medications.

84.4.1 Myocardial Stimulation Caused by the Catheter

During transcatheter closure of VSD, a VSD occluder is delivered to the VSD site with the help of guide wire and looper through the femoral arteriovenous cannulation. Transient episodes of tachycardia are quite common during this process due to the endocardial wall stimulation caused by violent or unskilled guide wire manipulations, which usually disappear after immediate cessation of intracardiac manipulation and do not need any treatments. Ventricular fibrillation is uncommon during transcatheter closure of VSD. Ventricular tachycardia occurs more commonly in patients with muscular VSD or perimembranous VSD extending to the muscle, which is usually related to the occluder stimulation of the ventricular muscle. If the ventricular rate is less than 100 beats per minute, transient cessation of intracardiac manipulation for observation is enough, and no further treatment is required. However, the arrhythmia causes unstable hemodynamics with a BP drop and cannot be maintained; the occlusion procedure must be terminated immediately beyond the symptomatic and antiarrhythmic treatments. If it is necessary, electrical cardioversion, electrical defibrillation, or even open chest removal of the occluder should be initiated for resuscitation.

84.4.2 Occluder Compression on the Conduction Bundle

Perimembranous VSD is the most common type of VSD, accounting for about 80% of all VSDs. Due to the anatomical location of the perimembranous VSD adjacent to the His-Purkinje system and the numeric anatomical variations of His-Purkinje system, the injuries of atrioventricular bundles and its bundle branches around VSDs, myocardial edema, and other conditions caused by the occluder friction and compression are more likely occur in this kind of patients, which will further cause atrioventricular conduction block, junctional rhythm, and other ECG changes. For those patients with persistent CLUB or high-degree atrioventricular block during the occlusion procedure, 5 mg of dexamethasone can be given intravenously based on expert consensus and clinical practice. The occlusion procedure can continue if the conduction block disappears after dexamethasone treatment. On the contrary, if the conduction block does not disappear after dexamethasone treatment, it should be considered to remove the occlude or open-chest surgical treatment. If Adams–Stokes syndrome occurs in these patients, the placement of a temporary cardiac pacemaker is required.

84.5 Discussion

84.5.1 Preoperative Assessment and Preparation

For children with VSD who are undergoing interventional closure, it is necessary to clarify the anatomical classification of VSD and the complications, such as pulmonary hypertension, before surgery. From a clinical practicality perspective, the Anderson VSD classification is commonly used, which is mainly divided into perimembranous, muscular, and doubly committed subarterial types. In this case, the patient was diagnosed with perimembranous VSD by preoperative echocardiography. Considering the anatomical characteristics of perimembranous VSD, there is a higher probability of conduction bundle block during surgery. Therefore, routine real-time 12-lead ECG monitoring should be provided to help early detection of premature ventricular contractions and ventricular tachycardia caused by manipulation. An external defibrillator and electrode plate should also be prepared in advance. Preoperative fluid imbalance and electrolyte disorders should be prevented and corrected, especially hypokalemia, which can easily cause the occurrence of malignant arrhythmias, and these malignant arrhythmias are difficult to correct. It is better to use anti-inflammatory drugs before surgery, such as corticosteroids and aspirin, to reduce the edema risk of the myocardium and other tissues caused by occluder compression.

84.5.2 Anesthetic Management During Cardiac Catheterization

For better respiratory management during transcatheter closure of VSD, general anesthesia with endotracheal intubation or laryngeal mask insertion is usually recommended. Routine monitoring of ECG, BP, SpO_2, $ETCO_2$, etc., and hemodynamic and respiratory parameters should be conducted. In addition to the optimization of the depth of anesthesia and anesthesia-related hemodynamic changes, close attention should be paid to the steps and process of transcatheter closure of VSD, whether the placement of the interventional guide wire is smooth, whether there is valvular traction, which can cause significant hemodynamic fluctuations. It is necessary to compare the ECG changes before and after the placement of the occlude since it may indicate or predict the occurrence of atrioventricular block, intracardiac conduction abnormalities, or other cardiac rhythm.

In this case, supraventricular tachycardia occurred during the procedure, which is characterized by heart rate at 150–250 beats/min, regular rhythm, and normal QRS complex duration and morphology. However, when intraventricular conduction disturbances or pre-existing bundle branch blocks occur, the QRS complex morphology can be abnormal. The P wave is retrograde, inverted on leads II, III, and avF. Based on the ECG features and the mild decrease in BP and SpO_2, this patient was preliminarily diagnosed with supraventricular tachycardia.

When the supraventricular tachycardia occurred, we first asked the cardiologist team to stop the manipulation, and then to ensure adequate oxygen supply, effective ventilation, and stable hemodynamics. Antiarrhythmic and symptomatic treatments should be initiated if there is no significant improvement after these treatments. Intravenous drugs such as adenosine, digoxin, and propafenone can be used for intraoperative supraventricular tachycardia control. In this case, propafenone was prescribed the supraventricular tachycardia. Propafenone is a class I antiarrhythmic drug with direct membrane stabilizing effects, which can reduce the maximum rate of rise of the myocardial action potential, prolong the conduction time and ventricular refractoriness, reduce the spontaneous excitability of the myocardium and block the reentrant of excitation. If the first dose of propafenone is not effective, then repeat it after 15 min. An intravenous bolus dose of propafenone can significantly reduce the ventricular rate even below 60 beats/min and prolong the Q-T interval. If the blood pressure is relatively stable, the slow ventricular rate can recover on its own without any special treatment. However, for those patients with prolonged cyanosis, hypotension, and any other signs of hemodynamic instability, immediate synchronized electrical cardioversion should be required if drug treatment is not effective. The initial energy dose is 0.5–1.0 J/kg, which can be increased to 2.0 J/kg if supraventricular tachycardia persists.

84.5.3 Postoperative Anesthetic Management

The peak of myocardial edema occurs on postoperative days 5–7 and maybe complicated with further arrhythmias and conduction bundle disorders. Therefore, postoperative continuous ECG monitoring and oxygen therapy are recommended. If III degree atrioventricular block or complete left bundle branch block occurs early after the procedure, glucocorticoids, albumin, and fructose diphosphate can be used to improve myocardial nutrition status. A temporary pacemaker can be implanted if it is necessary. If III degree atrioventricular block or complete left bundle branch block was not enhanced after 3–7 days of treatment, the occluder should be removed, and the VSD should be repaired directly by cardiac surgery. Late-onset III degree AV block could occur after surgery, drug treatment is usually not effective, and a permanent pacemaker is recommended to be implanted.

84.6 Shortcomings and Limitations

In this case, propafenone was chosen to control the supraventricular tachycardia. However, it should be noted that the negative inotropic action of propafenone can occur in children with cardiac dysfunction or severe cardiac structural abnormalities.

Current guidelines and expert consensus state that adenosine is the first choice for terminating supraventricular tachycardia. Intravenous administration of adenosine is a safe treatment for children of all age groups without any serious adverse events. However, if the patient has sinus node dysfunction or atrioventricular block or is taking drugs that affect atrioventricular conduction (such as β-receptor blockers, calcium channel blockers, and amiodarone), intravenous administration of adenosine can cause significant bradycardia. The current recommended dose for adenosine is 0.1 mg/kg.

84.7 Conclusion

The anesthetic management of pediatric transcatheter closure of VSD should focus on the assessment of VSD types and sizes and the comorbidities before surgery. Once arrhythmia occurs during surgery, active treatment or surgical strategy changes should be considered based on ECG characteristics and hemodynamic changes (Yingying Tao).

Anesthetic Management of Airway Bleeding During Transcatheter Occlusion of Major Aortopulmonary Collaterals in a Child with Fontan Circulation

85

Yanting Wang

Abstract

A 13-year-old girl was scheduled for transcatheter occlusion of major aortopulmonary collaterals under general anesthesia due to recurrent hemoptysis. She underwent a Fontan procedure 3 years ago. Massive airway bleeding occurred during cardiac catheterization intervention. After pure oxygen ventilation, high positive end-expiratory pressure ventilation, epinephrine spraying via endotracheal tube, and thorough cleaning of the airway blood, the airway bleeding was well-controlled. The transcatheter occlusion of major aortopulmonary collaterals was successful. The patient was returned to the cardiac intensive care unit with endotracheal intubation. The anesthetic management of such patients is to quickly and effectively control airway bleeding, timely assess the cardiac function and hemodynamic status, and follow the anesthetic management principles of patients with single ventricle physiology.

Y. Wang (✉)
The National Children's Medical Center (Shanghai), Department of Anesthesiology of Shanghai Children's Medical Center, Shanghai Jiao Tong University School of Medicine, Shanghai, China
e-mail: wangyanting@scmc.com.cn

Hemoptysis is one of the long-term complications of the Fontan procedure, which is mainly due to the widespread formation of major aortopulmonary collaterals (aortopulmonary collateral arteries, APCAs). These collateral vessels may have already existed before the Fontan procedure or may have compensatory proliferation caused by chronic hypoxia after the Fontan procedure. APCAs are an important source of left-to-right shunting, which further increases the load of the pulmonary circulation and causes excessive congestion and dilation of the vessels in the bronchi, bronchioles, and submucosal layer of the bronchi and bronchial arteries. Once this blood is ruptured, blood can enter the bronchial cavity and cause hemoptysis. Patients with Fontan circulation often present with a large volume of hemoptysis, which can cause severe hypoxemia or even suffocation. Once hemoptysis occurs in patients with APCAs, it is necessary to treat APCAs as soon as possible. This chapter reports the anesthetic management of airway bleeding during transcatheter occlusion of APCAs in a child with Fontan circulation.

85.1 Case Presentation

The patient was a 13-year-old girl with a height of 151 cm and a weight of 40.6 kg. She underwent a Fontan procedure 3 years ago; she was scheduled for transcatheter occlusion of APCAs

J. Zheng et al. (eds.), *Selected Pediatric Cardiovascular Surgery Anesthesia Cases*, https://doi.org/10.1007/978-981-96-5614-1_85

under general anesthesia due to recurrent hemoptysis. The patient's daily exertion tolerance was significantly decreased with NYHA heart function classification class III. She also has a history of recurrent respiratory tract infections. After she was admitted to our hospital, vasopressin and hemocoagulase was given to treat hemoptysis, but the effect of treat was not good. The patient still had hemoptysis every day with a hemoptysis volume of 100–150 mL, so she was scheduled for transcatheter occlusion of APCAs under general anesthesia.

Physical examination: The patient is conscious and oriented. The breathing sounds in both lungs were coarse, with a small amount of wet rale. An old surgical scar was seen in the precordial area. Pulse oxygen saturation (SpO_2) is 88% with nasal cannula oxygen therapy at 2 L/min.

Echocardiography: Post Fontan procedure for dextro-transposition of the great arteries (D-TGA, S.D.D)/ventricular septal defect (VSD)/atrial septal defect (ASD)/pulmonary stenosis (PS), the flow speed at the cavopulmonary anastomosis was 0.44 m/s and the blood flow waveform changes with respiration.

Preoperative CT angiography (CTA): Post Fontan procedure for D-TGA (S.D.D)/VSD/ASD/PS, multiple collateral vessels originate from the aortic arch, right subclavian artery, and vertebral artery.

85.2 Anesthetic Management

The patient was transported to the DSA examination room with a nasal cannula for oxygen therapy. When the patient was transferred to the operating table, she coughed and expectorated fresh blood of about 50–60 mL, bright red in color. After the patient's breathing was stabilized and the residual blood in the oral cavity was thoroughly cleaned, the basic monitoring was conducted in the supine position. The basic vital signs were heart rate (HR) 100 beats/min, blood pressure (BP) 130/76 mm Hg, SpO_2 90%. Rapid induction of anesthesia was conducted by intravenous bolus injection of midazolam 2.0 mg, propofol 80 mg, sufentanil 20 μg, and rocuronium 25 mg. The endotracheal intubation was smooth. Mechanical ventilation was initiated with pressure-controlled ventilation-volume guaranteed (PCV-VG) mode. The ventilation parameters were set as follows: oxygen flow rate of 2 L/min, a fraction of inspired oxygen (FiO2) of 80%, tidal volume (VT) of 400 mL, and respiratory rate of 12 breaths/min. The induction process of anesthesia was smooth. After intubation, a small amount of fresh bloody secretion was suctioned from the airway, and about 50 mL of old bloody secretion was suctioned from the stomach. When ascending aortic angiography started, the anesthesia machine suddenly alarmed for high airway pressure, and SpO_2 rapidly dropped to 40–50%. A large amount of bright red blood surged from the endotracheal tube. Immediate rapid fluid resuscitation and airway cleaning with negative pressure suction were conducted. Epinephrine (1:10,000) was sprayed via an endotracheal tube to control bleeding. In addition, pure oxygen, 10 cm H_2O positive end-expiratory pressure ventilation (PEEP), was used to conduct mechanical ventilation. At the same time, 3 U of vasopressin was intravenously injected. The airway bleeding was gradually controlled, and SpO_2 also gradually recovered to above 90%. The estimated blood loss was 200–300 mL, symptomatic supportive treatment with blood transfusion was given, and the operation continued. After the DSA angiography confirmed multiple systemic-pulmonary artery collateral vessel formation, collateral vessel occlusion was conducted. The operation was successful. The patient's vital signs were stabilized after the operation. The patient was returned to the pediatric Cardiac Intensive Care Unit (CICU) with endotracheal intubation.

85.3 Postoperative Outcome

The patient was transferred to the CICU with mechanical ventilation support after the operation and continued to be treated with vasopressin, bacitracin, and hemostatic agents to control airway bleeding. Cefuroxime was used to prevent infection, and diuretics were used to reduce cardiac load. The amount of bloody secretion in the airway was significantly reduced on the postoperative day 1. No obvious signs of active airway bleeding were found on postoperative day 2; then, the tracheal tube was successfully removed. The patient was supported with nasal cannula oxygen therapy. The patient was transferred out of the CICU with no longer coughing up blood 1 week later. She was discharged from the hospital 2 weeks later.

85.4 Review of Knowledge Points

85.4.1 Aortopulmonary Collateral Arteries

APCAs refer to vessels originating from the aorta or its branches, which can provide blood flow to the lung tissue, either alone or in conjunction with the inherent pulmonary arteries. They can be divided into the following three types according to the diameter of the vessels:

1. Large APCAs, with diameter > 2 mm.
2. Medium APCAs, with a diameter of 1–2 mm.
3. Small APCAs with a diameter < 1 mm.

They can be divided into the following three types according to their origin and connection with the pulmonary artery:

1. Bronchial artery type: These APCAs are the nutrient arteries of the bronchial lung, distributed in the lung parenchyma, supplying blood to the small branches of the pulmonary artery.
2. Direct aortopulmonary collateral type: These APCAs often originate from the upper middle segment of the descending aorta, directly connect to the pulmonary artery to provide blood supply.
3. Often originating from branches of the aorta, including the brachiocephalic artery, coronary arteries, and abdominal aorta.

The difficulty in dealing with APCAs is their wide range of origins and large anatomical variations. It is difficult to ligate them surgically. The preferred method is to use imaging angiography to clarify the number and direction of the vessels, and then perform occlusion under interventional conditions.

85.5 Discussion

85.5.1 Preoperative Assessment and Preparation

The preoperative assessment of children with Fontan circulation and hemoptysis should focus on the hemodynamic changes and whether there is active bleeding in the airway. Patients with Fontan circulation are extremely vulnerable to decreases in circulatory blood volume and acute increases in venous volume. So, it is better to avoid prolonging the preoperative fasting time. Infusing 10–15 mL/kg of fluid before the induction of anesthesia is beneficial to compensate for the blood volume loss caused by fasting, but the infusion speed should not be too fast. For patients with obvious symptoms of hemoptysis before surgery, preparations should be made to deal with reflux aspiration, even if strict fasting has been enforced due to the possible accumulation of blood or blood clots in the stomach.

85.5.2 Intraoperative Anesthetic Management

The goal of intraoperative management for children with Fontan circulation and hemoptysis is to optimize systemic oxygen supply and perfusion, maintain heart rate and myocardial contractility, and preload to maintain normal cardiac output. Considering the possible issue of a full stomach, the following recommendations of anesthetic management are made for these patients:

1. Rapid induction intubation should be performed for patients with good intubation conditions. For those suspected of difficult intubation, awake intubation under topical anesthesia or intubation with difficult airway equipment should be used.

2. Following the anesthetic protocol of full stomach. Preventive interventions such as nasogastric tube placement and negative pressure suction device preparation are widely accepted. For patients with clear preoperative hemoptysis location and a large amount of hemoptysis, the patient should be tilted toward the affected side during intubation to prevent blood from flowing to the healthy side. If conditions permit, a double-lumen endotracheal tube should be used to isolate the lungs.
3. Anesthetic induction should be smooth and rapid to avoid coughing to induce hemoptysis during the induction period.
4. Maintain an appropriate depth of anesthesia and actively replenish blood volume to ensure sufficient preload.
5. Maintain homeostasis and avoid risk factors such as hypoxia, hypercapnia, and metabolic acidosis that may increase pulmonary vascular resistance.

Severe hemoptysis can often happen in children with Fontan circulation. Once intraoperative airway bleeding occurs, it can cause severe asphyxia and hypoxia in a short time, which is life-threatening. Early detection and rapid treatment of intraoperative airway bleeding are extremely important for these patients. Under the DSA environment, anesthesiologists are often far away from the patient. When the patient cannot be directly observed, airway symptoms (high airway pressure, decreased tidal volume, etc.) often precede changes in heart rate, blood pressure, and SpO_2. If conditions permit, close attention should be paid to changes in the patient's intraoperative airway pressure, VTe, and $ETCO_2$ waveform. For patients who have already had airway bleeding, pure oxygen ventilation should be used, the accumulated blood in the airway should be cleaned, and epinephrine should be sprayed into the airway. In addition, it is better to use moderately high PEEP to facilitate hemostasis. It should be noted that each suction time should not be too long to avoid exacerbating hypoxia when the airway is cleaned.

85.6 Conclusion

The anesthetic management of children with Fontan circulation and airway bleeding for transcatheter occlusion of APCAs should consider the pathological physiology of Fontan circulation and the treatment strategies for airway bleeding. It is necessary to minimize the risk factors that adversely affect the balance of Fontan circulation and quickly deal with airway bleeding while the normal cardiac output is maintained (Yanting Wang).

MIX
Papier aus verantwortungsvollen Quellen
Paper from responsible sources
FSC® C105338

If you have any concerns about our products,
you can contact us on
ProductSafety@springernature.com

In case Publisher is established outside the EU,
the EU authorized representative is:
Springer Nature Customer Service Center GmbH
Europaplatz 3, 69115 Heidelberg, Germany

Printed by Libri Plureos GmbH
in Hamburg, Germany